MEDICAL RADIOLOGY
Radiation Oncology

Editors:
L. W. Brady, Philadelphia
H.-P. Heilmannn, Hamburg
M. Molls, Munich

Springer-Verlag Berlin Heidelberg GmbH

R. H. Sagerman · W. E. Alberti (Eds.)

Radiotherapy of Intraocular and Orbital Tumors

2nd Revised Edition

With Contributions by

D. A. Abramson · W. E. Alberti · L. L. Anderson · L. W. Brady · J. A. Bogart
S.-T. Chiu-Tsao · C. T. Chung · B. Damato · S. S. Donaldson · E. D. Donnenfeld
E. Egger · P. T. Finger · J. E. Freire · P. J. Fitzpatrick · G. Goitein · R. S. Gonnering
S. S. Hahn · G. F. Hatoum · A. Hassenstein · N. Hosten · H. J. Ingrahm · M. Isaac
J. L. Iwata · H. G. Journée-De Korver · J. E. E. Keunen · A.-J. Lemke · P. K. Lommatzsch
I. R. McDougall · B. Micaily · J. E. Munzenrieder · J. A. Oosterhuis · Z. Petrovich
G. Richard · S. B. Rudoler · R. H. Sagerman · J. Schipper · C. L. Shields · J. A. Shields
A. Walter · R. A. Weiss · C. Werschnik · A. Youssef · L. Zografos

Foreword by
L. W. Brady, H.-P. Heilmann, and M. Molls

Introduction by
A. P. Moulin, P. A. D. Rubin, and F. A. Jakobiec

With 142 Figures in 268 Separate Illustrations, 75 in Color and 49 Tables

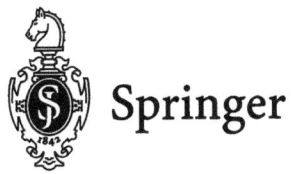 Springer

ROBERT H. SAGERMAN, MD, FACR
Professor, Department of Radiation Oncology
State University of New York
Upstate Medical University
750 East Adams Street
Syracuse, NY 13210
USA

WINFRIED E. ALBERTI, MD
Professor, Department of Radiotherapy and Radiooncology
University Hospital Hamburg-Eppendorf
Martinistrasse 52
20246 Hamburg
Germany

MEDICAL RADIOLOGY · Diagnostic Imaging and Radiation Oncology
Series Editors: A. L. Baert · L. W. Brady · H.-P. Heilmann · F. Molls · K. Sartor

Continuation of
Handbuch der medizinischen Radiologie
Encyclopedia of Medical Radiology

ISBN 978-3-642-63147-4

Library of Congress Cataloging-in-Publication Data

Radiotherapy of intraocular and orbital tumors / R. H. Sagerman, W. E. Alberti (eds.) ;
with contributions by D. H. Abramson ... [et al.] ; foreword by L. W. Brady, H.-P.
Heilmann, and M. Molls ; introduction by F. A. Jacobiec and A. Ahmadi. -- 2nd rev. ed.
      p. ; cm. -- (Medical radiology)
   Includes bibliographical references and index.
   ISBN 978-3-642-63147-4   ISBN 978-3-642-55910-5 (eBook)
   DOI 10.1007/978-3-642-55910-5
   1. Eye--Tumors--Radiotherapy 2. Eye-sockets--Tumors--Radiotherpy. I. Sagerman,
Robert H., 1930- II. Alberti, W. III. Abramson, David H. IV. Series.
   [DNLM: Eye Neoplasms--radiotherpy. WW 149 R129 2002]
   RC280.E9 R33 2002
   616.99'4840642--dc21   2002017023

httpllwww.springer.de
© Springer-Verlag Berlin Heidelberg 2003
Originally published by Springer-Verlag Berlin Heidelberg New York in 2003
Softcover reprint of the hardcover 2nd edition 2003
The use of general descriptive names, trademarks, etc. in this publication does not imply, even in the absence of a
specific statement, that such names are exempt from the relevant protective laws and regulations and therefore free for
general use.

Product liability: The publishers cannot guarantee the accuracy of any information about dosage and application
contained in this book. In every case the user must check such information by consulting the relevant literature.

Cover-Design and Typesetting: Verlagsservice Teichmann, 69256 Mauer

SPIN: 107 654 58   21/3130 – 5 4 3 2 1 0

Dedicated to my wife *Malyne,*
the keeper of the key to my soul

Robert H. Sagerman

Dedicated to my wife *Marion,*
and my children

Winfried E. Alberti

Foreword

Since the publication of the first edition of Radiotherapy of Intraocular and Orbital Tumors in 1993 the treatment programs for cure have changed from the dominance of surgical resection to the utilization of radiation therapy with preservation of the eye intact and preservation of vision.

In 2002 about 2,300 primary eye tumors will be diagnosed in the United states, 75% of which will be choroidal melanomas, 20% retinoblastomas, and the remainder a wide variety of tumors – malignant lymphoma, rhabdomyosarcomas, liposarcomas, meningiomas, malignant fibrous histiocytomas, etc. Even so, the majority of malignant tumors of the eye are metastatic, primarily from cancers of the lung or breast.

The impact of newer imaging studies, including computed tomography, magnetic resonance imaging, and ultrasound with and without contrast medium, have allowed for better tumor definition, more precise treatment techniques, and major improvement in local control, with preservation of the eye intact and excellent survival. The better histologic definition of the tumor has selected more appropriately the cases suitable for adjuvant chemotherapy particularly demonstrated by the combined integrated multimodal treatment of rhabdomyosarcoma without enucleation.

Surgical techniques are now being reserved for biopsy and for treatment failures, a dramatic change in treatment approaches since 1993.

The second edition by Sagerman and Alberti clearly demonstrates this major change in treatment. The volume explores the impact of diagnostic workup, the role of surgery, the role of external beam radiation therapy, the use of radioactive plaques, photocoagulation, cryotherapy, and other less major surgical procedures.

This book clearly demonstrates the importance of combined modality treatment and how it impacts on survival and vision preservation.

Philadelphia   LUTHER W. BRADY
Hamburg   HANS-P. HEILMANN
Munich   MICHAEL MOLLS

Preface

Preface of the First Edition

It is human nature to want to deal with well-defined situations which are pleasant and for which there is a favorable outcome. This is also true in the practice of medicine and, in radiation oncology, it is often left to the most inexperienced, junior physician to deal with those cancers for which radiation therapy has yielded poor results or led to severe complications. Tumors of the eye and orbit fell into this category 40 years ago. Ophthalmological oncology was but an embryonic specialty, radiations were known to be deleterious to the eye, and the late effects of irradiating a child were frightening. Independently, the editors learned to utilize irradiation in the management of tumors of the eye and orbit in two of the worlds most famous ophthalmological institutions, the Edward S. Harkness Institute of Ophthalmology at Columbia University's Columbia-Presbyterian Medical Center in New York City and at the Eye Clinic at the University of Essen, where Dr. Algernon B. Reese and Dr. Gerd Meyer-Schwickerath, respectively, fostered the development of ophthalmological oncology. *Radiotherapy of Intraocular and Orbital Tumors* is but a small downpayment for we can never adequately repay A.B. Reese and G. Meyer-Schwickerath, their colleagues and their disciples, who have taught us so much and with whom we have worked together to develop new and better treatments with improved results and fewer adverse reactions.

We undertook the task of editing *Radiotherapy of Intraocular and Orbital Tumors* in an attempt at collating what has been learned about the use of irradiation in the management of these lesions and to provide a current single reference. The first edition of *Tumors of the Eye* was published in 1956; in the third edition (1976), P. Tretter summarized "Radiotherapy of Ocular and Orbital Tumors" in five pages for Dr. Reese. Similarly, N. Tapley and M. Lederman described the use of irradiation for retinoblastorna and orbital tumors for M. Bonuik's *Ocular and Adnexal Tumors* (1964). Similar chapters are contained in many other texts and in the published proceedings of conferences, but the developing role of radiation therapy was best found in individual articles by a laborious search of the world's literature. Even today, one must search out radiotherapeutic techniques and results, often presented from an ophthalmologic viewpoint, among the several recent excellent oncologic treatises, among which are *Ocular and Adnexal Tumors* (F. A. Jakobiec, 1978), *Retino-blastoma* (J. Schipper, 1980), *Diseases of the Orbit* (J. Rootman, 1988), *Intraoculare Tumoren* (P. K. Lommatzsch, 1989), *Diagnosis and Management of Orbital Tumors* (J. A. Shields, 1989), *Clinical Ocular Oncology* (D. H. Char, 1989), *Intraocular Tumors* (J. A. Shields, C. L. Shields, 1992), and in adult and pediatric oncology texts as well as radiotherapy texts.

To the best of our knowledge, the only overview of radiotherapy for the eye, *L'Oeil et les Radiations Ionisantes* (C. Have, J. Jammet, N.A. M.-A. Dollfuss, 1965), was not translated from the French and is no longer in print. However, there have been great advances in surgical technique, knowledge of pathology, diagnostic and radiologic techniques and experience with radiotherapy in the subsequent 28 years and, at the urging of many colleagues, we decided to pool our resources and attempt to describe ocular and orbital tumors from a radiotherapeutic viewpoint. Recognizing the diversity of experience and technique, and that no one could speak as a world authority for all topics, our task was made easier by enlisting the help of 55 coauthors from Europe and North America who very kindly contributed their special knowledge. We have tried to provide an easy reading style by gentle editing and thank our coauthors for their gracious acceptance of suggestions. It is not their fault, but ours, for any inaccuracies and inconsistencies which occur. In addition, we must apologize for any omissions and for avoiding many fascinating discussions by taking a narrow radiotherapeutic view; there were already too many pages and illustrations. Nevertheless, as noted in scholarly fashion in the introduction, F. A. Jakobiec has pointed out several areas worthy of inclusion in a second edition.

We would like to express thanks to the Deutsche Forschungsgerneinschaft in Bonn, Germany, and the Deutsche Krebshilfe, Bonn, Germany, for supporting Dr. Alberti's experimental work with external beam therapy, plaque irradiation and hyperthermia (Chaps. 39, 40) of the eye which was done in cooperation with members of the Eye Clinic, University of Essen (Prof. Dr. med. M. H. Foerster, Prof. Dr. med N. Bornfeld). The authors express their thanks to the Altried Krupp van Bohlen unit Halbach-Stiftung, Essen, Germany, for their generous support, which made it possible to include so many color photographs. Thanks also to Ms. Ursula Davis, Mr. Rick Mills and Ms. Ingrid Haas, who did such an excellent job in preparing the book.

We also thank Andrea Roos-Detische and Maureen Knopp for typing so many manuscripts and for seeing to a myriad of chores. Without their excellent secretarial help, we could not have finished our task.

WINFRIED E. ALBERTI
ROBERT H. SAGERMAN

Preface of the Second Edition

Significant advances have been made in the management of tumors of the eye and orbit in the decade since publication of the first edition of "Radiotherapy of Intraocular and Orbital Tumors," consistent with the underlying philosophy of "cure with preservation of form and function". These involve (1) the role of magnetic resonance imaging in the depiction of the lesion and tissues affected, (2) clarification of cellular origin, classification, natural history, therapy, and results for the lymphomas, (3) the emergence of thermal therapy, (4) the use of chemotherapy, and (5) the importance of cooperative "combined modality treatment" utilizing the expertise of ophthalmologists, radiation oncologists, medical/pediatric oncologists, pathologists, physicists, and basic scientists.

In addition, we now have had more experience and longer follow-up for patients with melanoma, notably for plaque brachytherapy, proton beam irradiation, local resection, and thermotherapy, and confirmatory studies for choroidal hemangiomas, metastatic disease and rhabdomyosarcoma. We have defined better when to initiate treatment for optic nerve gliomas, Graves' disease, and just what tumor control rates can be expected from "monotherapies," especially chemotherapy and thermotherapy. This is best illustrated in the treatment of retinoblastoma, where the limitations of each monotherapy have been defined and the benefits of "combined modality therapy" have reduced the need for external beam irradiation, while indicating the role of plaque brachytherapy.

While maintaining the focus on the use of irradiation, we have obtained contributions from 43 authors, 21 of them new to this text, affecting diagnostic imaging, thermotherapy, surgery, plaque brachytherapy, and "combined modality therapy", incorporated new developments, especially involving chemotherapy, and updated results for treatments which remain current. We thank all authors for providing the most recent data in each area of expertise and urge the reader to seek out those references and texts, as well as the current literature, to keep up with this gratifyingly progressing field. We also express our gratitude to all those patients, adults and children, who have imparted so much knowledge, from their experience, to us.

We must acknowledge the invaluable help of U. Davis, J. Dodsworth, and the staff of Springer-Verlag, and the secretarial help provided by S. Kiehl in Syracuse and Anja Nitzchke in Hamburg.

<table>
<tr><td>Syracuse</td><td align="right">R. H. SAGERMAN</td></tr>
<tr><td>Hamburg</td><td align="right">W. E. ALBERTI</td></tr>
</table>

Introduction

A. P. MOULIN, P. A. D. RUBIN, F. A. JAKOBIEC

Introduction from the First Edition

Radiotherapy of Intraocular and Orbital Tumors fills a resource void that has existed for too long in both ophthalmology and radiation oncology. Beginning with the seminal clinical and pathologic investigations of the late Algernon B. Reese (Reese 1976) and his associates (one of whom was Dr. Robert Sagerman) at Columbia Presbyterian Medical Center in New York, ophthalmologic oncology has emerged over the past 40 years as a full-fledged subspecialty of ophthalmology, replete with modern molecular genetic insights into retinoblastoma (Dryja 1993) and lymphoproliferations (Neri et al. 1987; Jakobiec et al. 1987a; Knowles et al. 1989). Flourishing ocular oncologic clinical services are now found in many medical centers and eye institutes in the United States and Europe.

Because of the rarity of most classes of intraocular and adnexal (under the rubric of adnexa in ophthalmology are included the structures supporting the integrity and functioning of the globe – the eyelids, the conjunctiva, the tear production and drainage apparatuses, and the orbital soft tuissues and bones), certain clinical services have focused on specific families of entities, such as lesions of the orbit, intraocular tumors, conjunctival and eyelid tumors, and so on. It has, therefore, taken experts from many centers worldwide to assemble a comprehensive work on the subject of the radiotherapeutic management of patients with intraocular tumors, extraocular tumors, and simulating inflammatory conditions. My congratlation are consequently warmly extended to the co-editors, Dr. Alberti and Dr. Sagerman, who along with their other authoritative contributors have produced a magesterial treatise. ...

Introduction of the Second Edition

Radiotherapy has an essential role in the management of patients afflicted with intraocular or orbital tumors, and the present treatise covers this field in a remarkable manner, assembling contributors and experts with considerable experience in this domain. The role of radiotherapy is not limited to orbital and ocular tumors, but also encompasses inflammatory disorders. Alone, or in conjunction with surgery or chemotherapy, radiotherapy is one of the major tools allowing eradication or palliation of ocular and adnexal neoplastic or inflammatory disorders. In the last decade, evolution in technologies has allowed improvements in the appraisal and treatment of these diseases. The specific anatomy of the eye and orbit requires precise, powerful, efficient and localized treatment. Improvements in imaging making it capable of precise delineation of the target tumor, for example, have fostered the refinement of techniques such as conformational radiotherapy, allowing the

A.P. MOULIN, MD
David Cogan Eye Pathology Laboratory, Harvard Medical School, Massachusetts Eye and Ear Infirmary, 243 Charles Street, Boston, MA 02114, USA
P.A.D. RUBIN, MD
Assistant Professor, Department of Ophthalmology, Director, Ophthalmic Plastics and Orbital Surgery, Harvard Medical School, Massachusetts Eye and Ear Infirmary, 243 Charles Street, Boston, MA 02114, USA
F.A. JAKOBIEC, MD, DSc (Med)
Henry Willard Williams Professor of Ophthalmology, Professor of Pathology/Chairman of Ophthalmology, Harvard Medical School, Massachusetts Eye and Ear Infirmary, 243 Charles Street, Boston, MA 02114, USA

reduction of local side effects and further enhancing the efficacy of radiotherapy within oncological management. Refinements in charged-particle treatment for uveal melanoma have also helped to reduce the incidence of secondary neovascular glaucoma, with consequent sparing of the anterior segment.

The accumulation of a large body of data in the field of lymphomas has allowed a better understanding of their molecular biology, genetics, and pathology. The development of widely available antibodies has led to the adoption of new classifications. Ocular lymphoproliferative disorders can be divided into intraocular and adnexal disorders, the latter including conditions affecting the conjunctiva, the lacrimal gland, and the orbit.

Clinically, adnexal lymphoproliferative lesions often present in the conjunctiva as freely movable, plaque-like or nodular, often salmon-colored, masses, which can extend over the palpebral and bulbar regions. In a recent series (SHIELDS et al. 2001), conjunctival involvement at a forniceal or midbulbar site and an increasing number of conjunctival tumors were found to correlate with the risk of development of systemic lymphoma. The same authors also emphasize the importance of considering the diagnosis of lymphoma in patients aged 60 or over who have developed dry eye symptoms of irritation and levator dehiscence-related ptosis. Some recent reports (AKPEK et al. 1999c; LAUER 2000) have also stressed the need to consider the diagnosis of conjunctival lymphoma in cases of chronic conjunctivitis with a poor response to treatment and unexplained cicatrization and trichiasis.

An orbital lymphoid proliferation may manifest as a subcutaneous mass, typically with a rubbery consistency, with or without proptosis, and sometimes causing diplopia. Probably because of the lymphocytic population of the lacrimal gland, the superior and anterior orbit are frequently involved and a propensity to invade the superior rectus levator complex has been noted (HORNBLASS et al. 1987). In contrast to Graves' orbitopathy, the muscle contractility is relatively well preserved, which may be explained histologically by the paucity of collagen deposition. The lacrimal gland itself is involved in approximately 30% of cases, and this involvement may cause epiphora (SPECHT and LAVER 2000; JAKOBIEC 1982a,b; JAKOBIEC et al. 1982, 1987).

Radiologically, CT scans of these lymphoid tumors are characterized by unifocal, homogeneous, masses isodense with muscle and showing straight or angulated edges. As they grow, they mold to the orbital fascial planes, muscles and bones (COCKERHAM and JAKOBIEC 1997; YEO et al. 1982). In the orbital fat, which shows little resistance to their growth, they display fine, irregular serrations. Bone erosion and/or destruction is usually not a feature of low-grade lymphoproliferative tumors and is highly suggestive of a high-grade process, particularly in the orbital lobe of the lacrimal gland, where epithelial tumors with a firmer stroma tend to grow, causing a globular or round erosion of the orbital bone. Bone erosion has also been described in high-grade B-cell lymphomas (WHITE et al. 1995).

Adnexal lymphoproliferative lesions have been divided into benign lymphoid hyperplasias, atypical lymphoid hyperplasias, and lymphomas (KNOWLES et al. 1990). These lesions have been reappraised in the last decade with the aid of the REAL classification, which defines each disease according to morphologic, immunophenotypic, genetic, and clinical features and, when possible, also according to the postulated normal counterpart of the neoplastic cells (HARRIS et al. 1994; JENKINS et al. 2000; MANNAMI et al. 2001; AUW-HAEDRICH et al. 2001; WHITE et al. 1995; COUPLAND et al. 1998, 1999a, b; CAHILL et al. 1999; SASAI et al. 2001; NAKATA et al. 1999; McKELVIE et al. 2001).

Reactive lymphoid hyperplasia, which is difficult to distinguish clinically and radiologically from lymphoma, is defined histopathologically as a focal lymphoid collection displaying cellular poly-morphism with plasma cells, histiocytes and a variable number of polymorphonuclear leukocytes against a background of small lymphocytes that are often organized in discrete, poorly formed lymphoid follicles. T cells, mostly situated in the interfollicular zones, usually make up more than 40% of the cellular population (KNOWLES and JAKOBIEC 1992; COUPLAND et al. 1998). B cells, mostly situated in the follicular zone, produce many different immunoglobulins (polyclonality). In a recent series (MANNAMI et al. 2001), all reactive lymphoid hyperplasias appeared immunophenotypically and genetically to be polyclonal. However, other data have demonstrated that these lesions may harbor a small collection of monoclonal B cells (JAKOBIEC et al. 1987; POLITO et al. 1996; TAKANO et al. 1992; JAKOBIEC and KNOWLES 1989; JOHNSON et al. 1999). It has also been suggested that an excess T helper population in these lesions (JAKOBIEC and KNOWLES 1989) may trigger B cell proliferation (SPECHT and LAVER 2000). Indeed, persistent, antigenically driven, stimulation of B cells leading to hypermutation of the immunoglobulin genes may eventually result in monoclonality, which might suggest that reactive lymphoid hyperplasia can be regarded as one end of a continuous spectrum extending to low-grade lymphoma. This idea seems to be supported by the observation that the lesions classified as reactive lymphoid hyperplasia and small lymphocytic lymphomas have, over time, almost the same rate of systemic involvement (SPECHT and LAVER 2000; KNOWLES and JAKOBIEC 1992; KNOWLES et al. 1990; KELETI et al. 1992).

Since its description in the stomach in 1983 (ISAACSON and WRIGHT 1983), the concept of mucosa-associated lymphoid tissue lymphoma (MALT) has been extended, and similar tumors are now known to involve other sites, such as the salivary glands, lungs, thyroid, breast, skin, kidney, dura (BURKE 1999a, b) and ocular adnexa, though strictly speaking its designation does not appear entirely adequate for the orbit, which is normally devoid of epithelium, lymphoid aggregates, and lymphatic vessels (ISAACSON 1999). Clinically, MALT lymphomas are defined as extranodal lymphomas that are localized at presentation, have an indolent course, and are potentially curable with local therapy (HARRIS and ISAACSON 1999). MALT lymphoma is frequently preceded by an immunological stimulation such as *Helicobacter pylori* in the stomach, Sjögren syndrome in the salivary glands or Hashimoto thyroiditis in the thyroid. So far, such immunological stimulation has not been clearly defined in the ocular adnexa, and cases of orbital lymphoma arising in such a context are rare (NAGAKI et al. 1998; NASSIF and FELDON 1992; ELLIS et al. 1985). Nevertheless, recent studies (COUPLAND et al. 1999b; MANNAMI et al. 2001) have demonstrated that these tumors frequently use germline genes that are usually associated with autoantibody production, further underscoring the importance of autoimmunity in the pathogenesis of these disorders. In one of these reports (COUPLAND et al. 1999a) the authors also express the conclusion that the Ig heavy chain mutation pattern in these lymphomas supports the concept that most of them represent clonal expansion of postgerminal center memory B cells.

Histopathologically, MALT lymphomas are defined as neoplasms recapitulating the features of a Peyer's patch, including (1) reactive lymphoid follicles colonized by neoplastic cells, (2) marginal neoplastic zone or monocytoid B cells (centrocyte like) infiltrating the overlying epithelium, (3) small B lymphocytes, and (4) plasma cells (HARRIS and ISAACSON 1999). Centrocyte-like cells are medium-sized to small lymphocytes with relatively abundant pale cytoplasm and a slightly irregular nucleus resembling a small cleaved cell or a centrocyte. As in the thyroid, plasmacytoid cells with Dutcher bodies (PAS-positive herniations of the cytoplasm into the nucleus) may be seen and have been found to correlate with malignancy (MEDEIROS and HARRIS 1989; COUPLAND et al. 1998). These tumors display a B lymphocyte immunophenotype characterized by an absence of CD 5 reactivity and cyclin D1 reactivity (in contrast to mantle cell lymphomas) and an absence of CD 10 reactivity (in contrast to follicular lymphoma). They also lack rearrangement of the *bcl 2* locus, a feature usually observed in virtually all follicular center lymphomas and in approximately 20% of diffuse large cell lymphoma (FRIZZERA et al. 1999).

From an epidemiological point of view, extranodal lymphomas represent 26% of all lymphomas, and aggressive extranodal lymphomas predominate, especially large B cell lymphomas, which constitute 60–85% of all extranodal lymphomas (BURKE 1999b). However, in the ocular adnexa, where lymphomas represent between 3% and 28% of extranodal lymphomas (AKPEK et al. 1999c), the MALT-type lymphoma is preponderant and accounts for between 38% and 86% of the cases (AUW-HAEDRICH et al. 2001; MANNAMI et al. 2001). The ocular adnexa are involved in 12% of cases of MALT lymphoma. In reports of adnexal lymphoid tumors, MALT lymphomas most often show an indolent behavior with a favorable outcome and have the propensity to remain localized for long periods of time, the rate of systemic spread varying from 3% (MANNAMI et al. 2001) to approximately 30% (CAHILL et al. 1999; AUW-HAEDRICH et al. 2001; WHITE et al. 1995). Nevertheless, in a recent series (JENKINS et al. 2000) the 5-year risk of systemic spread of MALT lymphoma was estimated at about 47% and the 5-year lymphoma-related mortality, at about 12%. Thus, follow-up for periods even longer than 5 years is advisable.

The second most common lymphoma encountered in the ocular adnexa, accounting for 10–28% of cases, is the follicular center lymphoma (COUPLAND et al. 1998; WHITE et al. 1995), and this is defined as a neoplasm of the follicle center B cell, which has at least a partially follicular pattern, often with poorly defined follicles that are closely packed. These follicles are populated by small to intermediate-sized lymphocytes with cleaved nuclei (centrocytes) and large cells with round vesicular nuclei, often showing one to three peripheral nucleoli (centroblasts). These tumors are graded according to their proportion of centroblasts. Grade 3 tumors, containing more than 15 centroblasts per high-power field, have a more aggressive behavior, usually requiring combination chemotherapy (NATHWANI et al. 2001). Immunophenotypically, these tumors display CD 10 reactivity and express both the Bcl 2 antiapoptotic protein and the nuclear protein Bcl 6. In these tumors, the chromosomal rearrangement t(14;18) is believed to prevent the normal switching off of the antiapoptotic Bcl 2 protein. In a recent series (JENKINS et al. 2000), follicular center lymphomas were found to be more likely than MALT lymphomas to have a systemic spread at presentation and had a 5-year mortality rate of 22%.

Only a small proportion of adnexal lymphomas are mantle cell lymphoma [5.7% (MANNAMI et al. 2001); 3.7% (AUW-HAEDRICH et al. 2001); 3.1% (JENKINS et al. 2000); 7.1% (WHITE et al. 1995)].The diagnosis of this tumor is important in view of its aggressive behavior and the frequency of associated systemic disease. It is defined as a monomorphous B cell neoplasm composed of small to medium-sized lymphoid cells with slightly irregular nuclei. The immunophenotype is characteristically CD 5 reactive and usually CD 43 positive. All cases also express the bcl 2 protein but not bcl 6.The detection of the cylin D1 protein in the nuclei is the most specific diagnostic criterion (FRIZZERA et al. 1999).

Another type of lymphoma with an aggressive behavior, which is encountered with a frequency ranging from 9% (COUPLAND et al. 1998) and 10% (JENKINS et al. 2000) to 30% (CAHILL et al. 1999) in the ocular adnexa, is the diffuse large B cell lymphoma characterized by a diffuse proliferation of B lymphoid cells with nuclei more than twice the size that of a normal lymphocyte. Immunophenotypically, the neoplastic cells show panB markers, such as CD 20, CD 22 and CD79a, and 10% of the cases express CD 5. The estimated 5-year risk of systemic spread has been estimated at about 81% and the 5-year mortality rate, at about 48% (JENKINS et al. 2000).

For all types of adnexal lymphoma, the most important prognostic factor appears to be the stage at presentation. Localized stage I disease is associated with the most favorable outcome: 87% of 108 patients with stage I disease followed for at least for 6 months were free of systemic spread after a mean follow-up of 51 months (JAKOBIEC and KNOWLES 1989). More recent data have further confirmed the importance of the stage at presentation as a prognostic factor (AUW-HAEDRICH et al. 2001; MCKELVIE et al. 2001). As examples, 78–93% of cases with stage 1E had no extraocular spread during a median follow-up of 27–44.3 months (JOHNSON et al. 1999; COUPLAND et al. 1998). The location of the tumor has been found by several authors (JAKOBIEC and KNOWLES 1989; JOHNSON et al. 1999; SIGELMAN and JAKOBIEC 1978) to correlate with the outcome, tumors located in the eyelid bearing the worst prognosis with a 67% risk of systemic involvement. Nevertheless, other authors have failed to demonstrate such a correlation (MEDEIROS and HARRIS 1989; COUPLAND et al. 1998; ELLIS et al. 1985; MCKELVIE et al. 2001). Bilaterality itself does not appear to be linked to a more frequent systemic involvement, and tumors arising in both ocular adnexa share the same molecular genetic features, indicating an origin from the same clone (MCNALLY et al. 1987).The histological type of lymphoma appears to be clearly correlated with outcome, diffuse large B cell lymphomas bearing the gloomiest outcome (JENKINS et al. 2000; CAHILL et al. 1999; MANNAMI et al. 2001; COUPLAND et al. 1998; AUW-HAEDRICH et al. 2001; SMITT and DONALDSON 1993; NAKATA et al. 1999; McKELVIE et al. 2001). Other prognostic factors are the presence of cytologic atypias, the MIB1 proliferation index (COUPLAND et al. 1998; MEDEIROS and HARRIS 1990; AUW-HAEDRICH et al. 2001), overexpression of the tumor suppressor gene *p53* in high-grade lymphoma (COUPLAND et al. 1998), expression of the marker CD 5, which is more frequently associated with bone marrow involvement (FERRY et al. 1996), the serum level of LDH (NAKATA et al. 1999) and finally the presence of monoclonality (MEDEIROS and HARRIS 1989), a feature almost universally accepted as a criterion of malignancy (KURTIN 1999). Regarding monoclonality, cases of systemic involvement with polyclonal lesions have been described, but the possibility that these lesions harbor a monoclonal population has not been genotypically excluded (ROOTMAN et al. 1984). In a recent series (JOHNSON et al. 1999), molecular genetic analysis of gene rearrangement was not helpful in predicting the development of systemic lymphomas (patients without rearrangement had a 63% incidence of systemic disease, compared with a 52% incidence of systemic involvement in patients with gene rearrangements).

It appears clear that radiotherapy is the treatment of choice for localized adnexal lymphomas, and numerous recent reports have added more evidence in this direction (STAFFORD et al. 2001; ESIK et al. 1996; SMITT and DONALDSON 1993; BALDINI et al. 1998; BOLEK et al. 1999; KENNERDELL et al. 1999). Several authors (COUPLAND et al. 1998; AUW-HAEDRICH et al. 2001; ESIK et al. 1996) agree on the fact that surgery alone triggers a higher rate of recurrence, although some studies (HARDMAN-LEA et al. 1994) have found a good outcome for conjunctival lymphomas treated with surgery alone or with cryotherapy alone (EICHLER and FRAUNFELDER 1994). Although localized orbital lymphoma can respond to chemotherapy alone (BALDINI et al. 1998), several authors (ESIK et al. 1996; LETSCHERT et al. 1991; SIGELMAN and JAKOBIEC 1978) have found its role questionable in this condition. In this latter group of series (ESIK et al. 1996), chemotherapy did not influence the length of the disease-free interval and often failed to achieve permanent local control. Nevertheless, chemotherapy in conjunction with local radiotherapy has an important role in the management of more advanced stages of disease with systemic involvement (SPECHT and LAVER 2000) and in high-grade lymphomas (SMITT and DONALDSON 1993). Intensity-modulated radiotherapy might help to reduce the rate of treatment-induced complications, and recent data have succeeded in reducing the predicted risk of severe toxicity to less than 5% while treating the planned target volume in an optimal manner (MIRALBELL et al. 2000).

Although there is undoubtedly a correlation between pathologic findings and systemic involvement, this correlation does not appear to be strong enough to make systematic work-up unnecessary in any patient with an adnexal lymphoid lesion. The importance of this systematic work-up, including a full hematological evaluation with complete blood count, liver profile, serum immuno-electrophoresis, antinuclear antibodies, possible bone marrow biopsy, and radiographic studies comprising CT scans of the orbit, chest and abdomen, is also clearly underscored by the fact that the extent of disease at presentation appears to be the most important prognostic factor. Two systematic work-ups 6 months apart usually detect nonocular disease within the 1st year in most patients; nevertheless, an annual systematic work-up should be undertaken for at least 5 years after initial diagnosis.

Ocular lymphomas can be classified into primary central nervous lymphoma, which accounts for most of the cases, and reactive hyperplasia of the uveal tract, which appears, in the light of immunophenotypical (BEN-EZRA et al. 1989; JAKOBIEC et al. 1987) and some recent genotypical data (COCKERHAM et al. 2000), to be a low-grade lymphoma likely to be extramarginal in type (MALT) in most instances, with a diffuse infiltrate of lymphocytes, plasmacytoid lymphocytes, Dutcher bodies and interspersed germinal centers. The eye, and more specifically the uveal tract, can also be secondarily infiltrated by systemic lymphoma or leukemic processes that originate elsewhere.

Primary central nervous lymphoma, whose incidence has recently increased mainly as a consequence of the AIDS epidemic (PAULUS et al. 2001), becomes manifest in the eye as

multiple creamy subretinal and epithelial pigment infiltrates; these remain static for a prolonged period of time, but over 5–10 years the entire uvea becomes diffusely thickened,
frequently with evidence of extraocular episcleral extension behind the globe or into the
conjunctiva. Vitreous cells mimicking uveitis refractive to steroid treatment are the most
common clinical characteristic (66%), followed by pseudohypopyon (40%) (VELEZ et al.
2000; CHAR et al. 1988). Nonrhegmatogenous retinal detachment produced secondarily by
the subretinal pigmented epithelium tumoral infiltrates, scarring and atrophy of the retinal
pigment epithelium, necrotizing retinitis, infiltration of the retinal vasculature with arterial
or venous obstruction, and finally optic nerve invasion, have also been described
(BARDENSTEIN 1998; GILL and JAMPOL 2001). About 80% of the lesions will involve both
eyes at some point of the disease. Ocular symptoms such as floaters and painless visual loss
precede CNS symptoms in about 80% of patients.

Histopathologically, the most characteristic finding is that of collections of pleomorphic
cells with frequently indented nuclei and usually scant cytoplasm in the space between the
retinal pigment epithelium and Bruch's membrane. If the retinal pigment epithelium is
ruptured and the inner layers of the retina are invaded, the tumor cells tend to grow in an
angiocentric pattern with perivascular cuffs and concentric reticulin deposits. Immuno-
histochemically these tumors more often express B cell markers, and recent investigations
(DAIBATA et al. 2000) have shown the presence of Epstein-Barr virus and human herpes
virus-6 genome in these neoplastic cells, underscoring the possible importance of these viruses
as etiological factors. Vitreous cytology has proved to be a sensitive, reliable, and reproducible
method of diagnosing intraocular lymphoma in cases with a high index of suspicion based on
the clinical findings (AKPEK et al. 1999b; SCROGGS et al. 1990). Flow cytometry (DAVIS et al.
1997) and PCR (KATAI et al. 1997; WHITE et al. 1999) further enhance the accuracy of
diagnosis (DE LAEY 2001). Nevertheless, it must be emphasized that the absence of
neoplastic cells in specimen sampling in no way rules out the diagnosis of intraocular
lymphoma. One group found an elevated level of interleukin 10 in vitreous and CSF, with an
IL10-to-IL6 ratio greater than 1 in patients with primary CNS lymphoma but not in those
with nonneoplastic uveitis (WHITCUP et al. 1997). However, a recent prospective study
(AKPEK et al. 1999a) found an IL10-to-IL6 ratio greater than 1 in 8 of 14 vitreous biopsies
performed in 13 patients with nonneoplastic uveitis.

The outcome of patients with primary CNS lymphoma is dismal, with a survival of
1.5 months without treatment once debilitating neurological symptoms have occurred.
Although a correlation between survival and the histological subtype of lymphoma has
been described (HOCHBERG and MILLER 1988), most authors have found no correlation
(PAULUS et al. 2000). The treatment can be limited to vitrectomy in patients with only
vitreous involvement or with nonprogressive lesions without the threat of macular
invasion. When signs of progression are observed, whole-eye irradiation is
recommended, with the realiza-tion or recognition that complications such as retinal
vasculopathy and optic neuropathy may occur. When concomitant CNS involvement is
found, combination treatment based on chemo-therapy, including intrathecal
methotrexate and multiple systemic agents, and on radiotherapy has been
recommended (DEANGELIS et al. 1992; VALLURI et al. 1995). Methotrexate given prior to
radiotherapy helps to reduce the risk of leukoencephalopathy and cognitive defects.
Methotrexate, a drug that crosses the blood–brain barrier, given in high doses appears
to be the single most effective chemotherapeutic agent for primary CNS lymphoma (NASIR and
DEANGELIS 2000; BLAY et al. 1998), but some authors have expressed doubts about the role of
single-agent chemotherapy in the management of primary CNS lymphoma (NASIR and
DEANGELIS 2000; MCLAUGHIN 2000). In one study (FREILICH et al. 1996), a response rate of
92% and a median survival of 30 months was observed with chemotherapy using high-dose
methotrexate + vincristine + procarbazine or thiotepa. The incidence of neurotoxicity was
extremely low. In other studies there have been attempts to break down the blood–brain
barrier with mannitol in order to enhance the concentration of chemotherapeutic agents in

the brain (NEUWELT et al. 1991). With a multimodal treatment, a response rate of 85% is observed with a median survival of 17–45 months (PAULUS et al. 2000). Patients with AIDS show a poorer prognosis, with a median survival of 13.5 months, when treated with multimodal therapy (PAULUS et al. 2000). Highly active antiretroviral therapy (HAART) has been shown to be linked with a positive outcome in HIV patients with non-Hodgkin lymphomas (TIRELLI and BERNARDI 2001).

Systemic lymphoma may also involve the eye secondarily. In most such cases the choroid is characteristically involved, generating a progressive diffuse choroidal thickening. In other cases there may be signs of anterior uveitis or iris infiltration, or the lesion may be seen posteriorly as a focal choroidal mass simulating a primary ocular melanoma. T-cell lymphomas involving the eye secondarily have a poor prognosis. The treatment of secondary uveal lymphoma consists in ocular radiation therapy, which appears to be effective in combination with regional or whole-body regional lymph node irradiation and chemotherapy for advanced stage disease.

Pseudotumor, or idiopathic orbital inflammation, must be clinically differentiated from lymphoma, on one hand, and on the other from Graves' disease. In contrast to the indolent growth of orbital lymphomas, the presentation of orbital pseudotumor can be explosive and can mimic orbital cellulitis of acute onset, erythema of the eyelids, chemosis of the conjunctiva, motility disturbances and, rarely, progressive decline in vision. In children, the lesions are bilateral in 40% of cases. In other cases a subacute presentation is observed, with less significant inflammatory signs leading to proptosis and motility disturbances. The least common presentation of orbital pseudotumor is that of a progressive and inexorable congealing fibrosis of the entire orbit, ultimately with extension into the adjacent sinuses. These cases of idiopathic sclerosing orbital inflammation have histological and immunophenotypical features similar to those observed in retroperitoneal fibrosis (McCARTHY et al. 1993) and have been reported to occur in association with multifocal fibrosclerosis (AYLWARD et al. 1995). On CT scanning, pseudotumor can be distinguished from Graves' orbitopathy by the inflammatory involvement of both the extraocular muscles and their tendons, while Graves' orbitopathy characteristically involves the muscles but spares the tendons. The inflammation also usually invades the orbital fat or the Tenon tissue outside the sclera and may spread to the connective tissues around the dura of the optic nerve or to the lacrimal gland. Histopathologically, pseudotumors are hypocellular. The inflammatory cells that are present are mostly T lymphocytes, and lesser numbers of plasma cells, eosinophils and neutrophils. There is a fibrous stroma with numerous collagen bundles clinically giving the lesion a firm consistency, in contrast to the rubbery consistency of lymphomas, which are usually devoid of prominent fibrous tissue. If granulomatous inflammation or an angiocentric or angiodestructive pattern is noted histologically, a systemic disease such as Wegener's granulomatosis or polyarteritis nodosa should be considered and the appropriate clinical tests should be ordered. In cases with vasculitis, radiotherapy would not be recommended and may add more insult to the already destructive process triggered by the vasculitis itself.

A pseudotumor may show a dramatic and rapid response to high-dose corticosteroids, which usually relieve symptoms and signs rapidly. In order to prevent a rebound, corticosteroids should be tapered over a period of 4–6 weeks. If corticosteroid therapy sustained over several weeks fails to clear the symptoms, radiotherapy is then recommended, and doses ranging from 10 to 30 Gy have been reported (ROOTMAN and NUGENT 1982; KENNERDELL 1991a, b; LANCIANO et al. 1990; JEREB et al. 1984; ORDER and DONALDSON 1990). Low-dose radiotherapy has also been advocated (HENDERSON 1980; SERGOTT et al. 1981) and, in a more recent study, doses of 2–3 Gy fractionated over several weeks allowed resolution of the symptomatology in eight histologically proven pseudotumors (NOTTER et al. 1997). The same authors also suggested that the need for higher doses in the preceding studies might be linked with the difficulties in distinguishing pseudotumor from lymphoma in some cases. However, in cases of myositis, doses between

25 and 30 Gy are re-commended (SNEBOLD 2000) and when there is intracranial extension of the inflammation, doses ranging from 20 to 40 Gy have been recommended (FROHMAN et al. 1986; KAYE et al. 1984). In cases of idiopathic sclerosing inflammation of the orbit, aggressive multiagent immunosuppression with systemic cortocosteroids and cyclophosphamide or azathioprine has been recommended (ROOTMAN et al. 1994).

In Graves' orbitopathy, autoantibodies are targeted against TSH receptor in the orbital fibroblasts (HEUFELDER 1995) and extraocular muscles (BUSUTTIL and FRAUMAN 2001). The resulting recruitment and activation of lymphocytes leads to the production of cytokines, such as interferon gamma, that stimulate the orbital fibroblasts to produce glycosaminoglycans, leading to edema and chemosis. Interleukin 1 and TNF alpha, which are produced by stimulated macrophages, exacerbate the inflammation by allowing fibroblasts to act as antigen-presenting cells with aberrant expression of HLA DR (WARWAR 1999). Pentoxifylline, by inhibiting cytokine-induced expression of HLA DR (BALAZS et al. 1997), reduced the orbital swelling but not the proptosis and extraocular muscle involvement in 8 of 10 patients. Radiotherapy also modulates the expression by orbital fibroblasts of the interleukin 1 receptor antagonist. Low baseline values of IL1 RA have been found in smokers who have an unfavorable response to treatment (HOFBAUER et al. 1997). However, other investigators (KAHALY et al. 1999) have found no difference in clinical amelioration and response rate to radiotherapy between smokers and nonsmokers, suggesting that cigarette smoking is only one of the many factors involved in the progression of thyroid-associated ophthalmopathy.

Radiologically, in Graves' orbitopathy swelling of extraocular muscles is seen while their tendons are spared. The inferior rectus muscle is the more frequently involved. Radiotherapy has been used in Graves' disease for more than 50 years. Its beneficial effect may be linked to the suppression of the highly sensitive orbital lymphocytes and the orbital fibroblasts, which have intermediate sensitivity and whose premature terminal differentiation into postmitotic fibrocytes is also accelerated (KAHALY et al. 1989). Analysis of the literature is complicated by the absence of standardized protocols and consensus criteria on how to judge the results of radiotherapy. Several studies have shown an overall response rate of approximately 60% (SANDLER et al. 1989; ERICKSON et al. 1995; KAO et al. 1993). Radiotherapy appears to be effective in the early, inflammatory phase of the disease, but has little effect in the chronic fibrotic stages, in which surgery is indicated. Radiotherapy reduces the congestion and the inflammation, but there is little amelioration of proptosis (PRUMMEL et al. 1993; PRUMMEL and WIERSINGA 1993; DALLOW and NETLAND 2000; BECKENDORF et al. 1999). There are conflicting opinions on motility disturbances: some authors have suggested that radiotherapy produces little improvement in the treatment of strabismus associated with Graves' disease (DALLOW and NETLAND 1999), while others have found that radiotherapy should only be used to treat motility impairment in cases of moderately severe Graves' orbitopathy (MOURITS et al. 2000). Some authors claim that radiotherapy and corticosteroid treatment are equally effective in the treatment of Graves' disease (PRUMMEL et al. 1993), although radiotherapy is associated with less frequent and less severe side effects. Others (MARCOCCI et al. 1993) have found radiotherapy combined with steroids more effective than corticosteroid treatment alone. The generally accepted dose is 20 Gy delivered over 2 weeks (DONALDSON et al. 1973; see also chapter 15 in this volume), but recent data (KAHALY et al. 1999) have suggested that administration of 20 Gy in 20 weeks is better tolerated and more effective than 20 Gy in 2 weeks; visual acuity and muscle motility improved only in patients treated with 1 Gy/week. Controversies still persist about the management of thyroid ophthalmopathy, and the recent results of a prospective, randomized, double-blind, placebo-controlled study (GORAM et al. 2001) in 42 patients with mild to moderate ophthalmopathy have led to doubts about the role of radiotherapy in the treatment of Graves' disease. As emphasized by FELDON (2001), broader multicenter studies using carefully defined clinical progression as a criterion for eligibility should be performed.

Radiotherapy plays a central role in the management of orbital rhabdomyosarcoma (see chapter 13 in this volume), and recent results from different groups (CRIST et al. 2001; KODET et al. 1997; OBERLIN et al. 2001) have shown excellent overall survival when it has been given in combination with chemotherapy. However, late complications linked to the high radiation doses often occur (PAULINO et al. 2000; RANEY et al. 2000; FIORILLO et al. 1999). Improved techniques able to reduce such local side effects as cataracts, orbital hypoplasia, dry eyes, radiation retinopathy, and chronic keratoconjunctivitis will be important. In this context, conformational radiotherapy appears to have an important role. Conformational three-dimensional planning-assisted proton beam radiation has recently been successfully used to treat two patients with orbital rhabdomyosarcomas (HUG et al. 2000). Patients with recurrent rhabdomyosarcoma can be treated with implant brachytherapy administered by molds containing iodine-125 and generating highly localized radiation with minimal opportunity for damage to the brain (ABRAMSON et al. 1997).

Liposarcoma, the most common soft tissue sarcoma of adults, rarely infiltrates the orbit. In the orbit, histopathology usually reveals a well-differentiated or a myxoid type, and it has a better prognosis than the aggressive pleiomorphic or round cell variants. Myxoid liposarcoma, the commonest subtype encountered in the body, is composed of numerous lipoblasts proliferating among a stroma rich in mucopolysaccharides with a characteristic plexiform vascular network. Some authors (EVANS 1995) have suggested that round cell liposarcomas are actually cellular myxoid liposarcomas and that both tumors are associated with the same chromosomal translocation (KNIGHT et al. 1995). Primary orbital liposarcoma is difficult to excise completely because of its infiltrating behavior. Radiotherapy is often required postoperatively, especially with regard to the apparent radiosensitivity of this sarcoma (BASSO et al. 1992; EVANS 1995). In the few orbital cases described that had been treated with surgery alone, a recurrence rate of 85% was observed (COCKERHAM et al. 1998). In a series of a 112 liposarcomas, mostly situated in the lower extremities and treated by conservative surgery and radiation, the histological subtype appeared to correlate with the outcome in terms of local control, metastasis, and survival. Well-differentiated and myxoid liposarcoma had local control rates exceeding 90% at 10 years (ZAGARS et al. 1996).

The treatment of pilocytic astrocytoma of the optic nerve is controversial, but there seems to be a current trend toward surveillance of these patients. Primary resection appears to be indicated in the case of tumor progression and intracranial extension or progressive visual impairment. Numerous studies have demonstrated that postsurgical radiotherapy is more effective than surgery alone to reduce the treatment failure rate (GRABENBAUER et al. 2000; JENKIN et al. 1995; FLICKINGER et al. 1988; PACKER et al. 1983).The role of chemotherapy is controversial, but recent reports have included encouraging data in the management of progressive lesions or posterior lesions (MAHONEY et al. 2000; SILVA et al. 2000; AQUINO et al. 1999; CHAMBERLAIN and GRAFE 1995). Chemotherapy, though not devoid of side effects, also has the advantage in young patients of avoiding the late side effects sometimes associated with radiotherapy, such as endocrine dysfunction and intellectual decline (THOMPSON and LESSELL 1997; PIERCE et al. 1990). In this context, the advantage of conformational radiotherapy appears clear (LOEFFLER et al. 1999), and a recent report of the use of fractionated stereotactic radiotherapy for optic nerve glioma in ten children showed excellent tumor control with a follow-up ranging from 12 to 72 months (DEBUS et al. 1999). Further studies with longer follow-up times are needed to corroborate these findings.

Sebaceous carcinoma represents a neoplasm that is frequently encountered in the eyelid, where it can arise from the meibomian glands, from the glands of Zeiss, or even from the sebaceous glands in the caruncle. This tumor displays an aggressive behavior and shows a tendency to spread diffusely in a pagetoid fashion within the conjunctiva and towards the skin. Surgery with wide excision has been recommended. However, serial sections of surgical margins with microscopic control yielded better results in a recent study (SPENCER et al. 2001). Although sebaceous cell carcinoma is regarded as relatively radioresistant, some reports have shown no recurrences after high-dose radiotherapy (YEN et al. 2000; PARDO and BORODIE 1996; MATSUMOTO et al. 1995), but further studies with longer follow-up intervals are required to confirm the efficacy of this treatment.

Another eyelid tumor displaying an aggressive behavior and the ability for pagetoid spread and extensive invasion within the conjunctiva is the Merkel cell tumor, which usually affects patients in their seventies. Involvement of regional lymph nodes and metastatic disease are regarded as poor prognostic factors (FENIG et al. 1997). The radiosensitivity (FENIG et al. 1997; MARKS et al. 1990; MORRISON et al. 1990) and chemosensitivity (TAI et al. 2000; WYNNE and KEARSLEY 1988) of this tumor have been demonstrated. Immediate postoperative irradiation of the primary tumor site and the adjacent lymph nodes with the aim of achieving local control has been recommended on the basis of a recent series (BISCHOF et al. 1999). Adequate treatment of this aggressive tumor appears to be multimodal, requiring surgery, combination chemotherapy, and radiotherapy (FENIG et al. 1997; TAI et al. 2000).

In conclusion, it appears clear that radiotherapy is and remains one of the cornerstones of management of patients with intraocular and adnexal tumors. However, controversies persist, and the precise role of radiotherapy in the management of such rare and aggressive tumors as orbital angiosarcoma, leiomyosarcoma, osteosarcoma and alveolar soft tissue sarcoma still requires further worldwide cooperation. We are grateful for the extraordinarily fine and well-balanced coverage of the most common ocular conditions covered in this second edition and thank the chief editors, ophthalmic clinical oncologists, and radiotherapists who have made this valuable enterprise possible by sharing their knowledge for the benefit of patients and their less experienced colleagues.

Acknowledgements. We would like to thank Dr. Thaddeus P. Dryja for helpful suggestions on this text.

References

Abramson DH, Fass D, McCormick B et al (1997) Implant brachytherapy: a novel treatment for recurrent orbital rhabdomyosarcoma. J AAPOS 1:154–157

Akpek EK, Maca SM, Christen WG et al (1999a) Elevated vitreous interleukin-10 level is not diagnostic of intraocular-central nervous system lymphoma. Ophthalmology 106:2291–2295

Akpek EK, Ahmed I, Hochberg FH et al (1999b) Intraocular-central nervous system lymphoma: clinical features, diagnosis, and outcomes. Ophthalmology 106:1805–1810

Akpek EK, Polcharoen W, Ferry JA et al (1999c) Conjunctival lymphoma masquerading as chronic conjunctivitis. Ophthalmology 106:757–760

Aquino VM, Fort DW, Kamen BA (1999) Carboplatin for the treatment of children with newly diagnosed optic chiasm gliomas: a phase II study. J Neurooncol 41:255–259

Auw-Haedrich C, Coupland SE, Kapp A et al (2001) Long term outcome of ocular adnexal lymphoma subtyped according to the REAL classification. Revised European and American Lymphoma. Br J Ophthalmol 85:63–69

Aylward GW, Sullivan TJ, Garner A, Moseley I et al (1995) Orbital involvement in multifocal fibrosclerosis. Br J Ophthalmol 79:246–249

Balazs C, Kiss E, Vamos A, Molnar I et al (1997) Beneficial effect of pentoxifylline on thyroid associated ophthalmopathy (TAO): a pilot study. J Clin Endocrinol Metab 82:1999–2002

Baldini L, Blini M, Guffanti A, Fossati V et al (1998) Treatment and prognosis in a series of primary extranodal lymphomas of the ocular adnexa. Ann Oncol 9:779–781

Bardenstein DS (1998) Intraocular lymphoma. Cancer Control 5:317–325

Basso Ricci S, Milani F, Gramaglia A et al (1992) On extravisceral soft tissue sarcomas. Effectiveness of radiation treatment and problems of radiotherapy and radiosurgical treatment. Panminerva Med 34:69–76

Beckendorf V, Maalouf T, George JL, Bey P et al (1999) Place of radiotherapy in the treatment of Graves' orbitopathy. Int J Radiat Oncol Biol Phys 43:805–815

Ben-Ezra D, Sahel JA, Harris NL et al (1989) Uveal lymphoid infiltrates: immunohistochemical evidence for a lymphoid neoplasia. Br J Ophthalmol 73:846–851

Bischof M, Van Kampen M, Huber P et al (1999) Merkel cell carcinoma: the role of radiation therapy in general management. Strahlenther Onkol 175:611–615

Blay JY, Conroy T, Chevreau C et al (1998) High-dose methotrexate for the treatment of primary cerebral lymphomas: analysis of survival and late neurologic toxicity in a retrospective series. J Clin Oncol 16:864–871

Bolek TW, Moyses HM, Marcus RB Jr et al (1999) Radiotherapy in the management of orbital lymphoma. Int J Radiat Oncol Biol Phys 44:31–36

Burke JS (1999a) Are there site-specific differences among the MALT lymphomas – morphologic, clinical? Am J Clin Pathol 111 [1 Suppl 1]:S133–S143

Burke JS (1999b) Extranodal hematopoietic/lymphoid disorders. An introduction. Am J Clin Pathol 111 [1 Suppl 1]:S40–S45

Busuttil BE, Frauman AG (2001) Extrathyroidal manifestations of Graves' disease: the thyrotropin receptor is expressed in extraocular, but not cardiac, muscle tissues. J Clin Endocrinol Metab 86:2315–2319

Cahill M, Barnes C, Moriarty P et al (1999) Ocular adnexal lymphoma-comparison of MALT lymphoma with other histological types. Br J Ophthalmol 83:742–747

Chamberlain MC, Grafe MR (1995) Recurrent chiasmatic-hypothalamic glioma treated with oral etoposide. J Clin Oncol 13:2072–2076

Char DH, Ljung BM, Miller T et al (1988) Primary intraocular lymphoma (ocular reticular cell sarcoma) diagnosis and management. Ophthalmology 95:625–630

Cockerham GC, Jakobiec FA (1997) Lymphoproliferative disorders of the ocular adnexa. Int Ophthalmol Clin 37:39–59

Cockerham KP, Kennerdell JS, Celin SE et al (1998) Liposarcoma of the orbit: a management challenge. Ophthalmic Plast Reconstr Surg 14:370–374

Cockerham GC, Hiddayat AA, Bijwaard KE et al (2000) Re-evaluation of "reactive lymphoid hyperplasia of the uvea": an immunohistochemical and molecular analysis of 10 cases. Ophthalmology 107:151–158

Coupland SE, Krause L, Delecluse HJ et al (1998) Lymphoproliferative lesions of the ocular adnexa. Analysis of 112 cases. Ophthalmology 105:1430–1441

Coupland SE, Foss HD, Anagnostopoulos I et al (1999a) Immunoglobulin VH gene expression among extranodal marginal zone B-cell lymphomas of the ocular adnexa. Invest Ophthalmol Vis Sci 40:555–562

Coupland SE, Foss HD, Assaf C et al (1999b) T-cell and T/natural killer-cell lymphomas involving ocular and ocular adnexal tissues: a clinicopathologic, immunohistochemical, and molecular study of seven cases. Ophthalmology 106:2109–2120

Crist VM, Anderson JR, Meza JL et al (2001) Intergroup rhabdomyosarcoma study-IV: results for patients with nonmetastatic disease. J Clin Oncol 19:3091–3102

Daibata M, Komatsu T, Taguchi H (2000) Human herpesviruses in primary ocular lymphoma. Leuk Lymphoma 37:361–365

Dallow R.L, Netland P (2000) Management of thyroid associated orbitopathy. In: Albert DM, Jakobiec FA (eds) Principles and practice of ophthalmology. Saunders, Philadelphia, pp 3082–3099

Davis JL, Viciana AL, Ruiz P (1997) Diagnosis of intraocular lymphoma by flow cytometry. Am J Ophthalmol 124:362–372

De Laey JJ (2001) Intra-ocular non-Hodgkin's lymphoma. Diagnostic aspects. Bull Soc Belge Ophtalmol 279:81–89

DeAngelis, Yahalom J, Thaler T (1992) Combined modality therapy for primary CNS lymphoma. J Clin Oncol 10:635–643

Debus J, Kocagoncu KO, Hoss A et al (1999) Fractionated stereotactic radiotherapy (FSRT) for optic glioma. Int J Radiat Oncol Biol Phys 44:243–248

Donaldson SS, Bagshaw MA, Kriss JP (1973) Supervoltage orbital radiotherapy for Graves' ophthalmopathy. J Clin Endocrinol Metab 37:276–285

Drya T (1993) Fundamentals of ophthalmic genetics. In: Albert DM, Jakobiec FA (eds) Principles and practice of ophthalmology: basic siences. Sounders Philadelphia

Eichler MD, Fraunfelder FT (1994) Cryotherapy for conjunctival lymphoid tumors. Am J Ophthalmol 118:463–467

Ellis JH, Banks PM, Cambell RJ et al (1985) Lymphoid tumors of the ocular adnexa. Clinical correlation with the working formulation classification and immunoperoxidase staining of paraffin sections. Ophthalmology 92:1311–1324

Erickson BA, Harris GJ, Lewandowski MF et al (1995) Echographic monitoring of response of extraocular muscles to irradiation in Graves' ophthalmopathy. Int J Radiat Oncol Biol Phys 31:651–660

Esik O, Ikeda H, Mukai K et al (1996) A retrospective analysis of different modalities for treatment of primary orbital non-Hodgkin's lymphomas. Radiother Oncol 38:13–18

Evans HL (1995) Classification and grading of soft-tissue sarcomas. A comment. Hematol Oncol Clin North Am 9:653–656

Feldon SE (2001) Radiation therapy for Graves' ophthalmopathy: trick or treat? Ophthalmology 108:1521–1522

Fenig E, Brenner B, Katz A et al (1997) The role of radiation therapy and chemotherapy in the treatment of Merkel cell carcinoma. Cancer 80:881–885

Ferry JA, Yang WI, Zukerberg LR et al (1996) CD5+ extranodal marginal zone B-cell (MALT) lymphoma. A low grade neoplasm with a propensity for bone marrow involvement and relapse. Am J Clin Pathol 105:31–37

Fiorillo A, Migliorati R, Vassallo P et al (1999) Radiation late effects in children treated for orbital rhabdomyosarcoma. Radiother Oncol 53:143–148

Flickinger JC, Torres C, Deutsch M (1988) Management of low-grade gliomas of the optic nerve and chiasm. Cancer 1:635–642

Freilich RJ, Delattre JY, Monjour A et al (1996) Chemotherapy without radiation therapy as initial treatment for primary CNS lymphoma in older patients. Neurology 6:435–439

Frizzera G, Wu CD, Inghirami G (1999) The usefulness of immunophenotypic and genotypic studies in the diagnosis and classification of hematopoietic and lymphoid neoplasms. An update. Am J Clin Pathol 11 [1 Suppl 1]:S13–S39

Frohman LP, Kupersmith MJ, Lang J et al (1986) Intracranial extension and bone destruction in orbital pseudotumor. Arch Ophthalmol 104:380–384

Gill MK, Jampol ML (2001) Variations in the presentation of primary intraocular lymphoma: case reports and a review. Surv Ophthalmol 45:463–471

Gorman CA, Garitty JA, Fatourechi V et al (2001) A prospective, randomized, double-bind, placebo-controlled study of orbital radiotherapy for Graves' Ophthalmopathy. Ophthalmology 108:1523–1534

Grabenbauer GG, Schuchardt U, Buchfelder M et al (2000) Radiation therapy of optico-hypothalamic gliomas (OHG) – radiographic response, vision and late toxicity. Radiother Oncol 54:239–245

Hardman-Lea S, Kerr-Muir M, Wotherspoon AC et al (1994) Mucosal-associated lymphoid tissue lymphoma of the conjunctiva. Arch Ophthalmol 112:1207–1212

Harris NL, Isaacson PG (1999) What are the criteria for distinguishing MALT from non-MALT lymphoma at extranodal sites? Am J Clin Pathol 111 [1 Suppl 1]:S126–S132

Harris NL, Jaffe ES, Stein H et al (1994) A revised European-American classification of lymphoid neoplasms: a proposal from the International Lymphoma Study Group. Blood 84:1361–1392

Henderson JW (1980) Lymphocytic inflammatory pseudotumor. In: Henderson JW, Farrow GM (eds) Orbital tumors. Decker, New York, pp 512–526

Heufelder AE (1995) Involvement of the orbital fibroblast and TSH receptor in the pathogenesis of Graves' ophthalmopathy. Thyroid 5:331–340

Hochberg FH, Miller DC (1988) Primary central nervous system lymphoma. J Neurosurg 68:835–853

Hofbauer LC, Muhlberg T, Konig A et al (1997) Soluble interleukin-1 receptor antagonist serum levels in smokers and nonsmokers with Graves' ophthalmopathy undergoing orbital radiotherapy. J Clin Endocrinol Metab 82:2244–2247

Hornblass A, Jakobiec FA, Konig A et al (1987) Orbital lymphoid tumors located predominantly within extraocular muscles. Ophthalmology 94:688–697

Hug EB, Adams J, Fitzek M et al (2000) Fractionated, three-dimensional, planning-assisted proton-radiation therapy for orbital rhabdomyosarcoma: a novel technique. Int J Radiat Oncol Biol Phys 47:979–984

Isaacson PG (1999) Mucosa-associated lymphoid tissue lymphoma. Semin Hematol 36:139–147

Isaacson PG, Wright DH (1983) Malignant lymphoma of mucosa-associated lymphoid tissue. A distinctive type of B-cell lymphoma. Cancer 52:1410–1416

Jakobiec FA (1982a) Orbital inflammations and lymphoid tumors. Trans New Orleans Acad Ophthalmol 30:52–85

Jakobiec FA (1982b) Tumors of the lacrimal gland and lacrimal sac. Trans New Orleans Acad Ophthalmol 30:190–202

Jakobiec FA, Knowles DM (1989) An overview of ocular adnexal lymphoid tumors. Trans Am Ophthalmol Soc 87:420–442

Jakobiec FA, Yeo JH, Trokel SL et al (1982) Combined clinical and computed tomographic diagnosis of primary lacrimal fossa lesions. Am J Ophthalmol 94:785–807

Jakobiec FA, Sacks E, Kronish JW et al (1987a) Multifocal static creamy choroidal infiltrates: an early sign of lymphoid neoplasia. Ophthalmology 94:397–406

Jakobiec FA, Neri A, Knowles DM (1987) Genotypic monoclonality in immunophenotypically polyclonal orbital lymphoid tumors. A model of tumor progression in the lymphoid system. The 1986 Wendell Hughes lecture. Ophthalmology 94:980–994

Jakobiec FA, Sacks E, Kronish JW et al (1997) Multifocal static creamy choroidal infiltrates. An early sign of lymphoid neoplasia. Ophthalmology 94:397–406

Jenkin D, Greenberg M, Hoffman H et al (1995) Brain tumors in children: long-term survival after radiation treatment. Int J Radiat Oncol Biol Phys 31:445–451

Jenkins C, Rose GE, Bruce C et al (2000) Histological features of ocular adnexal lymphoma (REAL classification) and their association with patient morbidity and survival. Br J Ophthalmol 84:907–913

Jereb B, Lee H, Jakobiec FA et al (1984) Radiation therapy of conjunctival and orbital lymphoid tumors. Int J Radiat Oncol Biol Phys 10:1013–1019

Johnson TE, Tse DT, Byrne Ge Jr et al (1999) Ocular-adnexal lymphoid tumors: a clinicopathologic and molecular genetic study of 77 patients. Ophthal Plast Reconstr Surg 15:171–179

Kahaly G, Grubl M, Moncayo R et al (1989) Thyroid-stimulating and eye muscle antibodies in Graves' disease and Graves' orbitopathy. Dev Ophthalmol 20:68–78

Kahaly G, Roesler HP, Kutzner J et al (1999) Radiotherapy for thyroid-associated orbitopathy. Exp Clin Endocrinol Diabetes 107 [Suppl 5]:S201–S207

Kao SC, Kendler DH, Nugent RA et al (1993) Radiotherapy in the management of thyroid orbitopathy. Computed tomography and clinical outcomes. Arch Ophthalmol 111:819–823

Katai N, Kuroiwa S, Fujimori K et al (1997) Diagnosis of intraocular lymphoma by polymerase chain reaction. Graefes Arch Clin Exp Ophthalmol 235:431–436

Kaye AH, Hahn JF, Cracium A et al (1984) Intracranial extension of inflammatory pseudotumor of the orbit. Case report. J Neurosurg 60:625–629

Keleti D, Flickinger JC, Hobson SR et al (1992) Radiotherapy of lymphoproliferative diseases of the orbit. Surveillance of 65 cases. Am J Clin Oncol 15:422–427

Kennerdell JS (1991a) The management of sclerosing nonspecific orbital inflammation. Ophthalmic Surg 22:512–518

Kennerdell JS (1991b) Management of nonspecific inflammatory and lymphoid orbital lesions. Int Ophthalmol Clin 31:7–15

Kennerdell JS, Flores NE, Hartsock RJ (1999) Low-dose radiotherapy for lymphoid lesions of the orbit and ocular adnexa. Ophthal Plast Reconstr Surg 15:129–133

Knight JC, Renwick PJ, Cin PD et al (1995) Translocation t(12;16)(q13;p11) in myxoid liposarcoma and round cell liposarcoma: molecular and cytogenetic analysis. Cancer Res 55:24–27

Knowles DM, Jakobiec FA (1992) Malignant lymphoma and lymphoid hyperplasia occurring in the ocular adnexa. In: Knowles DM (ed) Neoplastic hematology. Williams and Wilkins, Baltimore, pp 1009–1046

Knowles DM, Jakobiec FA, McNally L et al (1990) Lymphoid hyperplasia and malignant lymphoma occurring in the ocular adnexa (orbit, conjunctiva, and eyelids): a prospective multiparametric analysis of 108 cases during 1977 to 1987. Hum Pathol 21:959–973

Knowles DM II, Athan E, Ubriaco A et al (1989) Extranodal noncutaneous lymphoid hyperplasias represented a continous spectrum of B-cell neoplasia: demontration by molecular genetics analysis. Blood 73:1635–1645

Kodet R, Newton Wa Jr, Hamoudi AB et al (1997) Orbital rhabdomyosarcomas and related tumors in childhood: relationship of morphology to prognosis – an Intergroup Rhabdomyosarcoma study. Med Pediatr Oncol 29:51–60

Kurtin PJ (1999) How do you distinguish benign from malignant extranodal small B-cell proliferations? Am J Clin Pathol 111 [1 Suppl 1]:S119–S125

Lanciano R, Fowble B, Sergott RC (1990) The results of radiotherapy for orbital pseudotumor. Int J Radiat Oncol Biol Phys 18:407–411

Lauer SA (2000) Ocular adnexal lymphoid tumors. Curr Opin Ophthalmol 11:361–366

Letschert JG, Gonzalezgonzalel D, Oskam J et al (1991) Results of radiotherapy in patients with stage I orbital non-Hodgkin's lymphoma. Radiother Oncol 22:36–44

Loeffler JS, Kooy HM, Tarbell NJ (1999) The emergence of conformal radiotherapy: special implications for pediatric neuro-oncology. Int J Radiat Oncol Biol Phys 44:237–238

Mahoney DH Jr, Cohen ME, Friedman HS (2000) Carboplatin is effective therapy for young children with progressive optic pathway tumors: a Pediatric Oncology Group phase II study. Neurooncology 2:213–220

Mannami T, Yoshimo T, Oshima K et al (2001) Clinical, histopathological, and immunogenetic analysis of ocular adnexal lymphoproliferative disorders: characterization of MALT lymphoma and reactive lymphoid hyperplasia. Mod Pathol 14:641–649

Marcocci C, Bartelana L, Bruno-Bossio G et al (1993) Orbital radiotherapy in the treatment of endocrine ophthalmopathy: when and why? Dev Ophthalmol 25:131–141

Marks ME, Kim RY, Salter MM et al (1990) Radiotherapy as an adjunct in the management of Merkel cell carcinoma. Cancer 65:60–64

Matsumoto CS, Nakatsuka K, Matsuo K et al (1995) Sebaceous carcinoma responds to radiation therapy. Ophthalmologica 209:280–283

McCarthy JM, White VA, Harris G et al (1993) Idiopathic sclerosing inflammation of the orbit: immunohistologic analysis and comparison with retroperitoneal fibrosis. Mod Pathol 6:581–587

McKelvie PA, McNab A, Francis IC et al (2001) Ocular and lymphoproliferative disease: a series of 73 cases. Clin Exp Ophthalmol 29:387–393

McLaughin P (2000) The Nasir/DeAngelis article reviewed. Oncology 14:244

McNally L, Jakobiec FA, Knowles DM Jr (1987) Clinical, morphologic, immunophenotypic, and molecular genetic analysis of bilateral ocular adnexal lymphoid neoplasms in 17 patients. Am J Ophthalmol 103:555–568

Medeiros LJ, Harris NL (1989) Lymphoid infiltrates of the orbit and conjunctiva. A morphologic and immunophenotypic study of 99 cases. Am J Surg Pathol 13:459–471

Medeiros LJ, Harris NL (1990) Immunohistologic analysis of small lymphocytic infiltrates of the orbit and conjunctiva. Hum Pathol 21:1126–1131

Miralbell R, Cella R, Weber D et al (2000) Optimizing radiotherapy of orbital and paraorbital tumors: intensity- modulated X-ray beams vs. intensity-modulated proton beams. Int J Radiat Oncol Biol Phys 47:1111–1119

Morrison WH, Peters LJ, Silva EG et al (1990) The essential role of radiation therapy in securing locoregional control of Merkel cell carcinoma. Int J Radiat Oncol Biol Phys 19:583–591

Mourits MP, Van Kempen-Harteveld ML, Garcia MBG et al (2000) Radiotherapy for Graves' orbitopathy: randomised placebo-controlled study. Lancet 355:1505–1509 [abstract by NJ Newman in: Am J Ophthalmol 130:382]

Nagaki Y, Hayasaka S, Kitagawa K (1998) Orbital lymphoma of mucosa-associated lymphoid tissue in a patient with rheumatoid arthritis. Jpn J Ophthalmol 42:223–226

Nakata M, Matsuno Y, Katsumata N et al (1999) Histology according to the Revised European-American Lymphoma Classification significantly predicts the prognosis of ocular adnexal lymphoma. Leuk Lymphoma 32:533–543

Nasir S, DeAngelis LM (2000) Update on the management of primary CNS lymphoma. Oncology 14:228–234; discussion 237–242, 244

Nassif PS, Feldon SE (1992) Orbital lymphoma in a patient with Felty's syndrome. Br J Ophthalmol 76:173–174

Nathwani BN, Harris NL, Weisenburger D, Isaacson PG, Piris MA, Berger F, Mueller-Hermelink HK, Swerdlow SH (2001) Follicular lymphoma. In: Jaffe ES, Harris NL, Stein H, Vardiman JW (eds) World Health Organization classification of tumours. Pathology and genetics of tumours of haematopoietic and lymphoid tissues. IARC Press, Lyon, pp 162–167

Neri A, Jakobiec FA, Pelicci PG et al (1987) Immunoglobulin and T-cell receptor beta chain gene rearrangement analysis of ocular adnexal lymphoid neoplasm: clinical and biologic implications. Blood 70:1519–1529

Neuwelt EA, Goldman DL, Dahlborg SA et al (1991) Primary CNS lymphoma treated with osmotic blood-brain barrier disruption: prolonged survival and preservation of cognitive function. J Clin Oncol 9:1580–1590

Notter M, Kern TH, Forrer A et al (1997) Radiotherapy of pseudotumor orbitae. In: Wiegel T, Bornfeld N, Foerster MH, Hinkelbein W (eds) Radiotherapy of ocular disease. (Frontiers of radiation therapy and oncology, vol 30) Karger, Basel, pp 180–191

Oberlin O, Rey A, Anderson J (2001) Treatment of orbital rhabdomyosarcoma: survival and late effects of treatment-results of an international workshop. J Clin Oncol 19:197–204

Order SE, Donaldson SS (1990) Lymphoid hyperplasia-pseudotumor. In: Order SE, Donaldson SS (eds) Radiation therapy of benign disease: a clinical guide. Springer, Berlin Heidelberg New York, pp 156–157

Packer RJ, Savino PJ, Bilaniuk LT et al (1983)Chiasmatic gliomas of childhood. A reappraisal of natural history and effectiveness of cranial irradiation. Childs Brain 10:393–403

Pardo FS, Borodic G (1996) Long-term follow-up of patients undergoing definitive radiation therapy for sebaceous carcinoma of the ocular adnexa. Int J Radiat Oncol Biol Phys 34:1189–1190

Paulino AC, Simon JH, Zhen W et al (2000) Long-term effects in children treated with radiotherapy for head and neck rhabdomyosarcoma. Int J Radiat Oncol Biol Phys 48:1489–1495

Paulus W, Jellinger K, Morgello S, Deckert-Schlueter M (2000) Malignant lymphoma. In: Kleinhues P, Sobin LH (eds) World Health Organisation classification of tumours. Pathology and genetics of tumours of the nervous system. IARC Press, Lyon, pp 198–203

Reese AB (1976) Tumors of the eye, 3rd edn. Harper and Row, Hagerstown

Pierce SM, Barnes PD, Loeffler JS et al (1990) Definitive radiation therapy in the management of symptomatic patients with optic glioma. Survival and long-term effects. Cancer 65:45–52

Polito E, Galieni P, Leccisotti A (1996) Clinical and radiological presentation of 95 orbital lymphoid tumors. Graefes Arch Clin Exp Ophthalmol 234:504–509

Prummel MF, Wiersinga WM (1993a) Smoking and risk of Graves' disease. JAMA 269:479–482

Prummel MF, Mourits MP, Blank L et al (1993b) Randomized double-blind trial of prednisone versus radiotherapy in Graves' ophthalmopathy. Lancet 342:949–954

Raney RB, Anderson JR, Kollath J et al (2000) Late effects of therapy in 94 patients with localized rhabdomyosarcoma of the orbit: report from the Intergroup Rhabdomyosarcoma Study (IRS) III, 1984–1991. Med Pediatr Oncol 34:413–420

Rootman J, Nugent R (1982) The classification and management of acute orbital pseudotumors. Ophthalmology 89:1040–1048

Rootman J, Patel S, Jewell L (1984) Polyclonal orbital and systemic infiltrates. Ophthalmology 91:1112–1117

Rootman J, McCarthy, White V et al (1994) Idiopathic sclerosing inflammation of the orbit. A distinct clinicopathologic entity. Ophthalmology 101:570–584

Sandler HM, Rubinstein JH, Fowble BL et al (1989) Results of radiotherapy for thyroid ophthalmopathy. Int J Radiat Oncol Biol Phys 17:823–827

Sasai K, Yamabe H, Dodo Y et al (2001) Non-Hodgkin's lymphoma of the ocular adnexa. Acta Oncol 40:485–490

Scroggs MW, Johnston WW, Klintworth GK (1990) Intraocular tumors. A cytopathologic study. Acta Cytol 34:401–408

Sergott RC, Glaser JS, Charyulu K et al (1981) Radiotherapy for idiopathic inflammatory orbital pseudotumor. Indications and results. Arch Ophthalmol 99:853–856

Shields CL, Shields JA, Carvalho C et al (2001) Conjunctival lymphoid tumors: clinical analysis of 117 cases and relationship to systemic lymphoma. Ophthalmology 108:979–984

Sigelman J, Jakobiec FA (1978) Lymphoid lesions of the conjunctiva: relation of histopathology to clinical outcome. Ophthalmology 85:818–843

Silva MM, Goldman S, Keating G (2000) Optic pathway hypothalamic gliomas in children under three years of age: the role of chemotherapy. Pediatr Neurosurg 33:151–158

Smitt MC, Donaldson SS (1993) Radiotherapy is successful treatment for orbital lymphoma. Int J Radiat Oncol Biol Phys 26:59–66

Snebold NG (2000) Non infectious orbital inflammation. In: Albert DM, Jakobiec FA (eds) Principles and practice of ophthalmology. Saunders, Philadelphia, pp 3100–3120

Specht CS, Laver NM (2000) Benign and malignant lymphoid tumors, leukemia, and hystiocytic lesions. In: Albert DM, Jakobiec FA (eds) Principles and practice of ophthalmology. Saunders, Philadelphia, pp 5146–5168

Spencer JM, Nossa R, Tse DT et al (2001) Sebaceous carcinoma of the eyelid treated with Mohs micrographic surgery. J Am Acad Dermatol 44:1004–1009

Stafford SL, Kozelski TF, Garrity JA et al (2001) Orbital lymphoma: radiotherapy outcome and complications. Radiother Oncol 59:139–144

Tai PT, Yu E, Winquist E et al (2000) Chemotherapy in neuroendocrine/Merkel cell carcinoma of the skin: case series and review of 204 cases. J Clin Oncol 18:2493–2499

Takano Y, Kato Y, Sato Y et al (1992) Clonal *Ig*-gene rearrangement in some cases of gastric RLH detected by PCR method. Pathol Res Pract 188:973–980

Thompson CR, Lessell S (1997) Anterior visual pathway gliomas. Int Ophthalmol Clin 37:261–279

Tirelli U, Bernardi D (2001) Impact of HAART on the clinical management of AIDS-related cancers. Eur J Cancer 37:1320–1324

Valluri S, Moorthy RS, Khan A et al (1995) Combination treatment of intraocular lymphoma. Retina 15:125–129

Velez G, de Smet MD, Whitcup SA et al (2000) Iris involvement in primary intraocular lymphoma: report of two cases and review of the literature. Surv Ophthalmol 44:518–526

Warwar RE (1999) New insights into pathogenesis and potential therapeutic options for Graves' orbitopathy. Curr Opin Ophthalmol 10:358–361

Whitcup SM, Stark-Vancs V, Wittes RE et al (1997) Association of interleukin 10 in the vitreous and cerebrospinal fluid and primary central nervous system lymphoma. Arch Ophthalmol 115:1157–1160

White WL, Rootman J, Quenville N et al (1995) Ocular adnexal lymphoma. A clinicopathologic study with identification of lymphomas of mucosa-associated lymphoid tissue type. Ophthalmology 102:1994–2006

Wynne CJ, Kearsley JH (1988) Merkel cell tumor. A chemosensitive skin cancer. Cancer 62:28–31

Yen MT, Tse DT, Wu X et al (2000) Radiation therapy for local control of eyelid sebaceous cell carcinoma: report of two cases and review of the literature. Ophthal Plast Reconstr Surg 16:211–215

Yeo JH, Jakobiec FA, Abbott GF et al (1982) Combined clinical and computed tomographic diagnosis of orbital lymphoid tumors. Am J Ophthalmol 94:235–245

Zagars GK, Goswitz MS, Pollack A (1996) Liposarcoma: outcome and prognostic factors following conservation surgery and radiation therapy. Int J Radiat Oncol Biol Phys 36:311–319

Contents

1 Diagnostic Approaches to Posterior Uveal Melanomas

J. A. SHIELDS, C. L. SHIELDS, L. W. BRADY, B. MICAILY

CONTENTS

Although ophthalmologists are generally familiar with the typical clinical features of posterior uveal melanoma, a specific approach is helpful in establishing the diagnosis. This chapter covers the application of these methods specifically to ciliary body and choroidal melanoma. The material is condensed from two recent textbooks on the subject of intraocular tumors, which cite numerous references on the subject (SHIELDS and SHIELDS 1991, 1999).

The diagnosis of posterior uveal melanoma may occasionally be difficult because of the several clinical variations this tumor can assume. Furthermore, a number of benign lesions can simulate a choroidal melanoma ophthalmoscopically. The problem is further compounded in eyes with opaque media, because the lesion cannot be visualized ophthalmoscopically. In such cases the clinician needs to carry out selected ancillary tests to arrive at an accurate diagnosis.

Although the frequency of erroneous diagnosis was quite high up to several years ago, clinicians have recently become more accurate in their ability to diagnose posterior uveal melanoma. This improved diagnostic accuracy has been attributed to increased familiarity with the clinical features of uveal melanomas and pseudomelanomas and the judicious use of selected ancillary diagnostic studies. The following approach to the diagnosis of posterior uveal melanoma is the one followed by the authors. We believe that adherence to these steps in each case will minimize diagnostic error and thus help prevent misdirected therapy. When the diagnosis can be made by ophthalmoscopy alone, we may not employ all the procedures listed below. In cases where the diagnosis is less certain, more ancillary studies may be utilized.

J.A. SHIELDS, MD
Thomas Jefferson University, Philadelphia and Ocular Oncology Service, Wills Eye Hospital, Ninth and Walnut Sts., Philadelphia, PA 19107, USA

C.L. SHIELDS, MD
Thomas Jefferson University, Philadelphia and Ocular Oncology Service, Wills Eye Hospital, Ninth and Walnut Sts., Philadelphia, PA 19107, USA

L.W. BRADY, MD
Department of Radiation Oncology, Hahnemann University, Philadelphia, Pennsylvania, USA

B. MICAILY, MD
Department of Radiation Oncology, Hahnemann University, Philadelphia, Pennsylvania, USA

1.1 History

A detailed history should be taken and recorded before direct examination of a patient with a suspected uveal melanoma. Any family history of ocular disease or cancer should be recorded. Although uveal melanoma is generally considered to be nonfamilial, we have seen several cases of uveal melanoma in first- or second-degree relatives of our patients with posterior uveal melanoma. The patient should be questioned about systemic illness, cancer, surgery, or ocular problems.

1.2
Systemic Evaluation

Each patient in whom a posterior uveal melanoma is suspected should undergo a medical evaluation to detect any distant metastases from the primary uveal melanoma. If a uveal melanoma metastasizes, there is at least a 95% chance that there will be early involvement of either the liver or the lung. Plasma lactate dehydrogenase (LDH), serum glutamic oxaloacetic transaminase (SGOT), alkaline phosphatase and gamma-glutamyl transpeptidase (GGTP) levels may be helpful in detecting early hepatic metastases. If these enzymes are elevated, then computed tomography (CT) or magnetic resonance imaging (MRI) of the liver can be performed. A chest roentgenogram should be done to rule out pulmonary involvement. In most patients with uveal melanoma these studies prove to be negative at the time of diagnosis of the primary intraocular tumor.

1.3
Examination of the Opposite Eye

Although primary uveal melanoma is almost always unilateral, we have seen several patients with bilateral involvement. Since several lesions that can simulate a melanoma, such as degenerative retinoschisis and macular degeneration, are usually bilateral, careful examination of the opposite eye is mandatory. In patients referred for suspected ciliary body or choroidal melanoma, our policy is to examine the opposite eye prior to performing ophthalmoscopy on the eye with the suspected tumor. This approach

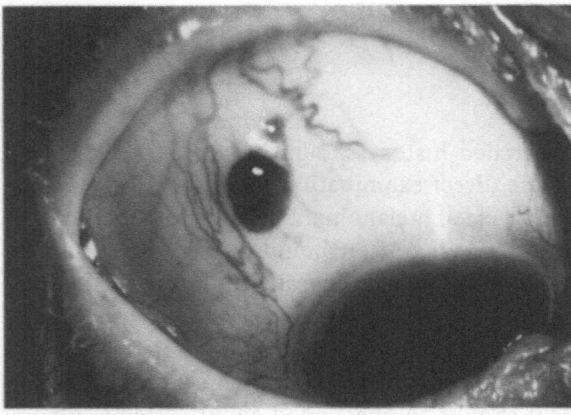

Fig. 1.1. Dilated episcleral vessels and nodule of extraocular extension of ciliary body melanoma

prevents the examiner from becoming preoccupied with the suspected tumor and overlooking pertinent pathologic changes in the fellow eye.

1.4
External Ocular Examination

An external ocular examination may occasionally provide clues that suggest the presence of a posterior uveal melanoma. Dilated episcleral vessels (sentinel vessels) or a pigmented nodule of extraocular extension are highly suggestive of an underlying melanoma (Fig. 1.1). Evidence of ocular melanocytosis also suggests that an intraocular mass is likely to be a melanoma.

1.5
Slit Lamp Biomicroscopy

Slit lamp evaluation may help detect anterior bulging of the iris, a subluxed lens, or a sector cataract, all of which are signs of a ciliary body melanoma. Melanomas that have invaded the retina or are necrotic may shed cells in the anterior vitreous, which also can be recognized with routine slit lamp biomicroscopy.

1.6
Indirect Ophthalmoscopy

Indirect ophthalmoscopy is the most important step in the evaluation of a fundus mass suspected to be a melanoma. A ciliary body or choroidal melanoma has ophthalmoscopic features that help differentiate it from simulating lesions (Figs. 1.2, 1.3A) (SHIELDS and SHIELDS 1991, 1999).

1.7
Gonioscopy

The fundus contact lens is useful for evaluating a suspected choroidal melanoma. Subtle changes over the tumor, such as orange pigment, cystoid retinal degeneration, and small amounts of subretinal fluid can be best appreciated with this technique. The

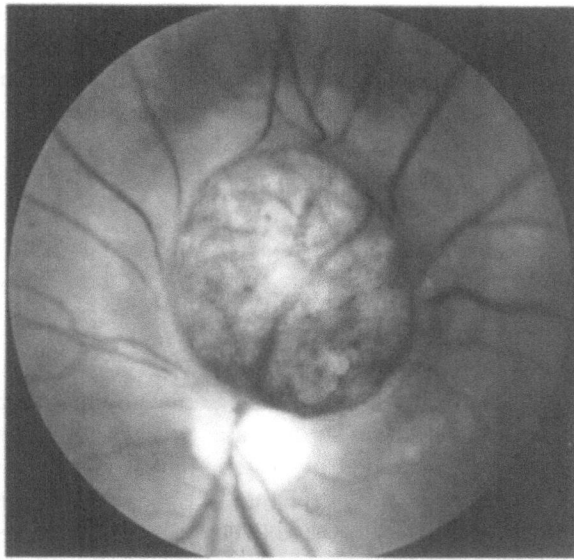

peripheral mirrors allow detection of anterior extension of posterior tumors into the ciliary body and anterior chamber angle. Hand-held 60-diopter and 90-diopter lenses are also employed to better evaluate posterior segment tumors.

Fig. 1.2. Pedunculated choroidal melanoma superior to optic disc

1.8
Transillumination

With transillumination techniques, hyperpigmented tumors and hemorrhages cast a shadow, whereas serous retinal detachments, serous choroidal detachments, and nonpigmented tumors permit transmission of light. Accurate transscleral transillumination is essential for determining the basal dimensions of a uveal melanoma that is to be treated with local resection or plaque radiotherapy.

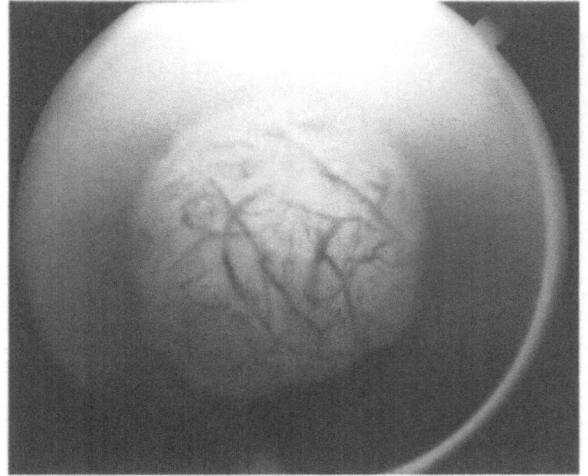

A

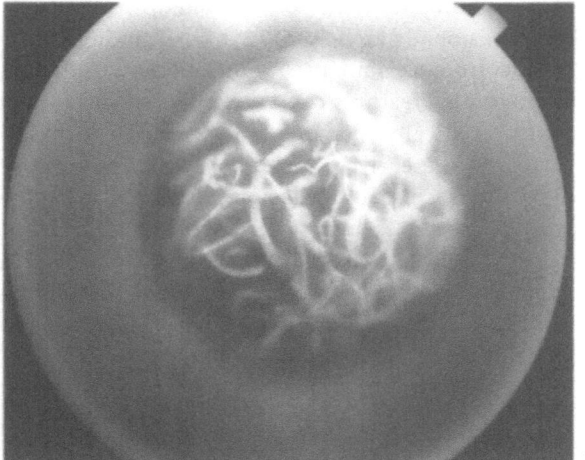

B

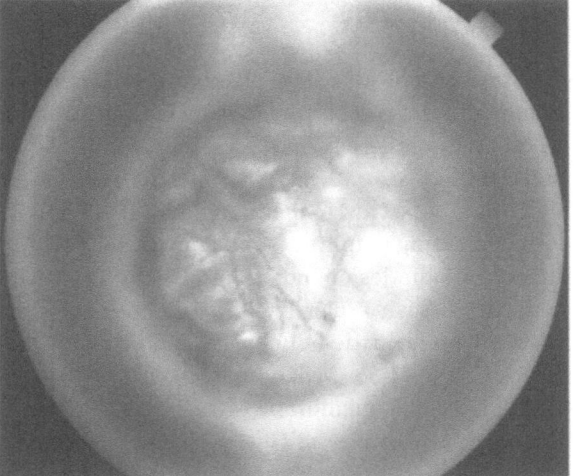

C

Fig. 1.3A–C. Fluorescein angiography of a dome-shaped choroidal melanoma. **A** Clinical appearance before fluorescein injection, showing prominent vessels within mass. **B** Angiogram in venous phase, showing linear hyperfluorescence of the vessels in the tumor. **C** Late angiogram showing diffuse hyperfluorescence of the tumor

1.9
Fundus Photography

Fundus photographs enable the ophthalmologist to better evaluate and monitor nevi and small malignant melanomas of the choroid. Comparison of serial photographs can be used to detect and document even subtle growth of lesions that are being followed by periodic observation. The use of stereoscopic photography allows better estimation of the elevation of such lesions. Photographs of 45° or 60° are often preferable for tumors whose margins will not fit into the standard 30° field. For even larger tumors the equator-plus camera may be preferable.

1.10
Fluorescein Angiography

Although fluorescein angiography shows no pattern that is pathognomonic for choroidal melanoma, it can occasionally be helpful in differentiating a melanoma from certain pseudomelanomas. Although angiographic features can vary, a sizable melanoma characteristically demonstrates prominent blood vessels in the early venous phase with late diffuse hyperfluorescence of the lesion (Fig. 1.3). During the late arterial or early venous phase, the prominent blood vessels in the dome of the tumor show relative hyperfluorescence caused by the presence of fluorescein within their lumina (SHIELDS and SHIELDS 1991, 1999).

1.11
Ultrasonography

Ultrasonography is a useful procedure in the diagnosis of choroidal and ciliary body melanomas and for differentiating these from the various simulating lesions. With A-scan, the typical melanoma shows a high initial spike, low to medium internal reflectivity with decreasing amplitude, and a prominent echo at the base of the lesion, corresponding to the sclera (Fig. 1.4). B-scan typically shows a choroidal mass pattern with acoustic hollowness and choroidal excavation (Fig. 1.5). Melanomas that have broken through Bruch's membrane show a classic mushroom shape with B-scan (Fig. 1.4), sometimes with an adjacent linear echo characteristic of a secondary retinal detachment. Ultrasonography can also demonstrate relatively small degrees of extraocular extension of posterior uveal melanomas. Extraocular extension appears as an acoustically empty area behind the sclera (SHIELDS and SHIELDS 1991, 1999).

1.12
Computed Tomography and Magnetic Resonance Imaging

In recent years computed tomography and magnetic resonance imaging have been used occasionally in the diagnostic evaluation of posterior uveal melanoma. These techniques can depict the size and extent of the tumor and can detect sizable nodules of extraocular extension. However, they are more expensive and time consuming than ultrasonography and provide little additional information. We no longer recommend these techniques except under unusual circumstances.

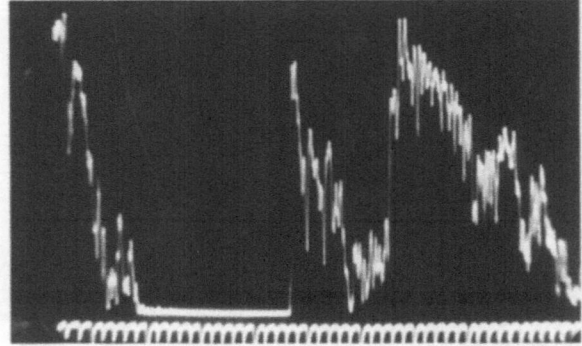

Fig. 1.4. A-scan ultrasonogram of a medium-sized choroidal melanoma

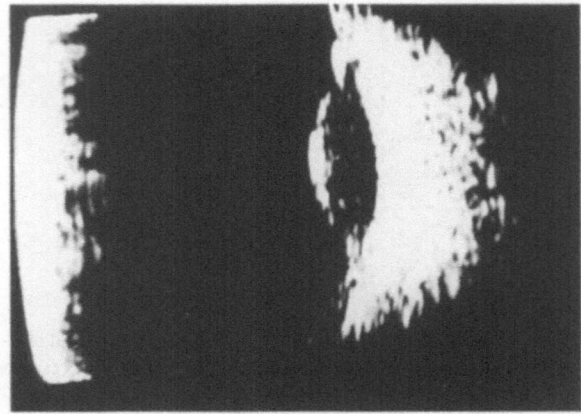

Fig. 1.5. B-scan ultrasonogram of a medium-sized choroidal melanoma

1.13
Radioactive Phosphorus Uptake Test

The radioactive phosphorus uptake (32P) test has been utilized as an aid in the diagnosis of a number of ocular tumors and related lesions, but its greatest value is in differentiating posterior uveal melanoma from benign simulating lesions (SHIELDS and SHIELDS 1991). In recent years it has been used less frequently because of improvements in fine-needle aspiration biopsy, which provides a tissue diagnosis.

1.14
Intraocular Biopsy

It may not be justified to perform a biopsy of a posterior uveal melanoma when the diagnosis can be made with a high degree of accuracy using noninvasive modalities. However, some form of biopsy may be employed when the diagnosis has not been clearly established by the aforementioned ancillary diagnostic procedures. We have occasionally employed either a fine-needle aspiration biopsy (FNAB) or a wedge biopsy technique. The fine-needle biopsy, which we most often recommend, is performed by a trans-pars plana, transvitreal approach, using indirect ophthalmoscopy (Fig. 1.6). These techniques are discussed in detail in recent textbooks (SHIELDS and SHIELDS 1991, 1999).

1.15
Summary

Malignant melanomas of the ciliary body and choroid have typical clinical features, and the correct diagnosis can usually be made by taking a thorough history and performing a complete ocular examination. The most important diagnostic modality is binocular indirect ophthalmoscopy. In addition, there are a number of ancillary techniques that are helpful in making a definitive diagnosis. These include transillumina-

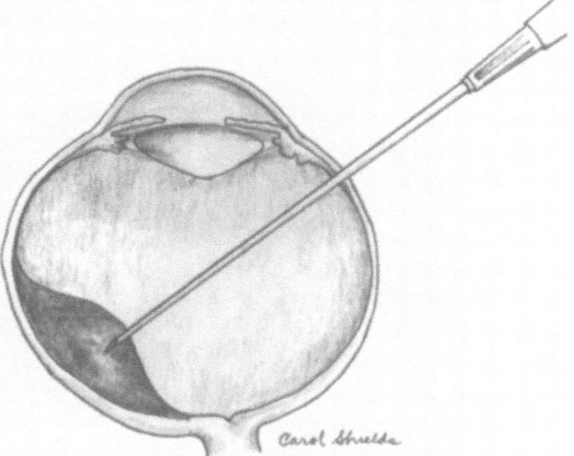

Fig. 1.6. Technique of fine-needle aspiration biopsy of an intraocular tumor

tion, fundus photography, fluorescein angiography, ultrasonography, CT, MRI, and the ^{32}P test.

Transillumination may be performed by any of several techniques. In general, pigmented tumors and hemorrhages transmit light poorly, whereas nonpigmented lesions transmit light readily. Fundus photographs and fluorescein angiograms permit a detailed magnified evaluation of the lesion and may be mailed to colleagues for further diagnostic opinions. Ultrasonography is of considerable value in melanoma diagnosis. B-scan techniques provide information regarding the overall shape and growth characteristics of the lesion, whereas A-scan provides additional data as to tissue reflectivity. The ^{32}P test is quite reliable in differentiating benign from malignant lesions. In cases where the diagnosis is more challenging, a transocular fine-needle aspiration biopsy with cytologic diagnosis may be of diagnostic value.

References

Shields JA, Shields CL (1991) Intraocular tumors. A text and atlas. Saunders, Philadelphia

Shields JA, Shields CL (1999) Atlas of intraocular tumors. Lippincott / Williams & Wilkins, Philadelphia

2 Histopathology of Uveal Malignant Melanoma and Other Uveal Tumors

C. L. SHIELDS and J. A. SHIELDS

CONTENTS

2.1
General Anatomy of the Eyeball

The size of the normal globe can vary, but it usually averages about 24 mm in diameter. The wall of the eye is composed of three ocular coats (Fig. 2.1). The outermost coat is fibrous and consists of the cornea and sclera. The middle, or vascular coat, is known as the uveal tract and consists of the iris, ciliary body, and choroid. The innermost, or sensory, coat consists of the retina and optic nerve head. The intraocular portion of the globe also may be divided anatomically into two main cavities: the aqueous cavity, consisting of the anterior and posterior chambers, and the vitreous cavity. Most intraocular tumors arise from

the uveal tract; less commonly they originate from the retina or optic disk.

2.1.1
Retina

The sensory retina is a thin, transparent tissue that lines the inner surface of the eye. The retinal arteries emerge from the optic disk and branch to supply the quadrants of the retina, with those on the temporal side arching around the avascular foveal region. The anterior termination of the retina is called the ora serrata. The fovea is the depressed central area of the retina and is about the size of the optic disk, being about 1.5 mm in diameter. The center of the fovea, known as the foveola, is about 300–400 μm in size. Destruction of the retina in this area is associated with significant loss of central vision. Histologically the sensory retina is composed of nine layers of neural tissue with vascular and glial tissue.

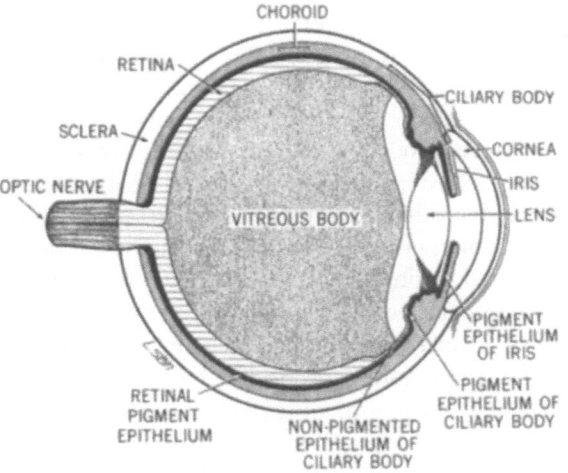

Fig. 2.1. Schematic diagram of the anatomy of the eyeball, showing the three coats of the eye and other structures

C.L. SHIELDS, MD
Thomas Jefferson University, Philadelphia and Ocular Oncology Service, Wills Eye Hospital, Ninth and Walnut Sts., Philadelphia, PA 19107, USA
J.A. SHIELDS, MD
Thomas Jefferson University, Philadelphia and Ocular Oncology Service, Wills Eye Hospital, Ninth and Walnut Sts., Philadelphia, PA 19107, USA

2.1.2
Retinal Pigment Epithelium

The retinal pigment epithelium is a monolayer of hexagonal, deeply pigmented cells that form a sheet between Bruch's membrane and the sensory retina. Each cell contains a round nucleus near its base and numerous elliptical melanosomes within the cytoplasm. Unlike the uveal melanocytes, which have a propensity to undergo neoplastic transformation, the retinal pigment epithelial cells have a greater tendency to undergo hyperplasia, particularly following ocular inflammation or trauma. True neoplasms of the retinal pigment epithelium are rare (SHIELDS et al. 1999a).

In the normal state the retinal pigment epithelium is in apposition to the sensory retina. In certain pathologic conditions serous fluid or blood may accumulate between these two layers, producing a retinal detachment. A variety of intraocular tumors can produce such a secondary retinal detachment.

2.1.3
Uveal Tract

As indicated above, the uveal tract can be divided anatomically into three portions: iris, ciliary body, and choroid. The uvea is a highly vascular structure with a large amount of loose connective tissue. The rich blood supply may increase the chances of hematogenous dissemination of tumor cells to and from the uvea, perhaps explaining why most tumors that metastasize to the eye lodge in this layer. There are no lymphatic channels in the uvea, explaining the lack of lymphatic dissemination of tumor cells.

Scattered throughout the uveal stroma are branching pigmented cells known as uveal melanocytes. These cells are derived from the neural crest and are the cells of origin of uveal nevi and melanomas. Tumors and related lesions that occur in the uvea may exhibit variable clinical behavior, depending on the portion of the uvea involved; therefore the anatomy of the iris, ciliary body, and choroid is considered separately.

The iris is a thin diaphragm that forms a central round opening, or pupil, which regulates the amount of light entering the eye. Clinically the iris varies from blue to brown, depending on the concentration and degree of pigmentation of uveal melanocytes within the stroma. Histologically the iris consists of an anterior border layer, the stroma, the dilator and sphincter muscles of the pupil, and the posterior pigment epithelium.

The ciliary body is a circular structure about 6 mm in anteroposterior length, which extends from the iris root to the anterior limit of the choroid. The anterior 2 mm contains the ciliary crests and is known as the pars plicata. The flat posterior 4 mm of the ciliary body is known as the pars plana and is continuous with the choroid posteriorly. Histologically the pars plicata consists of a vascular stroma with melanocytes and bundles of smooth muscle, while the pars plana is thin and avascular. Both have a pigmented and nonpigmented epithelium overlying them. Tumors arising from the ciliary body are hidden behind the iris in an area that is difficult to visualize clinically. Consequently such growths may become sizable before they are clinically detected.

The choroid, which comprises the posterior four-fifths of the uvea, is situated between the retina and the posterior sclera. Histologically the choroid has several ill-defined layers of closely packed vessels. Nutrients pass through the endothelial cells of the inner choroidal layer to supply the retinal pigment epithelium and the overlying retina. In the middle and outer layers of the choroid there is an abundance of loose connective tissue that contains branching uveal melanocytes.

Bruch's membrane is a thin elastic and collagenous structure between the choroid and retinal pigment epithelium. It is a dense, tough structure that tends to resist extension of choroidal tumors into the retina and the extension of retinal tumors into the choroid. Choroidal melanomas, however, can rupture Bruch's membrane and assume a mushroom configuration.

2.2
Uveal Tumors

2.2.1
Melanocytic Tumors of the Uvea

The incidence of choroidal nevi is estimated to range from 1% to 2% (SHIELDS and SHIELDS 1992). In contrast, the incidence of malignant melanomas of the choroid in the general population is much lower, generally ranging between 4.9 and 7 cases per million per year (CUTLER and YOUNG 1975; GANLEY and COMSTOCK 1973; WILKES et al. 1979). Melanocytic tumors of the choroid have a peculiar predisposition to occur in whites. Both nevi and malignant melanomas of the uvea are extremely rare in blacks and appear to be relatively rare in Orientals. Typical uveal nevi characteristically become clinically apparent at about the time of puberty. Most posterior uveal melanomas are diagnosed when the patient is over 50 years old, while iris melanomas are diagnosed somewhat earlier (SHIELDS et al. 2001). It is possible that many posterior uveal melanomas could have been growing slowly for many years before coming to clinical recognition, so that the age of onset is never determined. In general, uveal melanomas have no familial tendency.

2.2.1.1
Cytologic Classification of Uveal Melanomas

Melanocytic tumors of the uveal tract have been classified into several cytologic types. Four types of cells have been recognized in choroidal nevi: (a) plump, polyhedral nevus cell, (b) slender spindle nevus cell, (c) plump fusiform and dendritic nevus cell, and (d) balloon cells (NAUMANN et al. 1966). Three types of

cells are recognized to occur in uveal melanomas: spindle A, spindle B, and epithelioid. Spindle A cells are long and slender and contain elongated, flattened nuclei (Fig. 2.2). A dark 'chromatin' line, often seen extending longitudinally through the nucleus, has been demonstrated to represent a peculiar infolding of the nuclear membrane. The nuclei of spindle A cells rarely display evidence of mitoses. Spindle B cells are more oval or plump than spindle A cells (Fig. 2.3). The nuclei are likewise oval and are characterized by a more prominent nucleolus than is seen in the nuclei of spindle A cells. The cells are less compact than spindle A cells, and their nuclei occasionally show mitotic figures. Epithelioid cells are round to polyhedral cells with abundant eosinophilic cytoplasm (Fig. 2.4). The cell membrane is more clearly delineated, and the cells are less cohesive than spindle cells. Their nuclei are large and round and contain prominent nucleoli. Mitotic figures are frequently present. In all types of melanoma cells, pigmentation can vary.

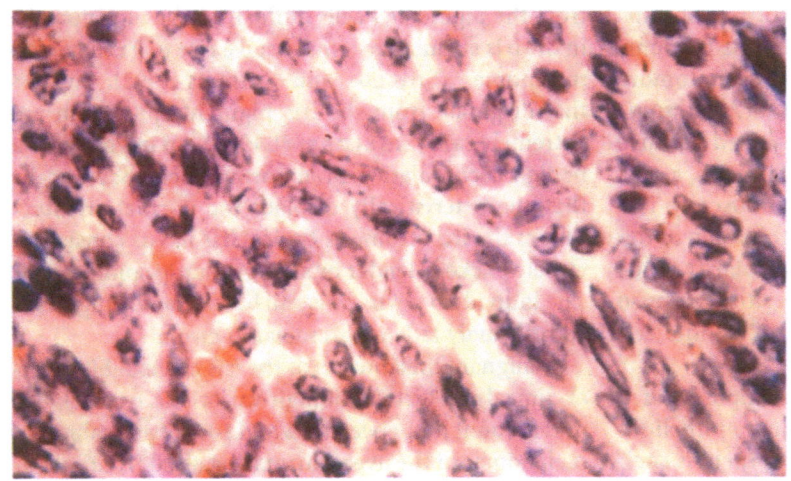

Fig. 2.2. High-power microscopy illustrating spindle A cells in a uveal melanoma. These cells are typically slender and have a prominent chromatin strip down the center of the cell. (H and E, ×100)

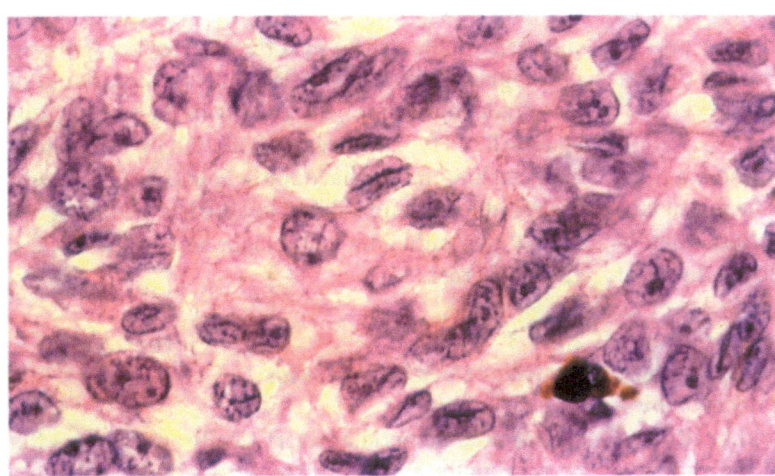

Fig. 2.3. High-power microscopy showing spindle B cells with rather homogeneous oblong nuclei. (H and E, ×100)

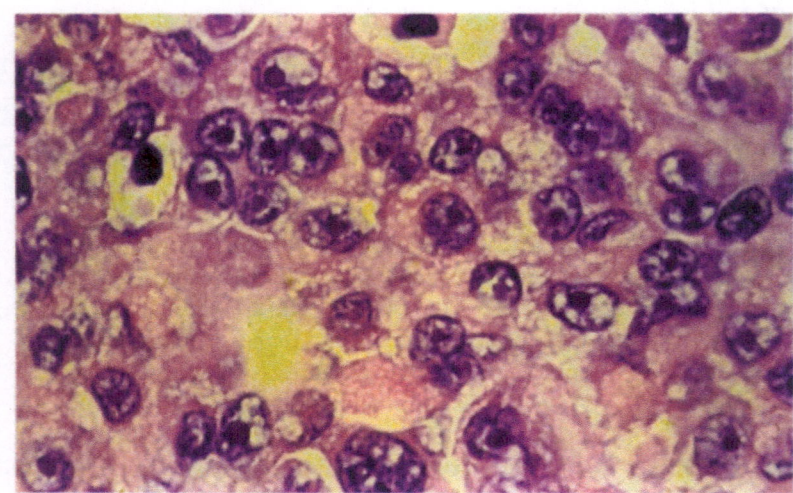

Fig. 2.4. High-power microscopy showing numerous epithelioid cells with abundant cytoplasm and large atypical nuclear detail. (H and E, ×100)

Callender Classification of Uveal Melanomas. In 1931, CALLENDER divided malignant melanomas of the uveal tract into six cell types: spindle A, spindle B, fascicular, mixed, necrotic, and epithelioid. A spindle A tumor is one composed almost entirely of spindle A cells, and a spindle B tumor contains predominantly spindle B cells. Most spindle cell tumors contain variable amounts of both spindle A and spindle B cells. Fascicular tumors are so named because the cells are arranged in ribbons or fascicles, a pattern best appreciated on low-power microscopy. The cells are spindle A, spindle B, or a combination of the two. Most authorities believe that fascicular type tumors do not deserve separate categorization because they have a similar prognosis to other spindle cell melanomas.

A mixed cell type tumor is one composed of a variable mixture of spindle cells and epithelioid cells. A tumor is classified as necrotic if there is such extensive necrosis that the cell type cannot be adequately determined. Such necrosis is most often seen in larger choroidal melanomas which have broken through Bruch's membrane. Epithelioid cell tumors are composed almost entirely of epithelioid cells.

McLean Classification of Uveal Melanomas. Although the Callender classification has been used for many years, a more recent classification, that of McLean and associates, is now employed in most ophthalmic pathology laboratories (MCLEAN et al. 1978). Melanomas are now divided into four groups: (a) spindle cell melanoma, (b) mixed cell melanoma, (c) epithelioid cell melanoma, and (d) necrotic melanoma. This revised classification should be utilized in the histologic classification of uveal melanomas.

2.2.1.2
Iris Melanomas

A number of benign and malignant tumors can arise from the pigmented cells of the iris. The melanocytes in the iris stroma presumably give rise to iris nevi and melanomas (SHIELDS and SHIELDS 1992). Tumors that originate from the iris pigment epithelium are extremely rare (SHIELDS et al. 1985). An iris nevus is a benign accumulation of abnormal melanocytic cells that characteristically displace the normal architecture of the iris stroma. A typical iris nevus consists of closely packed slender or slightly plump spindle cells. The individual nevus cells can be minimally pigmented or heavily laden with melanin granules.

Malignant melanomas of the iris can exhibit several clinical and histopathologic variations. Iris melanomas account for between 3% and 10% of all malignant melanomas of the uvea (SHIELDS et al. 2001; ZIMMERMAN 1972). Iris melanomas show considerable variation with low-power microscopy. These tumors typically arise in the stroma near the anterior border layer. Cytologically, most iris melanomas are composed of low-grade melanoma cells, usually of the spindle A or spindle B cell types (SHIELDS et al. 2001). An occasional iris melanoma will have epithelioid cells mixed with the spindle cells and will be classified as the mixed cell type. Pure epithelioid cell melanomas in the iris are extremely rare.

2.2.1.3
Posterior Uveal Melanomas

A choroidal nevus characteristically appears as a flat or minimally elevated slate-gray lesion. With low-power microscopy, a choroidal nevus characteristically appears as a variably pigmented, placoid lesion rarely more than 2 mm in thickness. It may have a fairly distinct margin or it may blend imperceptibly into the adjacent choroid. Choroidal nevi can have several cytologic variations, including polyhedral, spindle, fusiform, or balloon cells (SHIELDS and SHIELDS 1992, 1999).

Malignant melanomas of the ciliary body and choroid (posterior uvea) differ from melanomas of the iris in several respects. They usually produce more profound symptoms, are larger at the time of clinical recognition, are composed of more malignant cell types, and carry a worse prognosis (SHIELDS et al. 1991). Because the posterior uveal melanoma is the most frequently diagnosed primary intraocular malignancy, it has received more attention in the literature than any other intraocular tumor (SHIELDS and ZIMMERMAN 1973; SHIELDS et al. 1991).

Ciliary body melanomas that are small and hidden behind the iris are often asymptomatic and may be difficult to detect on routine ocular examination. Larger tumors, however, can produce a variety of symptoms, including painless blurred vision or a visual field defect. Melanomas of the ciliary body assume nodular or diffuse growth patterns or various combinations of the two. The nodular melanoma appears as a round, well-circumscribed mass, which is best seen through a dilated pupil. The diffuse melanoma of the ciliary body appears clinically as an irregular or diffuse thickening that may extend for 360° in the ciliary body (ring melanoma). The diffuse melanoma is usually more invasive and is characterized by more malignant cell types.

Although most ciliary body melanomas appear pigmented clinically, they are found on gross examination to range from deeply pigmented to amelanotic. Many of the amelanotic tumors probably appear pigmented clinically because the overlying ciliary epithelium imparts a dark appearance to the surface of the lesion.

Malignant melanomas arising from the choroid characteristically have symptoms, clinical variations, and effects on the adjacent ocular structures that differ from those of ciliary body tumors. Patients with choroidal melanomas may be asymptomatic or they may complain of blurred vision. With the widespread use of indirect ophthalmoscopy, choroidal melanomas are more frequently discovered during routine ocular examination of asymptomatic patients.

Choroidal melanomas grow in either a nodular or a diffuse form. Although there is great variation, a choroidal melanoma characteristically assumes a nodular configuration and grows as a fairly well-circumscribed thickening of the choroid (Fig. 2.5). With further growth, many tumors break through Bruch's membrane and assume a mushroom shape (Fig. 2.5). When this occurs, congested blood vessels appear within the dome of the tumor. Pigmentation within choroidal melanomas can vary considerably, so that they range from yellow amelanotic tumors to deeply melanotic brown tumors. With time, most choroidal melanomas lead to an overlying or adjacent detachment of the sensory retina. Choroidal melanomas can invade the sclera or extend through the sclera into the orbit.

The treatment of posterior uveal melanomas includes observation, photocoagulation, transpupillary thermotherapy, episcleral plaque radiotherapy, local tumor resection, enucleation, or exenteration. The choice of treatment depends upon several factors, such as the location and size of the tumor and the patient's status. The two most common forms of treatment are episcleral plaque radiotherapy and enucleation. Preliminary data have shown 10-year survival rates to be the same in patients treated with plaque radiotherapy and in those treated with enucleation.

Recent studies have shown that posterior uveal melanomas show a remarkable decrease in mitotic activity after episcleral plaque radiotherapy. In a large series, SHIELDS et al. (1989, 1990) found that most (64%) irradiated uveal melanomas that were later enucleated had no mitotically active cells. However, if the irradiated eye was enucleated for suspected tumor regrowth, the mitotic activity was much higher.

A number of factors that are recognized pathologically or clinically have been correlated with the prognosis for life in patients with posterior uveal melanomas. These include the age of the patient at the time of enucleation, location of the tumor, location of the anterior border of the tumor, largest tumor diameter in contact with the sclera, height of the tumor, integrity of Bruch's membrane, cell type, pigmentation, scleral infiltration by tumor cells, mitotic activity, vascular loops and networks within the tumor, and tumor infiltrating lymphocytes (DE LA CRUZ et al. 1990; FOLBERG et al. 1993; MCLEAN et al. 1977; SHAMMAS and BLODI 1977). Cytologic factors and genetic factors have also been found to have prognostic value for uveal melanoma.

Since there are no lymph channels in the eye, distant metastases from uveal melanoma occur by hematogenous routes. Metastases from iris melanomas are relatively rare, whereas metastases from choroidal and ciliary body melanomas are much more common. It is estimated that between 20% and 50% of patients with a posterior uveal melanoma will

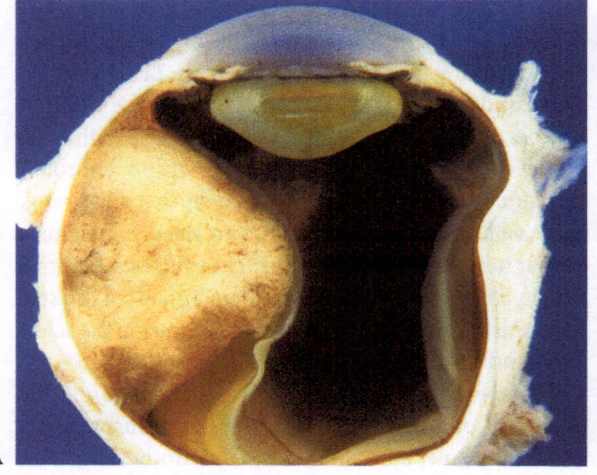
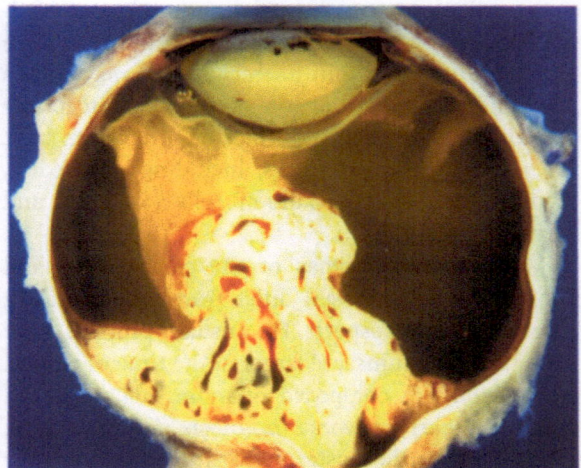

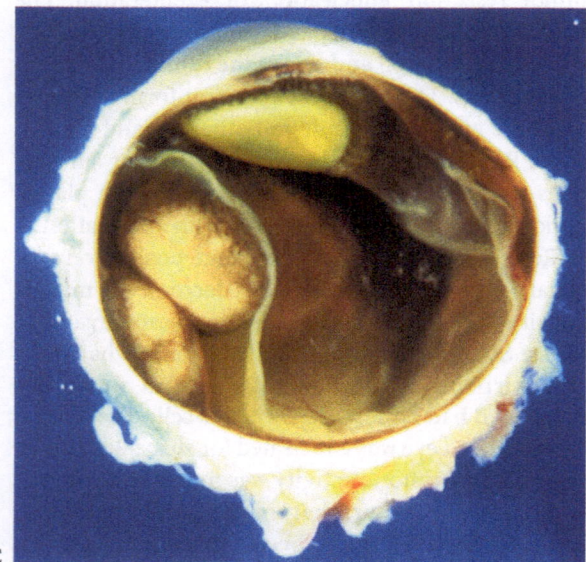

Fig. 2.5A–C. Pathology of various choroidal melanomas. A Amelanotic choroidal melanoma. B Amelanotic mushroom-shaped choroidal melanoma. C Variably pigmented choroidal melanoma

eventually die of metastatic disease (SHIELDS et al. 1991). Malignant melanomas of the uvea have an unusual propensity to metastasize to the liver. EINHORN et al. (1974) found that 88% of patients had hepatic involvement as the initial manifestation of metastatic disease. The second and third most common sites of metastases are lung and skin, respectively. The average interval between the treatment of the uveal melanoma (usually enucleation) and the clinical development of metastasis is approximately 33 months (EINHORN et al. 1974).

2.2.2
Uveal Metastases

Neoplasms that have metastasized to the intraocular structures compose a group of tumors which are im-

portant to ophthalmologists, internists, general surgeons, radiation oncologists, and other specialists. Since the intraocular structures have no lymphatic channels, metastatic tumors reach the uvea and retina solely by hematogenous routes (SHIELDS et al. 1997) Probably because of its marked vascularity with relatively slow blood flow, the uvea is the site of most ocular metastases. The posterior portion of the choroid, which contains the greatest number of blood vessels, is the most frequent location of metastatic disease. Metastatic tumors to the retina and optic disk are rare, and metastases to other intraocular structures are almost nonexistent. Most tumors that metastasize to the uvea are carcinomas. Sarcomas metastasize to the uvea extremely rarely (SHIELDS and SHIELDS 1992, 1999; SHIELDS et al. 1997). Metastatic tumors to the uvea typically occur in middle-aged or older patients, between the ages of 40 and 70 years.

The tumor that most frequently metastasizes to the uvea is carcinoma of the breast, which accounts for about 47% of uveal metastases in the series from the Ocular Oncology Service at Wills Eye Hospital, Philadelphia (SHIELDS et al. 1997). The second most common primary tumor is carcinoma of the lung, which accounts for 21% of uveal metastases. In 17% of cases, the location of the primary tumor remains unknown, in spite of an extensive systemic examination. Less commonly, the primary tumor is in the gastrointestinal tract, kidney, pancreas, or another organ.

In the aforementioned series, approximately 66% of patients report prior treatment for known cancer, usually a mastectomy for breast carcinoma (SHIELDS et al. 1997). In the remaining cases, the primary tumor was often diagnosed by breast examination or by chest radiograph at the time the suggestive ocular lesion was detected. In nearly 34% of patients, the patient presented with the uveal metastasis before the primary tumor was diagnosed. In these cases, the primary site most often is the lung (SHIELDS et al. 1997).

Most patients with a tumor that has metastasized to the iris are asymptomatic or have only mild visual symptoms in the involved eye. Clinically, in most cases an iris metastasis appears as a distinct yellow-white gelatinous iris mass with many vessels on its surface (SHIELDS et al. 1995). Metastatic tumors to the ciliary body are often difficult to detect clinically. Their appearance may be similar to that of a diffuse amelanotic melanoma of the ciliary body. Patients with tumors that metastasize to the choroid are often asymptomatic, but they may have painless blurred vision or, in some instances, pain caused by secondary glaucoma. Ophthalmoscopic examination of a choroidal metastasis characteristically reveals one or more creamy yellow placoid lesions in the posterior choroid (SHIELDS and SHIELDS 1999). Tumors that are slightly more elevated frequently produce a retinal detachment and retinal pigment epithelial changes.

Gross examination of an eye with metastatic carcinoma usually reveals one or more tumors that have a diffuse growth pattern in the uvea (Fig. 2.6). Some metastatic uveal tumors may be quite elevated, but even these usually have a diffuse growth pattern. The histopathologic appearance of a metastatic carcinoma depends partly upon the features of the primary tumor. With low-power magnification the tumor is characteristically placoid or diffuse in configuration, and an overlying serous detachment of the sensory retina is usually present. The smaller, diffuse tumors appear to infiltrate and replace the normal choroidal architecture. Multiple microscopic foci may be present. If a tumor that has metastasized to the uvea is poorly differentiated, it may be impossible to determine the site of the primary tumor on the basis of routine histopathologic evaluation, and special stains and electron microscopy may be necessary. When a metastatic tumor is better differentiated, it may retain certain histologic or histochemical features of the primary tumor.

2.2.3
Intraocular Lymphoid Tumors and Leukemias

Lymphoid tumors and the leukemias can affect almost any part of the eye or ocular adnexa. They occur more commonly in the orbit and conjunctiva and only rarely involve the intraocular structures. Clinically, intraocular lymphoid tumors mimic more common entities, such as amelanotic melanoma, metastatic tumor, or intraocular inflammation. Consequently, the clinical diagnosis is difficult and there is often a long delay before the correct diagnosis is established. The histologic diagnosis can also be difficult. Ocular lymphoid tumors are separated into three main categories based on their histopathologic features, and these are benign reactive lymphoid hyperplasia, atypical lymphoid hyperplasia, and malignant lymphoma. Recent emphasis has been placed upon immunologic characterization of ocular adnexal lymphoid neoplasms. Benign reactive lymphoid hyperplasias tend to be immunologically polyclonal, consisting of a mixture of T-lymphocytes and B-lymphocytes, while malignant lymphomas tend to be immunologically monoclonal, consisting of an almost pure B-lymphocyte proliferation with an absence or sparsity of T cells (KNOWLES and JAKOBIEC 1981).

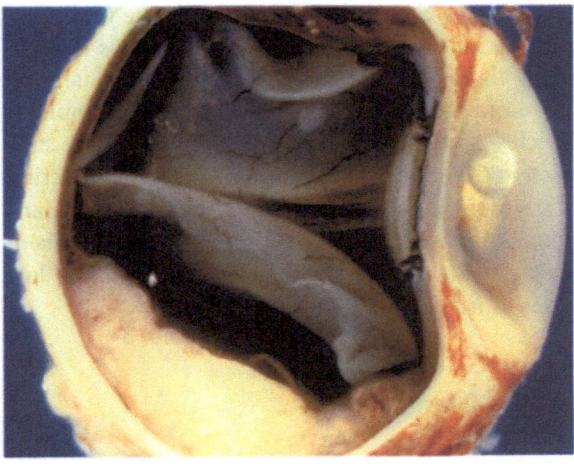

Fig. 2.6. Characteristic flat diffuse metastasis of the choroid with overlying retinal detachment

2.2.3.1
Benign Reactive Lymphoid Hyperplasia

Benign reactive lymphoid hyperplasia is a peculiar form of pseudotumor that can involve the uvea with or without simultaneous involvement of the conjunctiva and/or orbit. It is usually a disease of middle-aged or older individuals, with an average age at onset of 55 years. It is usually unilateral, although occasionally both eyes are involved. The patient characteristically has painless, blurred vision in the involved eye. If there is orbital involvement, the patient may complain of prominence of one or both eyes.

The ophthalmologic findings of benign reactive lymphoid hyperplasia vary with the extent of ocular involvement. The conjunctiva, uvea, and orbit are most frequently affected. Iris involvement is often characterized by a diffuse thickening of the iris stroma. In other instances, benign reactive lymphoid hyperplasia of the iris can occur as a localized nodular tumor, simulating an iris melanoma or a metastatic tumor (SHIELDS et al. 1981). Ciliary body involvement rarely, if ever, occurs as an isolated entity, but rather occurs as a part of panuveal affection. Posterior uveal involvement is characterized by a diffuse or nodular amelanotic thickening of the choroid. In cases with posterior uveal involvement, the finding of an associated salmon pink conjunctival mass in the same eye facilitates the diagnosis and provides accessible tissue for biopsy confirmation.

The histologic features of benign reactive lymphoid hyperplasia include mature lymphocytes, reticular lymphoblasts, plasma cells, and modified plasma cells termed Russell bodies and Dutcher bodies. Other histologic features include lymph follicles, germinal centers, periodic acid–Schiff-positive ground substance, and hyalinization. The finding of massive infiltration of mature lymphocytes is interesting in view of the fact that there is normally no lymphoid tissue in the eye or orbit. These lymphoid follicles often demonstrate germinal centers, supporting the concept that the eye is capable of acting as a lymph node under certain circumstances. Management of benign reactive lymphoid hyperplasia of the uvea includes systemic corticosteroids or low doses of irradiation.

2.2.3.2
Malignant Lymphoma

With the exception of large cell lymphoma (reticulum cell sarcoma), malignant lymphomas involving the intraocular structures are very rare. Intraocular large cell lymphoma is typically a disease of older people, often beginning unilaterally but frequently involving the second eye within weeks or months. The affected patient usually complains of painless, blurred vision. Examination characteristically reveals vitreous cells with or without retinal or choroidal involvement (SHIELDS and SHIELDS 1992, 1999). In some instances, these patients have yellow, deep retinal infiltrative lesions, while in other cases a solitary subretinal or choroidal mass occurs. The location of the ocular involvement in large cell lymphoma can vary with the type of systemic disease. In the case of primary central nervous system large cell lymphoma the retina and vitreous are more likely to be involved, whereas in systemic lymphoma, which is characterized by lymphadenopathy and visceral involvement, the uvea is more likely to be affected.

Histopathologically, intraocular large cell lymphoma can infiltrate the uvea (Fig. 2.7) or the retina, or extend under the retinal pigment epithelium. There are usually poorly differentiated mononuclear cells with large hyperchromic nuclei. In cases with severe vitreous involvement, the diagnosis can be made by cytologic examination of vitreous aspirations. In such preparations the cells are usually large and atypical with scanty cytoplasm, oval or bean-shaped nuclei, and prominent nucleoli. A characteristic feature is distinct lobulation of the nuclei with finger-like protrusions.

In cases in which the clinical diagnosis of intraocular large cell lymphoma is proven histologically, oc-

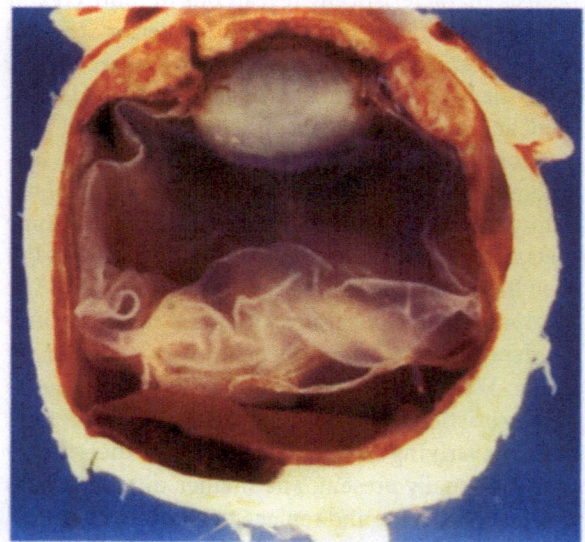

Fig. 2.7. Anterior uveal involvement with lymphoma

ular irradiation is the treatment of choice. If the diagnosis is not established on the basis of cytologic examination of ocular tissues, but large cell lymphoma is still strongly suspected clinically, then a cautious trial of irradiation still may be considered. The prognosis for vision is often poor in patients with ocular large cell lymphoma. The prognosis for life is poor, and most patients die of systemic complications within 2 years after the ocular diagnosis. Longer survivals have been reported after simultaneous irradiation to the central nervous system and the eye (CHAR et al. 1981).

2.2.3.3
Leukemia

Although leukemia does not occur primarily in the eye and adnexa, these structures are involved as part of the systemic disease in about half of the cases. Ocular changes are more frequent in the acute leukemias. Intraocular involvement is often subtle and is sometimes only recognized on postmortem examination of the eyes. There can be involvement of the iris, vitreous, retina, choroid, optic nerve head, and retinal pigment epithelium. Iris involvement in leukemia is characterized by a diffuse white thickening of the iris, often with small nodules at the pupillary margin. Retinal involvement in leukemia includes perivascular sheathing, venous tortuosity, nerve fiber layer infarcts (cotton-wool spots), hemorrhages, and Roth's spots. Preretinal and vitreous hemorrhages can occur secondary to the associated anemia and thrombocytopenia. Yellow infiltrates may be apparent in the retina, subretinal space, or choroid.

The pathologic findings in an eye with leukemic involvement can vary considerably. The uvea can be diffusely thickened with leukemic cells or it can show marked intravascular involvement with the neoplastic cells. Retinal involvement with leukemic cells is characterized by diffuse intravascular and extravascular infiltration of the neoplastic cells. The retinal 'hemorrhages' seen clinically and on gross examination often represent a combination of erythrocytes and leukemic blast cells (WALLACE et al. 1991).

The treatment of intraocular involvement with leukemia is ocular irradiation. If the optic nerve head is involved, prompt and adequate irradiation is mandatory to prevent irreversible visual loss. If irradiation is instituted early enough, the visual outcome is often favorable.

References

Callender GR (1931) Malignant melanotic tumors of the eye: a study of histologic types in 111 cases. Trans Am Acad Ophthalmol Otolaryngol 36:131–142

Char DH, Margolis L, Newman AB (1981) Ocular reticulum cell sarcoma. Am J Ophthalmol 91:480–483

Cutler SJ, Young JL Jr (1975) Third National Cancer Survey. Incidence data. (NCI monograph no 41) Government Printing Office, Washington, DC

De la Cruz PO, Specht CS, McLean IW (1990) Lymphocytic infiltration in uveal malignant melanoma. Cancer 65:112–115

Einhorn LH, Burgess MA, Gottlieb JA (1974) Metastatic patterns of choroidal melanoma. Cancer 34:1001–1004

Folberg R, Rummelt V, Parys-Van Ginderdeuren R et al (1993) The prognostic value of tumor blood vessel morphology in primary uveal melanoma. Ophthalmology 100:1389–1398

Ganley JP, Comstock GW (1973) Benign nevi and malignant melanomas of the choroid. Am J Ophthalmol 76:19–25

Knowles DM Jr, Jakobiec FA (1981) Quantitative determination of T cells in ocular lymphoid infiltrates: an indirect method for distinguishing between pseudolymphomas and malignant lymphomas. Arch Ophthalmol 99:309–316

McLean IW, Foster WD, Zimmerman LE (1977) Prognostic factors in small malignant melanomas of the choroid and ciliary body. Arch Ophthalmol 95:48–58

McLean IW, Zimmerman LE, Evans RE (1978) Reappraisal of Callender's spindle A type of malignant melanoma of the choroid and ciliary body. Am J Ophthalmol 86:557–564

Naumann G, Yanoff Y, Zimmerman LE (1966) Histogenesis of malignant melanomas of the uvea. I. Histopathologic characteristics of nevi of the choroid and ciliary body. Arch Ophthalmol 76:784–796

Shammas HF, Blodi FC (1977) Prognostic factors in choroidal and ciliary body melanomas. Arch Ophthalmol 95:63–69

Shields CL, Shields JA, Cook GR, von Fricken M, Augsburger JJ (1985) Differentiation of adenoma of the iris pigment epithelium from iris cyst and melanoma. Am J Ophthalmol 100:678–681

Shields CL, Shields JA, Karlsson U, Markoe AM, Brady LW (1989) Reasons for enucleation following plaque radiotherapy: clinical findings. Ophthalmology 96:919–924

Shields CL, Shields JA, Karlsson LL, Menduke H, Brady LW (1990) Enucleation following plaque radiotherapy for posterior uveal melanoma: histopathologic findings. Ophthalmology 97:1665–1670

Shields CL, Shields JA, Gross N, Schwartz G, Lally S (1997) Survey of 520 uveal metastases. Ophthalmology 104:1265–1276

Shields CL, Shields JA, Materin M, Gershenbaum E, Singh A, Smith A (2001) Iris melanoma: risk factors for metastasis in 169 consecutive patients. Ophthalmology 108:172–178

Shields JA, Shields CL (1992) Intraocular tumors. A text and atlas. Saunders, Philadelphia

Shields JA, Shields CL (1999) Atlas of intraocular tumors. Lippincott / Williams and Wilkins, Philadelphia

Shields JA, Zimmerman LE (1973) Lesions simulating malignant melanomas of the posterior uvea. Arch Ophthalmol 89:466–471

Shields JA, Augsburger JJ, Gonder JR, McLeod D (1981) Localized benign lymphoid tumor of the iris. Arch Ophthalmol 99:2147–2148

Shields JA, Shields CL, Donoso LA (1991) Management of posterior uveal melanomas. Surv Ophthalmol 36:161–195

Shields JA, Shields CL, Kiratli H, De Potter P (1995) Metastatic tumors to the iris in 40 patients. Am J Ophthalmol 119:422–430

Shields JA, Shields CL, Gunduz K, Eagle RC Jr (1999a) Neoplasms of the retinal pigment epithelium. (The 1998 Albert Ruedemann Sr Memorial Lecture, part 2) Arch Ophthalmol 117:601–608

Shields JA, Shields CL, Mercado G, Gunduz K, Eagle RC Jr (1999b) Adenoma of the iris pigment epithelium. A report of 20 cases. (The 1998 Pan-American Lecture) Arch Ophthalmol 117:736–741

Wallace RT, Shields JA, Shields CL, Ehya H, Ewing M (1991) Leukemic infiltration of the optic nerve. Arch Ophthalmol 109:1027

Wilkes SR, Robertson DM, Kurland LT, Cambell JR (1979) Incidence of uveal malignant melanoma in the resident population of Rochester and Olmsted County, Minnesota. Am J Ophthalmol 87:639–641

Zimmerman LE (1972) Histopathologic considerations in the management of tumors of the iris and ciliary body. Ann Inst Barraquer 10:27–57

3 Overview of Management of Posterior Uveal Melanoma

J. A. SHIELDS, C. L. SHIELDS, L. W. BRADY, B. MICAILY

CONTENTS

In the first edition of this textbook, we stressed the controversies in management of melanomas of the ciliary body and choroid (posterior uveal melanoma). Many of the controversies have been largely resolved, and there continue to be new developments related to the management of patients with posterior uveal melanoma. Therefore, it seems appropriate in this chapter to provide a brief overview of the current options in management of this important intraocular tumor. Other authors will discuss the details of radiation therapy of uveal melanoma.

The current methods of management include observation, photocoagulation, transpupillary thermotherapy, radiotherapy, local resection, enucleation,

J.A. SHIELDS, MD
Thomas Jefferson University, Philadelphia and Ocular Oncology Service, Wills Eye Hospital, Ninth and Walnut Sts., Philadelphia, PA 19107, USA
C.L. SHIELDS, MD
Thomas Jefferson University, Philadelphia and Ocular Oncology Service, Wills Eye Hospital, Ninth and Walnut Sts., Philadelphia, PA 19107, USA
L.W. BRADY, MD
Department of Radiation Oncology, Hahnemann University, Philadelphia, Pennsylvania, USA
B. MICAILY, MD
Department of Radiation Oncology, Hahnemann University, Philadelphia, Pennsylvania, USA

orbital exenteration, chemotherapy, and immunotherapy, depending on the clinical circumstances. The authors of a recent publication have identified the clinical risk factors for metastasis for small choroidal melanomas (SHIELDS et al. 1995). Consequently, there is a trend away from observation of some small melanocytic lesions and a trend toward earlier treatment of lesions that possess those risk factors for possible metastasis. Transpupillary thermotherapy has been introduced and is gaining in popularity as a method of treating selected small melanomas (SHIELDS et al. 1996, 1998). It is being used as a primary treatment for small tumors and as supplemental treatment to radiotherapy for medium-sized and some large melanomas. Updated results of treating uveal melanoma with plaque brachytherapy (SHIELDS et al. 1993b) and charged particles (CHAR et al. 1998; GRAGOUDAS et al. 1986) have been published. This chapter provides an overview of the methods of managing patients with ciliary body and choroidal melanoma, with emphasis on the newer developments related to each specific method.

3.1 General Considerations

Historically, enucleation of the affected eye was once considered to be the only appropriate management for the patient with a posterior uveal melanoma (SHIELDS and SHIELDS 1992; SHIELDS et al. 1991a). Several years ago, however, some authorities challenged the effectiveness of enucleation for preventing metastatic disease and even proposed that enucleation might somehow promote or accelerate metastasis (ZIMMERMAN and MCLEAN 1979; ZIMMERMAN et al. 1978). The validity of these arguments has been challenged by others (MANSCHOT and VAN PEPERZEEL 1980; SEIDEL et al. 1979), some of whom still believe that early enucleation offers the patient the best chance of a cure (MANSCHOT and VAN PEPERZEEL 1980). This controversy over enucleation has led to a trend away from enucleation and the increasing use of more conservative therapeutic methods (SHIELDS and SHIELDS 1992; SHIELDS et al. 1991a).

Depending upon a number of clinical factors, management alternatives to enucleation include observation, photocoagulation, thermotherapy, radiotherapy, local tumor resection, and occasionally others. The two treatment methods most frequently employed today are enucleation and episcleral plaque brachytherapy (SHIELDS and SHIELDS 1992). The Collaborative Ocular Melanoma Study (COMS) was organized to address some of the complex treatment questions, and some patients are being enrolled in this study (STRAATSMA et al. 1988). There are many complexities involved in conducting such a study, but is hoped that some useful therapeutic information will be gleaned from this clinical trial, since a large amount of money has been expended. Until more definitive data become available, one should recommend the treatment which, on the basis of the currently available information and clinical experience, seems to provide the best systemic prognosis while preserving as much useful vision as possible in the affected eye (SHIELDS 1988; SHIELDS and SHIELDS 1992; SHIELDS et al. 1991a). If possible, the patient should be referred to an ocular oncologist who has experience in managing patients with posterior uveal melanoma.

3.2
Periodic Observation

Until very recently, some authorities managed many small melanocytic lesions of the posterior uvea with periodic fundus photography and ultrasonography to document growth of the lesion before recommending definitive treatment (GASS 1980; SHIELDS and SHIELDS 1992). Recently identified risk factors for metastasis include greater tumor thickness, tumor proximity to the optic nerve, presence of visual symptoms from the melanoma, and prior documented growth (SHIELDS et al. 1995). Since documented growth may be associated with a worse systemic prognosis, there is a current tendency to treat patients who have the other risk factors without waiting for documentation of growth. Tumors that show highly suggestive features or unequivocal evidence of growth should generally have some form of active therapy, depending upon the factors mentioned previously.

3.3
Photocoagulation

Photocoagulation is still an acceptable method for treating selected small choroidal melanomas (SHIELDS et al. 1990; VOGEL 1972). It was originally done with xenon photocoagulation, but argon laser subsequently became more commonly employed. Studies showed that xenon photocoagulation achieved better tumor control but argon laser was associated with fewer complications (SHIELDS et al. 1990). Recently, transpupillary thermotherapy has largely replaced argon laser for treating selected small melanomas (OOSTERHUIS et al. 1995; SHIELDS et al. 1996, 1998). If thermotherapy is not available, photocoagulation is still an appropriate therapeutic option for selected tumors which are less than 3 mm in thickness and which are located more than 3 mm from the foveola (SHIELDS et al. 1990). Low-energy, long-exposure laser therapy has been advocated by some authorities in the management of selected small choroidal melanoma (FOULDS and DAMATO 1986b).

3.4
Transpupillary Thermotherapy

Transpupillary thermotherapy is a recently popularized method of treating selected small and medium-sized choroidal melanomas. It delivers heat to the tumor in the infrared range using a modified diode laser delivery system. It does not appear to produce as much damage to the sensory retina as does laser photocoagulation. The instrumentation and technique have been reported and will probably be modified in the future. Preliminary data have suggested that it achieves tumor control in over 90% of selected small and medium-sized choroidal melanomas (SHIELDS et al. 1996, 1998). It is currently the authors' treatment of choice for most melanomas that are located in posterior pole and are less than 10 mm in diameter and 3 mm in thickness. Long-term follow-up of cases treated by this method has not yet been reported.

3.5
Radiotherapy

Radiotherapy is still the most widely employed therapeutic modality for posterior uveal melanomas (SHIELDS and SHIELDS 1992; SHIELDS et al. 1982,

1991a, 1993b). There has been some controversy as to whether radiotherapy is superior to enucleation with regard to patient survival and as to which method of radiotherapy provides better therapeutic results and fewer complications.

The most commonly employed form of radiotherapy has been the application of a radioactive plaque (EARLE et al. 1987; SHIELDS and SHIELDS 1992; SHIELDS et al. 1982, 1993b). Iodine-125 and ruthenium-106 are currently the most frequently used isotopes. The type of plaque selected in a given case should depend upon close coordination between the ocular oncologist and the radiation oncologist. Recent studies have outlined the results of plaque radiotherapy for macular and ciliary body melanoma and for melanoma with extrascleral extension (GUNDUZ et al. 1999a, b, 2000).

Another method of radiotherapy is charged-particle irradiation (CHAR et al. 1998; GRAGOUDAS et al. 1980, 1986). Although this technique was originally believed to provide a collimated beam which would limit the radiotherapy to the precise area of the tumor, this theory has not been substantiated by clinical experience. In fact, there have been instances of radiation complications in the eye and adnexa, often remote from the irradiated tumor. Similar complications occurred with cobalt plaques, but our group believes that major complications are less frequent with the newer shielded iodine plaques (SHIELDS and SHIELDS 1992; SHIELDS et al. 1993b).

On the basis of currently available information, it appears that patients treated with radiotherapy have a survival rate similar to those treated by enucleation (SEDDON et al. 1985; SHIELDS and SHIELDS 1992). Furthermore, there is probably no significant difference between plaque radiotherapy and charged-particle radiotherapy with regard to short-term and long-term complications. Studies have shown that between 5% and 10% of patients treated with radiotherapy ultimately require enucleation of the affected eye because of tumor recurrence or radiation complications (SHIELDS et al. 1989, 1990).

3.6
Local Resection

Techniques of local resection of melanomas involving the ciliary body and choroid have been employed more frequently. On the Oncology Service, approximately 250 resections have been performed on melanomas involving the ciliary body and/or choroid.

We initially began using the technique of penetrating sclerouveoretinectomy (full-thickness eye-wall resection) as advocated by MEYER-SCHWICKERATH (1974) and later popularized by PEYMAN et al. (1984). Although there are a number of potential serious complications, the eye can tolerate fairly extensive resections. More recently, we have employed a partial lamellar sclerouvectomy, a modification of the technique popularized by FOULDS and DAMATO (1986a), in which the tumor is removed with the aim of leaving the retina and vitreous intact (SHIELDS and SHIELDS 1988, 1992; SHIELDS et al. 1991b, 1993a). Our surgical technique for this procedure is described elsewhere (SHIELDS and SHIELDS 1988).

Local resection of a posterior uveal melanoma offers several theoretical advantages over enucleation and radiotherapy. In contrast to enucleation, it is designed to preserve vision and to maintain a cosmetically normal eye. In contrast to radiotherapy, it has fewer long-term complications if the initial surgery is successful. However, it does have more potential immediate complications, such as vitreous bleeding, retinal detachment and cataract (SHIELDS et al. 1991b), while radiotherapy is almost never associated with such immediate complications. However, some degree of radiation retinopathy and cataract are common long-term complications of all forms of radiotherapy. There is no current evidence that local resection of posterior uveal melanomas is any different from enucleation or radiotherapy with regard to patient survival. There are fewer complications and better visual results for smaller, more anteriorly located tumors. More complications can be expected when larger, postequatorial tumors are managed in this manner. Local resection of posterior uveal melanomas will probably be used more frequently in the future, as the surgical technique becomes better developed.

3.7
Enucleation

As mentioned earlier, the traditional method of treating uveal melanomas by enucleation was challenged several years ago (ZIMMERMAN and MCLEAN 1979; ZIMMERMAN et al. 1978). Enucleation is generally indicated for advanced melanomas that occupy most of the intraocular structures and for those that have produced severe secondary glaucoma. Another relative indication for enucleation is a melanoma that has invaded the optic nerve. It is currently believed that radiotherapy eventually results in profound visual loss in such cases. Furthermore, the degree of invasion of the optic nerve cannot be easily assessed with ophthalmoscopy, ultrasonography, or computed tomography. Enucleation with a long section of the optic nerve seems more reasonable in such cases. However, many juxtapapillary melanomas that have not actually invaded the nerve can be managed by custom-designed notched radioactive plaques (DePotter et al. 1994).

The so-called no touch enucleation was introduced to minimize the amount of surgical trauma and theoretically, to lessen the chance of tumor dissemination at the time of surgery (Wilson and Fraunfelder 1978). An essential aspect of this technique is to freeze the venous drainage from the tumor prior to cutting the optic nerve. The "no touch" technique has recently fallen into disuse at most centers, because it is cumbersome and its benefits are only theoretical. However, a very gentle standard technique of enucleation should be employed, without clamping the optic nerve prior to cutting it (Shields and Shields 1992, 1992).

There have been recent advances in the types of orbital implants used following enucleation. The hydroxyapatite implant, designed to improve the ocular motility in patients undergoing enucleation, is still used widely, but other motility implants have been introduced (Shields et al. 1993). Preliminary results suggest that there are no significant complications and that patients have much better ocular motility when this method is employed (Dutton 1991; Shields et al. 1993).

Pre-enucleation radiotherapy (PERT) has recently been advocated by some authorities. In general this involves the use of 2,000 cGy of external beam radiotherapy to the affected eye and orbit prior to enucleation. Recent nonrandomized studies have suggested that PERT does not have any advantage over standard enucleation (Char et al. 1988). The COMS has recently confirmed that PERT is not effective in preventing metastatic disease.

3.8
Orbital Exenteration

The subject of orbital exenteration for uveal melanomas with extrascleral extension is also controversial. It seems that complete orbital exenteration should not be done in cases of mild degrees of extrascleral extension. However, in the rare instance of massive

orbital extension in a blind, uncomfortable eye, primary orbital exenteration is probably justified. PERT, as described above under enucleation, can be considered in such advanced cases. In most instances of orbital extension of uveal melanoma it is not necessary to sacrifice the skin of the eyelid. The eyelid-sparing exenteration skin provides a much better cosmetic appearance (Shields and Shields 1992; Shields et al. 1991c).

3.9
Chemotherapy and Immunotherapy

Once a uveal melanoma has metastasized to distant organs, the patient's prognosis is poor. There is no current evidence that chemotherapy or immunotherapy is effective in the primary management of uveal melanomas. The vast majority of affected patients have no detectable evidence of systemic metastasis at the time of diagnosis of the uveal melanoma. Consequently, clinicians have not been inclined to employ such treatment.

Likewise, the role of chemotherapy and immunotherapy is unproved in the treatment of patients with systemic metastasis from uveal melanomas. There have been reports of tumor regression after hepatic arterial chemoembolization with cisplatin and polyvinyl sponge (Mavligit et al. 1988). There is a possibility that such treatment may prolong survival for a few months, but it is unlikely that it will be curative. A recent report of a double blind study has indicated that intradermal injections of MER (methanol-extracted residue of BCG) do not alter the systemic prognosis in patients who are at high risk for developing metastasis after enucleation (McLean et al. 1990). The role of monoclonal antibodies in the detection and management of metastatic uveal melanoma is currently being investigated.

3.10
Summary

This chapter has provided an update on some general principles of management of posterior uveal melanomas. There is controversy as to whether enucleation or conservative treatment offers the best prognosis. Studies comparing the various therapeutic methods are currently under way. Small asymptomatic melanocytic tumors of the posterior uvea that exhibit dormant features can probably be observed periodically without any treatment until definite evidence of growth is documented. Some small choroidal melanomas that were previously treated with photocoagulation are now being treated with newer techniques of transpupillary thermotherapy.

Radiotherapy can be employed, using a variety of episcleral plaques or charged particle treatment. The two methods appear to be nearly equal with regard to the development of systemic metastasis. Plaques seem to be associated with fewer anterior segment complications. Selected melanomas of the ciliary body and peripheral choroid can be treated by local resection using partial lamellar sclerouvectomy. Local resection techniques have theoretical advantages, but the surgery takes longer and the immediate complications are potentially greater.

Enucleation is generally indicated for most large melanomas greater than 15 mm in diameter and greater than 10 mm in thickness. It is also generally indicated for tumors that have invaded the optic nerve. There is probably no practical role for the so-called no touch technique of enucleation. The value of pre-enucleation radiotherapy in improving patient survival is unproved, although this technique seems reasonable in selected advanced tumors where enucleation seems inevitable. Orbital exenteration is justified for very advanced uveal melanomas with massive extraocular extension. Its value in the management of smaller degrees of extraocular extension is uncertain. It currently appears that chemotherapy and immunotherapy do not provide a therapeutic cure for uveal melanomas, but their true effectiveness awaits the results of further studies.

References

Char DH, Phillips TL, Andejeski Y et al (1988) Failure of pre-enucleation radiation to decrease uveal melanoma mortality. Am J Ophthalmol 106:21–26

Char DH, Kroll SM, Castro JK (1998) Ten-year follow-up of Helium ion therapy of uveal melanoma. Am J Ophthalmol 125:81–89

DePotter, P, Shields CL, Shields JA, Cater JC, Tardio DJ (1994) The impact of enucleation versus plaque radiotherapy in the management of juxtapapillary choroidal melanoma on patient survival. Br J Ophthalmol 78:109–114

Dutton JJ (1991) Coralline hydroxyapatite as an ocular implant. Ophthalmology 98:370–377

Earle J, Kline RW, Robertson DM (1987) Selection of Iodine-125 for the collaborative ocular melanoma study. Arch Ophthalmol 105:763–764

Foulds WS, Damato BE (1986a) Alternative to enucleation in the management of choroidal melanoma. Aust NZ J Ophthalmol 14:19–27

Foulds WS, Damato BE (1986b) Low energy long-exposure laser therapy in the management of choroidal melanoma. Graefe's Arch Clin Exp Ophthalmol 224:26–31

Gass JDM (1980) Observations of suspected choroidal and ciliary body melanomas for evidence of growth prior to enucleation. Ophthalmology 87:523–528

Gragoudas ES, Goitein M, Verhey L, Munzenreider J, Suite HD, Koehler A (1980) Proton beam irradiation. An alternative to enucleation for intraocular melanomas. Ophthalmology 89:571–581

Gragoudas ES, Seddon JM, Egan K et al (1986) Long-term results of proton beam irradiated uveal melanomas. Ophthalmology 94:349–353

Gunduz K, Shields CL, Shields JA, Cater J, Freire J, Brady LW (1999a) Plaque radiotherapy of choroidal melanoma with macular involvement. Am J Ophthalmol 127:579–588

Gunduz K, Shields CL, Shields JA, Cater J, Freire J, Brady LW (1999b) Plaque radiotherapy of ciliary body melanoma. Arch Ophthalmol 117:170–177

Gunduz K, Shields CL, Shields JA, Cater J, Brady LW (2000) Plaque radiotherapy for management of ciliary body and choroidal melanoma with extrascleral extension. Am J Ophthalmol 130:97–102

Manschot WA, Van Peperzeel HA (1980) Choroidal melanoma – Enucleation or observation? A new approach. Arch Ophthalmol 98:71–77

Mavligit GM, Charnsangevej C, Carrasco H et al (1988) Regression of ocular melanoma metastatic to the liver after hepatic arterial chemoembolization with cisplatin and polyvinyl sponge. JAMA 260:974–976

McLean IW, Berd D, Mastrangelo MJ, Shields JA, Davidorf FH, Grever M, Makley TA, Gamel JW (1990) A randomized study of methanol-extraction residue of Bacille Calmette-Guérin as postsurgical adjuvant therapy of uveal melanoma. Am J Ophthalmol 110:522–526

Meyer-Schwickerath G (1974) Excision of malignant melanoma of the choroid. Mod Probl Ophthalmol 12:562–566

Oosterhuis JA, Journee-de Korver HG, Kakebeeke-Kemme HM, Bleeker JC (1995) Transpupillary thermotherapy in choroidal melanomas. Arch Ophthalmol 113:315–321

Peyman GA, Juarez CP, Diamond JG, Raichand M (1984) Ten years' experience with eye wall resection of uveal malignant melanomas. Ophthalmology 91:1720–1724

Seddon JM, Gragoudas ES, Albert DM, Hseih CC, Polivogianis L, Fridenberg GR (1985) Comparison of survival rates for patients with uveal melanoma after treatment with proton beam irradiation or enucleation. Am J Ophthalmol 99:282–290

Seigel D, Myers M, Ferris F, Steinhorn SC (1979) Survival rates after enucleation of eyes with malignant melanoma. Am J Ophthalmol 87:751–765

Shields CL, Shields JA, Karlsson U, Markoe AM, Brady LW (1989) Reasons for enucleation after plaque radiotherapy for posterior uveal melanoma. Ophthalmology 96:919–924

Shields CL, Shields JA, Karlsson U, Menduke H, Brady LW (1990) Enucleation following plaque radiotherapy: for posterior uveal melanoma. Histopathologic findings. Ophthalmology 97:1665–1670

Shields CL, Shields JA, De Potter P (1992) Hydroxyapatite

orbital implant after enucleation. Experience with 100 consecutive cases. Arch Ophthalmol 110:333–338

Shields CL, Shields JA, DePotter P (1993) Hydroxyapatite orbital implant after enucleation for intraocular tumors. In: Shields JA (ed) Update on malignant ocular tumors, vol 33. International Ophthalmology Clinics, Little Brown, Boston, pp 83–93

Shields CL, Shields JA, Kiratli H, Cater JR, De Potter P (1995) Risk factors for metastasis of small choroidal melanocytic lesions. Ophthalmology 102:1351–1361

Shields CL, Shields JA, DePotter P, Kheterpel S (1996) Transpupillary thermotherapy in the management of choroidal melanoma. Ophthalmology 103:1642–1650

Shields CL, Shields JA, Cater J, De Potter P, Lois N, Edelstein C, Mercado G, Gunduz K (1998) Transpupillary thermotherapy for choroidal melanoma. Tumor control and visual outcome in 100 cases. Ophthalmology 105:581–590

Shields JA (1988) Counseling the patient with a posterior uveal melanoma (editorial). Am J Ophthalmol 106:88–91

Shields JA, Shields CL (1988) Surgical approach to lamellar sclerouvectomy for posterior uveal melanomas. The 1986 Schoenberg Lecture. Ophthalmol Surg 19:774–780

Shields JA, Shields CL (1992) The management of posterior uveal melanoma. In: Shields JA, Shields CL (eds) Intraocular tumors. A text and atlas. Philadelphia, Saunders, pp 191–192

Shields JA, Augsberger JJ, Brady LW, Day J (1982) Cobalt plaque therapy of posterior uveal melanomas. Ophthalmology 89:1201–1207

Shields JA, Glazer LC, Mieler WF, Shields CL (1990) Comparison of xenon arc and argon laser photocoagulation in the treatment of choroidal melanomas. Am J Ophthalmol 109:647–655

Shields JA, Shields CL, DePotter P (1993a) Local resection of posterior uveal tumors. In: Shields JA (ed) Update on malignant ocular tumors, vol 33. International Ophthalmology Clinics, Little Brown, Boston, pp 137–142

Shields JA, Shields CL, DePotter P, Cu-Ujieng A, Hernandez C, Brady LW (1993a) Plaque radiotherapy for uveal melanoma. In: Shields JA (ed) Update on malignant ocular tumors, vol 33. International Ophthalmology Clinics, Little Brown, Boston, pp 129–135

Shields JA, Shields CL, Donoso LA (1991a) Management of posterior uveal melanomas. Surv Ophthalmol 36:161–195

Shields JA, Shields CL, Shah P, Sivalingam V (1991b) Partial lamellar sclerouvectomy for ciliary body and choroidal tumors. Ophthalmology 98:971–983

Shields JA, Shields CL, Suvarnamani C, Tantasira M, Shah P (1991c) Orbital exenteration with eyelid sparing: indications, technique and results. Ophthalmic Surg 22:292–297

Straatsma BR, Fine SL, Earle JD (1988) The Collaborative Ocular Melanoma Study Research Group. Enucleation versus plaque irradiation for choroidal melanoma. Ophthalmology 95:1000–1004

Vogel MH (1972) Treatment of malignant choroidal melanomas with photocoagulation. Evaluation of 10-year follow-up data. Am J Ophthalmol 74:1–10

Wilson RS, Fraunfelder FT (1978) „No touch" cryosurgical enucleation: a minimal trauma technique for eyes harboring intraocular malignancy. Ophthalmology 85:1170–1175

Zimmerman LE, McLean IW (1979) An evaluation of enucleation in the management of uveal melanomas. Am J Ophthalmol 87:741–760

Zimmerman LE, McLean IW, Foster WD (1978) Does enucleation of the eye containing a malignant melanoma prevent or accelerate the dissemination of tumour cells? Br J Ophthalmol 62:420–425

4 Local Resection and Radiotherapy for Uveal Melanoma

B. Damato

4.1
Introduction

Local resection of choroidal melanoma has hitherto been limited by excessive ocular morbidity, fears of inducing metastatic disease and concerns about profound hypotensive anaesthesia. These obstacles are gradually being overcome. Advances in surgical techniques have led to better prevention and treatment of retinal detachment and residual tumour. Follow-up studies have not shown survival after local resection to be worse than after enucleation (FOULDS et al. 1987). Techniques for profound hypotensive anaesthesia have become safer, and therefore more routine, thanks to developments in cerebral and cardiac monitoring. For these reasons, it is likely that local resection will be performed more widely in the future.

In the 1960s, Stallard described the technique of 'partial choroidectomy', which he performed in a

B. DAMATO, MD
Liverpool Ocular Oncology Centre, Royal Liverpool University Hospital, Prescot Street, Liverpool, L7 8XP, UK

small number of patients who had tumour recurrence after radiotherapy and who also each had poor vision in the fellow eye (STALLARD 1966). In 1970, Foulds started performing choroidectomy as a primary procedure irrespective of the status of the other eye (FOULDS 1973). In 1984, he was joined by the present author, who has further developed the technique and evaluated its results in terms of visual outcome (DAMATO et al. 1993), local tumour control (DAMATO et al. 1996a), metastatic disease (DAMATO et al. 1996b) and, recently, retinal detachment (B. Damato et al., personal communication, Jules Gonin meeting, 2000). Bornfeld has compared the results of local resection and of radiotherapy, providing evidence that in patients with a large tumour surgical resection may give a better functional outcome (BORNFELD et al. 1997). Others have also reported their experience with local resection (PEYMAN et al. 1984; SHIELDS et al. 1991).

This chapter gives a brief overview of transscleral local resection of choroidal melanoma and discusses its various relationships with radiotherapy.

4.2
Primary Transscleral Local Resection

4.2.1
Indications and Contraindications

In the few centres where it is performed regularly, local resection tends to be reserved for tumours that are deemed unsuitable for radiotherapy because of their large size. For example, we prefer local resection for tumours having a thickness greater than 5.5 mm. Contraindications include (1) tumour diameter greater than 16 mm; (2) extensive retinal invasion or perforation; (3) involvement of more than 3 h of the ciliary body, iris or angle; (4) optic disc invasion; (5) transscleral spread; and (6) poor general health precluding hypotensive anaesthesia. Several of these contraindications are only relative. For example, the introduction of adjunctive plaque radiotherapy has made it possible to resect tumours with intraretinal or orbital spread. Furthermore, the need for profound systemic hypotension has been lessened by cauterization of the short posterior ciliary arteries and other blood vessels supplying the tumour.

4.2.2
Surgical Technique

The technique of local resection has been described previously (DAMATO and FOULDS 1994). Briefly, a 180° conjunctival peritomy is performed. Any extraocular muscles overlying the tumour are dis-inserted. Two bridle sutures are placed in the sclera, 4 mm from the limbus. The tumour is localized by transpupillary transillumination, and its margins are marked on the sclera with a felt-tipped pen. A lamellar scleral flap is created, hinged posteriorly, the flap having approximately 75% of the thickness of the sclera. Any vortex veins in the operative field are closed with bipolar diathermy and then divided. The globe is decompressed by limited pars plana vitrectomy, which is performed through a single port, without infusion and using the illumination from the operating microscope. Long and short posterior ciliary arteries in the quadrant of the tumour are cauterized. The systolic blood pressure is lowered to approximately 40–50 mmHg, using appropriate cardiac and cerebral monitoring (TODD and COLVIN 1991). Deep scleral incisions are made, approximately 1.5 mm inside the superficial scleral incisions, so as to create a stepped wound edge, thereby facilitating closure. The choroid adjacent to the tumour is perforated by being grasped with two pairs of microforceps, which are then pulled apart. The uveal tissue is divided with corneo-scleral scissors while the tumour is gently lifted out of the eye (Fig. 4.1). Any adhesions between the tumour and the retina are divided by blunt dissection. The scleral flap is closed with interrupted 9/0 nylon sutures. The globe is reformed with balanced salt solution. A 20-mm ruthenium plaque is positioned over the resection area, secured with a mattress suture, and left in place for between 2 and 3 days until a dose of 100 Gy has been delivered to a depth of 2 mm (Fig. 4.2). The muscles are re-inserted or attached to the plaque sutures, using 6/0 polyglactin sutures. The conjunctiva is closed with 7/0 polyglactin sutures. Postoperatively, the patient is treated with topical and systemic antibiotics and steroids.

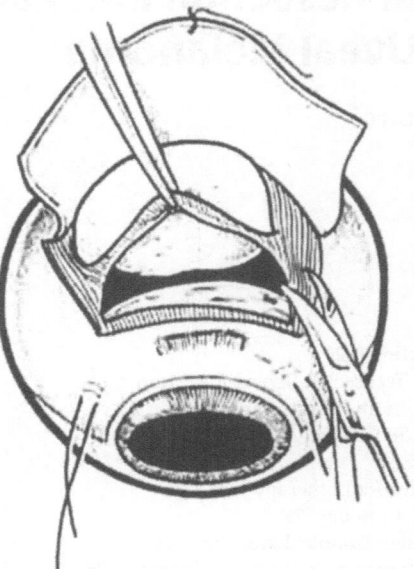

Fig. 4.1. Method of transscleral local resection of uveal melanoma

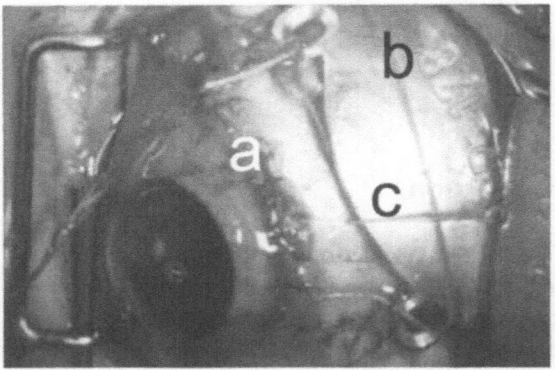

Fig. 4.2. Intraoperative photograph showing a 20-mm plaque after choroidectomy (*a* scleral flap, *b* mattress suture, *c* muscle sling)

4.2.3
Results

The main complications of local resection are residual tumour and retinal detachment. In the absence of either of these complications about 99% of eyes are retained, with 70% of eyes retaining vision of counting fingers (CF) or better, and about 30% having good vision of 6/12 or better, depending on the distance between tumour and fovea (Table 4.1, Fig. 4.3).

Table 4.1. Last known visual acuity according to residual tumour and retinal detachment in 156 patients treated in Liverpool between January 1993 and June 2000 (*CF* counting fingers, *HM* hand movement , *NLP* no light perception)

Last vision	Tumour recurrence and retinal detachment				Total
	Nil	Tumour	Detachment	Both	
6/5–6/12	36 (34%)	2 (9%)	1 (5%)	0 (0%)	39 (25%)
6/18–6/60	36 (34%)	6 (26%)	2 (10%)	0 (0%)	44 (28%)
3/60-CF	24 (23%)	1 (4%)	8 (38%)	0 (0%)	33 (21%)
HM-NLP	8 (8%)	0 (0%)	5 (24%)	1 (14%)	14 (9%)
Enucleated	1 (1%)	14 (61%)	5 (24%)	6 (86%)	26 (16%)
Total	105	23	21	7	156

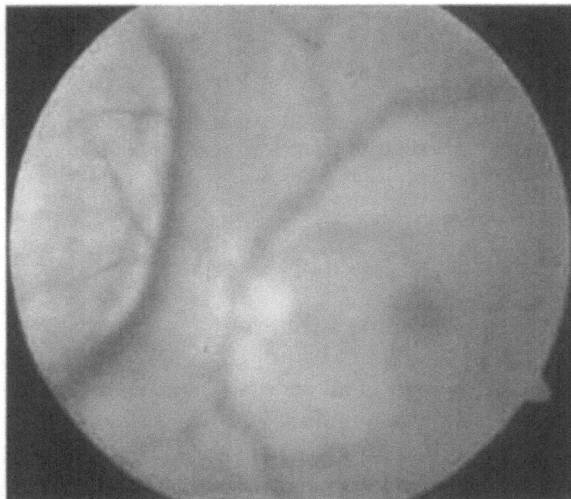
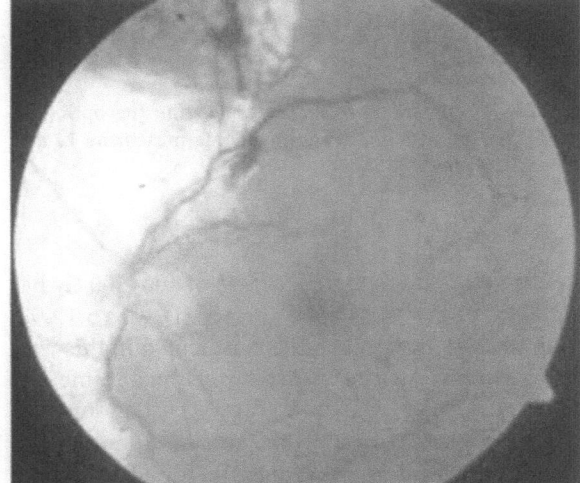

A   B

Fig. 4.3. Left eye of a 57-year-old man with a nasal choroidal melanoma measuring 16 mm×15 mm×7 mm, **A** preoperatively, and **B** after transscleral local resection. The visual acuity 30 months after resection, phototherapy and adjunctive plaque radiotherapy was 6/9

4.2.4
Adjunctive Radiotherapy

4.2.4.1
Residual Tumour

Visible residual tumour at the end of a local resection is rare, occurring in only about 3% of patients. A greater problem is tumour recurrence from invisible microscopic deposits. Such recurrences are usually located in the choroid at the margins of the surgical coloboma (Fig. 4.4), but they can also arise from intrascleral tumour remnants, becoming manifest either as a subretinal tumour within the coloboma or extraocularly. Rarely, recurrences develop in the uvea distant from the coloboma. Visible residual tumour at the end of surgery is related statistically to proximity of the posterior tumour margin to the optic disc or fovea (DAMATO et al. 1996a). Tumour recurrence after apparently complete resection is also related to posterior tumour extension, additional predictive factors being large tumour diameter and epithelioid cell type (DAMATO et al. 1996a). There are plausible explanations for all three risk factors. Resection of tumours extending far posteriorly is more difficult, so that safety margins are less likely to be adequate. Large tumours are more prone to have diffuse lateral and intrascleral extensions. Epithelioid tumours tend to be more aggressive.

In the early years of local resection, it was hoped that local tumour control could be achieved by performing local resection alone (DAMATO et al. 1996a). The margins of the resected tumour were examined histologically for clearance, and if incomplete excision was suspected then photocoagulation was applied. This policy was abandoned, however, when follow-up studies demonstrated unacceptable rates of local tumour recurrence even when tumour excision appeared to be complete both clinically and histologically. The role of adjunctive plaque radiotherapy

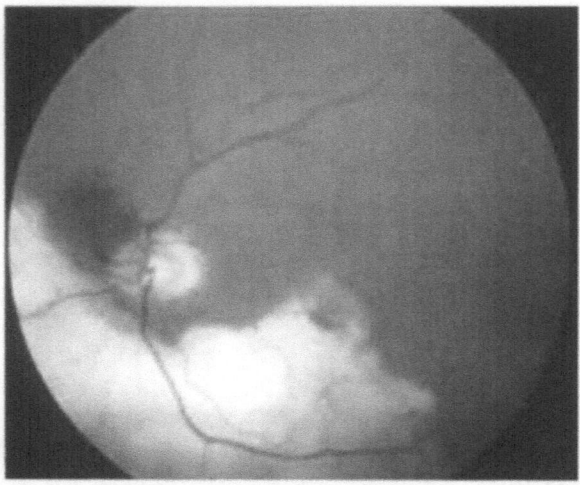

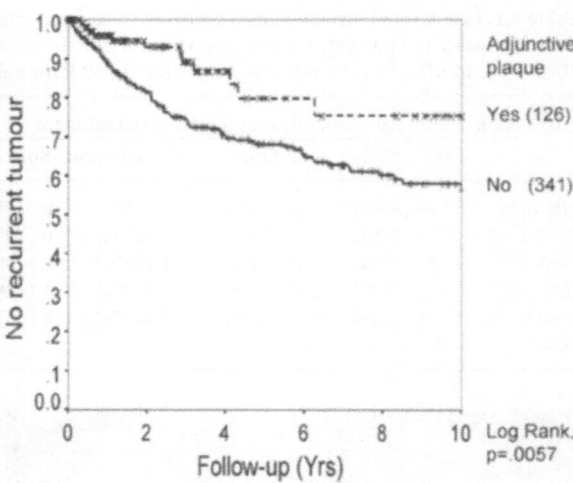

Fig. 4.4. Local tumour recurrence involving the optic disc after resection of a choroidal melanoma measuring 14 mm ×13 mm×7 mm

Fig. 4.5. Kaplan-Meier survival curves showing time to local recurrence according to whether patients had or had not received adjunctive plaque radiotherapy

was therefore investigated, a dose of 400–500 Gy being delivered to the scleral surface (DAMATO 1997). After about 50 patients had been treated in this way, complications such as optic neuropathy became evident and adjunctive radiotherapy was abandoned in favour of wider clearance margins and phototherapy. Further studies subsequently revealed significantly lower rates of local tumour recurrence in the series of patients receiving adjunctive radiotherapy, which was reintroduced, albeit with only 100 Gy to a depth of 2 mm (log rank, $P=0.0057$; Fig. 4.5). This practice has now become routine. A review of 467 choroidectomies without visible residual tumour showed that only 12 out of 126 patients receiving adjunctive plaque radiotherapy developed recurrent tumour. These comprised (1) 7 patients who had a large tumour, greater than 15.4 mm in diameter, so that the safety margin provided by a 20 mm plaque was inadequate, (2) 1 patient with a C-shaped tumour curving around the optic disc, so that only a part of the coloboma could be treated with the ruthenium plaque, and (3) 7 patients with recurrences in other parts of the eye, distant from the primary tumour, 4 of them also having a tumour diameter exceeding 15.4 mm. Only 1 of these 12 patients, therefore, developed tumour recurrence within the irradiated area. These results suggest that adjunctive radiotherapy with a 20-mm ruthenium plaque is effective for tumours less than 16 mm in diameter, although there may be the rare patient with extensive diffuse spread or intraocular metastases giving rise to recurrent disease.

4.2.4.2
Extraocular Tumour Extension

A further benefit of adjunctive plaque radiotherapy has been seen in tumours with transscleral extension. Previously, any extraocular tumour nodule was excised together with the intraocular tumour and the full thickness of sclera, the scleral defect being closed with a partial-thickness scleral graft taken from another part of the same eye (DAMATO and FOULDS 1994). In view of the difficulty of such en bloc excision, there was a tendency to abort the local resection and to proceed to enucleation if extraocular extension was detected. Today, with adjunctive plaque radiotherapy, it is possible to save such eyes by first treating any circumscribed extraocular tumour nodules with bipolar diathermy and then completing the local resection in the usual manner.

4.2.4.3
Rhegmatogenous Retinal Detachment

As mentioned above, the second main complication after local resection is rhegmatogenous retinal detachment. In the early years of local resection, the exposed retina tended to prolapse through the scleral window, pressing against the scissors as the posterior part of the tumour was resected, often resulting in a large retinal tear. To a large extent, this problem was solved by the introduction of ocular decompression, so that when the eye was opened the retina fell away from the tumour and the uvea, leaving more space for the scissors. Retinal tears therefore became less common, except when there was an unusually strong adherence of the tumour to the retina, which probably represented invasion. Previously, when local resection was performed without adjuvant radiotherapy, attempts to separate the tumour from the retina tended to result in large retinal breaks. Recently, the resection technique has been modified so that any tumour adherent to retina is left in situ, to be sterilized by the plaque radiotherapy (Fig. 4.6). It is still too soon to confirm the efficacy of this modification, but early results are encouraging.

4.2.4.4
Phthisis

Adjunctive plaque radiotherapy has also improved the outcome in patients with ciliochoroidal tumours. Previously, when local resection was performed alone, it was necessary to excise the tumour with wide clearance margins, sacrificing healthy ciliary body and iris, thereby resulting in a cosmetic defect, photophobia and an increased risk of phthisis (Fig. 4.7). Today, adjunctive plaque radiotherapy has eliminated the need for such safety margins, with better conservation of the ciliary body and iris. In several cases with ciliary body involvement it has been possible to perform cyclo-choroidectomy without disturbing the anterior chamber, greatly reducing morbidity.

4.2.4.5
Complications

Adjunctive plaque radiotherapy is not without its complications. These include: (1) optic neuropathy; (2) maculopathy (Fig. 4.9); (3) cataract; (4) wound dehiscence (Fig. 4.10); and (5) ocular hypotony. Optic neuropathy and maculopathy can be avoided by placing the plaque away from these structures and treating the posterior margin of the coloboma with phototherapy. Cataract is easily treatable with phacoemulsification, so that it should not influence adjunctive radiotherapy. Wound dehiscence is avoided by using nonabsorbable sutures, although if these become exposed they may need to be removed once wound healing has occurred (Fig. 4.11). Ocular hypotony, which tends to develop after cyclectomy, presumably occurs because the radiotherapy prevents adhesion of the uvea to the sclera, so that a cyclodialysis develops. This is an uncommon but serious complication, which can cause disc swelling, macular oedema, and eventually phthisis. The author has suc-

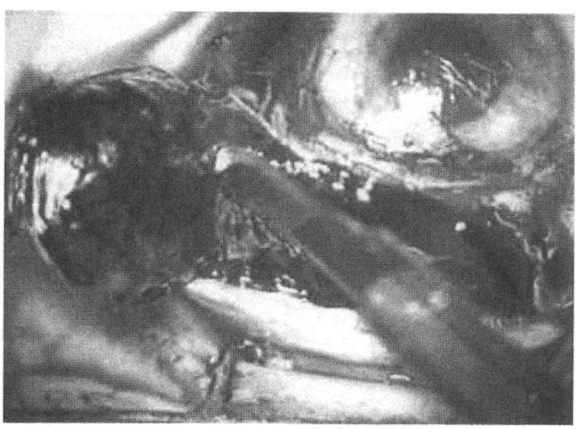

Fig. 4.6. Intraoperative photograph taken during cyclo-choroidectomy of a superotemporal choroidal and ciliary body tumour in the left eye. The apex of the tumour was adherent to retina and ciliary epithelium. It was therefore shaved off with a no. 15 Bard-Parker scalpel and left in situ for treatment with adjunctive plaque radiotherapy

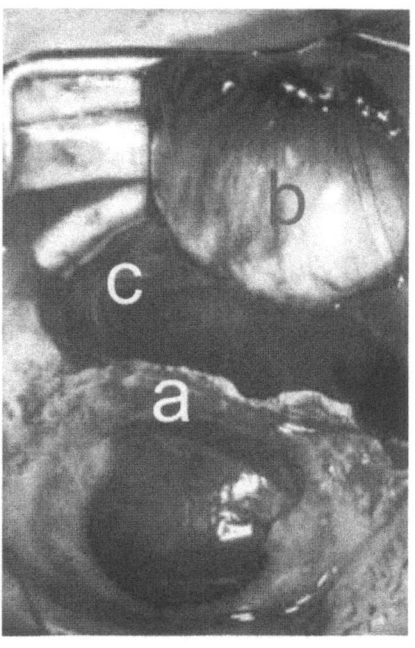

Fig. 4.7. Intraoperative photograph showing irido-cyclo-choroidectomy in 1986, with iridectomy (*a*), tumour (*b*), and edge of retina at ora serrata (*c*) seen

cessfully treated this complication with oral steroid therapy in two patients and by re-opening the scleral flap and suturing the edges of the coloboma to the sclera in another two patients. An alternative approach might be to perform vitrectomy, filling the eye with silicone oil to push the ciliary body against

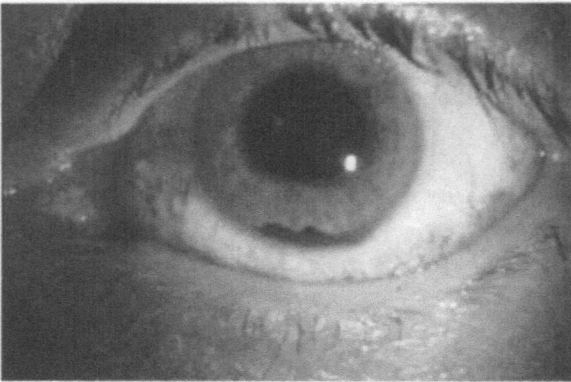

Fig. 4.8. Anterior segment after local resection and plaque radiotherapy of a ciliochoroidal melanoma measuring 14 mm×12 mm×7.6 mm. Three years postoperatively the patient's vision was 6/12. Without adjunctive radiotherapy it would have been necessary to perform a more extensive local resection, with broad iridectomy and inevitably a less satisfactory result

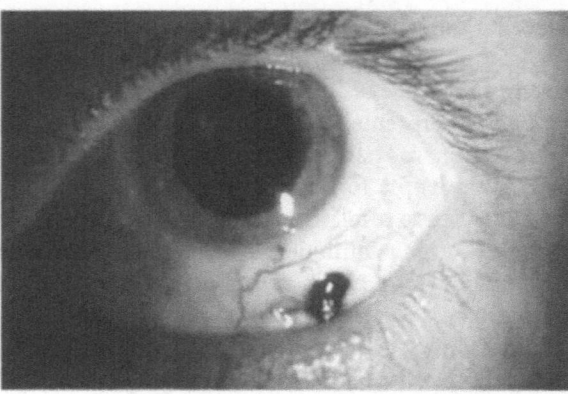

Fig. 4.10. Wound dehiscence after transscleral biopsy and adjunctive radiotherapy delivered with a 15-mm ruthenium plaque. The defect was repaired with a partial-thickness scleral graft taken from another part of the same eye

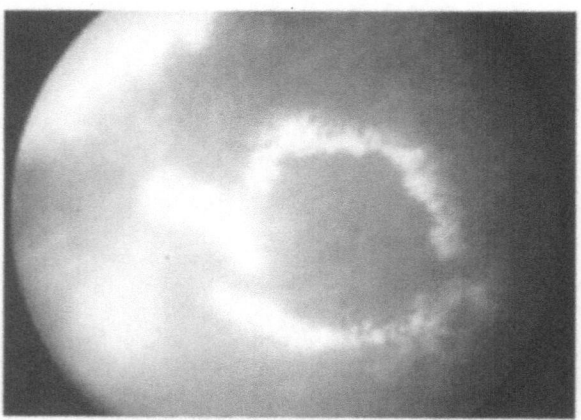

Fig. 4.9. Optic neuropathy and maculopathy after local resection and plaque radiotherapy of a superonasal choroidal melanoma in the left eye. The eye was conserved, but with light perception (LP) only

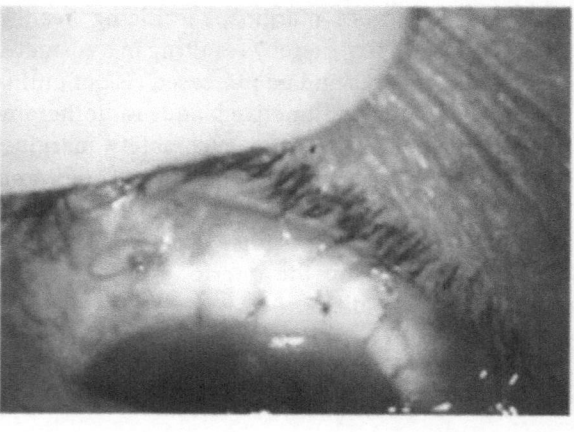

Fig. 4.11. Exposed nylon sutures after cyclo-choroidectomy

the sclera until adhesion occurs. There is also an argument in favour of performing the initial local resection alone and delaying the adjunctive plaque radiotherapy for a few weeks until the eye has healed.

4.2.5
Secondary Radiotherapy for Recurrent Tumour

Radiotherapy is the first choice of treatment for recurrent tumour after local resection, unless the recurrence is very small, in which case phototherapy may seem reasonable, especially if the tumour is close to the optic nerve or fovea. Plaque radiotherapy

would be the first choice of treatment at our centre. In selected cases, for example, if it is difficult to place a plaque over a tumour because of its proximity to the optic nerve or macula proton beam radiotherapy may be preferable (Fig. 4.12).

The technique of plaque insertion needs to be modified in eyes that have previously undergone local transscleral resection. First of all, there may be extensive fibrosis overlying the scleral flap, which can surround the extraocular muscles and cause adhesion of the conjunctiva to the sclera. The author's approach to this problem is to dissect conjunctiva, muscles and scar tissue away from the sclera using a no. 15 Bard-Parker scalpel. There is no need to iso-

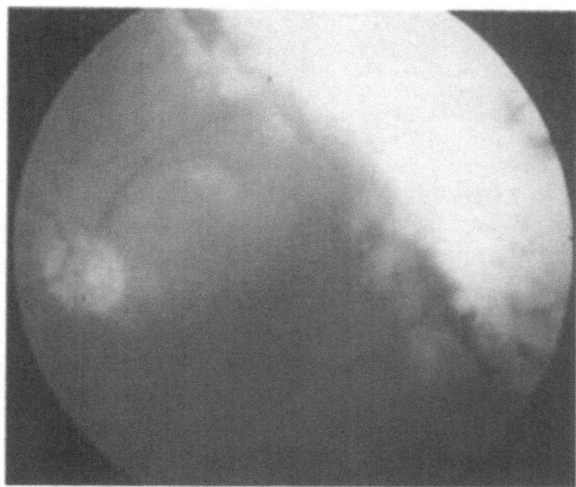

Fig. 4.12. Fundus photograph of the left eye in after local resection of a superotemporal choroidal melanoma measuring 14 mm×13 mm×11 mm, which was followed by photocoagulation and proton beam radiotherapy for residual tumour. Five years postoperatively, the patient's vision was 6/18

late or suture the extraocular muscles, as these should be repositioned accurately if the conjunctiva is replaced accurately in its original position. Secondly, when the plaque is sutured to the eye, great care must be taken to avoid perforating the scleral flap with the suture needles. This complication is avoided by locating the margins of the coloboma by transpupillary transillumination and marking them on the sclera with a pen so that any sutures are placed in normal sclera. The lugs of the plaque can be attached by slings if necessary, as long as a mattress suture is placed over the plaque itself. Thirdly, recurrent tumour is perhaps more likely than the primary tumour to have invisible lateral extensions, so that it is important to use a large plaque, thereby achieving wide safety margins. Finally, if over several years more than one recurrence develops in different parts of the same eye, it is possible to treat each of these with plaque radiotherapy, in view of the localized nature of the radiotherapy.

4.3
Secondary Transscleral Local Resection

4.3.1
Recurrent Tumour

Local resection can successfully conserve eyes with tumour recurrence after radiotherapy. The technique is the same as for primary local resection, except for the need to deal with episcleral fibrosis, as described above.

4.3.2
Exudative Retinal Detachment

As mentioned in other chapters, persistent exudative retinal detachment can develop after radiotherapy of large choroidal and ciliary body tumours. It is a serious complication, often leading to the development of rubeosis and neovascular glaucoma, which tend to result in a blind and painful eye requiring enucleation (Zografos et al. 1991). The author has attempted to deal with this problem in three patients who had previously received proton beam radiotherapy. The first patient, a 55-year-old woman, had rapidly developed a total retinal detachment with the retina touching the back of the lens. Local resection was performed 5 months after the radiotherapy. This was performed in the standard fashion, except that viscoelastic fluid was injected into the retinal funnel with a blunt cannula, which was passed through a small trapdoor over the pars plana. The retina was flat at the end of the operation and the patient did not develop any complications, although visual function was poor because of the retinal detachment. The second patient, a 37-year-old man, had a tumour measuring 15 mm×10 mm×7 mm in the left eye with retinal invasion, which was why he had had proton beam radiotherapy instead of local resection. Six months after the radiotherapy, he developed an extensive exudative retinal detachment and therefore underwent transscleral local resection. This was complicated by a retinal tear at the site of the invaded retina. He was treated by vitrectomy with silicone oil, which was successful, the retina remaining flat after oil removal (Fig. 4.13). The third patient, a 30-year-old man, developed progressive exudation and retinal detachment 4 years after proton beam radiotherapy to a superonasal melanoma measuring 13 mm×9 mm×6 mm in his left eye. Local resection was attempted but the retina adjacent to the tumour was thin and friable, so that a large retinal break developed. The resection was aborted and the eye was enucleated.

Several lessons can be learnt from these three patients. The first case suggests that exudative retinal detachment after radiotherapy is probably due to 'intratumoral radiation vasculopathy' and not neces-

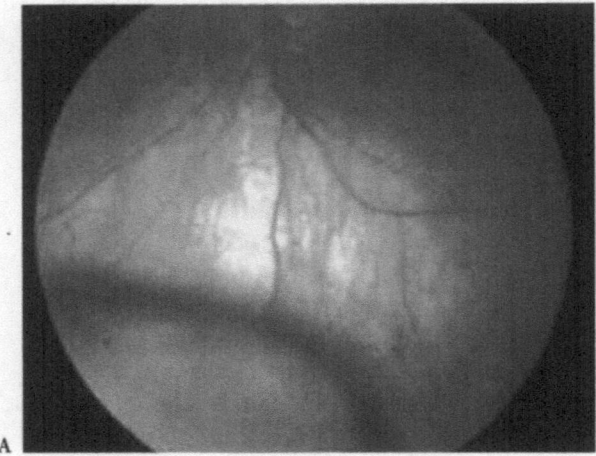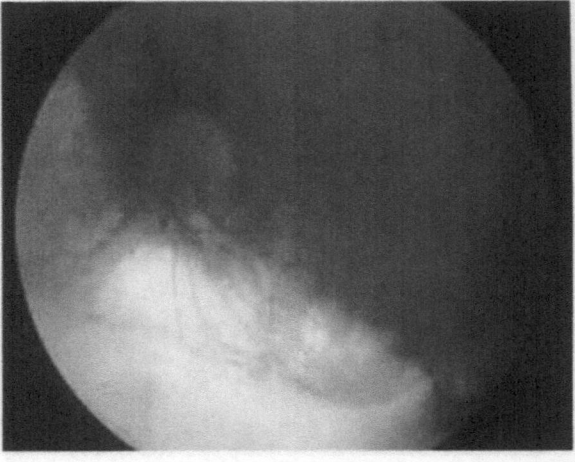

Fig. 4.13. Left eye **A** at presentation, and **B** after proton beam radiotherapy, local resection, retinal detachment surgery and removal of silicone oil. The vision was only counting fingers (CF), but the eye was comfortable with a flat retina

sarily to the effects of the radiation on normal tissues. This would mean that it should be possible to treat exudative retinal detachment by removing or debulking the offending tumour. The second patient, treated several years ago, would probably not have developed rhegmatogenous retinal detachment after the local resection if the intraretinal tumour had been left in situ, as is now current practice. The third case suggests that local resection of an irradiated tumour for exudative retinal detachment is less likely to succeed if performed long after the development of the retinal detachment, once atrophy has made the retina more delicate.

Finally, the author has seen resolution of rubeosis, neovascular glaucoma of 63 mmHg and exudative retinal detachment after local resection of a previously untreated choroidal melanoma measuring 8 mm×7 mm×8 mm in a 45-year-old man. This would suggest that the rubeosis developed because of retinal ischaemia attributable to separation of the detached retina from the choriocapillaris. It is well known that the outer retina is supplied by the choriocapillaris and not the retinal arteries. Neovascular glaucoma after radiotherapy may therefore regress in a similar fashion to that seen in this patient if the retinal detachment is treated successfully.

These anecdotal reports suggest that the presence of a large volume of irradiated tumour can cause severe ocular morbidity, which may be treatable by excising or debulking the tumour, as long as special precautions are taken not to damage the retina.

4.4 Conclusions

Transscleral local resection and radiotherapy are to some extent complementary, with some tumours being more suitable for surgical excision than radiotherapy, and vice versa. The two forms of treatment are also interdependent: adjunctive radiotherapy greatly improves the results of local resection. Conversely, although further studies are necessary, some anecdotal evidence suggests that local resection can eliminate exudative retinal detachment after radiotherapy, therefore preventing or reversing neovascular glaucoma. Each type of treatment therefore enhances the scope of the other, so that the prospects for conserving the eye and vision are improved.

Acknowledgements. I gratefully acknowledge the contributions of: Professor Wallace S. Foulds, who performed most of the local resections before 1989; Dr. Tom Barry, Mr. Carl Groenewald, Dr. H. Hammer, Mr. Jim McGalliard and Mr. David Wong, for performing the vitreoretinal surgery in patients with retinal problems; Dr. Doug Errington, Dr. Adrian Harnett, Dr. Helen Mayles and Dr. Philip Mayles, for radiotherapy advice; Dr. Paul Hiscott and Professor Bill Lee, for pathological studies; Sister Jane Humphreys, for nursing support; Mr. Gary Cheetham, for database management; and Mrs. Julie Sudlow, for secretarial support. The surgery was performed at the Tennent Institute of Ophthalmology in Glasgow until the end of 1992 and at the Royal Liverpool

University Hospital from 1993 onwards. The proton beam radiotherapy was delivered at Clatterbridge Centre for Oncology in collaboration with Dr. Andrzej and colleagues.

References

Bornfeld N, Chauvel P, Sauerwein W, Friedrichs W, Tiburtius T, Wessing A, Foerster MH (1997) Metastatic disease, eye retention and visual function in conservative treatment of uveal melanoma. In: Wiegel T, Bornfeld N, Foerster MH, Hinkelbein W (eds) Radiotherapy of ocular disease. (Frontiers of radiation therapy and oncology, vol 30) Karger, Basel, pp 97–110

Damato B (1997) Adjunctive plaque radiotherapy after local resection of uveal melanoma. In: Wiegel T, Bornfeld N, Foerster MH, Hinkelbein W (eds) Radiotherapy of ocular disease. (Frontiers of radiation therapy and oncology, vol 30) Karger, Basel, pp 97–110

Damato BE, Foulds WS (1994) Surgical resection of choroidal melanomas. In: Ryan SJ (ed) Retina. Mosby, St Louis, chap 47

Damato BE, Paul J, Foulds WS (1993) Predictive factors of visual outcome after local resection of choroidal melanoma. Br J Ophthalmol 77:616–623

Damato BE, Paul J, Foulds WS (1996a) Risk factors for residual and recurrent uveal melanoma after trans-scleral local resection. Br J Ophthalmol 80:102–108

Damato BE, Paul J, Foulds WS (1996b) Predictive factors for metastasis after trans-scleral local resection of uveal melanoma. Br J Ophthalmol 80:109–116

Foulds WS (1973) The local excision of choroidal melanomata. Trans Ophthalmol Soc UK 93:343–346

Foulds WS, Damato BE, Burton RL (1987) Local resection versus enucleation in the management of choroidal melanoma. Eye 1:676–679

Peyman GA, Juarez CP, Diamond JG, Raichand M (1984) Ten years' experience with eye wall resection for uveal malignant melanomas. Ophthalmology 91:1720–1725

Shields JA, Shields CL, Shah P, Sivalingam V (1991) Partial lamellar sclerouvectomy for ciliary body and choroidal tumors. Ophthalmology 98:971–983

Stallard H (1966) Partial choroidectomy. Br J Ophthalmol 50:660–662

Todd JG, Colvin JR (1991) Ophthalmic surgery. In: MacRae WR, Wildsmith JAW (eds) Induced hypotension. Elsevier Science, London, pp 257–259

Zografos L, Perret C, Gailloud C (1991) Conservative treatment of uveal melanomas by accelerated proton beam. In: Bornfeld N. Gragoudas ES, Hoepping W, Lommatzsch PK, Wessing A, Zografos L (eds) Tumors of the eye. Kugler, Amsterdam, pp 497–506

5 Brachytherapy in the Management of Uveal Melanoma

J. E. Freire, L. W. Brady, Z. Petrovich, A. Youssef, J. A. Shields, C. L. Shields

CONTENTS

5.1 Introduction

The most common primary intraocular tumor is uveal melanoma, with an incidence of 6 cases per million per year (SHIELDS and SHIELDS 1992a). In the United States, it represents less than 0.2% of all cancers (AMERICAN CANCER SOCIETY 1990).

This tumor is found at all ages, with a median age of 55 at the time of diagnosis. It is 8–20 times as common in Caucasians as in nonwhite races

J. E. FREIRE, MD; L.W. BRADY, MD
Department of Radiation Oncology, MCP – Hahnemann University Hospital, Broad & Vine Sts., Mail Stop 200, Philadelphia, PA 19102, USA
Z. PETROVICH, MD, FACR
Department of Radiation Oncology, University of Southern California, School of Medicine, Los Angeles, California, USA
A. YOUSSEF, MD
Department of Radiation Oncology, MCP – Hahnemann University Hospital, Broad & Vine Sts., Mail Stop 200, Philadelphia, PA 19102, USA
J.A. SHIELDS, MD; C.L. SHIELDS, MD
Thomas Jefferson University, Philadelphia and Ocular Oncology Service, Wills Eye Hospital, Ninth and Walnut Sts., Philadelphia, PA 19107, USA

(CALLENDER et al. 1942; CAMPBELL WILDER and PAUL 1951; CHALKELY 1980).

Uveal melanoma seems to lack an inheritance pattern; however, very rare cases of familial choroidal melanoma have been reported (SINGH et al. 1996).

Predisposing factors for uveal melanoma include pre-existing melanocytosis and nevus. It can also be associated with familial atypical mole-melanoma syndrome (FAM-M) and neurofibromatosis (SINGH et al. 1996). It has been estimated that 0.25% of patients with ocular melanocytosis develop uveal melanoma (SINGH et al. 1998) and only 1 in 5,000 patients with pre-existing uveal nevi progress to melanoma (GANLEY et al. 1973).

Factors that assist in identifying small (less than 3 mm) choroidal tumors include the presence of symptoms, subretinal fluid, orange pigment on the surface, location close to the optic disc, and tumor thickness of more than 2 mm (SHIELDS et al. 1995a, b, 1998).

The uvea or choroid is the site of a large conglomerate of melanocytes and is thus the selective location of origin for melanoma. The tumor appears as a pigmented or a nonpigmented mass (SHIELDS and SHIELDS 1992).

Uveal melanoma most often assumes a nodular or dome-shaped configuration, but occasionally the tumor is flat or diffuse, extending through the uvea with little elevation (SHIELDS et al. 1996). The tumor can also break through Bruch's membrane and develop a mushroom-shaped appearance (SHIELDS et al. 1998). Extrascleral extension occurs in approximately 8% of tumors (STAR et al. 1962; SHIELDS et al. 1987a, b, 1999).

Secondary glaucoma is associated with uveal melanoma as a result of different mechanisms: cataract, subluxated lens with ciliary body melanoma, serous retinal detachment, orange pigment on the tumor surface, and both vitreous and subretinal hemorrhage.

Symptoms and signs depend on the tumor location and size. Partial subjective loss of vision, blurred vision, ocular pain, photopsia, amaurosis, increased intraocular pressure, presence of a mass, fluid, or blood, and abnormal pupillary response are commonly found (FITTERMAN and McLEAN 1963).

5.2
Histopathology

CALLENDER et al. (1942) proposed a classification of uveal melanoma based on the cell type and other characteristics, such as pigment content, tumor necrosis and argyrophilic fibers. This was subsequently modified (McLEAN et al. 1983) to correlate cell type with mortality.

There are four cell types: spindle A and B, mixed, and epithelioid. Spindle cell A has been downgraded to benign tumor with no associated mortality (McLEAN et al. 1982; SINGH et al. 2001). In general, spindle cell types carry the best prognosis and epithelioid the worst, with mixed cell type suggesting an intermediate prognosis (McLEAN et al. 1982). It appears that the presence of argyrophilic fibers is an important factor correlated with prognosis; lack of fibers determines more aggressiveness and a poorer prognosis (McLEAN et al. 1983) (Table 5.1).

Table 5.1. Callender's classification of uveal melanoma

Cell characteristics	Pigment content	Argyrophilic fiber content
Spindle A	Light	Absent
Spindle B	Medium	Light
Epithelioid	Marked	Medium
Mixed fascicular	Heavy	Marked
Necrotic	Heavy	Heavy

5.3
Prognostic factors

An updated and detailed review of prognostic factors shows that cell type, mitotic activity, microcirculation networks, tumor-infiltrating lymphocytes (TIL), and extrascleral extension are of paramount importance (McLEAN et al. 1982; SINGH et al. 2001). According to these authors, a report from the Armed Forces Institute of Pathology showed that 56% of 3,432 cases of choroidal and ciliary body melanomas were of mixed cell type (McLEAN et al. 1982). Mixed-cell melanomas are characterized by the presence of spindle and epithelioid cells; the higher the concen-

tration of epithelioid cells, the poorer the prognosis. In a series of 267 patients, the 10-year mortality rate for tumors containing less than 0.5 epithelioid cells per high-power field (HPF) was 14%, compared with 70% for tumors with more than 0.5 epithelioid cells per HPF (SEDDON et al. 1983).

Similarly, mitotic activity was found to be associated with prognosis; thus, the more mitotic figures per HPF, the higher the mortality. Tumors with 0–1 per HPF had a 6-year mortality of 15%, whereas with 9–48 mitoses per HPF mortality rose to 56% (McLEAN et al. 1977).

Microcirculation architecture patterns had a more significant prognostic impact in terms of metastatic death than did tumor size, cell type or tumor location. The presence of vascular networks had a negative influence on patient survival. Tumors lacking vascular networks had a 10-year survival of 90%, as against those rich in vascular architecture, which dropped the survival rate to 50% (FOLBERG et al. 1993).

Tumor-infiltrating lymphocytes are present in approximately 5–12% of tumors. In a study of 27 tumors, T-suppressor/cytotoxic lymphocytes were found to predominate (DURIE et al. 1990). A report from the Armed Forces Institute of Pathology on 1,193 cases showed that tumors with more than 100 TILs per 20 HPFs were associated with a 15-year survival rate of 37% and those tumors containing fewer than 100 TILs per 20 HPFs had a survival rate of 70% (DE LA CRUZ et al. 1990).

Extrascleral extension is observed in 8% of enucleated eyes (MARKUS et al. 1990). The 10-year mortality rate is 75% in such cases, compared with 12% for melanomas with no extrascleral extension (SEDDON et al. 1983). Tumors arising from the ciliary body tend to be larger and are more likely to break through the sclera (SHAMMAS et al 1977a).

Cellular variables have also been investigated with reference to survival and prognostic characteristics. Such cytologic factors include: cell proliferation, nucleolar organizer regions, aneuploidy, and expression of Ki-67 and proliferating cell nuclear antigen (PCNA) (MARKUS et al. 1990; MEECHAM et al. 1986; MOOY et al. 1995).

5.4
Tumor Natural History

Excellent data on tumor behavior were reported from Denmark in a study of 302 patients diagnosed between 1943 and 1952. As expected, nearly all (97%) tumors originated in the choroid or choroid and ciliary body. The iris was involved in 3% (JENSEN 1982; SHIELDS et al. 2001). The tumor is thought to grow by local expansion with progressive invasion of ocular and orbital structures. In a study reported from Vancouver, Canada, local tumor spread was seen in nearly one-third of patients (FITTERMAN and MCLEAN 1963). Sclera, vascular structures, and orbit were most frequently involved by this local tumor spread, with involvement of optic nerve, iris, and lymphatic system seen less frequently (FITTERMAN and MCLEAN 1963; WRIGHT 1949). Vitreous involvement is seen in patients with large and necrotic tumors (SPENCER 1975). The presence of melanoma cells in the vitreous indicates a very poor prognosis (SHAMMAS and BLODI 1977a).

Local recurrence in the orbit is surprisingly uncommon. Its incidence has been reported at a low of 2.5%. A sharp increase to 12% is seen in patients with extrascleral tumor extension (JENSEN 1982; SHIELDS et al. 1985). The incidence of orbital recurrence was nearly twice as high following enucleation in patients with extrascleral extension (AFFELDT et al. 1980). Orbital recurrence is usually seen within 2 years of enucleation and is controlled in only 40% of cases. The presence of local recurrence correlated well with the presence of metastasis and death due to metastatic disease (AFFELDT et al. 1980; SHAMMAS and BLODI 1977b).

The primary mode of death in patients with uveal melanoma is metastatic disease, which is seen in 51% of patients. Metastases occur early, in less than 2 years, in the majority of patients (JENSEN 1982; MCLEAN et al. 1990). Occasionally, however, a patient may develop clinical evidence of metastatic disease more than 20 years after diagnosis (JENSEN 1982; SHIELDS et al. 1987a, b). The liver is the most common site of metastatic disease in patients with uveal melanoma, in contrast to those with malignant melanoma of other primary sites, where liver involvement is seen in 20% of patients (CHAR 1978; DONOSO et al. 1986; EINHORN et al. 1974a, b; JENSEN 1982; RAJPAL et al. 1983; WRIGHT 1949).

5.5
General Considerations

Management of uveal melanoma continues to be controversial. Several options for treatment and general management have been advocated, including periodic observation, laser photocoagulation, thermotherapy, plaque brachytherapy, charged particle radiotherapy, local resection and enucleation (SHIELDS et al. 1998).

Several considerations influence the therapeutic options in the management of uveal melanoma and include tumor size, activity, location, growth pattern, the patient's general health and age, and status of the opposite eye. All of these factors should be analyzed collectively when a treatment decision has to be made. In those cases where there is hope for useful vision, every attempt should be made to use an organ-conserving procedure; however, if the chance of functional visual acuity is nil or minimal, or if intraocular pressure is elevated, enucleation is warranted (SHIELDS et al. 1998).

Tumor size becomes a determining factor for treatment; small melanomas (less than 10 mm in diameter and less than 3 mm thick) are usually subjected to scheduled observation, with the exception of a subset of tumors that show clinical risks for metastasis (SHIELDS et al. 1995a, 2000), which are commonly managed with laser photocoagulation, thermotherapy, charged-particle radiotherapy, plaque brachytherapy and/or local resection.

Medium-size uveal melanomas (3–8 mm in thickness and 10–15 mm in diameter) can be managed with plaque brachytherapy, charged-particle radiotherapy, local resection or enucleation, depending on particular factors. At present these are usually treated with plaque radiotherapy.

Larger tumors (more than 8 mm in thickness and greater than 15 mm in base diameter) are managed with local resection, plaque brachytherapy or enucleation. Enucleation is the preferred method, owing to ocular intolerance of conservative methods (SHIELDS et al. 1998, 2002).

Tumors that display a fast growth pattern, are diffuse, and are observed to have extrascleral extension can be treated with enucleation; however, if there is less extensive disease, radiotherapy in the form of plaque brachytherapy should be employed.

Uveal melanoma can present with involvement of the iris, the ciliary body, or the posterior choroid, and is managed accordingly. Iris melanoma can be treated with excision, plaque brachytherapy or enucleation, depending on tumor size and/or location and other characteristics (SHIELDS et al. 1995a, b, 2001). Ciliary body and choroidal melanoma are treated by different methods, but the closer the lesion is to the optic disc and fovea, the higher is the risk of irreversible visual impairment as a result of radioactive plaque brachytherapy (DEPOTTER et al. 1994).

5.6
Diagnosis

The goals of pretreatment assessment include establishing the diagnosis of melanoma, defining the tumor's anatomical extent, location, and dimensions, and identifying its important characteristics, such as degree of pigmentation and echographic properties. Histological confirmation of the clinical diagnosis is usually established only following enucleation, and the role of fine-needle biopsy is limited to those rare cases in which there is strong doubt (SHIELDS and SHIELDS 1993). The pretreatment diagnosis of uveal melanoma can be established noninvasively with a high degree of accuracy in most patients (SHIELDS and SHIELDS 1992a, b). A detailed general and ophthalmic history is essential.

General physical examination is directed toward discovering clinical evidence of metastatic disease. This is followed by a detailed ophthalmic examination, which includes general eye examination, visual acuity, fundus photography, and biomicroscopy. Ultrasound examination, using A and B modes, is performed in all patients. Although nonspecific, this examination has a critical role in helping to establish the diagnosis as well as in obtaining accurate tumor dimensions. Computed axial tomography (CT scan) and magnetic resonance imaging (MRI) studies are not in routine use at this time. Their value in uveal melanoma has yet to be established (GOMORI et al. 1986). In some centers fluorescein angiography and indocyanine angiography are performed (SHIELDS et al. 1995a, b). The radioactive phosphorus uptake test is of little value at the present time.

Other studies include chest X-rays, complete blood count, serum alkaline phosphatase, and serum lactic acid dehydrogenase. These basic studies, with a judicial use of other tests and intelligent interpretation of information obtained from the history and physical examination, are usually sufficient to establish a diagnosis of uveal melanoma and the presence or absence of metastatic disease (EINHORN et al. 1974a; McLEAN et al. 1990; SHIELDS and SHIELDS 1993). It is imperative that suspected metastases be histologically confirmed with an image-directed needle biopsy, most commonly CT scan-guided needle biopsy.

The accuracy of clinical, noninvasive diagnostic accuracy used to be in the range of 80%, but has most recently risen to 98% (FERRY 1964). The Collaborative Ocular Melanoma Study Group (COMS) reported an accuracy of 99% in 413 cases (COLLABORATIVE OCULAR MELANOMA STUDY GROUP 1990; SHIELDS and SHIELDS 1992a).

Two staging systems are currently in use by ophthalmic oncologists. The first system is the one recommended by the AMERICAN JOINT COMMITTEE ON CANCER (1988) (Table 5.2). The second is recommended by the COMS (EARLE et al. 1987) (Table 5.3).

5.7
Treatment Modalities

Depending on the size and extent of a uveal melanoma, some investigators advocate periodic observation, photocoagulation, thermotherapy, cryotherapy, local resection, or plaque brachytherapy. Currently, the therapeutic methods most frequently used are enucleation and plaque radiotherapy (SHIELDS et al. 1992a, b).

The COMS was organized to address some of the complex questions, and several centers joined this group (STRAASTMA et al. 1988). Patients with a diagnosis of uveal melanoma who refuse to enter the clinical trial should be managed according to the ocular oncologist's recommendation, based on his/her experience, to provide the best systemic prognosis while preserving as much useful vision as possible in the affected eye (SHIELDS and SHIELDS 1993).

5.7.1
Surgery

Recommendations and surgical techniques are discussed in detail in chapters 3, 4 and 6. In general, three surgical modalities are considered in the management of uveal melanoma: local resection, enucleation, and orbital exenteration.

The most frequent procedure is enucleation, which is used in the treatment of 35% of patients (SHIELDS and Shields 1992b, 1993). There is virtually no surgical mortality, morbidity is low, and the long-term survival rates are good. In a compilation of nine reported series consisting of 2,024 enucleations, the 5- and 10-year survival rates were 63% and 43%, respectively (DIENER WEST et al. 1992). In a series of 292 enucleations with 99% long-term follow-up, the 25-year survival rate was 40% (JENSEN 1982). Some of the indications for enucleation are advanced tumor stage, secondary glaucoma, and optic nerve invasion (SHIELDS and SHIELDS 1993).

Table 5.2. Staging of uveal melanoma (T, N, M)[a]

T stage	N stage	M stage
$T_1 \leq 10$ mm diameter and ≤ 3 mm thickness	N_0, no regional lymph node metastasis	M_0, no distant metastasis
$T_2 > 10 \leq 15$ mm diameter and $> 3 \leq 5$ mm thickness	N_1, regional lymph node metastasis	M_1, distant metastasis
$T_3 > 15$ mm diameter and > 5 mm thickness		
T_4, tumor with extraocular extension		

[a]American Joint Committee Staging System (1988)

Table 5.3. Staging of uveal melanoma (Collaborative Ocular Melanoma Study)

Stage	Description	Dimensions
I	Small	≤ 3 mm thickness, ≤ 5 mm diameter
II	Intermediate	$\geq 3.1 \leq 8$ mm thickness, ≤ 16 mm diameter
III	Large	> 8 mm thickness, > 16 mm diameter

Optic nerve invasion and juxtapapillary tumor location are widely considered to be adverse prognostic factors, but are overshadowed by other factors, such as epithelial histology, vitreous invasion, or inadequate surgical margins (SPENCER 1975; WEINHAUS et al. 1985).

Patients with orbital tumor extension experience an almost tenfold increase in the incidence of postenucleation orbital recurrence (SHAMMAS and BLODI 1977a). Orbital exenteration, although controversial, has been recommended by some investigators for patients with this tumor presentation (NAQUIN 1954). Others, however, feel that orbital exenteration should be used judiciously for selected patients with extrascleral tumor extension (JENSEN 1982; SHIELDS and SHIELDS 1992b). The same investigators recommend the use of radiotherapy for medium-sized uveal melanomas with minimal extrascleral extension. Of the 12,000 patients with uveal melanoma treated over a 25-year period at the Wills Eye Hospital, only 10 had orbital exenteration (SHIELDS and SHIELDS 1992b).

In highly selected patients with a small tumor, favorable characteristics, and a favorable location in the eye, a full-thickness local resection of eye wall or a partial lamellar sclerouvectomy can be performed (FOULDS and DAMATO 1986; SHIELDS and SHIELDS 1988).

Once the uveal melanoma metastasizes, particularly to the liver, the prognosis becomes poor. At present there is no effective treatment to modify its dismal outcome. Chemotherapy regimens have failed to demonstrate a beneficial response. Selective hepatic arterial embolization with cisplatin and polyvinyl improves survival temporarily (MAVLIGIT et al. 1988) The use of immunotherapy with the use of BCG did not alter survival (MCLEAN et al. 1990). The use of monoclonal antibodies is currently being investigated.

5.7.2
Radiotherapy

Radioactivity is the energy generated from an unstable nucleus that contains an excess of neutrons. Radioactivity was discovered by Pierre and Marie Curie in 1898 while they were working with the element Polonium. Radioactive atoms are termed isotopes.

There are two basic types of radiation: ionizing and nonionizing radiation. When an atomic particle or an electromagnetic wave hits another atom or molecule, an electron or a nucleon (proton or neutron) is removed, transforming the particle into an ion. Ionizing radiation is biologically important because it causes damage to DNA strands, impairing the cells' capacity to regenerate and duplicate. These events form the basis of radiation therapy for cancer treatment. Nonionizing radiation or excitation occurs when the outermost electrons of an atom are stimulated by an electromagnetic force and remain vibrating or fluctuating within different levels of the same orbit. This type of radiation has less biologic effect on cancer cells.

The radioactive elements emit three types of radiation, including alpha particles with a positive electrical charge (helium nucleus), beta particles with a negative charge (electrons), and gamma rays with no electrical charge. Gamma rays are similar to X-rays, but gamma rays originate in the atomic nucleus and X-rays from the peripheral electrons.

Radiotherapy can be delivered from a remote distance (teletherapy), or from a site close to or within the target tissue (brachytherapy). Teletherapy is administered by a linear accelerator or cyclotron, and this technique is employed for external-beam radiotherapy and charged-particle radiotherapy. Brachytherapy is administered to the eye by applying a radioactive isotope directly to the surface of the eye, and this is the technique of plaque radiotherapy.

The major goal of radiotherapy for uveal melanoma is to destroy the intraocular tumor and prevent metastasis and death. Secondary goals are to preserve the eye and maintain vision. Radiotherapy results in relatively slow regression of uveal melanoma during a period of 6 months to 2 years. The initial sign of tumor regression is resolution of subretinal fluid, and this usually occurs in the first 6 months after treatment, depending on the amount of fluid. Next, ultrasonographically detectable tumor shrinkage is apparent. Most tumors demonstrate regression by a decrease in thickness while the basal dimension remains stable. The most dramatic tumor thickness decline occurs in the 1st year after treatment; thereafter, the decline is slower. Irradiated uveal melanoma appears as a homogeneous atrophic mass, often with surrounding radiation-induced alterations in the retina, retinal pigment epithelium, and choroid.

Most tumors regress to approximately 50% of their original thickness. Only occasionally does a tumor regress to a completely flat scar, unless it was 3.0 mm or less in thickness prior to treatment. The rate of tumor regression after radiotherapy provides an indication of the tumor's malignant potential. It has been found that a rapid early regression of irradiated choroidal melanoma in the first few months after treatment correlates with an increased risk for metastases as compared with those tumors that regressed slowly. Established radiotherapy techniques for uveal melanoma include plaque radiotherapy and charged-particle radiotherapy. Other radiotherapy techniques that are occasionally employed, but are not well established, include external beam radiotherapy and gamma knife radiotherapy.

5.7.2.1
External Beam Radiotherapy

An interesting study of 110 patients with uveal melanoma treated with 50 Gy of postoperative orbital irradiation was reported to have been inconclusive since it did not compare the treatment arms in a prospective randomized trial (SOBANSKI et al. 1972). The same applies to another study designed to prove the benefit of preoperative external beam radiotherapy using 20 Gy in five fractions of 4 Gy (AUGSBURGER et al. 1987; CHAR et al. 1988).

This led the COMS to initiate a prospective randomized trial comparing enucleation alone with-pre enucleation external beam radiotherapy. The last COMS report describes how 1,317 patients were randomized to enucleation (660) and/or to ^{125}I plaque brachytherapy (657). Most (1,072, or 81%) of the patients were followed up for 5 years, and 416 (32%), for 10 years. A total of 364 patients had died: 188 (28%) of 660 patients in the enucleation group and 176 (27%) of 657 patients in the brachytherapy arm. The unadjusted estimated 5-year survival rates were 81% and 82%, respectively. Five-year rates of death with confirmed metastasis were 11% and 9% following enucleation and brachytherapy, respectively; after adjustment, the estimated risk ratio was 0.91, 95% CI, 0.66–1.24 (COLLABORATIVE OCULAR MELANOMA STUDY GROUP 2001).

5.7.2.2
Charged-particle Radiotherapy

A proton beam or a helium alpha particle beam can be used in the treatment of uveal melanoma (see Chapters 7, 8). Both have the advantage that radiation is precisely focused onto the target owing to the penetrating capacity of the beam, and they release the maximum energy abruptly at a given depth (called the Bragg effect) and minimize radiation laterally (GRAGOUDAS et al. 1982; SEDDON et al. 1983). Tumor control is satisfactory, with a recurrence rate of 2% (GRAGOUDAS et al. 1982). This modality also has disadvantages, such as the high cost of the equipment and treatment and also associated intra- and extraocular morbidity (CHAR et al. 1989).

Stereotactic radiosurgery with the use of X-knife or Linac, and also with the gamma knife, which contains 201 cobalt-60 sources and requires a sophisticated mechanism for immobilization of the globe, has been shown to have a potentially beneficial effect on uveal melanomas; however, there have been severe ocular and orbital complications. Several European centers, particularly in Vienna, Austria, are working on improving these promising methods (ZAMBRANO et al. 1989; ZEHETMEYER et al. 1995).

5.8
Plaque Brachytherapy

The application of a radiation device to the eye (brachytherapy) was first reported in 1930 by MOORE, who used radon seeds implanted directly into a ciliochoroidal melanoma in the patient's only useful eye. Later, STALLARD (1961, 1966) used radon seeds and then cobalt-60 plaques. Later still, LOMMATZSCH (1983, 1986) popularized ruthenium-106 plaques, with satisfactory tumor control and visual results.

Various isotopes and designs have been employed since, including cobalt-60, iridium-192, ruthenium-106, gold-198, palladium-103, and iodine-125. There are advantages and disadvantages associated with various isotopes. Cobalt-60 and iridium-198 are more difficult to shield and present a relatively greater risk both to the ocular structures and to the surgeon and ancillary personnel, than iodine-125. For example, it would take 25 mm of lead to shield 90% of the radiation from cobalt-60, whereas less than 1 mm of lead adequately shields 90% of the radiation from iodine-125. In addition, iodine-125 has a moderate half-life of 59 days and can be reused in different plaques (Fig. 5.1).

At the Oncology Service at Wills Eye Hospital, we have employed various radioisotopes for plaque treatment during the past 24 years. Presently, we have placed over 4,000 plaques for intraocular tumors. Iodine-125 is now the most commonly used isotope in our department and across the United States on account of its accessibility, good tissue penetration, ease of adequate shielding, and options for custom designing. The iodine-125 plaque has evolved over the years to the present design of a shield consisting of gold, occasionally lead, and the radioisotope seeds set within a template (Fig. 5.2). For uveal melanoma, the seeds are distributed to provide a dose of 8,000–10,000 cGy (1 cGy = 1 rad) to the tumor apex and 35,000–40,000 cGy to the tumor base. Radiation seeds that are reused need to be replaced every few weeks.

Plaques can be customized in several shapes and sizes to fit various tumor dimensions and locations (Fig. 5.3). There are round, notched, deep-notched, postage stamp-shaped, boomerang-shaped, and doughnut-shaped plaques. Custom-designed notched plaques are used to treat tumors at the optic disc. Postage stamp-shaped (rectangular) plaques are employed for oblong tumors, and boomerang-shaped (curvilinear) and doughnut-shaped (ring) plaques are used to treat ciliary body and iris tumors. The doughnut-shaped plaque provides a ring of 360° distribution with a central hole to protect the cornea. The radiation distribution may occupy the full 360° ring or only a portion of it, depending on the extension of the tumor. Plaques are generally 10, 12, 15, 18, 20, or 22 mm in diameter.

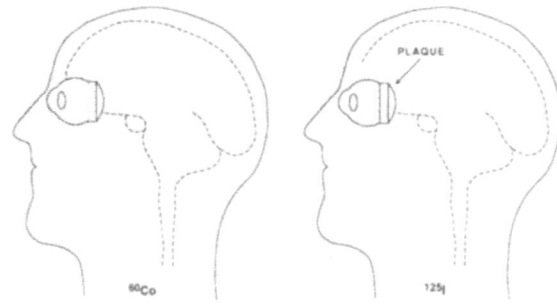

Fig. 5.1. A schematic representation of shielding efficiency with the use of a ^{125}I episcleral plaque compared with lack of this shielding effect for a ^{60}Co plaque. Note the far greater amount of intraocular and extraocular tissue exposed to high doses of radiation with the ^{60}Co plaque

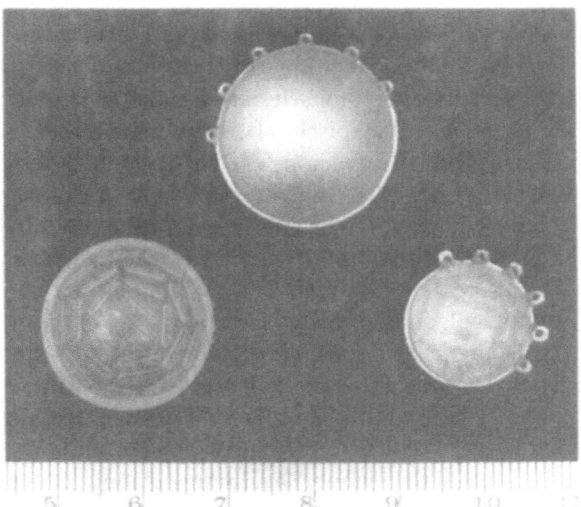

Fig. 5.2. Episcleral plaques used by the Collaborative Ocular Melanoma Study

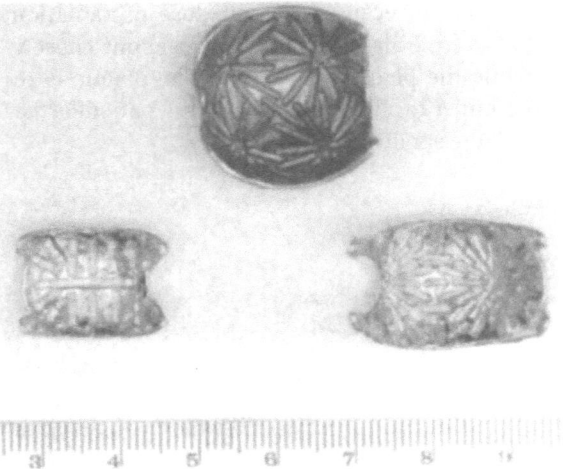

Fig. 5.3. Examples of episcleral plaques. Note the notch permitting effective dose delivery to tumors adjacent to the optic nerve

A detailed office evaluation with indirect ophthalmoscopy and ultrasonography is critical for accurate plaque placement, as the dimensions and features of the tumor are measured in the office and relayed to the radiation oncologist. The plaque design is then decided upon. Calculations for radiation dosimetry are made by the radiation physicist to allow adequate radiotherapy to the apex of the tumor during an acceptable period of time. In general, treatment is accomplished during a 4- to 5-day period.

5.8.1
Technique

Surgery is performed under local anesthesia in the operating room. A conjunctival peritomy is performed and the recti muscles are localized for traction purposes. The episcleral tissues are inspected for extraocular extension and scleral thickness (SHIELDS et al. 1999). Transillumination of the globe is performed through the sclera opposite (at 180°) to the tumor, and the tumor shadow is outlined with a marking pen on the sclera. A transparent acrylic (dummy) plaque is placed on the sclera precisely over the marked tumor shadow, allowing for a 2-mm overlap of the plaque on all margins of the tumor shadow. Loose sutures are placed through partial-thickness scleral incisions to correspond to the holes in the arms of the plaque. The dummy plaque is then removed and the radioactive plaque is placed and secured to the eye with the preplaced sutures.

While the plaque is on the eye, radiation precautions are observed. The patient is advised to wear a lead eye shield at all times. It is calculated that the patient's body receives a small dose of radiation, nearly the equivalent of that received at one chest X-ray, while the plaque is in place. The plaque is removed under local anesthesia and the patient is discharged the same day.

5.8.2
Dosimetry

The clear advantages of iodine-125 have made it the ideal isotope for plaque brachytherapy, by virtue of the physical properties previously discussed. Currently, model 6711 (3 M Co Medical Products Division, New Brighton, Minn.) is used, which contains a silver rod impregnated with iodine-125. The isodose distribution is more homogeneous than the distribution possible with the old model 6702, which had small spheres instead of a rod (see Fig. 25.1).

The complexity of iodine-125 seed dosimetry was applied to the optimization of treatment planning by ASTRAHAN et al. (1990a, b). These authors were able to substantially reduce the radiation dose to the important uninvolved structures of the eye, such as the macula, while leaving the tumor dose unchanged.

The anisotropy of the dose distribution from iodine-125 seeds enables the physical orientation of individual seeds to play a major part in the resulting treatment plan. Utilization of this property of I-125 seeds in clinical practice requires a 3-D treatment planning system. The system employed at the University of Southern California (USC) takes into account the location of important structures in relation to the plaque seeds, as well as processing a 2-D calculational model capability for radiation dose from individual seeds (ASTRAHAN et al. 1990a, b; LING et al. 1989). Additionally, it is useful to include the dose-modifying and shielding properties of the plaque itself (ASTRAHAN et al. 1990a, b).

5.8.3
Side Effects

The side effects of plaque radiotherapy involve the eyelid and conjunctiva as well as the anterior and posterior segments of the eye (CHAR et al. 1993; SHIELDS et al. 1998). Early side effects include transient diplopia, conjunctival chemosis, and irritation from the conjunctival sutures. Radiotherapy from an iodine-125 plaque does not typically cause the eyelid or cilia abnormalities seen with charged-particle radiotherapy.

Late side effects from plaque radiotherapy include persistent diplopia, dry eye symptoms, retinopathy, papillopathy, vitreous hemorrhage, uveitis, cataract, glaucoma, and scleral necrosis, all of which can affect the visual acuity. These problems appear to be considerably less frequent since lower energy radioactive plaques such as iodine-125 and ruthenium-106, rather than cobalt-60, have been employed (PACKER et al. 1992). Radiation-induced neovascular glaucoma was found in 47 of 630 eyes (7%) with macular melanoma, and in 21 of 136 eyes (15%) with ciliary body melanoma treated with plaque radiotherapy (GUNDUZ et al. 1998).

These side effects depend on the dose of radiation to the respective ocular structures, reflecting the location and size of the tumor. Tumors nearest the fovea and optic nerve receive a large dose of radiotherapy and are greatly at risk for radiation-induced papillopathy and maculopathy. Radiation retinopathy results from closure of the retinal vessels over the tumor, often with secondary exudation. This is an expected complication that develops in almost all cases, regardless of the type of radiotherapy employed. If the tumor is in the peripheral fundus, this problem is not visually significant.

Radiation retinopathy and papillopathy typically occur between 6 and 24 months after treatment (DE POTTER et al. 1996). Panretinal photocoagulation is used to treat proliferative radiation retinopathy, and grid laser photocoagulation is used to treat radiation-induced macular edema, with limited results (HYKIN et al. 1996). Radiation papillopathy is usually managed with observation. In rare instances, oral corticosteroids may reduce the visual loss from radiation papillopathy. Enucleation is performed for radiation-related problems or tumor regrowth after plaque radiotherapy in 6% of patients, a similar rate to that following charged-particle radiotherapy (MACFAUL and MORGAN 1977; SHIELDS et al. 1990).

Custom-designed plaque radiotherapy (SHIELDS et al. 1995c) can be employed for nonresectable iris melanomas, with reported tumor control of 93%. The cornea tolerates the radiation dose well. The main complication is the development of radiation cataract 1 year to several years after treatment. Cataract surgery is delayed until the regressed tumor site has been observed to be stable for at least 1 year. In addition, plaque design can be adjusted to cover melanomas in nearly all regions of the eye, including tumors in the macula, juxtapapillary region, and ciliary body and those with extraocular extension.

The cumulative 5-year survival rate after plaque radiotherapy (based on melanoma-related deaths) is approximately 85%. This survival rate compares favorably with matched eyes treated with enucleation for choroidal melanoma. Deaths appear to be more common among patients who fail plaque radiotherapy. However, these patients also tend to have large tumors (SHIELDS and SHIELDS 1999).

Those patients who demonstrate recurrence are treated with laser photocoagulation or thermotherapy if the recurrence is small, repeat plaque radiotherapy if the recurrence is medium sized, and enucleation if the recurrence is large and vision is poor. Tumor recurrence after radiotherapy has been correlated with a worse life prognosis. Presently, we generally supplement plaque treatment with ablative laser photocoagulation or thermotherapy to avoid recurrence, and preliminary data reveal that the recurrence rate has decreased substantially to approximately 3% (SHIELDS, HAMADA, KHETERPAL et al., unpublished data).

In a recently published report on 1,300 patients treated by plaque brachytherapy, 1,106 had a visual acuity of 20/100 or better at the time of treatment. Poor visual acuity (20/200 or worse) was found in 34% and 68% of these patients at the 5- and 10-year follow-up, respectively. Multiple factors that correlated with this outcome included: tumor thickness, proximity to the fovea (less than 5 mm away), notched plaques, isotopes, particularly cobalt-60, age older than 60 years, and subretinal fluid. Visual acuity was effectively preserved in patients with small tumors outside a radius of 5 mm from the fovea and optic disc (SHIELDS et al. 2000, 2002).

There is overwhelming evidence that malignant melanoma of the uveal tract can be treated safely with radioactive plaques, with long-term survival rates equal to those of enucleation.

Preservation of eye function is expected in the majority of plaque radiotherapy-treated patients. Application of low-energy isotopes, collimation of individual seeds, and routine use of 3-D dosimetry should help to further optimize episcleral plaque therapy.

In summary, the treatment of uveal melanoma continues to be a challenging problem; however, the therapeutic modalities described above, and particularly plaque brachytherapy, offer an excellent prognosis in those patients who have been carefully selected to benefit from this approach.

5.8.4
Results

Tumor control with plaque radiotherapy is satisfactory. In 86% of the patients, tumor control is achieved with clinical evidence of tumor regression.

References

Affeldt JC, Minckler DS, Azen SP et al (1980) Prognosis in uveal melanoma with extrascleral extension. Arch Ophthalmol 98: 1975–1979

American Cancer Society (1990) Cancer Statistics 1990. CA Cancer J Clin 4:9–26

American Joint Committee on Cancer (1988) Melanoma of

the uvea. In: Behrs OH (ed) Manual for staging of cancer. Lippincott, Philadelphia, pp 231–233

Astrahan MA, Luxton G, Jozsef G et al (1990a) An interactive treatment planning system for ophthalmic plaque brachytherapy. Int J Radiat Oncol Bioi Phys 18:679–687

Astrahan MA, Luxton G, Jozsef G et al (1990b) Optimization of I-125 ophthalmic plaque brachytherapy. Med Phys 17:1053–1057

Augsburger JJ, Eagle RC, Chiu M, Shields JA (1987) The effect of pre-enucleation radiotherapy on mitotic activity of choroidal and ciliary body melanomas. Ophthalmology 94:1627–1630

Callender GR, Wilder HC, Ash JE (1942) Five hundred melanomas of the choroid and ciliary body followed five years or longer. Am J Ophthalmol 25:962–967

Campbell Wilder H, Paul EV (1951) Malignant melanoma of the choroid and ciliary body: a study of 2535 cases. Milit Surg 109:370–378

Cappin JM (1973) Radiation scleral necrosis simulating early scleromalacia perforans. Br J Ophthalmol 57:425–428

Chalkely T (1980) Ocular Melanoma Task Force report. Am J Ophthalmol 90:728–733

Char DH (1978) Metastatic choroid melanoma. Am J Ophthalmol 86:76–80

Char DH, Phillips TL, Andejewski Y et al (1988) Failure of pre-enucleation radiation to decrease uveal melanoma mortality. Am J Ophthalmol 106:21–26

Char DH, Quivey JM, Castro JR et al (1989) Uveal melanoma radiation I-125 brachytherapy versus helium ion irradiation. Ophthalmology 96:1708–1715

Char DH, Quivey JM, Castro JR et al (1993) Helium ions versus iodine-125 brachytherapy in the management of uveal melanoma: a prospective randomized dynamically balanced trial. Ophthalmology 100:1547–1554

Collaborative Ocular Melanoma Study Group (1990) Accuracy of diagnosis of choroidal melanomas in the Collaborative Ocular Melanoma Study. (COMS report no 1) Arch Ophthalmol l08:1268–1273

Collaborative Ocular Melanoma Study Group (2001) The COMS randomized trial of iodine-125 brachytherapy for choroidal melanoma: III. Initial mortality findings. (COMS report no 18) Arch Ophthalmol 119:969–982

De la Cruz PO, Specht Cs, McLean IW (1990) Cancer 234:112–115

DePotter P, Shields CL, Shields JA et al (1994) Impact of enucleation versus plaque radiotherapy in the management of juxtapapillary choroidal melanoma on patient survival. Br J Ophthalmol 78:109–114

DePotter P, Shields CL, Shields JA et al (1996) Plaque radiotherapy for justapapillary choroidal melanoma: visual acuity and survival outcome. Arch Ophthalmol 114:1357–1365

Diener-West M, Hawkins BS, Markowitz JA et al (1992) AP. A review of mortality from choroidal melanoma. II. A meta-analysis of 5-year mortality rates following enucleation: 1966–1988. Arch Ophthalmol 110:245–250

Donoso LA, Augsburger JJ, Shields JA et al (1986) Metastatic uveal melanoma. Correlation between survival time and cytomorphometry of primary tumors. Arch Ophthalmol 104:76–78

Earle J, Kline RW, Robertson DM (1987) selection of iodine-125 for the Collaborative Ocular Melanoma Study. Arch Ophthalmol 105:763–764

Einhorn LH, Burgess MA, Gottlieb JA (1974a) Metastatic patterns of choroidal melanoma. Cancer 34:1001–1004

Einhorn LH, Burgess MA, Vallejos C et al (1974b) Advanced metastatic melanoma-prognostic correlations and response to treatment in 26 patients. Cancer Res 34:1994–2004

Ferry AP (1964) Lesions mistaken for malignant melanoma of the posterior uvea. Arch Ophthalmol 72:463–469

Fitterman HN, McLean JA (1963) Malignant melanoma: a fifteen year review. Am J Ophthalmol 56:90–97

Folberg, R, Rummelt V, Parys-van Ginderdeuren R et al (1993) Prognostic value of tumor blood vessel morphology in primary uveal melanoma. Ophthalmology 100:1389–1398

Foulds WS, Damato BE (1986) Alternatives to enucleation in the management of choroidal melanoma. Aust NZ J Ophthalmol 14:19–27

Ganley JP, Comstock GW (1973) Benign nevi and malignant melanoma of the choroids. Am J Ophthalmol 73:19–25

Gragoudas ES, Goitein M, Verhey L et al (1980) Proton beam irradiation: an alternative to enucleation for intraocular melanomas. Ophthalmology 87:571

Gunduz K, Shields CL, Shields JA et al (1999) Plaque radiotherapy of uveal melanoma with predominant ciliary involvement. Arch Ophthalmol 117:170–177

Hykin P, Shields CL, Arevalo F, DePotter P, Freire G, Shields JA (1996) The efficacy of focal laser treatment in radiation maculopathy. Paper presented to the Association for Research of Vision in Ophthalmology, Fort Lauderdale, Fla, 23 April 1996

Jensen OA (1982) Malignant melanomas of the human uvea in Denmark 1943–1952. Acta Ophthalmol 60:161–182

Ling CC, Chen GTY, Boothby JW et al (1989) Computer assisted treatment planning for I-125 ophthalmic plaque radiotherapy. Int J Radiat Oncol Biol Phys 17:405–410

Lommatzsch PK (1983) β-Irradiation of choroidal melanoma with ^{106}Ru/^{106}Rh applicators: 16 years experience. Arch Ophthalmol 101:713–717

Lommatzsch PK (1986) Results after β-irradiation ^{106}Ru/^{106}Rh) of choroidal melanomas: 20 years experience. Br J Ophthalmol 70:844–851

MacFaul P A, Morgan GL (1977) Histological changes in malignant melanomas of the choroid after cobalt plaque therapy. Br J Ophthalmol 61:221–228

MarkusDM, Minkowitz JB, Wardwell SD (1990) The value of nucleolar organizer regions in uveal melanoma. The Collaborative Ocolar Melanoma Study Group. Am J Ophthalmol 110:527–534

Mavligit GM, Charnsangavej C, Carrasco CH, Patt YZ, Benjamin RS, Wallace S (1988) Regression of ocular melanoma metastatic to the liver after hepatic arterial chemoembolization with cisplatin ans polyvinyl sponge. JAMA 260:974–976

McLean IW, Foster WD, Zimmerman LE (1977) Prognostic factors in small malignant melanomas of the choroid and ciliary body. Arch Ophthalmol 95:48–58

McLean IW, Foster WD, Zimmermann LE et al (1982) Uveal melanoma: location, size cell type and enucleation as risk factors in metastasis. Hum Pathol 13:123–132

McLean IW, Foster WD, Zimmerman LE et al (1983) Modifications of Callender's classification of uveal melanoma at the Armed Forces Institute of Pathology. Am J Ophthalmol 96:502–509

McLean IW, Berd D, Mastrangelo MJ et al (1990) A randomized study of methanol extraction residue of bacille Calmette-Guérin as post surgical adjuvant therapy of uveal melanoma. Am J Ophthalmol 110:522–526

Meecham WJ, Char DH, et al (1986) DNA content abnormalities and prognosis in uveal melanoma. Arch Ophthalmol 104:1626–1629

Moore RF (1930) Choroidal sarcoma treated by insertion of radon seeds. Br J Ophthalmol 14:145–152

Mooy CM, Luyten GPM, Luider TM et al (1995) An immunohistochemical and prognostic analysis of apoptosis and proliferationin uveal melanoma. Am J Pathol 147:1097–1104

Naquin HA (1954) Exenteration of the orbit. Arch Ophthalmol 51:850–862

Packer S, Stroller S, Lesser ML et al (1992) Long-term results of iodine-125 irradiation of uveal melanoma. Ophthalmology 99:767–774

Rajpal S, Moore R, Karakousis CP (1983) Survival in metastatic ocular melanoma. Cancer 52:334–336

Seddon JM, Albert DM, Lavin PT et al (1983) A prognostic factor study of disease-free interval and survival following enucleation for uveal melanoma. Arch Ophthalmol 101:1894–1899

Seddon JM, Gragoudas ES, Polivogianis L et al. (1986) Visual outcome after proton beam irradiation of uveal melanoma. Ophthalmology 93:666–674<reference>Shammas HF, Blodi FC (1977a) Prognostic factors in choroidal and ciliary body melanomas. Arch Ophthalmol 95:63–69

Shammas HF, Blodi FC (1977b) Orbital extension of choroidal and ciliary melanomas. Arch Ophthalmol 95:2002–2005

Shields CL, Shields JA, Yarian DL, Augsburger JJ (1987a) Intracranial extension of choroidal melanoma via the optic nerve. Br J Ophthalmol 71:172–176

Shields CL, Shields JA, Shields MB et al (1987b) Prevalence and mechanisms of secondary intraocular pressure elevation in eyes with intraocular tumors. Ophthalmology 94:839–846

Shields CL, Shields JA, Karlsson U et al (1990) Enucleation following plaque radiotherapy for posterior uveal melanoma: histopathologic findings. Ophthalmology 97:1665–1670

Shields CL, Shields JA, DePotter P, Singh AD (1993) Lack of complications of the hydroxyapatite orbital implant in 250 consecutive cases. Trans Am Ophthalmol Soc 91:177–189

Shields CL, Shields JA, DePotter P (1995a) Patterns of indocyanine green angiography of choroidal tumors. Br J Ophthalmol 79:237–245

Shields CL, Shields JA, Kiratli H, Cater JR, DePotter P (1995b) Risk factors for growth and metastasis of small choroidal melanocytic lesions. Ophthalmology 102:1351–1361

Shields CL, Shields JA, DePotter P, Singh AD, Hernandez JC, Brady LW (1995c) Treatment of nonresectable malignant iris tumors with custom designed plaque radiotherapy. Br J Ophthalmol 79:306–312

Shields CL, Shields JA, DePotter P, Cater J, Tardio D, Barrett J (1996) Diffuse choroidal melanoma: clinical features predictive of metastasis. Arch Ophthalmol 114:956–963

Shields CL, Shields JA, Gunduz K, Freire JE, Mercado G (1998) Radiation therapy for uveal malignant melanoma (surgical review). Ophthalmic Surg Lasers 29:397–409

Shields CL, Santos C, Shields JA, Singh AD, Eagle RC Jr (1999) Extraocular extension of unrecognized choroidal melanoma simulating a primary optic nerve tumor. Report of two cases. Ophthalmology 106:1349–1352

Shields CL, Cater JC, Shields JA, Singh AD, Santos MCM, Carvalho C (2000) Combination of clinical factors predictive of growth of small choroidal melanocytic tumors. Arch Ophthalmol 118:360–364

Shields CL, Shields JA, Materin M, Gershenbaum E, Singh AD, Smith A (2001) Iris melanoma: risk factors for metastasis in 169 consecutive patients. Ophthalmology 108:172–178

Shields CL, Shields JA, Cater J, Gunduz K, Miyamoto C, Micaily B, Brady LW (2002) Plaque radiotherapy for uveal melanoma. Long-term visual outcome in 1106 patients. Arch Ophthalmol 118:1219–1228

Shields CL, Naseripour M, Cater J, Shields JA, Youseff A, Freire J (2002) Plaque radiotherapy for large choroidal melanoma (8 mm in thickness) in 354 patients. Arch Ophthalmol (in press)

Shields JA, McDonald PR (1974) Improvements in the diagnosis of posterior uveal melanomas. Arch Ophthalmol 91:259–264

Shields JA, Shields CL (1988) Surgical approach to lamellar sclerouvectomy for posterior uveal melanomas. The 1986 Schoenberg Lecture. Ophthalmic Surg 19:774–780

Shields JA, Shields CL (1991) Massive orbital extension of posterior uveal melanoma. Ophthalmol Plast Reconstr Surg 7:238–251

Shields JA, Shields CL (1992a) Intraocular tumors: a text and atlas. Saunders, Philadelphia

Shields JA, Shields CL (eds) (1992b) Management of posterior uveal melanoma in intraocular tumors. Saunders, Philadelphia, pp 171–194

Shields JA, Shields CL (1993) Current management of posterior uveal melanoma. Mayo Clin Proc 68:1196–1200

Shields JA, Shields CL (1999) Atlas of intraocular tumors. Lippincott Williams and Wilkins, Philadelphia

Shields JA, Augsburger JJ, Donoso LA, Bernardino V, Portenar M (1985) Hepatic metastasis and orbital recurrence of uveal melanoma after 42 years. Am J Ophthalmol 100:666–668

Singh AD, Shields CL, DePotter et al (1996) Familial uveal melanoma. I. Clinical observations of 56 patients. Arch Ophthalmol 114:392–399

Singh AD, De Potter P, Shields CL et al (1998) Lifetime prevalence of uveal melanoma in white patients with oculo (dermal) melanocytosis. Ophthalmology 105:195–198

Singh AD, Shields CL, Shields CL (2001) Prognostic factors in uveal melanoma. Melanoma Res 11:1–9

Sobanski J, Zeydler-Gredzielewska L, Szusterowska Martinowa E (1972) Decreased mortality of patients with intraocular malignant melanoma after enucleation of the eyeball followed by orbit x-ray irradiation. Pol Med J 11:1512–1516

Spencer WH (1975) Optic nerve extension of intraocular neoplasms. Am J Ophthalmol 80:465–471

Stallard HB (1961) Malignant melanoma of the choroid treated with radioactive applicators. Ann R Coll Surg Engl 29:170–182

Stallard HB (1966) Radiotherapy for malignant melanoma of the choroid. Br J Ophthalmol 50:147–155

Star HJ, Zimmerman LE (1962) Extrascleral extension and

orbital recurrence of malignant melanomas of the choroid and ciliary body. Int Ophthalmol Clin 2:369–385

Straatsma BR, Fine SL, Earle JD et al (1998) Enucleation versus plaque irradiation for choroidal melanoma. Ophthalmology 95:1000–1004

Weinhaus RS, Seddon JM, Albert DM et al (1985) Prognostic factors: study of survival after enucleation for juxtapapillary melanomas. Arch Ophthalmol 103:1673–1677

Wright CJE (1949) Prognosis in cutaneous and ocular malignant melanoma: a study of 222 cases. J Pathol Bacteriol 61:507–525

Zambrano AD, Chinela AB, Bunge HJ et al (1989) Stereotactic radiosurgery for uveal melanomas: protocol for treatment. Arch Ophthalmol Buenos Aires 64:49–54

Zehetmeyer M, Menapace R, Kitz K (1995) Experience with a suction fixation system for stereotactic radiosurgery of intraocular malignancies. Stereotact Funct Neurosurg 64 [Suppl 1]:80–86

6 Radioactive Plaque Therapy with Iodine-125 and Palladium-103

P. T. FINGER

CONTENTS

6.1
The Evolution of Ophthalmic Plaque Brachytherapy

In 1930, Moore first used brachytherapy to preserve vision for a monocular patient with uveal melanoma (FINGER 1997a). He implanted radon seeds directly into the uveal melanoma. Stallard tried this technique, but went on to develop cobalt-60 (^{60}Co) plaque radiotherapy (FINGER 1997a). Since that time there have been multiple phase-I clinical trials describing the use of a variety of brachytherapy sources [primarily ruthenium-106 (^{106}Ru), iodine-125 (^{125}I), iridium-192 (^{192}Ir), and palladium-103 (^{103}Pd)] for eye plaques (FINGER 1997a).

Iodine-125 seeds in gold eye-plaques have replaced ^{60}Co plaque therapy in North America, while ^{106}Ru plaques have been introduced in Europe (STANNARD et al. 1987). By 1986, the Collaborative Ocular Melanoma Study (COMS) picked ^{125}I plaques as their eye-sparing alternative to enucleation for the medium-sized choroidal melanoma trial. Used widely, ^{125}I plaque radiation therapy has now gained worldwide acceptance (MAMEGHAN et al. 1992; ROBERTSON et al. 1981).

In July 2001, the COMS reported that with 5-years follow-up, ^{125}I plaque radiation therapy was as good as enucleation for the prevention of metastasis for medium-sized choroidal melanomas (DIENER-WEST et al. 2001). This finding will probably increase the use of plaque radiation therapy for intraocular tumors. But a persistent question arises: why was there an evolution away from ^{60}Co to ^{125}I and ^{106}Ru, and why the switch to ^{103}Pd (FINGER et al. 1993)?

Packer, Sealy and Robertson introduced ^{125}I, and Lommatszch ^{106}Ru, as safer alternatives to ^{60}Co plaque radiation therapy (STANNARD et al. 1987; ROBERTSON et al. 1983; PACKER and ROTMAN 1980). The use of these new radionuclides was clearly associated with improvements in radiation safety (FINGER 1997a; ROBERTSON et al. 1983; LAUBE et al. 2000). For example, radiation from ^{125}I and ^{103}Pd seeds is blocked by the gold seed carrier, eliminating almost all of the radiation to the sides and posterior to the plaque (Fig. 6.1). Plaques containing ^{106}Ru primarily emit beta particles, which travel only 4–5 mm (LOMMATZSCH 1986). With both radionuclides, significantly less radiation is delivered to normal ocular structures on the opposite side of the eye from the tumor/plaque (FINGER 1997a). With low-energy plaques, patients, surgeons and health care personnel were no longer exposed to the high-energy, unshielded radiation associated with ^{60}Co plaques.

P.T. FINGER, MD
Department of Ophthalmology, New York University School of Medicine, The New York Eye Cancer Center, 115 East 61st Street, New York City, NY 10021, USA

This work was supported (in part) by The EyeCare Foundation, Inc., NYC, USA; website: http://www.eyecarefoundation.org

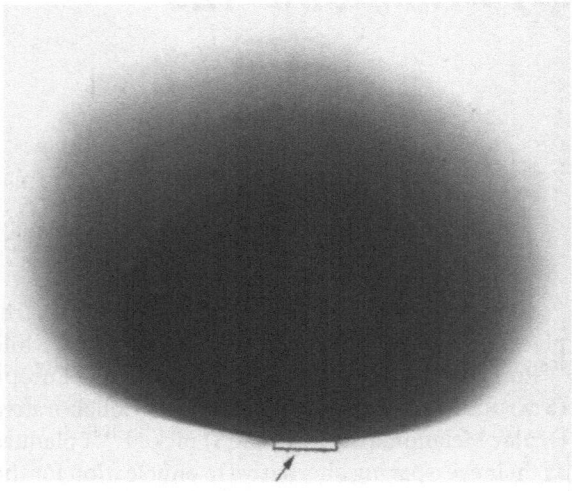
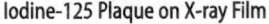
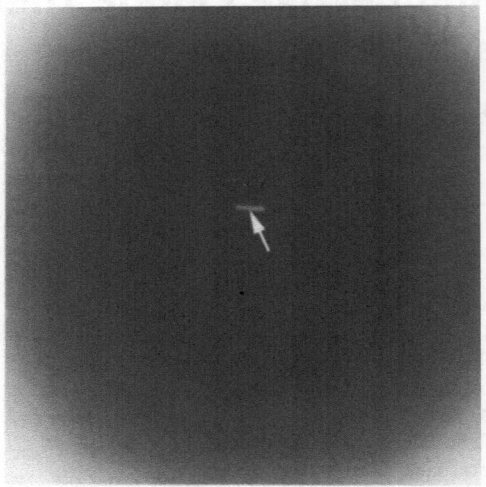

Iodine-125 Plaque on X-ray Film　　　　　　　　　　　Cobalt-60 Plaque on X-ray Film

Fig. 6.1. *Left*: [125]I plaque radiation is blocked by the gold seed carrier, resulting in a bowl-shaped directional radiation distribution (*arrow*). *Right*: [60]Co plaque irradiation (*arrow*) is not blocked, yielding a 360° or spherical radiation distribution

The intraocular distribution of radiation also changed. Compared with ^{60}Co, the use of low-energy radionuclides increased irradiation to the tumor's base and immediately surrounding tissue. The main disadvantage of using shielded and low-energy sources ([106]Ru, ^{125}I and [103]Pd) has been the necessity for more accurate plaque localization (FINGER et al. 1991, 1993, 1994, 1999c; PACKER et al. 1992; LOMMATZSCH et al. 1999; LOMMATZSCH and LOMMATZSCH 1991).

This chapter reviews the methods of and results obtained with the use of ^{125}I and [103]Pd ophthalmic plaque brachytherapy for treatment of intraocular tumors.

6.2
Methods

Before treatment, patients are examined for evidence of metastatic disease and for the ability to tolerate anesthesia. Patients are informed of the reported incidence of tumor regrowth, secondary enucleation, and potential treatment-associated complications. Patients with anterior tumors are told they are more likely to develop a cataract, while patients with posteriorly located tumors are informed that they are more likely to develop radiation retinopathy.

Anterior tumors are typically treated under local anesthesia with sedation. Most posterior choroidal melanomas are more difficult to localize and are plaqued under general anesthesia. Patients with low-

energy ^{125}I and [103]Pd plaques are allowed to be at home during radiotherapy.

6.2.1
Plaque Design and Placement

Low-energy plaque radiotherapy requires very accurate plaque-tumor localization. This is because when the radioactive sources (seeds) are affixed within a gold bowl-shaped plaque, the gold (high-"Z" metal) typically blocks greater than 99.5% of the radiation to the sides of and posterior to the plaque (Fig. 6.2) (WU and KRASIN 1990; FINGER 2000a; FINGER et al. 1998). In order to include possible microscopic extension beyond the tumor's edge, and to compensate for plaque movement, gold-plaque diameters are typically chosen at 2 mm larger than the tumor's largest basal diameter to include a "tumor-free" margin within the targeted zone (FINGER et al. 1998). For example, a 14-mm plaque diameter (targeted zone) would be used for treatment of a tumor clinically determined to have a largest basal diameter of 10 mm. Depending upon the radionuclide (isotope), the use of metallic plaques with sidewalls, the way the radioactive seeds are distributed within the plaque, Compton scatter, and the photoelectric effect, there is a variable amount of lateral spread beyond the targeted zone (FINGER 1997a; LUXTON et al. 1988). A standard set of gold COMS-type eye plaques consists of plaques with five diameters (12, 14, 16, 18 and 20 mm).

Surgical implantation requires a conjunctival peritomy. Tenon's fascia is opened in at least the two adjacent quadrants. Illumination of the globe typically reveals a dark tumor shadow on the eye wall. If the tumor's shadow extends beneath a rectus muscle, the muscle is isolated on a suture, transected from its insertion and allowed to retract. When the intraocular tumor's episcleral shadow is optimally visualized it is marked with a surgical pen. A surgical caliper is used to confirm the size of the tumor's base, mark a 2-mm tumor-free peripheral margin, and thus create the targeted zone. Typically, a minimum of four sutures are used to anchor the plaque onto the sclera, so as to cover the targeted zone. If disinserted, the rectus muscle is replaced into its insertion or given a temporary location until treatment is completed. After the plaque is sewn into position, the conjunctiva is closed. Iodine-125 or ^{103}Pd plaque radiotherapy is typically administered over 2–7 days (retinoblastoma and melanoma) (FINGER et al. 1999c; BOSWORTH et al. 1988).

6.2.2
Treatment of Posterior and Juxtapapillary Tumors

The transillumination shadow of small posterior, amelanotic tumors and retinoblastomas may not be visible to the surgeon. In these cases, scleral indentation along the edges of the inserted plaque can be used to confirm proper localization. Diode-light transillumination and 2D and 3D intraoperative ultrasonography allow for imaging of the plaque-tumor position (Fig. 6.3) (FINGER et al. 1998, 1999a,b; HARBOUR et al. 1996; ROBERTSON et al. 1987). Plaque-mounted diode lights can be visualized at the perimeter of the targeted zone (Fig. 6.4).

When an intraocular tumor touches the optic nerve head, it is physically impossible for an eye-plaque to be placed over the tumor's posterior margin (Fig. 6.5). The most common approach to this problem is the use of "notched" plaques. A notch, or cutout, is fashioned for the optic nerve at the plaque's most posterior (juxtapapillary) aspect. Using a notched plaque eliminates blocking from the sidewall, so that radiation "escapes" out of the plaque in the direction of the optic nerve. In addition, juxtapapillary plaques usually "tilt" back as they are pushed against the optic nerve (FINGER et al. 1998). Such plaque tilting will increase the dose to the tumor's posterior margin, but will simultaneously decrease the dose to the tumor's apex. Three-dimensional ultrasound offers the potential for measuring

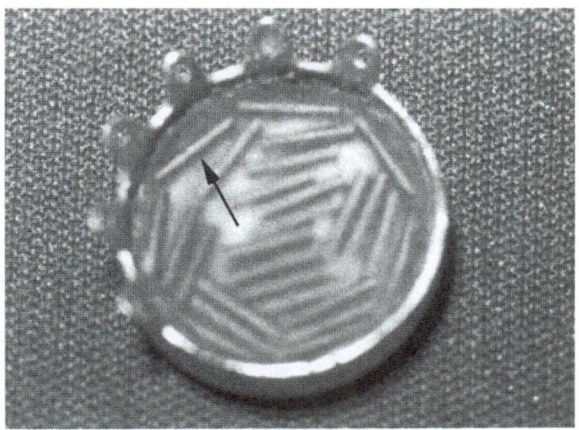

Fig. 6.2. Palladium-103 seeds (*arrow*) can be seen through the acrylic fixative used to hold them within the plaque

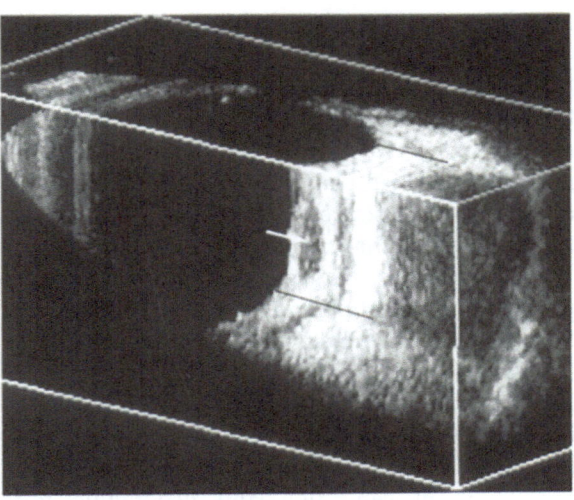

Fig. 6.3. Three-dimensional ultrasound has been used to confirm proper plaque localization. *Lines* have been added to demonstrate the plaque's edges. The *white arrow* points toward the melanoma. Note the volume of orbital shadowing seen in 3D

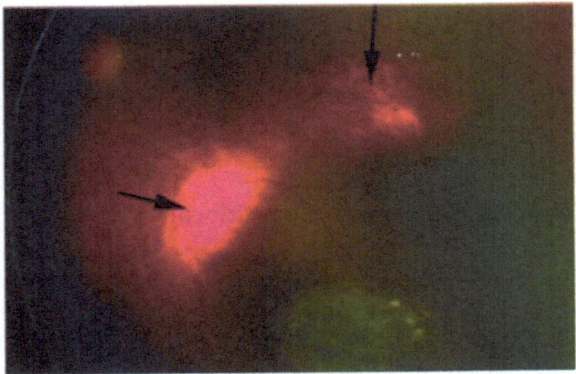

Fig. 6.4. Two diode-lights (*arrows*) were attached to the gold eye plaque prior to insertion. When turned on, they allow for a direct image of the plaques position behind the eye

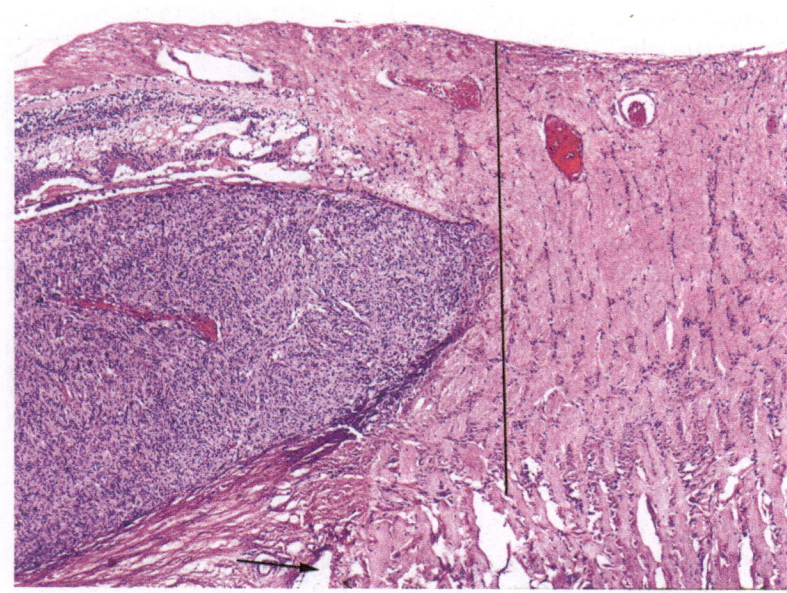

Fig. 6.5. The posterior margin of a juxtapapillary tumor is marked with a *black line*. The *black arrow* points toward the optic nerve sheath. Clearly a plaque placed up against the optic nerve sheath cannot "cover" the posterior tumor margin

the distance from the radioactive seeds to the tumor's apex in vivo (FINGER et al. 1998). Measurements of the tilted plaque's position relative to the tumor will increase the reliability of ophthalmic dosimetry in these challenging cases.

Enucleation or charged-particle therapy may be preferred for treatment of choroidal melanomas with greater than 180° contact with the optic nerve margin (FINGER 1997a; LOMMATZSCH and LOMMATZSCH 1991; MOSHFEGHI et al. 2000). This is because most studies suggest that small tumors adjacent to the optic nerve carry the greatest risk for eye-plaque malcentration and geographic miss (FINGER 1997a). Clearly, these cases should be reserved for surgeons with extensive experience with posterior plaque placement. Informed consent should include a statement which indicates that the use of notched plaques and charged-particle radiotherapy in the treatment of juxtapapillary tumors is associated with a higher risk of local treatment failure and loss of vision.

6.2.3
Treatment of Anterior and Iridociliary Tumors

Anterior intraocular tumors (posterior to the ciliary body and anterior to the equator) are the most accessible to eye-plaque radiation therapy. In these cases, transillumination shadows are easily seen, marked and covered.

When tumors involve the ciliary body and iris, definition of the tumor's base and localization of the eye-plaque become more difficult (REMINICK et al. 1998). In these cases, the tumor shadow merges with the ciliary body band and the tumor's shape becomes irregular. In treatment of iridociliary melanomas, the possibility of ring melanoma should always be suspected. High-frequency ultrasound has been particularly helpful in these cases (REMINICK et al. 1998; FINGER 2001). Iodine-125 and ^{103}Pd transcorneal plaque radiotherapy have been employed in the treatment of iridociliary melanomas. The cornea has been found to be relatively radiation resistant (Fig. 6.6) (FINGER 2001; SHIELDS et al. 1995).

Surgical placement of eye-plaques onto the cornea presents a unique challenge. The eye-wall is slightly indented at the limbus, the metallic plaque

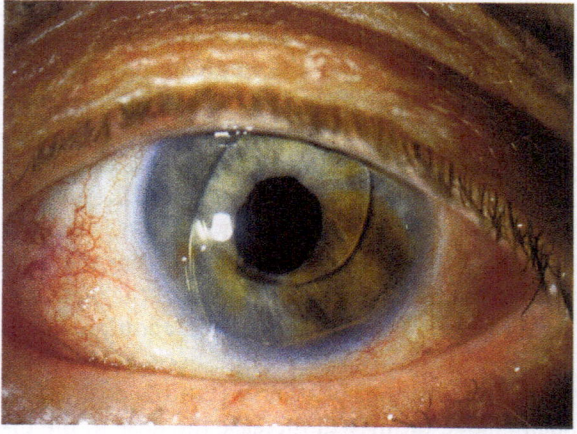

Fig. 6.6. Transcorneal ^{103}Pd plaque radiation therapy resulted in flattening of this iridociliary tumor, secondary cataract formation, and excellent visual acuity

can be irritating to the cornea, and movements of the eyelids can affect an epicorneal plaque. In these cases, the plaque should be attached "backwards" in such a way that the eyelets do not come in contact with the cornea and the conjunctiva must be drawn over so as to cover the back of the plaque. Extra sutures are required to prevent retraction of the surgically displaced conjunctiva. This conjunctival covering allows the lids to slide over the plaque, decreases the chance of displacement, and makes it more difficult to examine the eye during treatment.

6.2.4
Plaque Dosimetry

While ^{125}I and ^{103}Pd photon energy absorption is affected by Compton scattering and the photoelectric effect (resulting in the production of fast electrons which ionize atoms, break chemical bonds, and cause biological damage), the dominant factor affecting the distribution of plaque irradiation within the eye is the inverse-square law. As the radiation travels from the seed into the eye, it is absorbed by the tissue at an exponential rate ($1/x^2$ where x = distance).

Characteristics of the radioactive seeds increase both the flexibility and the uncertainty of dosimetry. These include: seed position within the plaque, anisotropy (radioactive seeds give off more radiation in the direction perpendicular to their long axis), backscatter (reflection of low-energy radiation from the inner aspect of the gold plaque), and also the use of collimation slots and seed holders (FINGER 1997a; LUXTON et al. 1988; ALBERTI et al. 1991). Clearly, the physics of plaque radiotherapy is complex and worthy of study (see chapter 26).

6.2.5
The Dose Gradient

Within the targeted volume, most of the radiation is deposited in the sclera beneath the eye-plaque, with progressively less delivered to the tumor's base, middle and apex. With this "dose gradient," the tumor's apex is both the prescription point and the site of minimum tumor dose (FINGER 1997a). In contrast, the tumor's base (at the inner scleral surface) is closest to the low-energy plaque and typically receives 2–4 times as much radiation as the apex.

The historical prescription, or minimum tumor dose (apex dose), for plaque radiotherapy has been near or equivalent to 70–100 Gy. Owing to radiation

absorption at a rate in proportion to the inverse-square law, when the tumor's apex is targeted to receive 100 Gy all other parts of the melanoma receive more than 100 Gy. In fact, the closer to the plaque one measures, the higher is the absorbed dose. This is the dose gradient.

The steepness of this dose gradient varies depending on the size of the tumor, the radionuclide selected for plaque therapy, and its specific energy. For example, if one treats two choroidal melanomas with ^{125}I ophthalmic plaque radiotherapy to an equivalent 100 Gy apex dose, and one tumor is 10 mm high while the other is 3 mm tall, the average doses absorbed by these two tumors are quite different. The dose gradient becomes particularly important in the treatment of tumors near the fovea and/or optic nerve. For example, both tumors may receive an equivalent 100 Gy apex dose, but the dose to the base of each tumor may vary by more than 200% (Table 6.1).

The choice of radionuclide can also affect the dose gradient. For example, the dose gradient is much steeper with ^{106}Ru plaques than with either ^{125}I or ^{103}Pd. In treatment of a 5-mm-high tumor, with ^{106}Ru the dose at the inner sclera can be 2–3 times that with ^{125}I or ^{103}Pd. In comparison with ^{125}I, ^{103}Pd has a slightly steeper dose gradient but the difference

Table 6.1. Relative dose distributions for three radiation sources. All three tumors measure 10×10 mm (base) and 5 mm in height, and all are centered at the vertical midline

Site[a]	Iodine-125 Dose or [% of dose]	Palladium-103 Dose or [% of dose]	Ruthenium-106 Dose or [% of dose]
Posterior			
Lens	14%	9%	0%
Fovea	124%	136%	216%
Optic nerve	103%	106%	140%
Apex	8,000 cGy	8,000 cGy	8,000 cGy
Base	384%	463%	946%
Equatorial			
Lens	25%	18.80%	0.04%
Fovea	21.60%	16.30%	0.01%
Optic nerve	19.80%	14.10%	0.01%
Apex	8,000 cGy	8,000 cGy	8,000 cGy
Base	384%	463%	946%
Anterior			
Lens	59%	55%	15%
Fovea	11%	6.70%	0%
Optic nerve	10.50%	6.30%	0%
Apex	8,000 cGy	8,000 cGy	8,000 cGy
Base	384%	463%	946%

Anterior centered at the ora serrata, *Equatorial* centered at the equator, *Posterior* 2 mm from the fovea and optic nerve

is nothing like that between ^{125}I and [106]Ru. The difference between [125]I (av. 28 keV photons) and [103]Pd (av. 21 keV photons) is related to the relative difference in these specific photon energies (Fig. 6.7).

High radiation doses, and dose rates, to the sclera and choroid are more likely to cause uveal effusions, tumor edema (pseudo-growth), and secondary retinal detachments. It has been my experience that the higher the radiation dose to the fovea, the faster the onset of radiation retinopathy, chorioretinal atrophy and loss of central vision. Most research intended to decrease irradiation of normal ocular structures has focused on reducing the apex dose by adding adjuvant hyperthermia, reducing the dose gradient, and blocking the radiation as it exits the tumor (FINGER 1997b; FINGER et al. 1990, 1993, 1999c).

There is always a percentage of low-energy photons that are not absorbed within the tumor during plaque radiation therapy. These unabsorbed photons emerge from the tumor's surface and are absorbed by the vitreous humor and by normal ocular tissues as a small percentage exit the eye. For example, in [103]Pd plaque treatment of a posterior choroidal melanoma (10×10 mm base and 5 mm high), the anterior segment typically receives less than 10% of the tumor's apex dose (FINGER 1997a).

6.3
Results

6.3.1
[125]I and [103]Pd Local Control and Metastasis

Local control is typically defined as cessation of growth or tumor shrinkage as determined by ophthalmoscopy and ultrasonography (Fig. 6.8). Local control rates of radiation-treated intraocular tumors are dependent on radiation dose, dose rate, tumor location, and length of follow-up (FINGER and MURPHREE 2001). Other, intrinsic tumor-specific factors (cell-type, melanin content, oxygenation, and pH) are also thought to affect tumor radiosensitivity (FINGER 1997a). Despite these factors, there is no current way to predict the radiosensitivity of any individual tumor. Local control rates for ^{125}I and [103]Pd for uveal melanomas have been published by PACKER et al. (1992), FONTANESI et al. (1993), KREISSIG et al. (1993), GIBLIN (1988), and FINGER et al. (1999c) (Table 6.2). From these series, the mean local control rate after ^{125}I plaque radiation therapy for choroidal melanoma was 94%.

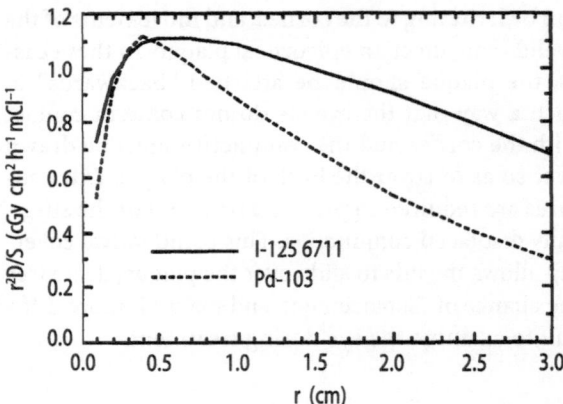

Fig. 6.7. Palladium-103-generated photons are known to be more rapidly absorbed in tissue: r^2D/S (cGy cm^2 h^{-1} mCi^{-1}), where r = radial distance perpendicular to the long axis of the source; D = dose; S = source strength normalization; cGy = centigray; h = hour. (From CHIU-TSAO and ANDERSON 1991)

The COMS standardized methods of diagnosis, plaque radiotherapy, and follow-up in more than 40 centers. Having selected ^{125}I as their radionuclide of choice, for the first time in medical history 40 centers utilized gold eye-plaques of the same size and shape with protective side walls and radioactive seed placement. COMS established a unique protocol to standardize each patient's dose and dose rate calculations.

There were significant differences in the methods used at all non-COMS centers using [125]I. Therefore, any two patients treated at two different institutions were not directly comparable. In Table 6.2, six case-series using ^{125}I, [103]Pd, and [106]Ru were selected for evaluation based on the author's treatment methods, duration of patient follow-up, and inclusion of a broad spectrum of reported results. At an average of 58 months after irradiation, a pooled analysis of the data reveals an average radiation dose of 80 Gy and a local control rate of 93%. Twelve percent were found to require secondary enucleation, and at least 41% of patients retained a visual acuity equal to or better than 20/200. Several authors have noted decreased local control after treatment of juxtapapillary tumors (FINGER 1997a). In this review, a mean metastatic death rate of 12% after plaque radiotherapy of choroidal melanoma appears favorable (as opposed to enucleation).

6.3.2
Prognosis for Vision

Secondary and co-existing ocular conditions are found prior to irradiation and can affect a patient's

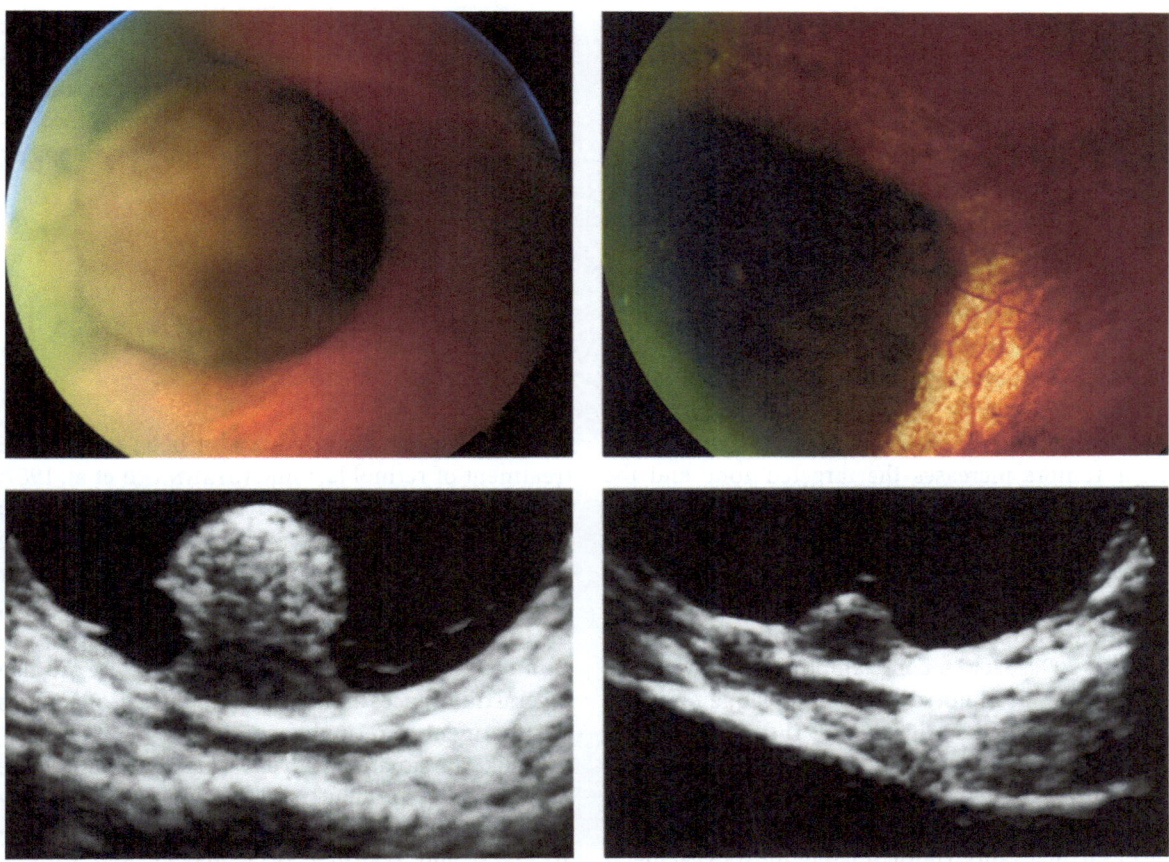

Fig. 6.8. Composite photograph demonstrates local regression of a collar-button choroidal melanoma treated with [103]Pd ophthalmic plaque radiation therapy. *Top* and *bottom left* show the tumor prior to regression. *Top* and *bottom right* show its response to treatment, as observed by ophthalmoscopy, evaluated by photography and measured by ultrasonography (*bottom*)

Table 6.2. Low-energy plaque radiation therapy for choroidal melanoma

Reference	Radiation	Apex dose	Follow-up	Recur-rence	Enucle-ation	Meta-stasis	Neo-vascular glaucoma	Cataract	Retinal detachment, secondary	Scleral melt	Retino-pathy	Visual acuity
		(mean)	(months)	(%)	(%)	(%)	(%)	(%)	(%)	(%)	(%)	
PACKER et al. (1992)	[125]I Results	91	64	7.8	17.2	15.6	10.9	6.3	n/a	n/a	23.4	45% better or = 20/100
FONTANESI et al. (1993)	[125]I Results	79	46	2.3	9.7	5.5	5.5	30	15.3	2.7	21.5	41% better or = 20/200
GIBLIN (1988)	[125]I Results	97	60	7.2	8.8	6.1	9.5	35	n/a	n/a	50	47% better or = 20/2000
KREISSIG et al. (1993)	[125]I Results	70	60	10	0	15.7	15.7	89	n/a	0	89	100% severe loss of vision
FINGER et al. (1999c)	[103]Pd Results	81	38	3.7	5	8.3	1.2	n/a	1.4	0	16.6	77% better or = 20/200
[125]I and [103]Pd series	**Mean results**	84	54	6	8	10	9	40	–	–	40	–
FINGER (1997b)	[125]I,[103]Pd and hypertermia, per the original submission	56	60	6	15	8	6.3	n/a	0	0	12.5	69% better or =20/200
LOMMATZSCH	[106]Ru Results	100	80	15	26	20	1.3	5.7	Present	0.4	35	n/a
All 7 trials	**Mean results**	82	58.3	7.4	11.7	11.3	7.2	33.2	–	1.4	35	–

outcome after treatment. For example, any one patient's vision can be improved when a pre-existing retinal detachment or vitreous hemorrhage resolves, or is corrected by cataract extraction after a tumor has been successfully irradiated. Other conditions (e.g., neovascular glaucoma, secondary cataract, vitreous hemorrhage, tumor under the fovea, radiation retinopathy, optic neuropathy) and secondary enucleation can all affect a patient's vision (Finger 1997a). Also consider that radiation damage tends to occur after years of functional vision, making it a challenge to report visual outcomes after ophthalmic radiation therapy.

Trends do emerge from the literature. Treatment of larger tumors increases the targeted zone and the amount of radiation delivered to the eye, and is associated with a poorer prognosis for vision. Treatment of nasal and anterior tumors shifts the targeted zone away from the macula, which decreases the incidence of radiation maculopathy and optic neuropathy (Finger 2000b, 2001). For example, no radiation retinopathy has been noted after [103]Pd plaque radiation therapy of iridociliary melanomas (Finger 2001).

In general, both ^{125}I and [103]Pd plaque brachytherapy offer a good visual prognosis in treatment of small anterior tumors, particularly those located in the nasal quadrants. Unfortunately, most uveal melanomas are located in the temporal posterior pole (Diener-West et al. 2001).

6.4
Radiation Complications

Complications are affected by both radiotherapy-specific factors (e.g. total dose, dose rate, and dose-volume) as well as tumor-related factors (e.g. tumor size, location, and its biologically variable response to irradiation) (Finger 1997a, 2000b, 2001; Lommatzsch 1986; Packer et al. 1992; Lommatzsch and Lommatzsch 1991; Lommatzsch et al. 1986). Radiation effects are often delayed, so that complications have been noted to increase over time (follow-up). Adnexal radiation complications are rarely associated with ^{125}I and [103]Pd plaque radiotherapy. Transient eyelid edema and iridocyclitis have been noted. Late anterior segment complications have included dry eye, iris neovascularization, secondary glaucoma, and cataract. Acute posterior segment or intraocular radiation complications have included secondary retinal detachment and hemorrhage (vitreous, retinal and/or choroidal). Common late posterior segment compli-

cations include both radiation retinopathy and optic neuropathy. Less common complications include strabismus, scleral atrophy, and cystoid macular edema. Radiation therapy of choroidal melanomas can induce exudative or hemorrhagic retinochoroidopathy (Finger 1997a).

6.5
Plaque Radiation Therapy for Retinoblastoma

Plaque radiation therapy has also been used in the treatment of retinoblastoma (Stannard et al. 1987; Finger and Murphree 2001; Amendola et al. 1989; Kiratli et al. 1998; Lommatzsch 1970; Murphree et al. 1996; Shields et al. 1993). Following a similar history as plaque therapy for choroidal melanoma, the first experience was with ^{60}Co followed by a transition to ^{125}I plaque radiation therapy. There are also several differences associated with the use of plaques for treatment of retinoblastoma.

Unlike the situation with choroidal melanoma, there is some concern about radiation-induced secondary cancers after treatment of retinoblastoma (Lommatzsch and Werner 1975; Finger and Packer 1993). Plaque radiation therapy, particularly that based on ^{125}I seed gold plaque delivery systems, limits the amount of irradiation to the orbit and adnexal structures. The even greater dosimetric advantages offered by [103]Pd plaque radiation therapy exist for retinoblastoma; unfortunately, there are no current published reports on utilization of this technique.

Plaque localization is more difficult in the case of retinoblastoma. These tumors are nonpigmented and do not create a transillumination shadow. Therefore, dummy plaques and scleral depression are more likely to be used for plaque localization. Scleral depression is typically performed around the "dummy" plaque and repeated after the "hot" plaque is in place.

Plaque radiation therapy is most commonly employed in the treatment of solitary retinoblastomas centered anterior to the equator, which are less than 15 mm in base and less than 10 mm in height. Posterior tumors have also been treated. If retinoblastoma seeds are present, they should be within 2 mm of the tumor's surface and the child concerned should not be receiving concurrent chemotherapy for the fellow eye. Plaques have also been used as treatment for recurrent retinoblastomas. Murphree has noted that these eyes have often failed external beam radiation therapy or chemotherapy, contain tumors that are likely to be radiation resistant, and are at higher risk for radiation retinopathy because of the cumulative radiation dose (FINGER and MURPHREE 2001; MURPHREE et al. 1996; WILSON et al. 2001; HERNANDEZ et al. 1993). The typical apical dose used for a previously untreated retinoblastoma currently ranges from 2,500 to 4,000 cGy. Because of chemo-sensitization, this number is diminished should systemic carboplatin be used.

6.5.1
Local Control After [125]I Plaque Therapy for Retinoblastoma

HERNANDEZ et al. (1993) reported on 103 eyes treated with ^{125}I plaque therapy for retinoblastoma. When ^{125}I plaque therapy was used as primary treatment, 5 of 31 patients (16%) had recurrences. When it was used as salvage therapy after external beam radiation therapy, 8 of 72 (11%) experienced recurrence.

6.6
New Applications: Hyperthermia

Enhancement of radiotherapy by the addition of the known radiation sensitizer, hyperthermia, may lead to a reduction in the amount of ionizing radiation used to treat intraocular tumors (FINGER 1992, 1997b; FINGER et al. 1984; LIGGETT et al. 1991). It would be reasonable to assume that these dose reductions would decrease the incidence of ionizing radiation-associated complications for currently employed plaque radiotherapy.

Plaque-like antennas have been fashioned for placement on the sclera beneath intraocular tumors (FINGER et al. 1984, 1985, 1989; LIGGETT et al. 1991). Two large clinical case-series have used hyperthermia together with plaque radiotherapy, resulting in similar local control and rates of metastasis. Heat-related complications have included chorioretinal infarctions anterior to the tumor's base and lowered intraocular pressure after treatment of anterior tumors. At our last review, 69% of our microwave thermoradiotherapy patients kept better than or equal to 20/200 vision (mean of 5 years' follow-up). This result may have been related, in part, to the lower plaque radiotherapy dose (average 56 Gy – apex) given to those patients who received adjuvant microwave hyperthermia (FINGER 1992, 1997).

Lagendijk and Murphree have described the use of adjuvant hyperthermia in the treatment of retinoblastoma (FINGER and MURPHREE 2001; LAGENDIJK 1982). There are no clinical studies proving the efficacy of hyperthermia as an adjuvant to radiation therapy.

6.7
Discussion

A review of the literature on ^{125}I plaque radiation therapy reveals that the only standardized methods of tumor classification, radiotherapy, or follow-up appear in the COMS study (DIENER-WEST et al. 2001a,b). The advantage of standardization is that the results are reproducible within the framework of the study. Unfortunately, since the other clinical studies largely used different methods (tumor-size classifications, radiation doses, visual assessments, and definitions of local failure), it is difficult to compare them. Overall, these studies have clearly given us methods to preserve eyes from enucleation and maintain visual acuity (FINGER 1997a). Recent results from COMS suggest there is no difference between eye removal (enucleation) and plaque radiation therapy as treatment so far as prevention of metastatic choroidal melanoma is concerned (DIENER-WEST et al. 2001a).

We have found clinical evidence that is corroborated by current knowledge of radiation physics and resultant dosimetric calculations (FINGER 2000b, 2001). Local tumor control, as well as the incidence and location of ocular complications, can be correlated to total radiation dose and its distribution within the eye and ocular adnexa. Compared with the treatment of small or medium-sized intraocular tumors, radiotherapy of large uveal melanomas (greater than 10 mm in apical height or 16 mm in basal dimension) is associated with worse outcomes for vision and eye retention (GUNDUZ et al. 1999). Irradiated eyes with large tumors are more likely to develop scleral thinning, neovascular glaucoma, cataract, vitreous hemorrhage, retinal detachment, radiation retinopathy, and radiation optic neuropathy (PACKER et al. 1992). Also, plaque radiotherapy of anterior uveal melanomas is more likely to induce cataract, while irradiation of posterior tumors is more likely to cause retinopathy (FINGER 2000b).

In summary, this review suggests that both ^{125}I and [103]Pd plaque radiotherapy can be used to control the growth of intraocular tumors. Comparative dosimetry suggests that the use of [103]Pd increases irradiation within the targeted zone while decreasing secondary irradiation of most normal ocular structures (FINGER et al. 1993). This dose shift should decrease the incidence of most radiation complications. Clearly a large prospective study comparing the different radionuclides for ophthalmic plaque radiation therapy is both needed and currently unavailable. Hopefully this review has revealed information that is helpful for patient education and informed consent.

6.8
Summary

The purpose of this chapter was to summarize the current results and indications for iodine-125 (^{125}I) and palladium-103 (^{103}Pd) radioactive plaque therapy. A review and analysis of the history, methods, and results after low-energy plaque radiation therapy of uveal melanoma and retinoblastoma is given. This review includes descriptions both of new localization techniques (3D ultrasound, diode light) and of ^{103}Pd plaque radiation therapy. Investigators using ^{125}I and ^{103}Pd have reported data on their methods, local control, visual acuity and metastasis. A compilation of these findings indicates a mean radiation dose of 84 Gy, a local control rate of 94%, 8% secondary enucleations, 9% neovascular glaucoma, and a 10% metastatic rate at a mean of 54 months. In most series, a large number of patients maintained 20/200 or better visual acuity. A recent report from the Collaborative Ocular Melanoma Study indicates that ^{125}I plaque radioactive plaque therapy is equivalent to enucleation for the prevention of metastases at 5 years of follow-up. Finger et al. have reported a 7-year study of ^{103}Pd for ophthalmic plaque radiation therapy. A comparison of clinical results and dosimetry is presented and favors the use of ^{103}Pd in preference to ^{125}I. In conclusion, both ^{125}I and ^{103}Pd plaque radiation therapy are eye- and vision-sparing alternatives to enucleation. The use of plaque therapy has resulted in complications, which often require subsequent treatment. Most irradiated patients have maintained useful vision as well as the cosmetic use of their eye.

References

Alberti W, Pothmann B, Tabor P, Muskalla K, Hermann KP, Harder D (1991) Dosimetry and physical treatment planning for iodine eye plaque therapy. Int J Radiat Oncol Biol Phys 20:1087–1092

Amendola BE, Markoe AM, Augsburger JI, Karlsson UL, Giblin M, Shields JA, Brady LW, Woodleigh R (1989) Analysis of treatment results in 36 children with retinoblastoma treated by scleral plaque irradiation. Int J Radiat Oncol Biol Phys 17:63–70

Bosworth JL, Packer S, Rotman M, Ho T, Finger PT (1988) Choroidal melanoma: I-125 plaque therapy. Radiology 169:249–251

Chiu-Tsao ST, Anderson LL (1991) Thermoluminescent dosmietry for ^{103}Pd seeds (model 200) in solid water phantom. Med Phys 18:449–452

Diener-West M, Earle JD, Fine SL, Hawkins BS, Moy CS, Reynolds SM, Schachat AP, Straatsma BR (2001) The COMS randomized trial of iodine 125 brachytherapy for choroidal melanoma. II. Characteristics of patients enrolled and not enrolled. COMS report no 17. Arch Ophthalmol 119:951–965

Diener-West M, Earle JD, Fine SL, Hawkins BS, Moy CS, Reynolds SM, Schachat AP, Straatsma BR (2001) The COMS randomized trial of iodine 125 brachytherapy for choroidal melanoma. III. Initial mortality findings. COMS report no 18. Arch Ophthalmol 119:969–982

Finger PT (1992) Microwave plaque thermoradiotherapy for choroidal melanoma. Br J Ophthalmol 76:358–364

Finger PT (1997a) Radiation therapy for choroidal melanoma. Surv Ophthalmol 42:215–232

Finger PT (1997b) Microwave thermoradiotherapy for uveal melanoma: results of a 10-year study. Ophthalmology 104:1794–1803

Finger PT (2000a) Intraoperative echographic localization of iodine-125 episcleral plaque for brachytherapy of choroidal melanoma. Am J Ophthalmol 130:539–540

Finger PT (2000b) Tumour location affects the incidence of cataract and retinopathy after ophthalmic plaque radiation therapy. Br J Ophthalmol 84:1068–1070

Finger PT (2001) Plaque radiation therapy for malignant melanoma of the Iris and Ciliary body. Am J Ophthalmol 132:328–335

Finger PT, Murphree AL (2001) Ophthalmic brachytherapy: treatment of choroidal melanoma and retinoblastoma. In: Peyman M, Meffert SA, Conway MD, Chou F (eds) Vitreoretinal surgical techniques. Dunitz, London, pp 403–418

Finger PT, Packer S (1993) Plaque radiotherapy of retinoblastoma. Ophthalmology 100:1277–1278

Finger PT, Packer S, Svitra PP, Paglione RW, Chess J, Albert DM (1984) Hyperthermic treatment of intraocular tumors. Arch Ophthalmol 102:1477–1481

Finger PT, Packer S, Svitra PP, Paglione RW, Anderson LL, Kim JH, Jacobiec FA (1985) Thermoradiotherapy for intraocular tumors. Arch Ophthalmol 103:1574–1578

Finger PT, Packer S, Paglione RW, Gatz JF, Ho TK, Bosworth JL (1989) Thermoradiotherapy of choroidal melanoma. Clinical experience. Ophthalmology 96:1384–1388

Finger PT, Ho TK, Fastenberg DM, Hyman RA, Stroh EM, Packer S, Perry HD (1990) Intraocular radiation blocking. Invest Ophthalmol Vis Sci 31:1724–1730

Finger PT, Moshfeghi DM, Ho TK (1991) Palladium 103 ophthalmic plaque radiotherapy. Arch Ophthalmol 109:1610–1613

Finger PT, Lu D, Buffa A, DeBlasio DS, Bosworth JL (1993) Palladium-103 versus iodine-125 for ophthalmic plaque radiotherapy. Int J Radiat Oncol Biol Phys 27:849–854

Finger PT, Buffa A, Mishra S, Berson A, Bosworth JL, Vikram B

(1994) Palladium 103 plaque radiotherapy for uveal melanoma. Clinical experience. Ophthalmology 101:256–263

Finger PT, Romero JM, Rosen RB, Iezzi R, Emery R, Berson A (1998) Three-dimensional ultrasonography of choroidal melanoma: localization of radioactive eye plaques. Arch Ophthalmol 116:305–312

Finger PT, Iezzi R, Estevo ML, Szechter A, Rosen RB, Berson A (1999a) Diode-light transillumination for ophthalmic plaque localization around juxtapapillary choroidal melanomas. Int J Radiat Oncol Biol Phys 44:887–890

Finger PT, Iezzi R, Romero JM, Rosen RB, Szechter A, Hegde H (1999b) Plaque-mounted diode-light transillumination for localization around intraocular tumors. Arch Ophthalmol 117:179–183

Finger PT, Berson A, Szechter A (1999c) Palladium-103 plaque radiotherapy for choroidal melanoma: results of a 7-year study. Ophthalmology, 106:606–613

Fontanesi J, Meyer D, Xu S, Tai D (1993) Treatment of choroidal melanoma with I-125 plaque. Int J Radiat Oncol Biol Phys 26:619–623

Giblin M (1988) Iodine-125 plaque radiation therapy for choroidal melanoma. In: Proceedings of the annual scientific meeting of the Royal Australian College of Ophthalmology

Gunduz K, Shields CL, Shields JA, Cater J, Freire JE, Brady LW (1999) Radiation retinopathy following plaque radiotherapy for posterior uveal melanoma. Arch Ophthalmol 117:609–614

Harbour JW, Murray TG, Byrne SF, Hughes JR, Gendron EK, Ehlies FJ, Markoe AM (1996) Intraoperative echographic localization of iodine 125 episcleral radioactive plaques for posterior uveal melanoma. Retina 16:129–134

Hernandez JC, Brady LW, Shields CL, Shields JA, DePotter P (1993) Conservative treatment of retinoblastoma. The use of plaque brachytherapy. Am J Clin Oncol 16:397–401

Kiratli H, Bilgic S, Atahan IL (1998) Plaque radiotherapy in the management of retinoblastoma. Turk J Pediatr 40:393–397

Kreissig I, Rose D, Jost B (1993) Long-term follow-up of iodine-125 brachytherapy for choroidal melanomas, part I. Anatomical results and life expectancy. Eur J Ophthalmol 3:121–126

Lagendijk JJ (1982) A microwave heating technique for the hyperthermic treatment of tumours in the eye, especially retinoblastoma. Phys Med Biol 27:1313–1324

Laube T, Fluhs D, Kessler C, En Fisica L, Bornfeld N (2000) Determination of surgeon's absorbed dose in iodine 125 and ruthenium 106 ophthalmic plaque surgery. Ophthalmology, 107:366–368; discussion 368–369

Liggett PE, Ma C, Astrahan M, Pince KJ, Green R, McDonnell J, Petrovich Z (1991) Combined localized current field hyperthermia and irradiation for intraocular tumors. Ophthalmology 98:1830–1835; discussion 1836

Lommatzsch PK (1970) Employment of beta-rays with 106Ru-106Rh applicators in the therapy of retinoblastoma. Klin Monatsbl Augenheilkd 156:662–669

Lommatzsch PK (1986) Results after beta-irradiation (106Ru/106Rh) of choroidal melanomas: 20 years' experience. Br J Ophthalmol 70:844–851

Lommatzsch PK, Lommatzsch R (1991) Treatment of juxtapapillary melanomas. Br J Ophthalmol 75:715–717

Lommatzsch PK, Werner W (1975) Radiation-induced sarcoma 12 years after high dosage x-ray treatment of a bilateral retinoblastoma. Ophthalmologica 171:109–118

Lommatzsch PK, Weise B, Ballin R (1986) Optimization of irradiation time in the treatment of malignant melanoma of the choroid with beta applicators (106Ru/106Rh). Klin Monatsbl Augenheilkd 189:133–140

Lommatzsch PK, Werschnik C, Schuster E (2000) Long-term follow-up of Ru-106/Rh-106 brachytherapy for posterior uveal melanoma. Graefes Arch Clin Exp Ophthalmol 238:129–137

Luxton G, Astrahan MA, Liggett PE, Neblett DL, Cohen DM, Petrovicn Z (1988) Dosimetric calculations and measurements of gold plaque ophthalmic irradiators using iridium-192 and iodine-125 seeds. Int J Radiat Oncol Biol Phys 15:167–176

Mameghan H, Karolis C, Fisher R, Mameghan J, Billson FA, Donaldson EJ, Giblin ME, Hunyor AB (1992) Iodine-125 irradiation of choroidal melanoma: clinical experience from the Prince of Wales and Sydney Eye Hospitals. Aust Radiol 36:249–252

Moshfeghi DM, Moshfeghi AA, Finger PT (2000) Enucleation. Surv Ophthalmol 44:277–301

Murphree AL, Villablanca JG, Deegan WF 3rd, Sato JK, Mallogolowkin M, Fisher A, Parker R, Reed E, Gomer CJ (1996) Chemotherapy plus local treatment in the management of intraocular retinoblastoma. Arch Ophthalmol 114:1348–1356

Myers CA, Abramson DH (1988) Radiation protection. Choroidal melanoma and iodine-125 plaques. J Ophthalmic Nurs Technol 7:103–107

Packer S, Rotman M (1980) Radiotherapy of choroidal melanoma with iodine 125. Int Ophthalmol Clin 20:135–142

Packer S, Stoller S, Lesser ML, Mandel FS, Finger PT (1992) Long-term results of iodine 125 irradiation of uveal melanoma. Ophthalmology 99:767–773; discussion 774

Reminick LR, Finger PT, Ritch R, Weiss S, Ishikawa H (1998) Ultrasound biomicroscopy in the diagnosis and management of anterior segment tumors. J Am Optom Assoc 69:575–582

Robertson DM, Fountain KS, Anderson JA, Posthumus GW (1981) Radioactive iodine-125 as a therapeutic radiation source for management of intraocular tumors. Trans Am Ophthalmol Soc 79:294–306

Robertson DM, Earle J, Anderson JA (1983) Preliminary observations regarding the use of iodine-125 in the management of choroidal melanoma. Trans Ophthalmol Soc UK 103:155–160

Robertson DM, Fuller DG, Anderson RE (1987) A technique for accurate placement of episcleral iodine-125 plaques. Am J Ophthalmol 103:63–65

Shields CL, Shields JA, DePotter P, Hernandez C, Brady LW (1993) Plaque radiotherapy for retinoblastoma. Int Ophthalmol Clin 33:107–118

Shields CL, Shields JA, DePotter P, Singh AD, Hernandez C, Brady LW (1995) Treatment of non-resectable malignant iris tumours with custom designed plaque radiotherapy. Br J Ophthalmol 79:306–312

Stannard C, Sealy R, Shackleton D, Hill J, Korrubel J (1987) The use of iodine-125 plaques in the treatment of retinoblastoma. Ophthalmic Paediatr Genet 8:89–93

Wilson MW, Czechonska G, Finger PT, Rausen A, Hooper ME, Haik BG (2001) Chemotherapy for eye cancer. Surv Ophthalmol 45:416–444

Wu A, Krasin F (1990) Film dosimetry analyses on the effect of gold shielding for iodine-125 eye plaque therapy for choroidal melanoma. Med Phys 17:843–846

7 Particle Treatment of the Eye

J. E. MUNZENRIDER

CONTENTS

7.1
Introduction

The most common primary adult ocular tumor is uveal melanoma, with approximately 1,500 new cases being diagnosed annually in the United States. Approximately equal proportions of males and females are affected. These melanomas are much less common than cutaneous melanomas, and occur infrequently in blacks. For most of the twentieth century, enucleation was the standard treatment, providing both effective treatment and an accurate histologic diagnosis. However, immediate blindness was the price paid for these benefits.

J.E. MUNZENRIDER, MD
Department of Radiation Oncology, Massachusetts General Hospital, Harvard University Medical School, Cox Building, Room 341, Boston, MA 02114, USA

Current noninvasive diagnostic techniques (indirect ophthalmoscopy, fundus photography, fluorescein angiography, and ultrasonography) have sufficiently high diagnostic accuracy that treatment decisions can routinely be based on clinical evaluation only. In a multi-institutional study, 1,532 eyes with a clinical diagnosis of choroidal melanoma were enucleated, and histology was independently reviewed by three independent ophthalmic pathologists. Diagnosis of melanoma was confirmed in 99.7% (1,527 eyes). Metastatic adenocarcinoma was present in four of the five patients with a false positive clinical diagnosis, and hemangioma was diagnosed in the fifth (THE COLLABORATIVE OCULAR MELANOMA STUDY GROUP 1990). A recent analysis of tumor location with respect to retinal topography and light dose distribution on the retinal sphere studied 420 Massachusetts residents with uveal melanomas diagnosed between 1984 and 1993. Analysis of fundus drawings and/or photographs suggested that tumor initiation occurred nonuniformly: tumors decreased monotonically with distance from the macula to the ciliary body, and were concentrated in the macular area. Pattern of tumor distribution correlated positively with the solar light distribution on the retina (LI et al. 2000). Sunlight exposure to the retina, determined in an epidemiological case-control study, has been implicated in the development of uveal melanomas (SEDDON et al. 1990b), although that suggestion has been questioned (DOLIN et al. 1994). A recent review has discussed the natural history of uveal melanomas, as well as their possible causes and treatment (ALBERT 1997).

7.2
Techniques for Eye Conservation

The potential for conservative treatment of uveal melanomas was first demonstrated by STALLARD and associates, who reported eye preservation in almost two-thirds of surviving patients treated with episcleral cobalt-60 plaque brachytherapy (STALLARD 1966). During the latter decades of the twentieth century, clinicians treating patients with ocular tumors generally accepted conservation treatment of the eye. Radiotherapy has been most commonly employed, using either external beam charged particle therapy, primarily with proton beams (BONNET et al. 1993; BROVKINA and ZARUBEI 1986; CASTRO et al. 1997, 1998; CHAR et al. 1998; DAFTARI et al. 1997; DESJARDINS et al. 1997; EGGER et al. 2001; GRAGOUDAS et al. 1987; SLATER et al. 1992; TSUNEMOTO et al. 1987; WILSON and HUNGERFORD 1999; ZOGRAFOS et al. 1990), or brachytherapy with episcleral radionuclide plaques (AUGSBURGER et al. 1999; FINGER et al. 1999; GARRETSON et al. 1997; GUNDUZ et al. 1999a, b; LOMMATZSCH et al. 2000; MARKOE et al. 1985; ROTMAN et al. 1997; STALLARD 1966; WILSON and HUNGERFORD 1999). Other treatment modalities have been employed in selected patients, including transpupillary thermotherapy (OOSTERHUIS et al. 1998; SHIELDS et al. 1998), internal resection (DAMATO et al. 1998; KERTES et al. 1998), microwave thermotherapy (FINGER 1997), stereotactic radiosurgery (LEUNG et al. 1999), and stereotactic radiotherapy (DIECKMANN et al. 2001; TOKUUYE et al. 1997).

The most commonly employed radiation modalities, proton therapy or plaque brachytherapy, are advantageous for treating ocular tumors because of the highly conformal dose that each can deliver. Choice of which radiation modality to employ is determined by the physical dose distribution characteristics of that modality, the size and location of the tumor to be treated, and the local availability of the treatment. The proton beam delivers a homogeneous dose to the tumor, while dose to the tumor base with a radionuclide plaque may be significantly greater than dose to the tumor apex, especially for taller tumors. The homogeneity of the proton beam may be advantageous for tumors abutting or involving the optic disc or the macula, because of the dose gradient from the tumor base to its apex seen with the plaque technique. The proton beam conforms the dose to an irregularly shaped tumor more readily than can the standard plaques. Proton beams deliver almost full dose to normal tissues in the entrance path of the beam; radiation dose from the plaque to normal structures in the forward direction from the tumor decreases relatively rapidly with increasing distance from the plaque. The proton beam dose to tissues in the distal path of the beam falls off rapidly; with currently employed plaques, there is little or no dose to tissues

behind the plaque. Proton beams can treat tumors of any size located anywhere within the eye. Adequate plaque placement may be difficult with posterior tumors due to both scleral accessibility because of the narrowing of the orbit posteriorly, and the anatomic difficulty presented by the optic nerve exiting the eye in patients with peripapillary tumors. Other factors may also influence the choice of treatment modality, such as the experience and expertise of the ophthalmologists and radiation oncologists with one modality or the other, and the geographic availability of the proton beam facility.

In summary, both radiation modalities offer advantages for treating eye tumors, by allowing the prescribed radiation dose to be conformed to the tumor, and the potential for relative sparing of uninvolved ocular and orbital structures. This chapter will discuss proton planning and treatment techniques for uveal melanomas, and treatment results with that modality.

7.3
Charged Particle Conservation Treatment

More precise focusing of the radiation dose in the target can be achieved with charged particle beams than with X-ray beams. This ability to better spare noninvolved ocular and orbital structures makes charged particle beams ideal for treating ocular tumors. Charged particle beams were first used to treat uveal melanomas over a quarter of a century ago, in what continues to be a most fruitful collaborative effort between the Radiation Oncology Department of Massachusetts General Hospital (MGH) and the Retina Service of the Massachusetts Eye and Ear Infirmary (MEEI). Patients were treated at the Harvard Cyclotron Laboratory (HCL) in Cambridge from 1975 through February, 2002. The program has continued at the MGH Northeast Proton Therapy Center since April 1, 2002. A similar collaboration was established between the Radiation Oncology Department and the Ocular Oncology Unit of the University of California-San Francisco (UCSF), and the Lawrence Berkeley Laboratory (LBL), using helium ions (CASTRO et al. 1997, 1998; CHAR et al. 1998). That program ended in 1992, when the accelerator at LBL was shut down. The UCSF group currently collaborates with the Douglas Cyclotron at the University of California-Davis in treating uveal melanomas with protons (DAFTARI et al. 1997). Proton beam therapy for uveal melanomas is also available in the former USSR (BROVKINA and ZARUBEI 1986), at Clatterbridge, UK (BONNET et al. 1993), at the Paul Scherrer Institute (PSI, formerly the Swiss Institute for Nuclear Research, SIN) in Villigen, Switzerland (EGGER et al. 2001; ZOGRAFOS et al. 1990), at the Gustav Werner Institute in Upsala, Sweden, in Brussels, Belgium, in both Nice and Orsay, France (DESJARDINS et al. 1997), in Chiba in Japan (TSUNEMOTO et al. 1987), at TRIUMF in Vancouver, BC, and at Loma Linda University in California (SLATER et al. 1992).

Well in excess of 10,000 patients have been treated with charged particle radiation throughout the world (SISTERSON 2000), using techniques and doses similar to those developed by the MGH-MEEI-HCL group. Preclinical studies, clinical indications, planning and treatment techniques, current treatment protocols, and treatment outcomes in the MGH-HCL uveal melanoma patients will be discussed below. Selected references regarding treatment outcomes at other particle therapy centers and with radionuclide plaque therapy will also be presented.

7.3.1
Preclinical Studies

Ocular tumor treatments were simulated by delivering single proton doses of 50–100 Gy through 7- or 10-mm-diameter apertures to normal monkey eyes. Within 20 h after irradiation, areas of edematous retina and choroid developed in the treated eyes, while outside the irradiated area the retina and choroid remained entirely normal (CONSTABLE et al. 1975). A marked effect of fractionation was demonstrated: 125 Gy in five fractions produced the same effect at 24 h and at 1 year as 30 Gy in a single pulse (CONSTABLE et al. 1976). Chorioretinal changes persisted within the irradiated area at 42–51 months, while normal retinal architecture was preserved immediately outside the discrete retinal scar produced by the proton beam (GRAGOUDAS et al. 1979).

7.3.2
Clinical Studies

Through February 2002, 2,971 uveal melanoma patients had been treated in the MGH-HCL-MEEI program; 1,405 (49.9%) were males, and 1,410 (50.1%), females. Patients ranged in age from 13 to 92

years (mean 58 years); 9 (0.3%) were £18 years of age. Using the Collaborative Ocular Melanoma Study (COMS) size categories (THE COLLABORATIVE OCULAR MELANOMA STUDY GROUP 1990), approximately 20% had small, 50% medium, and 30% large tumors.

7.3.3
Planning and Treatment Techniques

Treatment planning for all patients was performed with a program developed at MGH (GOITEIN and MILLER 1983). Input data for the planning program include axial eye length and tumor height as determined from A- and B-mode ultrasonography, tumor drawings by the ophthalmologist, and fundus photography. The tumor base is drawn manually on the computer screen, depicting the tumor as shown on sketches drawn by the ophthalmologist and/or fundus photographs. Most uveal melanoma patients undergo surgical tumor localization (GOITEIN and MILLER 1983; GRAGOUDAS et al. 1977, 1980), at which time the base of the tumor, as defined by transillumination and/or scleral depression and indirect ophthalmoscopy, is outlined on the sclera by suturing 2-mm-diameter tantalum rings (T-rings) to the sclera around the perimeter of the tumor. Orthogonal radiographs of the eye in the treatment position are taken on the second or third day after surgery. T-ring position for planning is determined from measurements of ring position made during surgery, and from simulation radiographs taken on the second or third day after surgery. A transparency with appropriate magnification shows the desired clip position when the eye is positioned at the angle chosen for treatment, and can be overlaid on a radiograph taken in the treatment position at treatment set-up. A transparency of the light field projection of the proton beam through the treatment aperture onto the front of the eye is also used as a final check on patient alignment. Anterior ciliary body or iris tumors, and other ocular lesions such as angiomas, hemangiomas, and choroidal metastases, can be planned for treatment with a light field set-up only. In those cases, tumor location is determined by transillumination of anterior melanomas, or from fundus photography in patients with other lesions. Dose volume histograms for the globe, lens, ciliary body, retina, macula, and disc are also routinely made available. An individualized brass aperture is fabricated for each patient by a computer-controlled milling machine to specifications defined by the planning program. Treatment portals are relatively small, ranging from 10 to 35 mm in diameter. Tissue compensators have not been used for the ocular treatments in the MGH-MEEI program.

Treatment is given in the seated position, with the patient's head immobilized with an individually molded face mask and bite block. Eye position for treatment is established and maintained by voluntary patient fixation on a light positioned to define the prescribed fixation angle. That angle is chosen so that the beam enters the eye to the extent possible through the sclera, reducing or eliminating direct irradiation of the cornea, anterior chamber, and lens. Eye position for treatment in patients who have had clips placed for tumor localization is determined radiographically, and verified by visualization of the light field as projected through the treatment aperture onto the front of the eye. A light field set-up only, with projection of a light through the aperture onto the front of the eye, is used for patients who have not undergone surgical localization. Irradiation of the eyelid is reduced or eliminated by lid retraction. Treatment set-up is routinely accomplished in 5–10 min, with irradiation times being 1–2 min. During treatment, eye position is monitored by a video camera. Mean movement during treatment was 0.5±0.3 mm, as determined during 41 treatments in 11 patients; maximum movement was 1.2 mm (VERHEY et al. 1982).

7.3.4
Dose and Follow-up

The standard dose, 70 CGE (cobalt Gy equivalents, CGE = proton Gy times RBE 1) (MILLER 1995; URANO et al. 1984; YASHKIN et al. 1995), was given to 94% of patients. Ninety-nine percent received five fractions, and 94% completed treatment in 7–9 days. Patients have generally been seen at MEEI or by the referring ophthalmologist 6 weeks after completion of treatment, every 3 months during the first year, and on a semiannual or annual schedule thereafter.

7.3.5
Treatment Outcome: Local Control and Survival

Local tumor control, defined as absence of increase in height on serial ultrasonography, or lateral growth seen on ophthalmoscopy or fundus photography, was achieved in 96.3%±1.5% and 95.4%±3.3% at 60 and 84 months: 236 and 82 patients were available for

follow-up at those intervals. Two failures were noted after 48 months. In ten of 12 patients, tumors recurred at the margin of the irradiated volume, with the other two patients having recurrence in the full dose (70 CGE) volume (MUNZENRIDER et al. 1989).

Survival at 5 years after proton beam treatment has been approximately 80% (GRAGOUDAS et al. 1986, 1988). This is at least as good as observed survival rates in patients treated primarily with enucleation, as determined by survival comparisons made between 556 proton-treated patients and two groups treated with enucleation. Two hundred thirty-eight patients were enucleated during the same 10-year period that the proton treatments were being given (July 1975 to December 1984), and 275 patients had been enucleated during the preceding decade (January 1965 to June 1975). Kaplan-Meier survival rates at 5 years were estimated to be 81%±2%, 68%±3%, and 74%±3% for irradiated patients, patients enucleated in the later period, and those enucleated in the earlier period, respectively. Estimated survival rates at 10 years were 63%±5%, 53%±4%, and 50%±3%, respectively. Median follow-up time for the three patient groups was 5.3, 8.8, and 17.0 years, respectively (SEDDON et al. 1985). Significant prognostic factors previously defined for both irradiated (GRAGOUDAS et al. 1986) and enucleated (SEDDON et al. 1983a) patients were used to classify patients in each treatment group. Lower risk patients were younger and had relatively small posterior tumors, while higher risk patients were older and had larger tumors involving the ciliary body. Intermediate risk patients had tumors extending anterior to the equator which did not involve the ciliary body, and were intermediate in terms of both tumor size and age. In each risk category, estimated survival probabilities were better for proton-treated patients than for either enucleated group. This study also demonstrated that patients receiving conservation therapy with protons did not have a worse outcome in terms of survival than those undergoing enucleation (SEDDON et al. 1990a). A retrospective study was similarly structured to compare survival in 103 enucleated patients with that in 345 patients receiving conservation therapy with isotope plaque brachytherapy. Results were similar to those obtained when comparing proton therapy with enucleation: there was no survival disadvantage for the irradiated patients. At 15 years, metastasis-free survival rates were 57.1% (SE 6.4%) and 61.8% (SE 3.3%) for the enucleated and the plaque-treated patients, respectively (AUGSBURGER et al. 1999).

7.3.6
Eye Retention and Survival

Probability of eye retention was found to depend largely on tumor size, with an estimated 97%, 93%, and 78% of patients with small, intermediate, and large tumors, respectively, retaining the eye at 5 years. Eye loss probability was significantly greater in patients with large tumors (tumor height >8 mm, tumor diameter >16 mm) and those with ciliary body tumor involvement (P=<0.0001 for all factors). Independent risk factors associated with greater likelihood of eye loss by multivariate analysis were ciliary body involvement, tumor height >8 mm, and distance between the posterior tumor edge and the fovea. Patients with the greatest risk of eye loss were those with two or more risk factors (238 patients). Eye loss risk was intermediate for those with one risk factor (569 patients), and least for patients with none of the risk factors (213 patients). Eye retention rates at 5 years were 99%±1% and 92%±2% for the low and intermediate risk groups, respectively. Only 76%±7% of patients in the highest risk group retained the eye at 5 years (EGAN et al. 1989). Pathological changes have been described in eyes enucleated after proton therapy (KINCAID et al. 1988; SEDDON et al. 1983b; ZINN et al. 1981).

The probability of eye retention at 10 years was 89%±2%, in 1,541 patients with a median follow-up of 8 years. In patients losing the eye after proton treatment, a relationship has been documented between the reason for enucleation and death from metastatic disease. Thirty-four patients enucleated for tumor growth were almost 4 times as likely to die from metastasis as were 103 patients in whom the eye was removed because of treatment complications (rate ratios 3.8 vs 0.9, 95% confidence limits 2.3–6.3 and 0.6–1.4, respectively) (EGAN et al. 1998).

7.3.7
Treatment-Related Morbidity and Visual Function

Visual acuity is unchanged or improved in more than 50% of treated eyes. Visual loss after treatment in patients with useful vision (visual acuity 20/200 or better) before treatment can be attributed to cataract progression, retinal detachment, and radiation retinopathy. Visual prognosis is significantly associated both with preexisting factors and with radiation dose. Preexisting factors significantly related to posttreatment visual acuity include initial visual acuity, tumor height, distance from the posterior tumor margin to the optic disc and/or fovea, and presence of a pretreatment retinal detachment involving the macula. Posttreatment vision is also related to radiation dose to the optic disc, fovea, and lens (SEDDON et al. 1986). Useful vision was preserved in 67% of 199 patients with posterior tumor edge >3 mm from both the optic disc and the fovea; 91% of that group received <35 CGE to those structures. In contrast, useful vision was preserved in only 39% of 363 patients with tumor edge ≤3 mm from the optic disc and/or fovea; 83% of that group received >35 CGE to either or both of those structures (SEDDON et al. 1987).

The only acute reaction was moist eyelid desquamation, which occurred in patients whose lids could not be completely retracted from the irradiation field. The lid segment involved was relatively small, typically ranging in size from 2–5 mm by 8–15 mm. This acute reaction heals in 4–6 weeks, and is followed by permanent eyelash loss, late eyelid atrophy, and scarring within the desquamated area.

Late radiation injury to anterior ocular structures includes rubeosis iridis with neovascular glaucoma and cataract formation. Vision can be preserved or restored in some patients developing these complications. Lens changes after proton therapy were studied in 388 patients with clear lenses initially. Posterior subcapsular opacities (PSC) developed in 42% within 3 years of treatment, with the probability of PSC formation being related to lens dose, tumor height, and older age (GRAGOUDAS et al. 1992). Lens opacities were present in 494 of the 1,171 patients (42%) treated through December 1987. Eighty-four such patients underwent cataract extraction between 2 months and 11 years after treatment. One year after surgery, approximately one-half of those patients had visual acuity 20/100 or better; in one-third of patients, it was 20/40 or better. Less good visual outcome after cataract extraction was highly correlated with larger tumor size. Enucleation was ultimately performed in six patients: in one patient because of a "ring melanoma" diagnosed after surgery, and in five owing to the development of painful blind eyes following surgery (GRAGOUDAS et al. 1995).

Significant visual loss can result from radiation-induced macular edema, maculopathy, papillopathy, and optic atrophy. Generally similar complication patterns are seen in radionuclide plaque-treated patients (GUNDUZ et al. 1999a, b). Few if any treatment options exist for patients with late radiation injury to posterior ocular structures, although focal laser therapy may be beneficial in the short term for some patients (HYKIN et al. 1998).

7.4
Clinical Trials

7.4.1
Dose-Searching Trial to Decrease Radiation Morbidity

A prospective randomized dose de-escalation trial was conducted between October 1989 and July 1994, in an attempt to reduce visual morbidity in patients at high risk of experiencing significant visual loss with the standard dose of 70 CGE. Patients studied had tumors ≤15 mm in greatest diameter and ≤5 mm in height, which were located within 6 mm of the optic disc and/or fovea. One hundred eighty-eight patients meeting the study criteria were randomly assigned to receive either the standard dose of 70 CGE or the experimental dose of 50 CGE. Both dose groups received five fractions over 7–9 days. The trial was planned with the expectation that most patients would be available for follow-up, since patients chosen for the study had prognostically favorable characteristics which predicted a relatively low risk of death from metastasis, or of eye loss due to radiation complications. Visual loss, retinopathy, and local control were the end points for the trial.

Baseline median visual acuity was 20/32 for both groups. The control group had a larger proportion of male patients (63% vs 44%, $P=0.04$), a smaller average largest tumor diameter (10 mm vs 11 mm, $P=0.03$), and a smaller proportion of patients with tumor extending anterior to the equator (6% vs 16%, $P=0.04$). The average dose to the optic disc and the macula was 31.2 and 45 CGE, respectively, for the 50-CGE group, and 42 and 67.9 CGE, respectively, for the 70-CGE group.

A progressive decline in median visual acuity was observed in both groups at each annual follow-up interval from 12 to 48 months, from a baseline value of 20/32 to 20/100 at 48 months. Median acuity at 60 months declined further, to 20/160 for the 50-CGE group, but remained stable at 20/100 for the higher dose group. Approximately 55% of patients in both groups had visual acuity of 20/200 or better at 5 years ($P=0.81$). Similar radiation maculopathy rates were seen in each dose group, occurring in approximately 75% of patients with tumors ≤1.5 mm from the macula and in 40% of patients with tumors ≥1.5 mm from the macula, respectively. A nonsignificant decrease in radiation papillopathy rates was observed in the lower dose group ($P=0.20$). A significantly less visual field deficit did occur in patients receiving the lower dose. Local recurrence occurred in two and three patients, and metastasis in seven and eight patients at the lower and higher dose levels, respectively ($P>0.99$ and 0.79, for the two comparisons). Four and five patients in the lower and higher dose groups, respectively, underwent enucleation for radiation complications following treatment. Other radiation complications were not significantly different in the two groups. Declines in mean tumor heights were similar for both dose groups, from initial values of 3.05 and 3.04 mm to 1.59 and 1.54 mm at 60 months for the lower and higher dose groups, respectively (GRAGOUDAS et al. 2000).

The somewhat disappointing finding that a 30% reduction in dose was not associated with a greater degree of visual preservation indicated that even the lower dose (50 CGE) given in five fractions over 7–9 days exceeded the radiation tolerance of the macula. However, a lesser degree of visual field loss and possibly a decrease in the rate of radiation papillopathy with the lower dose did suggest some visual benefit for the lower radiation dose. Since local tumor failure rates were not increased by the significantly lower dose employed, justification exists for further dose de-escalation, in another attempt to reduce visual morbidity. Such a study must be undertaken with great care, since further dose reductions could result in increased local failure rates, which might lead to greater rates of eye loss and possibly to increased rates of distant failure. We are currently planning to investigate an altered fractionation program in this patient population, in which the study group would receive a smaller radiation dose per fraction and a larger number of treatment fractions. This approach might reduce the biologic dose delivered to normal ocular structures because of the smaller dose per fraction, while still preserving a high degree of local tumor control.

7.4.2
Adjuvant Interferon in Patients at High Risk for Metastasis

Significantly greater median survival and median relapse-free survival rates were demonstrated in cutaneous melanoma patients at high risk for recurrence who were randomized to receive interferon-α-2b (INF), relative to patients randomized to observation only (KIRKWOOD et al. 1996). In a nonrandomized clinical trial done at MEEI, 130 patients with one or more risk factors for metastasis (tumor ≥15mm diameter, ciliary body involvement, and age over 65) have been offered INF following standard dose proton beam radiotherapy. Survival rates in the INF-treated patients will be compared to a historical control group of patients matched for known prognostic factors who were treated with protons only. An interim report on this study is planned for the latter part of 2002.

7.4.3
Particle Beam Therapy vs Radionuclide Plaque Brachytherapy

Uveal melanoma patients with tumors <10 mm in height and <15 mm in diameter were randomized by the LBL-UCSF group to receive either 70 GyE in five treatments with helium ions, or 70 Gy to the tumor apex with iodine-125 episcleral plaque brachytherapy. Local control rates were 100% and 87% with helium ions and with iodine-125 plaque therapy, respectively. Anterior segment complications were more common in particle-treated patients, while enucleation rates were significantly higher in plaque-treated patients (CHAR et al. 1993).

Treatment outcome was compared for patients treated with proton beam therapy (PBRT) and with radionuclide plaque brachytherapy, using two different isotopes in a retrospective study. Patients treated with ruthenium-106 had a significantly greater risk of local recurrence than those treated with either iodine-125 or PBRT (WILSON and HUNGERFORD 1999).

7.5
Discussion and Summary: Indications for Conservation Therapy of Uveal Melanomas

Preservation of the eye can be achieved in uveal melanoma patients with both external beam charged particle (proton) therapy and episcleral radionuclide plaque brachytherapy. Tumor size and location significantly impact upon the probability of visual preservation and of eye retention with either technique. Experience with proton beam therapy has shown that even very large tumors can be treated in patients with poor or absent vision in the fellow eye. The probability of eye salvage approximates 75%–80% in such patients, a portion of whom may preserve some level of visual function in the treated eye.

Local control is achieved in a large proportion of eyes treated with either technique, probably because large radiation doses can safely be delivered to these relatively small tumors with these techniques. Survival clearly has not been compromised in patients treated with radiation (AUGSBURGER et al. 1999; SEDDON et al. 1985, 1990a). Indeed, achieving local control may also contribute to improved survival in some patients (EGAN et al. 1998). Preservation of useful vision can be expected in eyes with tumors occurring in a favorable location with respect to the optic disc and/or macula (GUNDUZ et al. 1999a; SEDDON et al. 1987). At least one dose-searching trial has been completed, in an effort to improve visual outcome in patients with unfavorably located tumors (GRAGOUDAS et al. 2000). Although no improvement in vision was observed in patients receiving a significantly lower dose than the standard dose in that trial, its results are proving useful in planning future trials.

Successful treatment of uveal melanomas with preservation of the involved eye is one of the major oncologic triumphs of the latter part of the twentieth century. Either heavy charged particle external beam radiotherapy or radionuclide plaque brachytherapy can result in high rates of local control and preservation of a functionally useful eye in many patients. The excellent results achieved in uveal melanoma patients treated with external beam proton therapy have also proven that almost all patients can successfully position their tumor for treatment by voluntarily fixating the eye upon a particular point. The conservative treatment techniques have achieved local control rates similar to or superior to those achieved with radiation therapy alone in other commonly treated solid tumors, including early stage carcinomas of the breast, vocal cord, and prostate. Enhanced knowledge of radiation effects on uveal melanomas and on normal ocular structures will result from ongoing careful follow-up of conservatively treated patients.

That these gains have not been achieved at a cost of increased mortality is also impressive: survival rates in irradiated patients are at least as good as after enucleation (SEDDON et al. 1985, 1990a; AUGSBURGER et al. 1999; THE COLLABORATIVE OCULAR MELANOMA STUDY GROUP 2001a). Continuing follow-up observations will reveal whether these initial dramatic and encouraging results will be maintained. THE COLLABORATIVE OCULAR MELANOMA STUDY (COMS) has provided additional data regarding relative survival after enucleation and iodine-125 plaque brachytherapy (THE COLLABORATIVE OCULAR MELANOMA STUDY GROUP 2001a). However, that study does not allow direct comparison of the acute and chronic ocular effects of brachytherapy and charged particle therapy, nor will it clarify indications for use of those different modalities. The UCSF-LBL trial mentioned above, which compared helium ion therapy with iodine-125 plaque treatment has documented the superiority of charged particle therapy over plaque therapy in terms of local tumor control and eye retention, and also contrasted differences in morbidity between the techniques (CHAR et al. 1993). In this regard, it is of interest that a recent survey reported that choice of treatment for uveal melanoma did not seem to be associated with large differences in quality of life, when assessed at long-term follow-up (CRUICKSHANKS et al. 1999).

The morbidity and ultimate death from metastatic disease in uveal melanoma patients, occurring more commonly in older patients with larger and more anteriorly located tumors, are most distressing. Unfortunately, response rates to systemic therapy in patients with metastatic melanoma are poor, and elective treatment of patients at risk for metastases has not been systematically studied. The recent report of improved survival with elective interferon treatment in cutaneous melanoma patients at high risk for metastasis is encouraging (KIRKWOOD et al. 1996), and led to the initiation of the nonrandomized study described above, in which interferon was electively given to patients with increased risk of metastasis following proton eye irradiation. Clearly, clinical trials in this area would be indicated if more effective systemic therapies become available.

References

Albert DM (1997) The ocular melanoma story. LIII Edward Jackson Memorial Lecture. Part II. Am J Ophthalmol 123:729–741

Augsburger JJ, Schneider S, Freire J, et al. (1999) Survival following enucleation versus plaque radiotherapy in statistically matched subgroups of patients with choroidal melanomas: results in patients treated between 1980 and 1987. Graefes Arch Clin Exp Ophthalmol 237:558–567

Bonnet DE, Kacperek A, Sheen MA, et al. (1993) The 62 MeV proton beam for the treatment of ocular melanoma at Clatterbridge. Br J Radiol 66:907–914

Brovkina AF, Zarubei GD (1986) Ciliochoroidal melanomas treated with a narrow medical proton beam. Arch Ophthalmol 104:402–404

Castro JR, Char DH, Petti PL, et al. (1997) 15 years experience with helium ion radiotherapy for uveal melanoma. Int J Radiat Oncol Biol Phys 39:989–996

Castro JR, Petti PL, Blakely EA, et al. (1998) Particle radiation therapy. In: Leibel SA, Phillips TL (eds) Textbook of radiotherapy. Saunders, New York

Char DH, Quivey JM, Castro JR et al. (1993) Helium ions versus iodine-125 brachytherapy in the management of uveal melanoma, a prospective randomized dynamically balanced trial. Ophthalmology 100:1547–1554

Char DH, Kroll SM, Castro JR (1998) Ten-year follow-up of helium ion therapy for uveal melanoma. Am J Ophthalmol 125:81–89

Constable IJ, Koehler AM, Schmidt RA (1975) Proton irradiation of simulated ocular tumors. Investig Ophthalmol 14:547–555

Constable IJ, Goitein M, Koehler AM, et al. (1976) Small field irradiation of monkey eyes with protons and photons. Radiat Res 65:304–314

Cruickshanks KJ, Fryback DG, Nondahl DM, et al. (1999) Treatment choice and quality of life in patients with choroidal melanoma. Arch Ophthalmol 117:461–467

Daftari IK, Char DH, Verhey LJ, et al. (1997) Anterior segment sparing to reduce charged particle radiotherapy complications in uveal melanoma. Int J Radiat Oncol Biol Phys 39:997–1010

Damato B, Groenwald C, McGalliard J, et al. (1998) Endoresection of choroidal melanoma. Br J Ophthalmol 82:213–218

Desjardins L, Levy C, d'Hermies F (1997) Initial results of proton therapy in choroidal melanoma at the d'Orsey Ceter for proton therapy: the first 464 patients. Cancer Radiother 1:222–226

Dieckmann K, Bogner J, Georg D, et al. (2001) A LINAC-based stereotactic irradiation technique of uveal melanoma. Radiother Oncol 61:49–56

Dolin P, Foss A, Hungerford J (1994) Uveal melanoma: is solar UV radiation a risk factor? Ophthalmic Epidemiol 1:27–30

Egan K, Gragoudas ES, Seddon JM, et al. (1989) The risk of enucleation after proton beam irradiation of uveal melanoma. Ophthalmology 96:1377–1383

Egan KM, Ryan LM, Gragoudas ES (1998) Survival implications of enucleation after definitive radiotherapy for choroidal melanoma. An example of regression on time-dependent covariates. Arch Ophthalmol 116:366–370

Egger E, Schalenbourg A, Zografos L, et al. (2001) Maximizing local tumor control and survival after proton beam radiotherapy of uveal melanoma, Int J Radiat Oncol Biol Phys 51:138–147

Ferry AP, Blair, CJ, Gragoudas ES, et al. (1985) Pathologic examination of ciliary body melanoma treated with proton beam irradiation. Arch Ophthalmol 103:1849–1853

Finger PT (1997) Microwave thermoradiotherapy for uveal melanoma: results of a 10-year study. Ophthalmology 104:1794–1803

Finger PT, Berson A, Szechter A (1999) Palladium-103 plaque radiotherapy for choroidal melanoma: results of 7-year study. Ophthalmology 106:606–613

Garretson BR, Robertson DM, Earle JK (1987) Choroidal melanoma treatment with iodine-125 brachytherapy. Arch Ophthalmol 105:1394–1397

Goitein M, Miller T (1983) Planning proton therapy of the eye. Med Phys 10:275–283

Gragoudas ES, Goitein M, Koehler AM, et al. (1977) Proton irradiation of small choroidal malignant melanomas. Am J Ophthalmol 83:655–673

Gragoudas ES, Zakov NZ, Albert DM, et al. (1979) Long term observations of proton-irradiated monkey eyes. Arch Ophthalmol 97:2184–2191

Gragoudas ES, Goitein M, Verhey LJ, et al. (1980) Proton beam irradiation. An alternative to enucleation for intraocular melanoma. Ophthalmology 87:571–581

Gragoudas ES, Seddon JM, Polivogianis LL, et al. (1986) Prognostic factors for metastasis following proton beam irradiation of uveal melanomas. Ophthalmology 93:675–680

Gragoudas ES, Seddon JM, Egan K, et al. (1987) Long-term results of proton beam irradiated uveal melanomas. Arch Ophthalmol 94:349–353

Gragoudas ES, Seddon JM, Egan KM, et al. (1988) Metastasis from uveal melanoma after proton beam irradiation. Ophthalmology 95:992–999

Gragoudas ES, Egan KM, Arrigg PG, et al. (1992) Cataract extraction after proton beam irradiation for malignant melanoma of the eye. Arch Ophthalmol 110: 475–479

Gragoudas ES, Egan KM, Walsh SM, et al. (1995) Lens changes after proton beam irradiation for uveal melanoma. Am J Ophthalmol 119:157–164

Gragoudas ES, Lane AM, Regan S et al. (2000) A randomized controlled trial of varying radiation doses in the treatment of choroidal melanoma. Arch Ophthalmol 118:773–778

Gunduz K, Shields CL, Shields JA, et al. (1999a) Radiation complications and tumor control after plaque radiotherapy of choroidal melanoma with macular involvement. Am J Ophthalmol 127:579–589

Gunduz K, Shields CL, Shields JA, et al. (1999b) Radiation retinopathy following plaque radiotherapy for posterior uveal melanoma. Arch Ophthalmol 117:609–614

Hykin PG, Shields CL, Shields JA, et al. (1998) The efficacy of focal laser therapy in radiation-induced macular edema. Ophthalmology 105:1425–1429

Kertes PJ, Johnson JC, Peyman GA (1998) Internal resection of posterior uveal melanomas. Br J Ophthalmol 82:1147–1153

Kincaid MC, Folberg R, Torczynski E, et al. (1988) Complications after proton beam therapy for uveal malignant melanoma. Ophthalmology 95:982–991

Kirkwood JM, Strawderman MH, Ernstoff MS, et al. (1996) Interferon alpha-2b adjuvant therapy of high risk resected cutaneous melanoma: The Eastern Cooperative Oncology Group Trial EST 1684. J Clin Oncol 14:7–17

Leung SW, Hsiung CY, Chen HC, et al. (1999) Management of choroidal melanomas with linear accelerator-based stereotactic radiosurgery. Acta Ophthalmol 77:62–65

Li W, Judge H, Gragoudas ES, et al. (2000) Patterns of tumor initiation in choroidal melanoma. Cancer Res 60:3757–3760

Lommatzsch PK, Werschnik C, Schuster E (2000) Long-term follow-up of Ru-106/Rh-106 brachytherapy for posterior uveal melanoma. Graefes Arch Clin Exp Ophthalmol 238:129–137

Markoe AM, Brady LW, Shields J, et al. (1985) Radioactive eye plaque therapy versus enucleation for the treatment of posterior uveal malignant melanoma. Radiology 156:801–803

Miller DW (1995) A review of proton beam radiotherapy. Med Phys 22:1943–1954

Munzenrider JE, Verhey L, Gragoudas ES, et al. (1989) Conservative treatment of uveal melanoma: dose distribution to tumors with local recurrence after proton beam therapy. Int J Radiat Oncol Biol Phys 17:493–498

Oosterhuis JA, Journec-de-Korver HG, Keunen JE (1998) Transpupillary thermotherapy: results in 50 patients with choroidal melanoma. Arch Ophthalmol 116:157–162

Rotman M, Long RS, Packer S, et al. (1977) Radiation therapy of uveal melanomas. Trans Ophthalmol Soc UK 97:431–435

Seddon JM, Albert DM, Lavin P, et al. (1983a) A prognostic factor study of disease-free interval and survival following enucleation for uveal melanoma. Arch Ophthalmol 101:1894–1899

Seddon JM, Gragoudas ES, Albert DM (1983b) Ciliary body and choroidal melanomas treated by proton beam irradiation: histopathologic study of eyes. Arch Ophthalmol 101:1402–1408

Seddon JM, Gragoudas ES, Albert DM, et al. (1985) Comparison of survival rates for patients with uveal melanoma after treatment with proton beam irradiation or enucleation. Am J Ophthalmol 99:282–290

Seddon JM, Gragoudas ES, Polivogianis L, et al. (1986) Visual outcome after proton beam irradiation of uveal melanoma. Ophthalmology 93:666–674

Seddon JM, Gragoudas ES, Egan KM, et al. (1987) Uveal melanomas near the optic disc or fovea. Visual results after proton beam irradiation. Ophthalmology 94:354–361

Seddon JM, Gragoudas ES, Egan KM, et al. (1990a) Relative survival rates after alternative therapies for uveal melanoma. Ophthalmology 97:769–777

Seddon JM, Gragoudas ES, Glynn RJ, et al. (1990b) Host factors. UV radiation and risk of uveal melanoma: a case-control study. Arch Ophthalmol 108:1274–1280

Shields CL, Shields JA, Carter J, et al. (1998) Transpupillary thermotherapy for choroidal melanoma: tumor comtrol and visual results in 100 consecutive cases. Ophthalmology 105:581–590

Sisterson J (2000) Ion beam therapy: overview of the world experience. Application of Acdelerators in Research and Industry. Proceedings of the Sixteenth International Conference, Denton, Texas, November 3, 2000

Slater JM, Archambeau JO, Miller DW, et al. (1992) The proton treatment at Loma Linda University Medical Center: rationale for and description of its development. Int J Radiat Oncol Biol Phys 22:383–389

Stallard HB (1966) Malignant melanoblastoma of the choroid. Mod Prob Ophthalmol 7:16–38

The Collaborative Ocular Melanoma Study Group (1990) Accuracy of diagnosis of choroidal melanomas in the Collaborative Ocular Melanoma Study. COMS Report No. 1. Ophthalmology 108:1268–1273

The Collaborative Ocular Melanoma Study (COMS) (2001a) Randomized trial of I-125 brachytherapy for medium choroidal melanoma. III. Initial mortality findings. COMS report no. 18. Arch Ophthalmol 119:969–982

The Collaborative Ocular Melanoma Study (COMS) (2001b) Randomized trial of I-125 brachytherapy for medium choroidal melanoma. I. Visual acuity after 3 years COMS report no. 16. Ophthalmology 108:348–366

Tokuuye K, Akine Y, Sumi M (1997) Fractionated stereotactic radiotherapy for choroidal melanoma. Radiother Oncol 43:87–91

Tsunemoto H, Morita S, Kawachi K, et al. (1987) Clinical results of proton radiotherapy in Japan. Proceedings of the 8th International Cong of Rad Research, Edinburgh, 1987, pp 922–927

Urano M, Goitein M, Verhey LJ, et al. (1984) Relative biological effectiveness of modulated proton beams in various murine tissues. Int J Radiat Oncol Biol Phys 10:509–514

Verhey LJ, Goitein M, Munzenrider JE, et al. (1982) Precise positioning of patients for radiation therapy. Int J Radiat Oncol Biol 8:289–294

Wilson MW, Hungerford JL (1999) Comparison of plaque and proton beam radiation therapy for treatment of choroidal melanoma. Ophthalmology 106:1579–1587

Yashkin PN, Silin DI, Zolotov VA, et al. (1995) Relative biologic effectiveness of proton medical beam at Moscow Synchotron determined by the Chinese hamster cells assay. Int J Radiat Oncol Biol Phys 31:535–540

Zinn KM, Stein/Pokorny K, Jakobiec F, et al. (1981) Proton beam irradiated epithelial cell melanoma of the ciliary body. Ophthalmology 88:1315–1321

Zografos L, Perret C, Egger E, et al. (1990) Proton beam irradiation of uveal melanomas at Paul Scherrer Institute (former SIN). Strahlenther Onkol 166:114

8 Proton Beam Irradiation of Choroidal Melanoma: Technique and Results

E. Egger, L. Zografos, G. Goitein

CONTENTS

8.1 Introduction

Since March, 1984, proton beam radiotherapy (PBRT) has been used at the Paul Scherrer Institute (PSI) in a project being conducted jointly with the University Ophthalmological Hospital in Lausanne (Hôpital Ophtalmique Jules Gonin) for the treatment of patients with ocular tumors. Up to now we have treated over 3,000 patients. Among 2,705 cases treated by the end of 1998, there were 2,435 cases of uveal melanoma, 11 of melanoma of the iris, 50 of recurrence of melanoma (some of which had previously been exposed to brachytherapy with Ru-106 or Co-60 plaques), 77 of choroidal hemangioma, 50 of

E. Egger, PhD; G. Goitein, MD
Division of Radiation Medicine, Paul Scherrer Institute, 5232 Villigen–PSI, Switzerland
L. Zografos, MD
Hôpital Ophtalmique Jules Gonin, Avenue de France 15, 1004 Lausanne, Switzerland

melanoma of the conjunctiva, 32 of intraocular metastases, 34 of age-related macular degeneration, 8 of vascular tumor of the retina, 2 of tumor of the eyelids, and 6 of miscellaneous ocular tumors.

When we introduced PBRT into western Europe in 1984, this technique was regarded as a possible alternative to enucleation for large tumors and tumors located close to the optic disc and/or the macula (Gragoudas et al. 1977, 1980, 1982, 1984). At this time it was debated whether a conservative treatment would increase the risk of metastases over that with enucleation (Seddon et al. 1985).

Meanwhile, the long-term results obtained with proton and helium beam irradiation in terms of patient survival, local tumor control, eye retention, and visual outcome (Castro et al. 1997; Char et al. 1996, 1997, 1998; Egger et al. 1997; Gragoudas et al. 1987; Linstadt et al. 1990; Munzenrider et al. 1988, 1989) have led to wide acceptance of PBRT and resulted in a reduction of the number of patients now treated with enucleation. While in 1985 only 70 uveal melanoma patients underwent PBRT in western Europe, over 700 patients per year are benefiting from this treatment 15 years later. The number of facilities offering PBRT for ocular tumors in Western Europe increased from one center in 1984 to six in 1999. New centers are planned or will begin patient treatment soon.

The aim of this article is to describe the treatment technique and review the 2,435 cases of uveal melanoma. We will present our results in terms of survival, local tumor control, salvage of the eye, radiation-induced complications, and postirradiation visual acuity.

8.2 Treatment Technique

PBRT allows for precise irradiation of the target volume, which requires accurate knowledge of the tumor position. This requirement is satisfied by placing tantalum clips around the tumor and suturing them to the outer sclera to delimit the tumor border. This intervention is performed by an oph-thalmologist and can be compared to positioning an episcleral plaque for brachytherapy. No planning computed tomography (CT) is done, as it would be now for conventional radiotherapy. The precision of the whole treatment depends on the ocular mod-el of the treatment planning software, which starts with the input of the clip coordinates to build a model of the eye and of the tumor. The technique was developed to allow precise irradiation of the tumor without the requirement for CT scans. How-ever, because no image showing both clips and tu-mor simultaneously is created, it is essential to po-sition the clips very close to the tumor and so that they surround the whole of it (not only the part in the anterior part of the eye) to make optimal use of the precision that can be offered by PBRT. The orig-inal technique was developed in Boston in a joint project between the Eye and Ear Infirmary of the Massachusetts General Hospital and the Harvard Cyclotron Laboratory (GRAGOUDAS et al. 1977).

8.2.1
Ophthalmological Workup and Clip Surgery

The ophthalmological workup is performed at the University Eye Clinic in Lausanne. In order to gath-er the precise data on tumor size and location that are necessary to drive the eye and tumor during the treatment planning procedure, the eye length is measured by A-scan ultrasound, the tumor profile is illustrated with B-scan ultrasound pictures, and, if appropriate, wide-angle fundus photographs are taken to show the location of the posterior tumor margin relative to the optic disc and the macula. The best corrected visual acuity of the affected eye and of the fellow eye is recorded, as are the intraoc-ular pressure, the degree of retinal detachment, the presence of ocular melanocytosis, and all other current symptoms. Systemic examinations, includ-ing liver function tests and liver ultrasonography, are performed to exclude the presence of metastas-es. Generally, patients are accepted for PBRT if the tumor thickness is smaller than 15 mm and if the retina is not totally detached. Exceptions are made to these rules when patients refuse enucleation and when the melanoma is in a patient's only functional eye. Patients accepted for PBRT undergo a surgical procedure for the precise demarcation of the tumor margins. Generally under general anesthesia, the base of the tumor is localized by transillumination of the globe and indirect ophthalmoscopy. Depend-

ing on tumor size, shape and location, three to sev-en tantalum clips (diameter 2.5 mm, thickness 0.5 mm) are sutured to the outer surface of the sclera to mark the border of the tumor base as seen from the tumor shadow during the transillumination proce-dure. Normally, patients leave the Eye Clinic 1 day after the clip surgery and travel to the Paul Scherrer Institute (PSI) for the next treatment steps.

8.2.2
Molding and Simulation

At PSI, a customized bite block and a thermoplastic head mask are manufactured for each patient to im-mobilize the head during treatment. Then, before the patient enters the treatment room for a simulation, anesthetic drops are applied to the affected eye. The patient is positioned on the treatment chair, and the head mask is fixed on a frame; the patient fits his face into the mask and his upper jaw onto the bite block (see Fig. 8.1). Once the appropriate sitting position is found, the patient's motion is restricted by applying gentle pressure to the back of the head using a foam pad and drop weight. Upper and lower eyelid retrac-tors are applied. The chair is then rotated and placed in front of the beam line. Then, the tumor eye is cen-

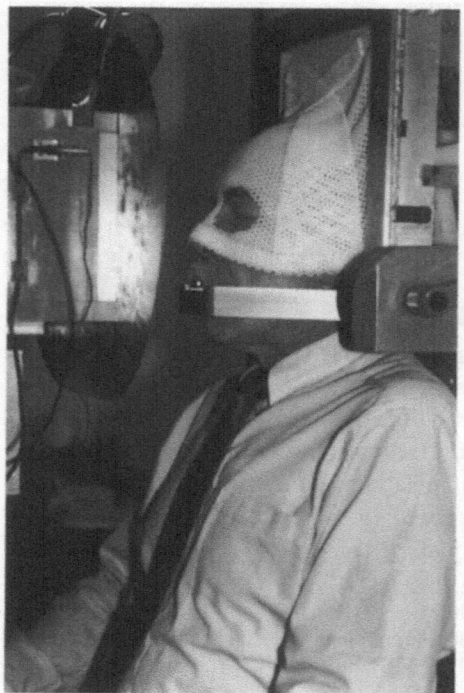

Fig. 8.1. Patient installed in the treatment chair; with the fixa-tion mask, the patient's head movement is restricted. Eyelid retractors are not yet in place

tered in the beam axis. The patient is asked to gaze at a light point appearing at the center of the beam axis with this eye. A pair of orthogonal X-ray pictures (one axial and one lateral) showing the clips in a beam coordinate frame are taken. If the patient is unable to fix the light with the tumor eye, a light is placed at an appropriate position on the coordinate frame surrounding the beam axes (see Fig. 8.2), so that the patient can fix his gaze with the fellow eye. In this case, the distance between the two eyes is measured to allow calculation of the light coordinates for both eyes by the treatment planning software.

Two additional pairs of X-ray pictures are taken, with the patient gazing at a light point placed at two different positions on the coordinate frame. The thickness and the position of the eyelids are measured according to the needs of the treatment planning procedure (SHEEN 1995).

For the rare cases when the patient is unable to fix the positioning light with either the affected eye or the fellow eye, we have developed a suction cup fixation system, which allows mechanical positioning and immobilization of the eye. This system is rarely used, however (approximately once in 300–400 cases).

8.2.3
Treatment Planning

Treatment planning is performed using the EYE-PLAN program developed originally by GOITEIN and MILLER (1983) and modified later by PERRET (1987) and by SHEEN (1995). Starting with the introduction of the clip coordinates as measured on the axial and lateral X-ray simulation pictures, followed by the eye

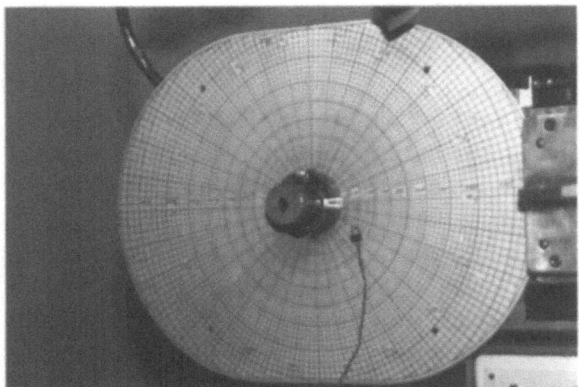

Fig. 8.2. Coordinate frame surrounding the beam line. The light point is placed at 20° (polar coordinate)/210° (azimuthal coordinate). The collimator shaped to the tumor profile of the patient is visible in the center

length measured by ultrasound, the EYEPLAN program builds a two-sphere model of the eye fitted into the coordinates defined by the clips. The eye axis is defined by the coordinates of the light point. The shape of the tumor base as defined by the position of the clips and the fundus photographs is drawn into this eye model, as is the tumor profile provided by the B-scan ultrasound. The treatment planning program calculates an eye fundus view, which can be compared with the eye fundus pictures in which the position of the posterior tumor border relative to the optic disc and the macula can be verified. In case of discrepancies between model and reality, the position of the model tumor has to be adjusted to coincide with the fundus picture. Such adjustments are required especially in cases of myopic and hypermetropic eyes. After construction of an adequate model of the eye and tumor, an optimal treatment position is determined, i.e. a position allowing irradiation of the tumor surrounded by a safety margin while minimizing irradiation to the optic disc and nerve, macula, ciliary body, and lens in declining order of priority. The penetration depth of the proton beam, the required width of the spread out Bragg peak (SOBP), and the shape of the aperture corresponding to the tumor shape in the treatment position surrounded by a safety margin (usually 2 mm) are also determined using the EYEPLAN program. The beam range is usually selected to place the 90% isodose of the distal fall-off 2.5 mm beyond the tumor. The 90% isodose of the proximal SOBP is placed 2.5 mm in front of the tumor. The lateral 90% isodose is placed 1.5 mm to each side of the tumor. At the distal edge and the lateral borders of the target volume the dose falls from 100% to 0% within 2 mm.

In cases requiring irradiation of the optic nerve, the length of nerve irradiated is minimized by the use of a wedge-shaped aluminum absorber placed in the beam proximal to the frontal surface of the eye in order to compensate partially for the eye's spherical surface. These wedges are also used in cases of large tumors to reduce the volume of the eye that receives irradiation.

Every treatment plan is discussed with the ophthalmologist who performed the clip surgery and a radiation oncologist before a patient is treated. Before a treatment plan is definitively accepted, a second simulation is performed in the calculated treatment position to verify that the patient is able to maintain the chosen gaze angle for the duration of the treatment. In 1 of 50 cases the plan has to be modified because the patient is not able to adopt and/or hold the calculated position. In such cases a position that is close to the calculated one but can be held by the patient is determined during the simulation. Then a new plan is calculated for this position and compared with the original plan. If it does not mean that irradiation to healthy structures is increased significantly, the new plan will be chosen over fixation with the suction cup. An acceptable increase in irradiation to healthy structures is a higher percentage of lens irradiation, while the dose received by the optic disc/nerve and the macula is still to be kept to a minimum.

The metallic lid retractors allow verification of the position of the eyelids on the positioning radiographs. If the lids cannot be retracted completely outside the irradiation field they are included in the model.

8.2.4
Irradiation

Treatment is delivered in four fractions, usually on 4 consecutive days. Most of the patients have been treated with a proton dose of 54.5 Gy, which corresponds to 60 CGE (Co-60 Gy equivalent) using a relative biological effectiveness (RBE) of 1.1 (GRAGOUDAS et al. 1977). Before each irradiation, a depth–dose distribution curve is measured using a Markus type ionization chamber and a Perspex phantom, to verify that the range and modulation have been adjusted correctly.

For treatment, the patient is positioned in the treatment chair according to the same procedure as described above for the simulation. The patient's individual collimator is placed in the beam line. The patient is then asked to gaze at the fixation light. A pair of X-ray pictures showing the clips and, additionally on the axial view, the collimator, is taken. A theoretical reference X-ray picture provided by the treatment planning program allows the detection of positioning errors of 0.1 mm or more. A light field simulating the proton beam allows us to verify that, where possible, the eyelids have been retracted from the irradiation field, or where not, that the position of the eyelid within the irradiation field corresponds to the treatment plan. After proper positioning of the eye, a video camera is directed at the eye to show the pupil on the monitors inside and outside the treatment room. The position of the pupil is delineated on the monitor. The pupil appears magnified 40 times on the monitor so that any movement of the eye can be detected immediately. If the patient should move the eye during irradiation, the therapist immediately

stops delivery of the proton beam. Only after correction of all positioning errors, i.e., when the positions of the tantalum clips are within 0.2 mm of those seen in the reference X-ray pictures, is the treatment applied. Irradiation lasts approximately 15–30 s.

8.2.5
Follow-up

After treatment, the patients are asked to return to the University Eye Clinic of Lausanne for follow-up examinations at 6 months, 1.5 years, 3 years, 5 years and then every 2.5 years, or at shorter intervals if required by the individual situation. Systemic examinations are recommended twice a year during the first 5 years, then once a year for 5 years, and then every 2.5 years. When patients are unable to return to Lausanne for their follow-up examinations (mainly patients who live more than 500 km from Lausanne), follow-up data are collected by contacting the referring ophthalmologist. Follow-up data include ultrasound measurement of the tumor thickness and wide-angle fundus pictures to judge the evolution of the tumor, best corrected visual acuity, measurement of the intraocular pressure, evaluation of retinal detachment, inflammation of the eye, lens opacity, hemorrhage, exudations, and presence of other irradiation-induced complications, such as maculopathy and papillopathy.

8.3
Results

8.3.1
Patients and Methods

We treated 2,435 cases of uveal melanoma between March 1984 and December 1998. For the presentation of our results, we have excluded 12 bilateral cases, 81 patients treated with a dose higher then 60 CGE, 20 patients treated with a reduced dose, 28 patients treated with a reduced safety margin, and 27 with invisible eye fundus. We have also excluded 9 patients with large tumors who received adjuvant chemotherapy immediately after PBRT. The remaining 2,258 cases are the subject of this analysis. Each of these received a total dose of 60 CGE, usually delivered on 4 consecutive days. Follow-up data available through September 1999 were used in this analysis. Follow-up times ranged from 0 to 167 months (mean 43.8 months, median 37 months). There were 147 patients (6.5%) who were lost to follow-up, who were censored at the last available examination. Eight patients refused any further follow-up examinations, but were still living at the time; they were considered only in the survival analysis.

Of the 2,258 patients, 1,169 were women (51.8%) and 1,089 were men (48.2%). The patients' ages ranged from 9 to 89 years (mean 54.3 years, median 56 years). There were 1,106 tumors (49.0%) located in left eyes, and 1,152 (51.0%) in right eyes. Visual acuity of the affected eye ranged from NLP (no light perception) to 150/100. The details of pretreatment visual acuity are given in Table 8.1. Intraocular pressures measured were between 4 and 56 mm Hg (mean 14.0 mm Hg, median 14 mm Hg). There was a known history of glaucoma in 29 patients (1.3%). No lens opacity was found in 1,850 cases (81.9%). Hemorrhage was found in 231 patients (10.2%); in 2 cases this was located in the anterior chamber and in 160 cases, in the tumor; 64 hemorrhages were vitreous hemorrhages and 68 were subretinal (more than one location per patient possible). Seventy-three patients (3.2%) presented with ocular melanocytosis. Retinal detachment was present in 1,594 patients (70.6%). The details are given in Table 8.2.

Tumor growth had been documented before treatment in 336 cases (14.9%). The tumor diameter was between 4.0 and 26.0 mm (mean 16.05 mm, median 16.0 mm). Tumor thickness ranged from 0.9 to 15.6 mm (mean 6.04 mm, median 5.7 mm). The anterior tumor margin was located posterior to the equator in 948 cases (42.0%), in the anterior choroid in 620 cases (27.5%), within the ciliary body in 606 cases (26.8%), and within the iris in 84 cases (3.7%). The location of the posterior tumor border relative to the macula and the optic disc is presented in more detail in Table 8.3. Extrascleral extensions were present in 110 cases (4.9%). There were 133 patients (5.9%) who had already been diagnosed with another cancer when they came for the treatment of their uveal melanoma.

A wedge-shaped bolus was used in 419 cases (18.6%) to reduce the length of optic nerve or volume of the eye irradiated. The safety margin was increased in 301 cases (13.3%), mainly cases of large, flat unpigmented tumors and large melanomas infiltrating the ciliary body.

The endpoint events assessed in each patient included death from any cause, ocular-tumor-related death only, local tumor control, eye retention, persistence of retinal detachment, appearance of total retinal detachment, radiation-induced complications such as papillopathy and maculopathy, rubeosis, glaucoma, neovascular glaucoma, lens opacity, and development of a total cataract. Visual acuity was investigated in terms of loss of 3 lines or more, 6 lines or more, and 9 lines or more. For patients having a visual acuity of 10/100 and better at the time of treatment, time to loss of visual acuity to less than 10/100 was analyzed.

Local recurrence after initial PBRT was defined as a persisting, documented increase of at least 1.0 mm in tumor basal diameter, as determined by comparison of initial and follow-up fundus photographs, or in tumor thickness, as measured by ultrasound, or both. If the increase of tumor volume was associated with a vitreous hemorrhage, tumor bleeding, or an exudative retinal detachment the patient was observed for several months to confirm the suspected tumor growth.

Table 8.1. Visual acuity at treatment time

Visual acuity	No. of patients	Proportion
<0.1	247	10.9%
0.1–0.3	262	11.6%
0.4–0.8	488	21.6%
>0.8	1,261	55.8%

Table 8.2. Retinal detachment before treatment

	No. of patients	Proportion
Absent	664	29.4%
<25%	597	26.4%
25%	409	18.1%
50%	525	23.3%
75%	60	2.7%
Total	3	0.1%

Table 8.3. Distance between posterior tumor border and optic disc or macula, respectively

		No. of cases	Proportion
Optic disc	Infiltration	138	6.1%
	0 mm	286	12.7%
	0<d≤3 mm	594	26.3%
	>3 mm	1,240	54.9%
Macula	Infiltration	356	15.8%
	0 mm	195	8.6%
	0<d≤3 mm	617	27.3%
	>3 mm	1,090	48.3%

Survival, local tumor control, eye retention, complication rates, and loss of visual acuity were estimated using the Kaplan-Meier method (KAPLAN and MEIER 1958). Cox's proportional hazards modeling was used to assess the prognostic value of the various demographic, ophthalmologic, and radiotherapeutic parameters (Cox 1972). The Kaplan-Meier method was used to estimate event-free survival in the subgroups of patients for the different endpoints. In these cases, the event-free survival rates were compared using the log rank test. All statistical analyses were calculated with the SPSS software package, version 7.5.

8.3.2
Survival

Of the 2,258 included in this study, 318 patients died: 258 of ocular-tumor-related causes, 18 of causes related to other tumors, 4 from some other cause but with known ocular tumor metastases, 24 from some other cause and without metastases, and 14 from causes that could not be determined. When all 318 deaths were taken into consideration, the overall survival rate was 81.9±1.1% at 5 years and 61.9±2.4% at 10 years. When only the 258 ocular-tumor-related deaths were taken account of, cause-specific survival was 84.3±1.1% at 5 years and 69.5±2.2% at 10 years. Both overall and cause-specific survival are shown in Fig. 8.3.

Metastases were found during follow-up examinations in 252 patients. In another 46 patients metastases were diagnosed at death. At the end of the study period, 35 (of the 252) patients were still alive with known metastases. One patient was lost to follow-up after detection of metastases. Four patients died from other causes but with known metastases from the uveal melanoma. The site of metastases in the 258 patients who died from metastatic disease is shown in Table 8.4.

Multifactorial analysis with the Cox proportional hazard model identified larger tumor diameter, older age, location of anterior tumor margin within the ciliary body, large retinal detachment, presence of an extrascleral extension of the tumor, and greater tumor thickness as statistically significant indicators of a lower chance of survival ($P<0.01$). The Kaplan-Meier ocular-tumor-related survival rate at 10 years is shown in Table 8.5 for all patients, as a function of age, largest tumor diameter (LTD), tumor thickness (H), location of the anterior tumor border, and absence or presence of extrascleral extension, and by gender. The number of tumor-related deaths and the number of patients in each group are also shown.

The average 10-year Kaplan-Meier survival rate is 70%. It can vary from over 90% for cases with a good prognosis (small tumors) to less than 30% (tumors with extrascleral extension).

We also analyzed whether survival was influenced by the evolution of the tumor, that is to say whether recurrent tumors were associated with poorer survival rates and whether patients who had to have their eye enucleated during follow-up had a different survival rate than those whose eye had been spared. The results of this analysis are shown in Table 8.6. They clearly show that the 10-year Kaplan-Meier mortality rate is significantly increased ($P=0.0001$) for patients with recurring tumors. These findings confirm that failing to achieve local tumor control also leads to lower survival in patients with melanoma (SUIT 1992; SUIT and WESTGATE 1986). KARLSSON also found lower survival rates for patients with recur-

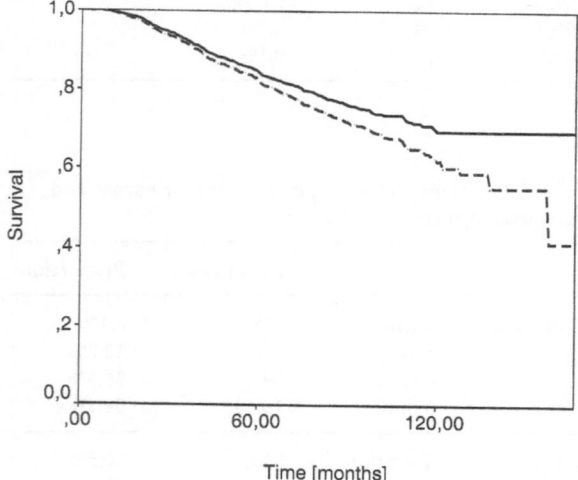

Fig. 8.3. Survival following proton beam radiotherapy (- - - all deaths, —— ocular-tumor-related deaths alone)

Table 8.4. Site of metastatic disease

	No.	Proportion[a]
Liver	240	93.0%
Lung	37	14.3%
Bone	29	11.2%
Skin	16	6.2%
CNS	15	5.8%
Lymph nodes	9	3.5%
Other	20	7.7%

[a]Multiple locations are possible

Table 8.5. Ocular-tumor-related deaths and survival rates at 10 years (*LTD* largest tumor diameter, *H* tumor thickness)

Parameter	No. of ocular-tumor-related deaths / patients in this group	Ocular-tumor-related survival rates at 10 years (Kaplan-Meier)
All patients	258/2258	69.5±2.2%
Age ≤55 years	111/1117	73.1±3.0%
Age >55 years	147/1141	65.5±3.3%
LTD≤10 mm	6/184	92.5±3.0%
10 mm<LTD≤15 mm	45/796	86.5±2.1%
15 mm<LTD≤20 mm	115/906	54.6±5.6%
20 mm<LTD	92/372	40.7±5.4%
H≤3 mm	15/355	90.8±2.5%
3 mm<H≤5 mm	37/612	81.0±3.6%
5 mm<H≤10 mm	161/1056	58.1±3.9%
10 mm<H	45/235	54.6±6.7%
Anterior tumor border posterior to equator	55/948	85.6±2.3%
Anterior tumor border anterior to equator	78/620	65.4±4.7%
Anterior tumor border in ciliary body	116/606	42.4±5.9%
Anterior tumor border in iris	9/84	75.4±8.4%
No extrascleral extension	229/2148	71.3±2.3%
With extrascleral extension	29/110	27.7±9.9%
Women	122/1169	71.5±2.9%
Men	136/1089	67.1±3.4%

Table 8.6. Ocular-tumor-related survival at 10 years as a function of evolution of the tumor

Parameter	Ocular-tumor-related deaths / patients in this group	Ocular-tumor-related survival (Kaplan-Meier)
Tumor controlled	235/2203	70.4±2.4%
Recurrent tumors	23/55	48.1±7.9%
Eye saved	230/2094	69.0±2.5%
Eye enucleated	28/164	72.2±5.0%

rent tumors than for patients whose tumors were controlled following Co-60 episcleral plaque brachytherapy (KARLSSON et al. 1989).

The survival rates of patients whose eyes were enucleated after PBRT are not significantly different from those of patients who kept their eye (log rank test *P*=0.7433). These results confirm previous findings of other groups (CHAR et al. 1996; LOMMATZSCH et al. 2000; SEDDON et al. 1985).

8.3.3
Local Tumor Control

Among the 2,258 patients considered in this analysis, 55 were prescribed a second treatment because local

tumor control had failed: 25 of them were managed by enucleation, 19 received a second PBRT (2 of these later had their eyes enucleated because their tumors were still uncontrolled), 5 were treated with episcleral plaque brachytherapy, 1 patient received photocoagulation, and 5 patients received no treatment because they had advanced metastatic disease and were in poor general health. The local tumor control rate was 96.2±0.5% after 5 years and 95.1±0.7% after 10 years. The dose distribution calculation, dosimetry, and position control X-ray pictures kept in the treatment records of the patients with recurring tumors were analyzed to determine whether, in retrospect, some aspect of the treatment planning, dosimetry, or positioning of these patients might have been inadequate. In 2 cases, the diagnosis of recurrence and the enucleation were performed by the referring ophthalmologist and no further information was made available to us. In 17 cases the eyelid was within the treatment field and its real thickness was found to be greater than the thickness modeled with EYEPLAN. In 19 cases tumors of the ciliary body recurred as ring melanomas. In 3 cases, the position of the clips relative to the tumor was found to be inadequate. In 10 cases the tumor model was inaccurate, i.e. an insufficient PTV was determined. In 1 case the ultrasound measurement of the eye length was too short, and in the remaining 3 cases we could not identify a probable cause of local tumor control failure.

These problems had already been identified in 1993. Consequently, we increased the safety margin in the ciliary body for those tumors infiltrating the ciliary body and introduced a new model of the eyelid into the TPS, allowing more precise modeling of the eyelid within the irradiation field. The number of recurrences could be notably reduced with these measures: only 3 recurrences have occurred in patients treated since the implementation of these changes at the end of 1993. The local tumor control rates for the patients treated before and after January 1994 are shown in Fig. 8.4. Thanks to these changes, the 5-year local tumor control rate was increased from 95.7±0.6% for patients treated before 1994 (52 recurrences among 1,304 patients), to 98.8±0.7% (3 recurrences among 954 patients) for the patients treated later. The log rank test supports a statistically significant difference with a P-value of 0.01.

8.3.4
Eye Retention

Following PBRT, 164 (7.3%) patients had their eyes enucleated. The causes for enucleation were unknown in 3 cases, because the enucleations were performed elsewhere and we were unable to obtain any further information. In 9 cases, the eye was removed on suspicion of recurrence, which was not, however, confirmed. Glaucoma was the reason in 108 cases, often associated with functional loss (112 cases). In 25 cases, recurrence was the cause for enucleation. In 19 cases it was total retinal detachment, while 1 patient underwent enucleation for psychological reasons, and 4 because it was not possible to control the evolution of the tumor. (The total number of causes listed can exceed the number of enucleations because more than one problem occurred in some patients.) Five years after treatment, 88.8±0.9% of the patients had retained their eye; at 10 years the rate of eye retention was 85.4±1.3%. Tumor thickness, amount of retinal detachment at treatment, and patient's gender were identified as significant predictors of enucleation following PBRT. Eyes containing very thick tumors associated with large retinal detachment in men were more subject to enucleation. The eye retention rate for tumors above and below 8 mm thickness is shown in Fig. 8.5. Numbers of enucleations and eye retention rates at 10 years according to Kaplan-Meier are shown in Table 8.7 for the different statistically significant parameters.

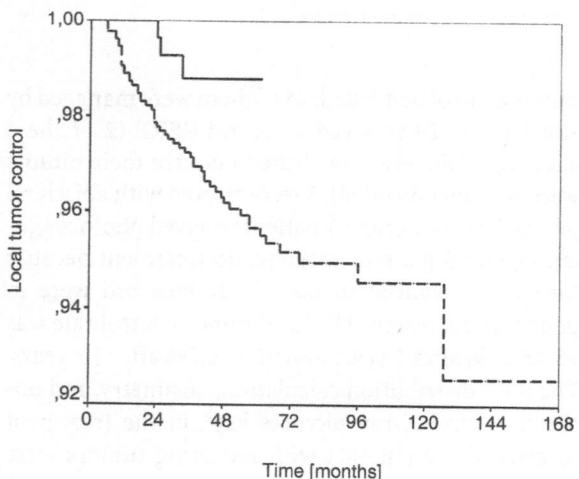

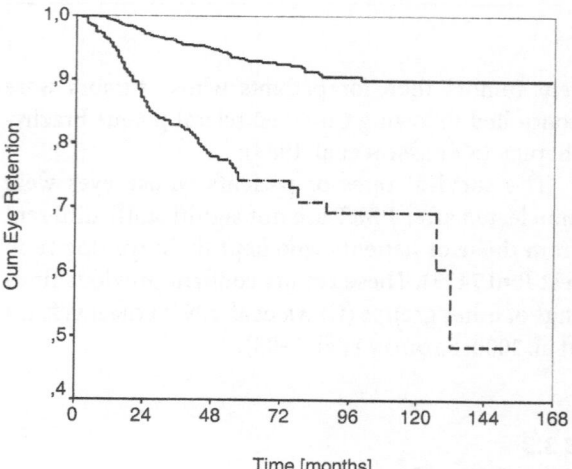

Fig. 8.4. Local tumor control following PBRT. Note that the "local control" axis begins at 0.92 (__ patients treated after January 1994, -- patients treated before January 1994)

Fig. 8.5. Eye retention following PBRT. Note that the "eye retention" axis begins at 0.4 (__ tumor thickness ≤8 mm, -- tumor thickness >8 mm)

Table 8.7. Eye retention as a function of different parameters

Parameter	Enucleations / patients	Eye retention at 10 years (Kaplan-Meier)
Tumor thickness ≤8.0 mm	78/1719	89.9±1.3%
Tumor thickness >8.0 mm	86/539	69.3±3.5%
Retinal detachment <50%	63/1670	91.1±1.3%
Retinal detachment ≥50%	101/588	71.8±2.8%
Men	108/1169	78.6±2.3%
Women	56/1089	91.1±1.4%

8.3.5
Complications

8.3.5.1
Retinal Detachment

Some degree of retinal detachment was found at the beginning of treatment in 1,594 (70.6%) patients (see Table 8.2). At 5 years the Kaplan-Meier rate of patients with some retinal detachment had fallen to 16.3%, and at 10 years only 9.9% of the patients were still suffering any amount of retinal detachment.

Among the 2,258 patients treated, 125 developed total retinal detachment. Larger tumors and larger degrees of retinal detachment at treatment correlate closely with development of a total retinal detachment. The proportion of patients who had developed total retinal detachment at 5 years was 2.9±0.6% in patients with an initial retinal detachment smaller than 50%, and 22.9±2.3% for those with 50% or more initial retinal detachment. These proportions increased to 4.4±1.1% and 38.8±5.8%, respectively, for the two groups at 10 years. In the group of 1,670 patients with initial retinal detachment smaller than 50%, 29 developed a total retinal detachment, while 96 of 587 patients in the group of patients with a retinal detachment equal to or larger than 50% presented with a total retinal detachment.

8.3.5.2
Radiation-induced Papillopathy

Radiation-induced papillopathy appeared only in patients who received some irradiation to the optic disc and nerve. This group was made up of 937 of the 2,258 patients, and 301 of them developed radiation-induced papillopathy. Among these 937 patients, complication-free survival was 45.2±2.4% at 5 years and 36.5±3.5% at 10 years. The irradiation of the optic disc and nerve was the only factor found to induce this complication.

8.3.5.3
Radiation-induced Maculopathy

Radiation-induced maculopathy appeared only in patients whose macula was irradiated. This concerned 1,221 of the 2,258 patients, 428 of whom developed radiation-induced maculopathy. Complication-free survival was 41.2±2.1% at 5 years and 24.9±2.9% at 10 years. For this complication too, no factor other than irradiation of the macula was found to be of statistical significance.

8.3.5.4
Rubeosis, Glaucoma, and Neovascular Glaucoma

Among the 2,258 patients treated, there were 334 cases of rubeosis. The rubeosis-free survival rate was 78.4±1.2% at 5 years and 72.2±1.8% at 10 years. Factors favoring the appearance of rubeosis were tumor thickness over 8 mm, large degree of retinal detachment (≥50%), tumors close to or infiltrating the optic disc, and older age (>60 years).

We identified 427 cases of glaucoma; 68 of them were in patients who had already been diagnosed before treatment and were excluded from the analysis. Glaucoma-free survival was therefore 76.9±1.2% at 5 years and 70.3±1.8% at 10 years. Tumor thickness greater than 8 mm, invasion of the iris by the tumor, proximity or infiltration of the optic disc, older age, and large degree of retinal detachment are the parameters identified as favoring the development of glaucoma following PBRT.

Neovascular glaucoma (NVG) was diagnosed in 219 cases. The NVG-free survival rates were 83.7±1.1% at 5 years and 77.5±2.0% at 10 years. Great tumor thickness, close proximity of the tumor to the optic disc or tumor infiltration of the disc, large degree of retinal detachment and older age are the parameters identified as significantly favoring development of NVG.

The complication-free survival rate at 10 years is shown in Table 8.8 as a function of tumor thickness for rubeosis, glaucoma and NVG.

Table 8.8. Rubeosis, glaucoma and neovascular glaucoma as a function of tumor thickness (H)

		No. of complications	Complication-free survival at 10 years
Rubeosis	H≤8.0 mm (1,719 patients)	158	81.7±1.8%
	H>8.0 mm (538 patients)	176	33.7±4.7%
Glaucoma	H≤8.0 mm	239	75.8±1.9%
	H>8.0 mm	188	36.3±3.9%
Neovascular glaucoma	H≤8.0 mm	102	84.2±2.1%
	H>8.0 mm	117	49.6±5.1%

8.3.5.5
Lens Opacity

Lens opacity was present before treatment in 393 of the 2,258 patients. During the follow-up period, lens opacity was found in 1,107 patients, including those with pretreatment lens opacity . Lens-opacity-free survival was 42.6±1.3% at 5 years and 22.8±1.9% at 10 years. Greater tumor thickness, older age, infiltration of the iris and ciliary body by the tumor, presence of ocular melanocytosis, inflammation of the anterior chamber, and large degree of retinal detachment were the parameters that favored the development of lens opacity.

Lens-opacity-free survival for patients with tumor thickness ≤8 mm was 29.2±2.4% at 10 years, while 730 of 1,719 patients developed opacity of the lens. In the group of patients with larger tumors, 377 of 538 patients developed lens opacity and their complication-free survival rate was 3.4±1.8% at 10 years; in other words, nearly all patients with large tumors had developed some degree of lens opacity within 10 years after treatment.

8.3.6
Visual Acuity

While saving the eye alone was considered to be important 15 years ago, posttreatment visual acuity has become an increasingly important factor today. Pretreatment visual acuity is listed in Table 8.1. Among the 2,258 patients considered in this report, 90% had useful vision at treatment, i.e. a visual acuity equal to or better than 20/200. Five years after treatment, the Kaplan-Meier rate of patients who retained useful vision was 36.7±1.3% (i.e. acuity + 20/200). After 10 years the rate had dropped to 27.7±1.5%. In total, 970 patients had a loss in visual acuity to less than 20/200.

There were 423 patients who experienced a loss of vision of 9 lines or more. The rate of loss of that much vision was 25.2±1.3% at 5 years and 37.3±2.4% at 10 years.

There were 928 patients who experienced a loss of vision of 6 lines or more. The rate of loss of vision for these cases was 51.3±1.3% at 5 years and 63.9±2.4% at 10 years.

And, finally, 1,311 patients experienced a loss of vision of 3 lines or more. The rate of loss of vision for these patients was 69.5±1.2% at 5 years and 80.2±1.7% at 10 years.

We used the Cox proportional hazard model to identify the following parameters that influenced the deterioration of vision: reduced visual acuity at treatment, large tumor thickness, close proximity of the posterior tumor margin to the optic disc and to the macula, a detached retina, and older age of the patient.

Figure 8.6 shows the Kaplan-Meier plot of the percentage of patients maintaining a visual acuity equal to or better than 20/200 as function of tumor thickness. Of 1,719 patients with a tumor thickness of 8 mm or less, 680 experienced a loss of visual acuity to less than 20/200, while 290 of 538 patients with larger tumors experienced the same loss of vision. The rate of patients retaining useful vision at 10 years was 37.1±2.1% for the group of patients with smaller tumors, versus 12.1±3.4% for those with larger tumors.

In the group of patients with tumor thickness smaller than 8 mm, 856 experienced a loss of visual acuity of 3 lines or more, 563 lost 6 lines or more and 304 lost 9 lines or more. The rates of loss of visual acuity at 10 years were 74.8±2.2%, 56.8±2.6%, and 35.7±2.6%, respectively.

In the group of patients with larger tumors, 291 experienced a loss of visual acuity of 3 lines or more, 201 lost 6 lines or more, and 119 lost 9 lines or more. The respective 10-year loss rates were 82.1±3.5%, 60.1±4.2%, and 42.4±5.4%.

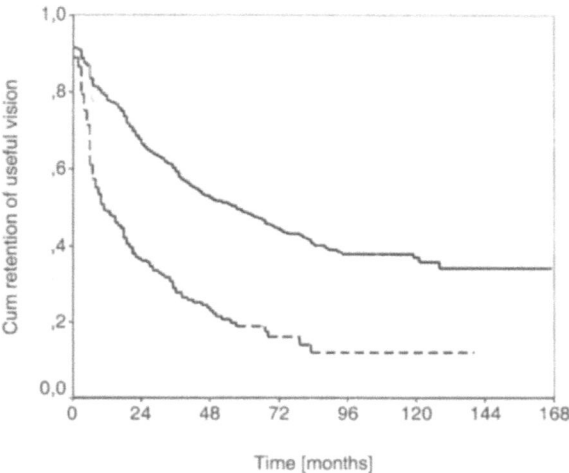

Fig. 8.6. Percentage of patients retaining useful visual acuity (__ tumor thickness ≤8 mm, -- tumor thickness >8 mm

We now give an example with the aim of illustrating the possibilities of proton beam radiotherapy. A woman of 52 presented with a large melanoma. Her visual acuity at treatment was 70/100 and the ocular tension, 13 mmHg; no lens opacity was found, and there was no hemorrhage. Retinal detachment was <25%, the macula was detached, and there was no ocular melanocytosis. The largest tumor diameter was 22.0 mm and the tumor thickness, 10.2 mm. The tumor was classified as very large or T3, depending on the system used. It was located in the posterior and anterior choroid and in the ciliary body. The distance to the optic disc was 6.0 mm and the distance to the macula, 9.0 mm. Tumor growth had been documented before treatment. The treatment plan applied is shown in Figs. 8.7–8.9.

At 3 months after treatment, the tumor thickness was reduced to 8.5 mm, and at 6 months to 7.2 mm. The retinal detachment decreased steadily and was absent at the 1.5 year follow-up examination. Lens opacity began to appear, reducing visual acuity to 0.6. Tumor thickness was 6.9 mm. At 3 years, visual acuity was reduced to 0.3, a cataract being the cause of vision loss. The tumor thickness was now constant at 6.9 mm. At 5 years cataract surgery was performed. After the intervention, visual acuity increased to 0.4. Tumor thickness was still constant at 6.9 mm. At 7 years, the last available follow-up examination, no complications were present, visual acuity had increased to 80/100, and residual tumor thickness was 5.6 mm. No metastases had been detected in this patient, who was doing very well.

8.4
Discussion

In a recently published paper, LOMMATZSCH et al. analyzed the results of Ru-106/Rh-106 brachytherapy for posterior uveal melanoma (LOMMATZSCH et al. 2000). All tumors included in their analysis were less than 12 mm in diameter and 7.0 mm in thickness. Since this excellent article is one of the rare publications with long-term follow-up data (more than 10 years), we will try to compare the results published in it with our results. However, since it makes no sense to compare the outcome of patients presenting with large and very large tumors with that of patients with small tumors, we will be considering only PBRT patients presenting with tumor thickness £8.0 mm. This value is often considered as a limit for the use of Ru-106/Rh-106 plaques.

The cause-specific survival rate in the article of LOMMATZSCH et al. (compared with *our data*, given in *italic in parentheses*) at 10 years was 81% (*76%*), local tumor control was 71% (*97%*) at 5 years and 66% (*96%*) at 10 years. The eye retention rate was 77% (*93%*) at 5 years and 72% (*90%*) at 10 years. Among the patients who had a pretreatment visual acuity better than 20/200, 51% (*52%*) had maintained that level of vision at 5 years, and 37% (*39%*) at 10 years.

Survival following PBRT or Ru-106/Rh-106 brachytherapy is comparable. The somewhat poorer

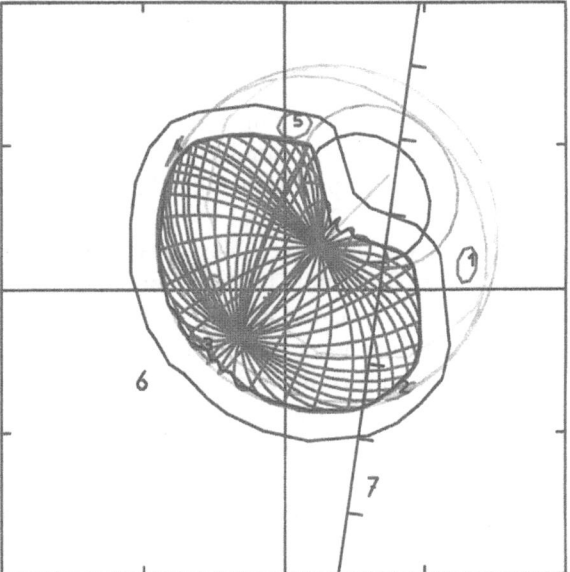

Fig. 8.7. Beam's eye view (*1, 2, 3, 4, 5* tantalum clips, *6* collimator shaped to the profile of the tumor with a safety margin of 2 mm, *7* position of the aluminum wedge

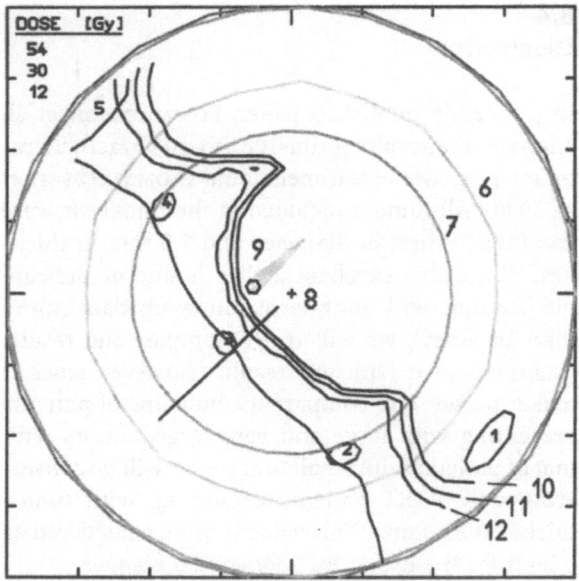

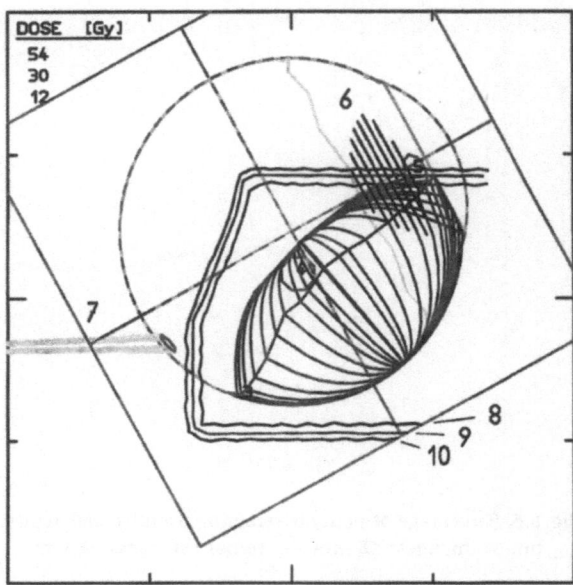

Fig. 8.8. Eye fundus view (*1, 2, 3, 4, 5* tantalum clips, *6* ora serrata, *7* equator, *8* macula, *9* optic disc and nerve, *10* 20% isodose, *11* 50% isodose, *12* 90% isodose)

Fig. 8.9. Plane through the eye (*1, 2, 3, 4, 5* tantalum clips, *6* lens, *7* optic nerve, *8* 20% isodose, *9* 50% isodose, *10* 90% isodose

survival following PBRT is probably due to the fact that in the study of Lommatzsch only posterior tumors were considered, while our study also includes tumors infiltrating the ciliary body, which are well known to have a poorer survival prognosis (GRAGOUDAS et al. 1986, 1988). Survival following PBRT is within the range of survival rates published for the different treatment modalities available today (AUGSBURGER et al. 1998, 1999; CHAR et al. 1989, 1993; POTTER et al. 1997; SEDDON et al. 1990).

PBRT has been demonstrated many times to be an excellent means of achieving local tumor control (GRAGOUDAS et al. 1992). Similarly high rates of local control have been published following helium ion beam radiotherapy (CHAR et al. 1997). Local control rates comparable to those achieved by PBRT have been published for tumors that are more than 3 mm distant from the optic disc following brachytherapy, while tumors close to or in contact with the optic disc are not easily controlled with brachytherapy (KLEINEIDAM et al. 1993; PETROVICH et al. 1992). This is probably due to the difficulties involved in placing the applicator appropriately close to the optic nerve, which is necessary to deliver adequate irradiation to the part of the tumor that is in contact with the optic disc.

As mentioned previously, the eye retention rate is influenced by the local tumor control rate. Approximately 50% of eyes with recurring tumors are enu-

cleated, and the others receive a second conservative treatment. However, some of those will later also have to be enucleated because of radiation-induced complications leading to complete loss of vision and painful eyes (EGAN et al. 1989; SHIELDS et al. 1989). This explains why the eye retention rate is much higher after PBRT than after brachytherapy.

One important goal following a conservative treatment is the preservation of vision. The data published by LOMMATZSCH et al. and our own data restricted to comparable tumors suggest that there is no difference between brachytherapy and PBRT in achieving this goal. Our results are also comparable to those of other groups (SEDDON et al. 1986, 1987). Preservation of useful vision has become a main concern over the last years, because the number of patients receiving PBRT has greatly increased, while the number of eyes enucleated has decreased. The authors are convinced that a further reduction in complication rates following PBRT is possible, which would increase the number of patients who retain useful vision.

At present, PBRT is mainly applied in physics research centers, where an accelerator is shared with experimental physicists and is usually available for medical applications for only 1 week per month. This has led to the fractionation scheme used in western Europe, with four fractions applied on 4 consecutive days. However, uveal melanoma is a slow-growing tumor. Tumor cell doubling times of several months have been published in the literature (MANSCHOT and VAN STRIK 1992). From the viewpoint of radiation biology there is no need to deliver the whole dose to this type of tumor within such a short time. It can be expected that a larger number of fractions applied over a longer time, which would mean a lower dose per fraction, might reduce the complication rate, thus increasing the proportion of patients who retain useful visual acuity without jeopardizing the excellent local tumor control rate. Such a study, though, would not be possible without the availability of an accelerator within a hospital environment, allowing the treatment of patients during 50 weeks per year.

8.5 Summary

There is evidence that malignant uveal melanoma can be safely treated with PBRT and long-term survival rates comparable to those of brachytherapy and enucleation can be achieved by this means. Local 5-year tumor control rates as high as 99% can be achieved. Tumors with a thickness in excess of 8 mm cannot be safely treated with brachytherapy, and tumors in contact with or close proximity to the optic disc are well known to have a reduced local control rate following brachytherapy. The advantage that PBRT has over brachytherapy is that local control is independent of tumor size and location. In many cases, where a treatment with brachytherapy is no longer possible PBRT is the only remaining possibility for conservative treatment. Preservation of the eye is achieved in the majority of cases. Preservation of eye function can be achieved in many cases despite unfavorable situations such as large tumors close to or in contact with the optic disc or the macula, or both.

Changes in the fractionation scheme are expected to improve these excellent results further.

References

Augsburger JJ, Correa ZM, Freire J et al (1998) Long-term survival in choroidal and ciliary body melanoma after enucleations versus plaque radiation therapy. Ophthalmology 105:1670–1678

Augsburger JJ, Schneider S, Freire J et al (1999) Survival following enucleation versus plaque radiotherapy in statistically matched subgroups of patients with choroidal melanomas: results in patients treated between 1980 and 1987. Graefes Arch Clin Exp Ophthalmol 237:558–567

Castro JR, Char DH, Petti PL et al (1997) 15 years' experience with helium ion radiotherapy for uveal melanoma. Int J Radiat Oncol Biol Phys 39:989–996

Char DH, Castro JR, Quivey JM et al (1989) Uveal melanoma radiation. 125-I brachytherapy versus helium ion irradiation. Ophthalmology 96:1708–15

Char DH, Quivey JM, Castro JR et al (1993) Helium ion versus iodine 125 brachytherapy in the management of uveal melanoma. Ophthalmology 100:1547–1554

Char DH, Kroll S, Quivey J, Castro J (1996) Long term visual outcome of radiated uveal melanomas in eyes eligible for randomisation to enucleation versus brachytherapy. Br J Ophthalmol 80:117–124

Char DH, Kroll SM, Castro J (1997) Long-term follow-up after uveal melanoma charged particle therapy. Trans Am Ophthalmol Soc 95:171–187

Char DH, Kroll SM, Castro J (1998) Ten-year follow-up of helium ion therapy for uveal melanoma. Am J Ophthalmol 125:81–89

Cox D (1972) Regression models and life-tables. J R Stat Soc Ser 34:187–220

Egan KM, Gragoudas ES, Seddon JM et al (1989) The risk of enucleation after proton beam irradiation of uveal melanoma. Ophthalmology 96:1377–1382

Egger E, Zografos L, Munkel G et al (1997) Results of proton radiotherapy for uveal melanomas. In: Wiegel T, Bornfeld N, Foerster MH, Hinkelbein W (eds) Radiotherapy of ocular disease. (Frontiers of radiation therapy and oncology, vol 30) Karger, Basel, pp 111–122

Goitein M, Miller T (1983) Planning proton therapy of the eye. Med Phys 10:275–283

Gragoudas ES, Goitein M, Koehler AM et al (1977) Proton irradiation of small choroidal malignant melanomas. Am J Ophthalmol 83:665–673

Gragoudas ES, Goitein M, Verhey L et al (1980) Proton beam irradiation: an alternative to enucleation for intraocular melanomas. Ophthalmology 87:571–581

Gragoudas ES, Goitein M, Verhey L et al (1982) Proton beam irradiation of uveal melanomas. Results of 5 1/2-year study. Arch Ophthalmol 100:928–934

Gragoudas ES, Goitein M, Seddon J et al (1984) Preliminary results of proton beam irradiation of macular and paramacular melanomas. Br J Ophthalmol 68:479–485

Gragoudas ES, Seddon JM, Egan KM et al (1986) Prognostic factors for metastasis following proton beam irradiation of uveal melanomas. Ophthalmology 93:675–680

Gragoudas ES, Seddon JM, Egan K et al (1987) Long-term results of proton beam irradiated uveal melanomas. Arch Ophthalmol 94:349–353

Gragoudas ES, Seddon JM, Egan KM et al (1988) Metastasis from uveal melanoma after proton beam irradiation. Ophthalmology 95:992–999

Gragoudas ES, Egan KM, Seddon JM et al (1992) Intraocular recurrence of uveal melanoma after proton beam irradiation. Ophthalmology 99:760–766

Kaplan E, Meier P (1958) Nonparametric estimation from incomplete observation. J Am Stat Assoc 53:457–481

Karlsson UL, Augsburger JJ, Shields JA et al (1989) Recurrence of posterior uveal melanoma after ^{60}Co episcleral plaque therapy. Ophthalmology 96:382–388

Kleineidam M, Guthoff R, Bentzen SM (1993) Rates of local control, metastasis, and overall survival in patients with posterior uveal melanomas treated with ruthenium-106 plaques. Radiother Oncol 28:148-56

Linstadt D, Castro J, Char D et al (1990) Long-term results of helium ion irradiation of uveal melanoma. Int J Radiat Oncol Biol Phys 19:613-618

Lommatzsch PK, Werschnik C, Schuster E (2000) Long-term follow-up of Ru-106/Rh-106 brachytherapy for posterior uveal melanoma. Graefes Arch Clin Exp Ophthalmol 238:129-137

Manschot WA, van Strik R (1992) Uveal melanoma: therapeutic consequences of doubling times and irradiation results; a review. Int Ophthalmol 16:91-99

Munzenrider JE, Gragoudas ES, Seddon JM et al (1988) Conservative treatment of uveal melanoma: probability of eye retention after proton treatment. Int J Radiat Oncol Biol Phys 15:553-558

Munzenrider JE, Verhey LJ, Gragoudas ES et al (1989) Conservative treatment of uveal melanoma: local recurrence after proton beam therapy. Int J Radiat Oncol Biol Phys 17:493-498

Perret C (1987) The therapy planning program EYE (internal report). Swiss Institute for Nuclear Research, Villigen

Petrovich Z, Luxton G, Langholz B et al (1992) Episcleral plaque radiotherapy in the treatment of uveal melanomas. Int J Radiat Oncol Biol Phys 24:247-251

Potter R, Janssen K, Prott FJ et al. (1997) Ruthenium-106 eye plaque brachytherapy in the conservative treatment of uveal melanoma: evaluation of 175 patients treated with 150 Gy from 1981-1989. In: Wiegel T, Bornfeld N, Foerster MH, Hinkelbein W (eds) Radiotherapy of ocular disease. (Frontiers of radiation therapy and oncology, vol 30) Karger, Basel, pp 143-149

Seddon JM, Gragoudas ES, Albert DM et al (1985) Comparison of survival rates for patients with uveal melanoma after treatment with proton beam irradiation or enucleation. Am J Ophthalmol 99:282-290

Seddon JM, Gragoudas ES, Polivogianis L et al (1986) Visual outcome after proton beam irradiation of uveal melanoma. Ophthalmology 93:666-674

Seddon JM, Gragoudas ES, Egan KM et al (1987) Uveal melanomas near the optic disc or fovea. Visual results after proton beam irradiation. Ophthalmology 94:354-361

Seddon JM, Gragoudas ES, Egan KM et al (1990) Relative survival rates after alternative therapies for uveal melanoma. Ophthalmology 97:769-777

Sheen M (1995) EYEPLAN proton therapy planning program (internal report). Clatterbridge Centre for Oncology, Bebington UK

Shields CL, Shields JA, Karlsson U et al (1989) Reasons for enucleation after plaque radiotherapy for posterior uveal melanoma. Clinical findings. Ophthalmology 96:919-923

Suit HD (1992) Local control and patient survival. Int J Radiat Oncol Biol Phys 23:653-660

Suit HD, Westgate SJ (1986) Impact of improved local control on survival. Int J Radiat Oncol Biol Phys 15:453-458

9 Clinical Features and Management of Choroidal Hemangiomas, Including Those Occuring in Association with Sturge-Weber Syndrome

W. E. ALBERTI and R. H. SAGERMAN

CONTENTS

9.1 Introduction

Choroidal hemangioma is a benign vascular tumor that can occur as a circumscribed lesion at the posterior pole or as a diffuse lesion associated with encephalofacial angiomatosis (Sturge-Weber syndrome). This chapter considers the clinical features and management of choroidal hemangioma. A more extensive discussion can be found in ophthalmology texts (SHIELDS 1983; CHAR 1989; LOMMATZSCH 1989).

9.2 Clinical Features and Diagnosis

Choroidal hemangiomas are relatively rare. The tumor starts at an early age and grows slowly. Cases associated with Sturge-Weber syndrome seem to progress more rapidly than isolated forms. The circumscribed type is diagnosed at a median age of 39 years and the diffuse type, at a median age of 8 years (WITSCHEL and FONT 1976).

More than 200 histopathologically confirmed cases have been reported in the Anglo-American and West European literature (WITSCHEL and FONT 1976). About 50% have been in patients with Sturge-Weber syndrome, which renders the diagnosis easy. Formerly, hemangiomas were incidental findings in eyes enucleated for absolute glaucoma or suspected malignant melanoma. In recent years improved diagnostic methods such as binocular ophthalmoscopy, fluorescein angiography, ultrasonography, and thin-section computed tomography (CT) have made it possible to detect more angiomas clinically (MACKENSEN and MEYER-SCHWICKERATH 1980; WESSING 1977; OSSOINIG 1974; JOHN et al. 1983).

9.2.1 Symptoms

Symptoms are related to the size and site of the tumor. A circumscribed hemangioma close to the optic disk or macula can cause blurred vision or metamorphopsia secondary to either a serous, nonrhegmatogenous retinal detachment or macular involvement, respectively.

9.2.2 Diagnosis and Differential Diagnosis

Ophthalmoscopically, a circumscribed hemangioma appears as a round or oval, non-pigmented, elevated mass at the posterior pole. The colors described vary from gray through yellow to salmon pink or raspberry red (MACKENSEN and MEYER-SCHWICKERATH 1980). Size ranges from 3 to 12 mm in diameter and 1 to 6 mm in thickness. Often, subretinal fluid can be detected adjacent to the

W. E. ALBERTI, MD
Professor, Radiologische Klinik, Abteilung für Strahlentherapie und Radioonkologie, Universitäts-Klinikum, Hamburg-Eppendorf, Martinistrasse 52, 20246 Hamburg, Germany
R. H. SAGERMAN, MD, FACR
Professor, Department of Radiation Oncology, SUNY Upstate Medical University, 750 E. Adams Street, Syracuse, NY 13210, USA

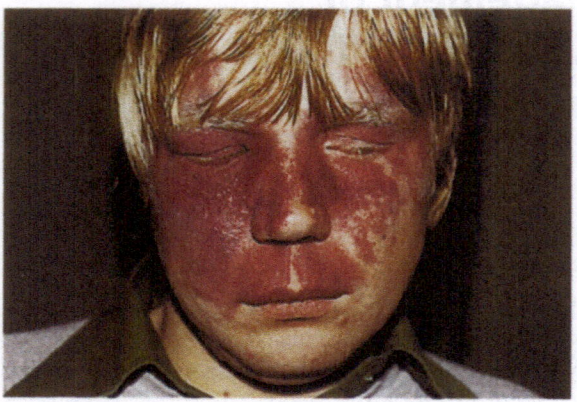

Fig. 9.1. Thirteen-year-old boy with a bilateral facial and diffuse choroidal hemangioma (Sturge-Weber syndrome)

9.2.3
Pathology

WITSCHEL and FONT (1976) classified choroidal hemangiomas histologically, according to the prevailing type of blood vessels, into predominantly capillary, predominantly cavernous, and mixed. The distribution of histology differed between solitary (*n*=45) and diffuse (*n*=17) lesions.

All Sturge-Weber hemangiomas in Witschel and Font's study were of the mixed type, whereas solitary lesions showed an equal distribution between the cavernous (20 tumors) and mixed (22 tumors) types. Capillary cases (only solitary lesions) were rare (3/45).

hemangioma, resulting in visual disturbance when close to the optic disk or macula. Retinal detachment can become total. Glaucoma is the almost inevitable outcome unless the tumor can be destroyed.

In contrast to the solitary type, diffuse hemangiomas are associated with Sturge-Weber syndrome, which consists of facial hemangioma (nevus flammeus, Fig. 9.1), buphthalmos, seizures, and intracranial vascular malformation.

As emphasized by SHIELDS (1983) and reported by GIOVANNINI and CAPONETTI (1984), most patients have a forme fruste rather than the entire syndrome. In the series of 42 patients reported on by GIOVANNINI and CAPONETTI (1984), only 6 (14%) had the classic form; 18 patients (43%) had only a facial hemangioma, and the rest of the patients had a combination of two signs. The ocular, cutaneous, and cerebral features are always ipsilateral; moreover, they can be unilateral or bilateral.

In the presence of a facial hemangioma, diagnosis of a diffuse hemangioma is usually easy. In contrast, the diagnosis of circumscribed lesions requires more effort, involving binocular ophthalmoscopy, fluorescein angiography, ultra-sonography, and, in the case of total retinal detachment, thin-section CT with contrast.

Choroidal hemangioma must be clinically differentiated from an amelanotic choroidal melanoma, choroidal metastasis, central serous chorioretinopathy, posterior scleritis, choroidal osteoma, central exudative hemorrhagic chorioretinopathy, retinoblastoma and, occasionally, other conditions (SHIELDS 1983).

9.3
Management

9.3.1
Photocoagulation

The choice of treatment modality for choroidal hemangiomas depends on the location of the tumor and the severity of symptoms and signs, such as decreased vision, retinal detachment, and secondary glaucoma. Photocoagulation, developed and first reported for the treatment of choroidal hemangiomas by MEYER-SCHWICKERATH in 1956, is the treatment of choice for circumscribed lesions. According to his experience, the entire surface of the tumor should be coagulated (MACKENSEN and MEYER-SCHWICKERATH 1980). Treatment of the surrounding blood supply, which is required for malignant melanoma, is not necessary. Regression of the associated retinal detachment is the significant criterion for the effect of coagulation therapy. If retinal detachment recurs, treatment can be repeated. In general, three or four coagulation treatments at monthly intervals are sufficient for tumor inactivation and resorption of the subretinal fluid. The size of the tumor does not decrease significantly after photocoagulation.

The success of photocoagulation may be explained by its effect in reducing the permeability of the superficial blood vessels, which are the source of the subretinal fluid (NORTON and GUTMAN 1968; MACKENSEN and MEYER-SCHWICKERATH 1980), or in producing a chorioretinal adhesion so that the retina reattaches and the subretinal fluid resorbs

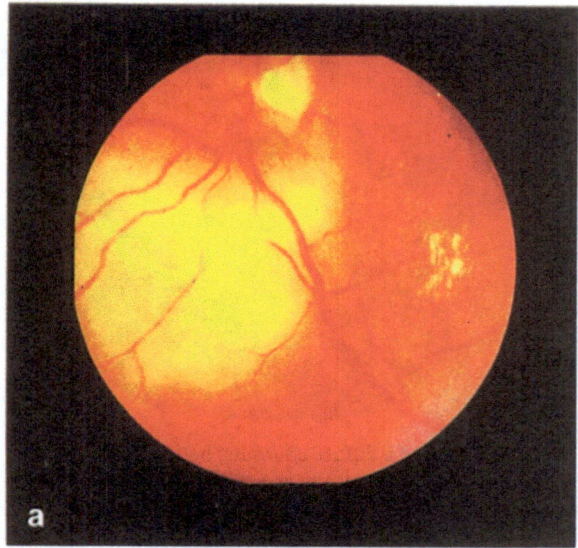

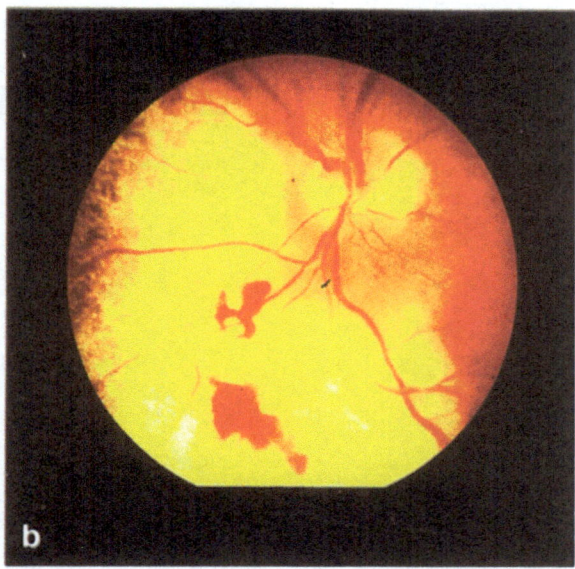

Fig. 9.2. a Hemangioma close to the optic disk before treatment; **b** fundus 5 years after xenon photocoagulation. Vision: 1.0 (LOMMATZSCH 1989)

(SHIELDS 1983). Figure 9.2 demonstrates a solitary hemangioma successfully treated with photocoagulation.

9.3.2
Radiation Therapy

Experience with radioactive plaque therapy or radon seeds sutured to the sclera over the tumor is anecdotal (MACLEAN and MAUMENEE 1959; R. LONG 1980, personal communication, cited by SHIELDS 1983, p. 273). Two patients have been coagulated by transscleral diathermy followed by irradiation with radon seeds. The first patient retained his eye, in which he had slightly improved vision 18 months after treatment. The second patient, whose lesion was in the area between the macula and the disk, developed a chorioretinal scar but had evidence of residual tumor 6 months after the combined treatment. One year later photocoagulation was performed, resulting in tumor inactivation and preservation of the eye, but with poor vision. There are no other reports of plaque therapy for hemangioma.

As far as we know, external beam irradiation for choroidal hemangiomas was first used in the Clinic for Radiotherapy in Essen (ALBERTI et al. 1983; GREBER et al. 1984; ALBERTI 1986). Between 1977 and 1984, 21 patients (22 eyes) were irradiated, 16 of whom presented with localized and 5 with diffuse involvement of the choroid (Table 9.1). All patients with circumscribed hemangiomas had decreased visual acuity. This was significant in 3 patients with amblyopia (2) or blindness (1) of the fellow eye. Two of 5 patients with Sturge-Weber syndrome presented with total retinal detachment, 1 of them with bilateral involvement. Total retinal detachment was present in 19 eyes. Two other eyes with solitary hemangiomas also had bullous retinal detachment. Secondary glaucoma was seen in 3 eyes in patients with Sturge-Weber syndrome.

Photocoagulation was considered to be too risky in some eyes because of total retinal detachment or involvement of or proximity to the optic disk or macula. Photocoagulation in lesions too close to the disk and macula may result in an irreversible

Table 9.1 Characteristics of 21 patients with choroidal hemangiomas who had irradiation treatment at the University of Essen between 1977 and 1984. (ALBERTI 1986)

Patients (total)	21 patients
Solitary hemangiomas	16 patients
Diffuse hemangiomas	5 patients
(Sturge-Weber syndrome)	(6 eyes involved)
Median age (years)	32 (7.5–60)
Male/female	18/3
Retinal detachment	
Partial	15 eyes
Complete	4 eyes
Secondary glaucoma	3 eyes
Impaired vision	22 eyes
Amblyopic fellow eye	2 patients
Blind fellow eye	1 patient

scotoma. In the past, these eyes were enucleated because of secondary glaucoma leading to a blind and
painful eye. Irradiation has been performed with ce-
sium-137 (8 eyes) and 5.7 MV photons (14 eyes) with
a temporal approach. The radiation beam was angled 10° posteriorly to spare the contralateral eye.
Total doses were 20 Gy (10 fractions, 2 weeks) in lesions without severe complications and 30 Gy (15
fractions, 3 weeks) in bullous retinal detachment
and absolute glaucoma. One patient with a suspected
melanoma received 42 Gy before the diagnosis of
hemangioma was established. At that time, patients
with centrally located choroidal melanomas in a
single functional eye and patients who refused
enucleation and could not be treated with a
radioactive plaque were irradiated using linac
photons (BORNFELD et al. 1983).

Results of irradiation were quite favorable in our
series (Table 9.2). All eyes were preserved.
Ultrasonography showed regression in all tumors.
Visual acuity improved in 8 eyes and was
unchanged in 7. In 7 eyes vision decreased: 5 of
them showed tumor-related maculopathy at the
time of diagnosis. The retina reattached in all 19
involved eyes. Reattachment in limited retinal
detachments occurred within a few weeks after
treatment, as against several months in eyes with
extensive retinal detachment (so-called bullous
retinal detachment up to the posterior pole of the
lens). The median follow-up was 24 months (range
12–108 months).

One of the patients, a 12-year-old boy with
Sturge-Weber syndrome, was referred to our clinic
for removal of a painful, glaucomatous eye. The
cause of the elevated intraocular pressure (50
mmHg) was a large diffuse hemangioma of the
posterior choroid with a maximal elevation of
about 7 mm (Fig. 9.3) and a complete exudative

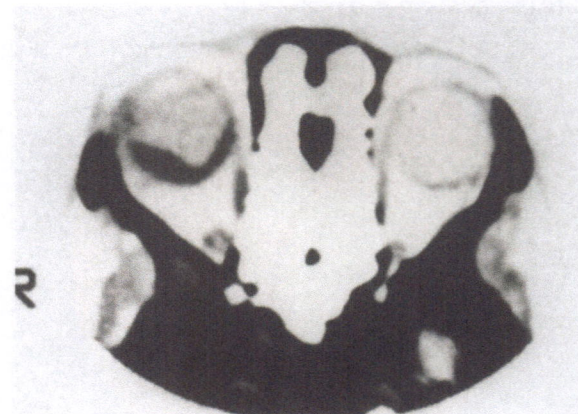

Fig. 9.3. CT scan of a diffuse choroidal hemangioma (Sturge-Weber syndrome) of the right eye of a 12-year-old boy before radiation therapy. The tumor at the posterior pole is shown by contrast enhancement. Exudative retinal detachment results in a higher density of the right eye than in the left. (ALBERTI et al. 1987)

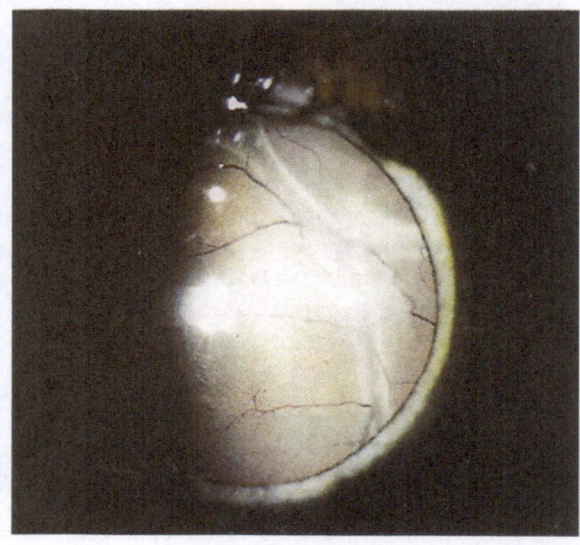

Fig. 9.4. Slit-lamp photograph of the same patient as in Fig. 9.3. Exudative, bullous retinal detachment up to the posterior pole of the lens (GREBER et al. 1984)

retinal detachment (Fig. 9.4). The eye was
irradiated with cesium-137 through a temporal
field with 30 Gy (15 fractions, 3 weeks). At the end
of external beam irradiation, intraocular pressure
had decreased to 26 mmHg. Seven weeks after
treatment the retina had partially reattached (Fig.
9.5) and intraocular pressure had normalized (10
mmHg). One year after irradiation the retina was
completely reattached, and a flat, pigmented
chorioretinal scar was visible (Fig. 9.6). Vision
improved from light perception without projection

Table 9.2. Clinical results after irradiation of 21 patients (22 treated eyes) between 1977 and 1984 at the University of Essen. (Alberti 1986)

Findings	No. of eyes
Preservation of eyes	22/22
Tumor regression	22/22
Retinal reattachment	19/19
Visual acuity	
Improved	8/22
No change	7/22
Impaired	7/22
Secondary glaucoma improved (Sturge-Weber syndrome)	3/3

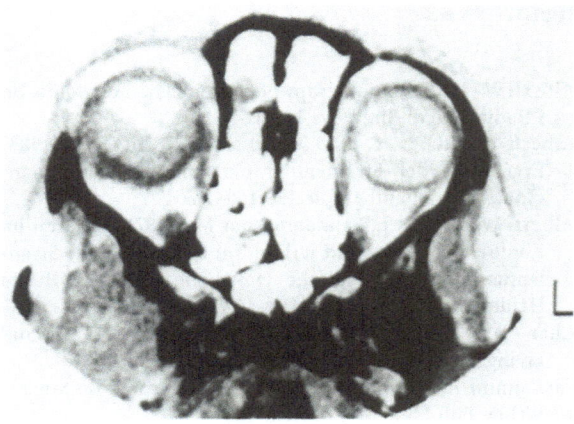

Fig. 9.5. Same patient as in Figs. 9.3 and 9.4. CT 7 weeks after radiation therapy. Retina is partially reattached (ALBERTI et al. 1987)

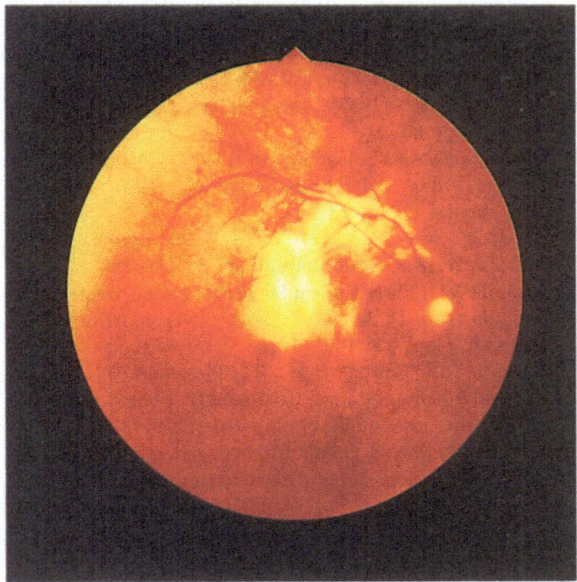

Fig. 9.6. Same patient as in Figs. 9.3–9.5. Flat pigmented chorioretinal scar 1 year after external beam therapy with 30 Gy (15 fractions, 3 weeks). Retina is completely reattached (GREBER et al. 1984)

to light perception with projection (GREBER et al. 1984). Ten years later the intraocular pressure remains normal and the retina is still attached.

ZOGRAFOS et al. (1998) reported a large series of choroidal hemangiomas (54 eyes in 53 patients) treated with proton beam irradiation in a dose range of 16.4–27.3 Gy in four daily fractions. Forty-seven eyes received 16.4–18.2 Gy, 3 received 22.7 Gy, and 4 received 27.3 Gy. There were 48 circumscribed hemangiomas and 6 diffuse hemangiomas in patients with Sturge-Weber syndrome.

The retina reattached within 6 months in all 54 eyes and remained stable during a follow-up period of 6 months to 9 years. Of 31 eyes treated with 16.4–18.2 Gy and followed up for more than 1 year, visual acuity improved in 22 eyes and was unchanged in 9 eyes. Although there was more rapid tumor resolution with higher doses, optic neuropathy developed in all 4 eyes receiving 27.2 Gy and retinal telangiectasia in 1 of the 3 eyes receiving 22.7 Gy. The authors recommend 16.4–18.2 Gy in four daily fractions, given as early as possible, in hemangiomas producing symptoms.

SCHILLING et al. (1997) reported a large series of 51 symptomatic eyes (48 patients) with both circumscribed (36 eyes) and diffuse angiomas (15 eyes) treated with linear accelerator photons (20 Gy/ 10 fractions over 2 weeks) and followed up for 4.5–5.3 years. There was complete resolution of subretinal fluid in 23 eyes and residual serous detachment distal to the fovea in 13 eyes in the circumscribed hemangioma group. Visual acuity improved in 14 eyes, stabilized in 14 and decreased in 8 eyes. Similar results were found in the diffuse hemangioma group. The improvement in vision was inversely related to the interval between onset of symptoms and referral for treatment. However, there was a late deterioration of visual acuity after initial improvement attributable to formation of subretinal fibrosis involving the fovea, and secondary glaucoma in those with Sturge-Weber syndrome. In the case of total retinal detachment, radiotherapy will not restore vision but may allow preservation of the eye (PLOWMAN and HUNGERFORD 1997).

MADREPERLA et al. (1997) reported a retrospective series of 23 patients with circumscribed choroidal hemangioma (CCH) treated with photocoagulation (13), plaque brachytherapy (8), and external beam irradiation (EBRT) (2), and 5 patients with diffuse choroidal hemangioma (DCH) treated with external beam therapy. At 1 year, subretinal fluid had resolved in 8 of 8, 6 of 13, and 1 of 2 of the CCH patients treated by plaque brachytherapy, photocoagulation, and EBRT, respectively, and in all 5 DCH patients. Visual acuity at 1 year was 6/12 or better for 6 of the 8 plaqued patients, 5 of 13 photocoagulation patients and neither of the 2 EBRT patients. Acuity improved in 2 and stabilized in 3 of the DCH patients. The authors concluded that plaque brachytherapy was effective for circumscribed hemangiomas, and external beam therapy for Sturge-Weber diffuse-type lesions.

MADREPERLA (2001) has recently reported on three patients treated with photodynamic therapy using verteporfin. Subretinal fluid resolved within 2 weeks; fluorescein angiography showed no leakage, the tumor flattened, and visual acuity improved in all. There were no complications and the average follow-up was 5.3 months.

9.4
Conclusions

With binocular ophthalmoscopy, fluorescein angiography, ultrasonography, and thin-section CT, the diagnosis of a circumscribed choroidal hemangioma can be established with high accuracy. Diagnosis of the diffuse type is easy because of the associated Sturge-Weber syndrome.

Management depends on the size and site of the tumor and on accompanying tumor-related complications. The treatment of choice for circumscribed lesions is photocoagulation according to MEYER-SCHWICKERATH. In eyes with extensive retinal detachment coagulation treatment is not possible, and in the case of hemangiomas close to the optic disk or macula it may cause an irreversible scotoma. In diffuse hemangiomas involving more than half of the choroid photocoagulation is less successful. In these cases, lens-sparing external beam irradiation with 20–30 Gy (10–15 fractions 2–3 weeks), proton beam therapy, or plaque brachytherapy is indicated. More experience and longer follow-up will determine the place of photodynamic therapy. In my experience (Alberti), eyes can be preserved, even those with massive glaucoma and extensive retinal detachment. Vision can be improved or stabilized if the fovea is not involved by the disease. In young patients, the hazard of radiation exposure must be weighed against the benefits to be achieved, namely preservation of the eye and possible improvement in vision. This is especially important in the case of single functional single eyes, when the fellow eye is amblyopic or blind, and in cases of bilateral diffuse hemangiomas. Because of the good long-term results reported by ALBERTI (1986), ALBERTI et al. (1987), ZOGRAFOS et al. (1998), SCHILLING et al. (1997), MADREPERLA et al. (1997), and PLOWMAN and HUNGERFORD (1997), we continue to recommend low-dose external beam therapy, in both circumscribed and diffuse hemangiomas, delivered with a lens-sparing technique.

References

Alberti W (1986) Radiotherapy of choroidal hemangioma. Int J Radial Oncol Biol Phys 12:122–123

Alberti W, Greber H, John V, Wessing A, Scherer E (1983) Ergebnisse der Strahlentherapie von Aderhauthämangiomen. Strahlentherapie 159:160–167

Alberti W, Halama J, Wannenmacher M (1987) Tumoren im Kopfbereich. Auge und Orbita. In: Scherer E (ed) Strahlentherapie. Radiologische Onkologie. Springer, Berlin Heidelberg New York, pp 412–467

Char DH (1989) Clinical ocular oncology. Churchill Livingstone, New York, pp 91–149

Giovannini A, Caponetti A (1984) Le syndrome de Sturge-Weber. Bull Mem SFO 95:484–487

Greber H, Wessing A, Alberti W, et al (1984) Die erfolgreiche Behandlung eines Aderhauthämangioms mit Sekundärveränderungen bei Sturge-Weber-Syndrom. Klin Monatsbl Augenheilkd 185:276–278

John V, Greber H, Alberti W (1983) Computertomographische Kontrastmittelstudien zum Nachweis und zur Therapiekontrolle angiomatoser Tumoren des Auges am Beispiel der okularen Manifestation des Morbus Sturge-Weber. Strahlentherapie 159:173–175

Lommatzsch PK (1989) Intraokulare Tumoren. Enke, Stuttgart, pp 80–86

Mackensen D, Meyer-Schwickerath G (1980) Diagnostik und Therapie des Aderhauthämangions. Klin Monatsbl Augenheilkd 177:16–23

MacLean AL, Maumenee AE (1959) Hemangioma of the choroid. Trans Am Ophthalmol Soc 57:171–194

Madreperla SA (2001) Choroidal hemangioma treated with photodynamic therapy using verteporfin. Arch Ophthalmology 119:1606–1610

Madreperla SA, Hungerford JL, Plowman PN (1997) Choroidal hemangiomas: treatment by photocoagulation or radiotherapy. Ophthalmology 104:1773–1778

Meyer-Schwickerath G (1956) Erfahrungen mit der Lichtkoagulation der Netzhaut und der Iris. Doc Ophthalmol 10:91

Norton EWD, Gutman F (1968) Fluorescein angiography and hemangiomas of the choroid. Mod Probl Ophthalmol 7:68–75

Ossoinig K (1974) Quantitative echography: the basis of tissue differentiation. J Clin Ultrasound 2:33–46

Plowman PN, Hungerford JL (1997) Radiotherapy for ocular angiomas. Br J Ophthalmol 81:258–259

Schilling H, Sauerwein W, Lommatzsch A, et al (1997) Long-term results after low dose ocular irradiation for choroidal hemangiomas. Br J Ophthalmol 81:267–273

Shields JA (1983) Diagnosis and management of intraocular tumors. Mosby, St Louis, pp 255–277

Wessing A (1977) Fluorescein angiography and the differential diagnosis of choroidal tumors. Bull Soc Belge Ophtalmol 175:5–14

Witschel H, Font RL (1976) Hemangioma of the choroid: a clinicopathologic study of 71 cases and a review of the literature. Surv Ophthalmol 20:415–431

Zografos L, Egger E, Bercher L, et al (1998) Proton beam irradiation of choroidal hemangiomas. Am J Ophthalmol 126:261–268

10 Radiation Therapy of Uveal and Orbital Metastases

S. B. RUDOLER, C. L. SHIELDS, J. A. SHIELDS

CONTENTS

10.1 Introduction

Metastatic deposits in every subsite of the eye and orbit have been described in the literature. It is now widely accepted that metastatic lesions are the most common intraocular malignancy (ELIASSI-RAD et al. 1996; FERRY and FONT 1974; SHIELDS et al. 1997b). Autopsy studies estimate the incidence at 4–12% in patients with solid tumors of all histologies, and greater than one third in breast cancer patients (BLOCH and GARTNER 1971; ELIASSI-RAD et al. 1996; FERRY and FONT 1974; NELSON et al. 1983). This chapter will exclude discussion of childhood cancers and ocular manifestations of systemic cancers such as lymphoma, leukemia and myeloma, focusing on metastatic disease from distant solid tumors.

S.B. RUDOLER, MD
Thomas Jefferson University, Bodine Center for Cancer Treatment, 111 S. 11th Street, Philadelphia, PA 19107-5098, USA
C.L. SHIELDS, MD; J.A. SHIELDS, MD
Thomas Jefferson University, Philadelphia and Ocular Oncology Service, Wills Eye Hospital, Ninth and Walnut Sts., Philadelphia, PA 19107, USA

10.2 Epidemiology

The overall incidence of metastases to the eye and orbit is difficult to quantify, since many patients may remain asymptomatic and succumb to their cancer before clinical detection of the ocular disease. However, with improvements in systemic therapy and general oncologic care, patients may be living longer with metastatic cancer and may, therefore, manifest intraocular and orbital metastases more frequently than in the past. For this reason, it is important to get a general sense of the extent of ocular spread of disease so that patients can be diagnosed and treated in a timely and effective manner.

A number of autopsy and prospective screening studies have shown an overall incidence of metastases to the eye in the range of 4–12%. BLOCH and GARTNER (1971) studied 230 cancer patients who were chosen randomly to undergo postmortem ocular examination, without prior history of clinical symptoms. They found the incidence of ocular involvement by distant solid primary tumor to be 12%. NELSON et al. (1983) studied at least one eye in every patient undergoing autopsy for cancer death over a 9-year period. Excluding patients with lymphoma or leukemia, 376 eyes were examined, with an overall incidence of ocular metastases of 4.0%. This figure might have been higher had both eyes been examined in all patients. In a prospective cohort of patients with disseminated breast cancer, WIEGEL et al. (1998) noted an overall incidence of asymptomatic choroidal metastases of 5% of all patients studied. The incidence rose dramatically to 11% in the subgroup of patients with more than one other site of known metastasis. At the Wilmer Institute (ELIASSI-RAD et al. 1996), postmortem examination was performed on eyes from 510 patients dying of carcinoma in the absence of clinical ocular symptoms. The incidence of intraocular metastases was 6.5% (5.1% microscopic, 1.4% gross).

Characteristics of patients with ocular metastases have been compiled from the data published by FERRY and Font (1974) and Shields et al. (1997b) and are shown in Table 10.1. The median age of patients is in the fifth and sixth decades of life. Ocular metastases are more commonly seen in female patients, since breast cancer is the primary tumor most likely to spread to the eye, followed by lung cancer. However, ocular metastases from nearly every type of solid tumor have been at least anecdotally reported. The most common subsite of metastatic deposits within the eye is in the posterior uveal tract, particularly in the choroid. Ferry and Font (1974) and Shields et al. (1997b) have published the most comprehensive report describing the clinical findings in patients with

uveal metastases (see Tables 10.1, 10.2). Metastases to every part of the eye and orbit have been described, however, including the anterior chamber, iris, conjunctiva, eyelid, lid, retina, optic disc, and orbit (Kiratli et al. 1996; Shields and Shields 1992, 1999; Shields et al. 1995, 1997b, 2000, 2001). Ocular metastases are bilateral in one third of patients, and are equally distributed in the right and left eyes (Bloch and Gartner 1971; Ferry and Font 1974; Shields et al. 1997b). Approximately 30% of patients have more than one metastatic deposit per eye (Shields et al. 1997b; Ferry and Font 1974). Presenting symptoms of uveal metastases are noted in Table 10.2 (Ferry and Font 1974; Shields et al. 1997b). They include blurred vision, loss of vision or a visual field deficit (70–80%), flashers or floaters (12%), pain (7–22%), and secondary glaucoma (4%). Secondary retinal detachment is frequently present with uveal metastases. Orbital metastases can present with pain, proptosis, and visual loss (Shields et al. 2001). Iris metastases can often present with uveitis or a visible mass (Shields et al. 1995). Interestingly, uveal metastases can become apparent before the primary tumor is recognized in 28–46% of patients (Shields et al. 1997b; Ferry and Font 1974).

Table 10.1. Characteristics of patients with uveal metastases

	Ferry and Font (1974)	Shields et al. (1997b)
Age, median (years)	53	58
Gender (%)		
Male	49	33
Female	51	67
Primary cancer (%)		
Breast	39.7	47
Lung	29.5	21
GI	3.5	4
Renal	4.0	2
Prostate	1.3	2
Sarcoma	0	<1
Skin melanoma	0	2
Unknown	18.3	17
Other	3.5	4
Sentinel finding (%)	46.3	34

Table 10.2. Characteristics of uveal and orbital metastases

	Ferry and Font (1974)	Shields et al. (1997b)
Site (%)		
Choroid/posterior segment	56.5	96
Iris/Anterior segment	18.6	8
Orbit	17.6	<1
Laterality (%)		
Unilateral	90	76
Bilateral	10	24
Involved eye (%)		
Right	38.8	48
Left	38.8	52
Presenting symptom		
Vision loss/field deficit	79.9	70
Flashers/floaters	0	12
Pain	22.4	7
Proptosis	11.4	0
Asymptomatic	0	11

10.3
Diagnosis and Workup

A careful history and ophthalmologic examination is generally sufficient to make the diagnosis of ocular metastasis. Complete ophthalmologic examination should include slit lamp examination, funduscopy, and ultrasonography. Detailed descriptions of the classic appearance of intraocular metastatic deposits to all ocular subsites have been published, and are summarized below (Kiratli et al. 1996; Shields and Shields 1992, 1999; Shields et al. 1995, 1997b, 2000, 2001). Choroidal metastases generally appear as creamy yellow subretinal masses, often with associated serous retinal detachment (Figs. 10.1, 10.2). Iris metastases are usually visualized as white or yellow, raised lesions, but may appear orange when the primary is lung carcinoid or renal cell carcinoma (Fig. 10.3). When primary cutaneous melanomas metastasize to the iris such metastases generally appear brown.

Classic ultrasonographic findings can usually differentiate choroidal metastases from primary choroidal melanomas (Sobottka and Kreissig 1999). These features include a combined pattern of high internal reflectivity and low height-to-base ratio. Other ultra-

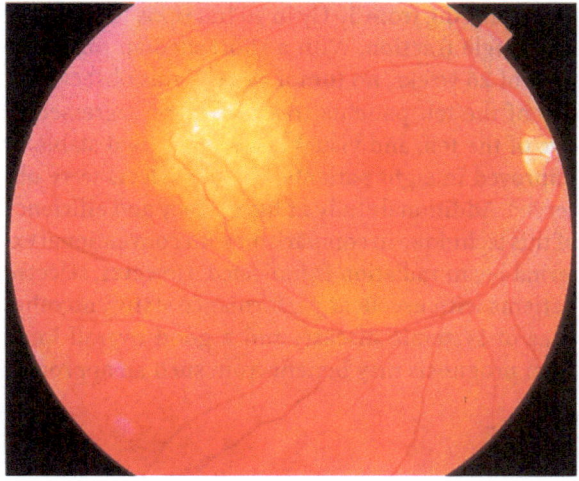

Fig. 10.1. Choroid metastasis from primary lung cancer in a 48-year-old woman. (Photo courtesy of Shields and associates, Ocular Oncology Service, Wills Eye Hospital, Philadelphia, Pennsylvania)

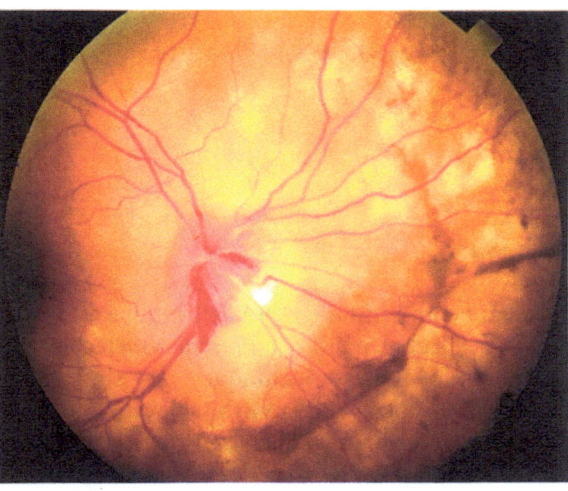

Fig. 10.2. Posterior uveal metastasis involving the optic disc in a 64-year-old man. (Photo courtesy of Shields and associates, Ocular Oncology Service, Wills Eye Hospital, Philadelphia, Pennsylvania)

sound features that are suggestive of, but not pathognomonic for, metastases include lack of spontaneous vascular movements, absence of choroidal excavation, and a plateau or domed shape rather than the mushroom shape that is typical of primary melanoma.

Computerized tomography or magnetic resonance imaging may be helpful in the case of orbital metastases. It is rare for a tissue diagnosis to be required, but this can be useful when the clinical findings and history do not allow the diagnosis. When the patient has no prior history of cancer, systemic workup should be performed to identify the primary and other sites of metastatic disease.

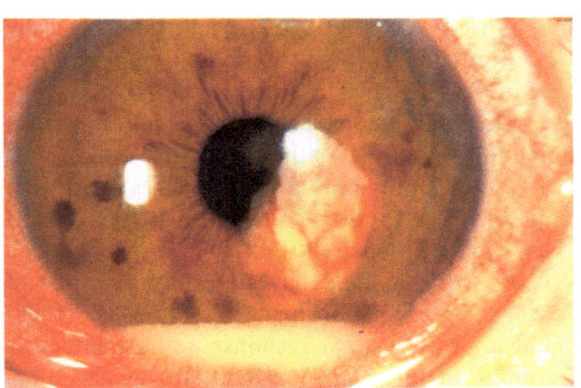

Fig. 10.3. This white, raised lesion is characteristic of carcinoma metastatic to the iris. (Photo courtesy of Shields and associates, Ocular Oncology Service, Wills Eye Hospital, Philadelphia, Pennsylvania)

10.4
General Management

The diagnosis of ocular metastases generally carries a poor prognosis. The median survival time from the date of ocular involvement is 9 months, with a reported range in the literature of 4–13 months (Chu et al. 1977; Jaeger et al. 1971; Maor et al. 1977; Mewis and Young 1982; Ratanatharathorn et al. 1991; Reddy et al. 1981; Rudoler et al. 1997b; Stephens and Shields 1999; Thatcher and Thomas 1975). These results vary depending on the primary diagnosis. For example, patients with breast cancer or carcinoid live longer, on average, than do patients with other malignancies. In addition, adult patients with orbital metastases, as opposed to intraocular metastases, may have a slightly prolonged median survival (McCormick and Harrison 1993). The overall goals of treatment of ocular and orbital metastases are palliative, the intention being to enhance patients' quality of life by improving or preserving vision and avoiding the development of a painful eye, which might require enucleation. Treatment options include observation, systemic therapy (chemotherapy and/or hormonal therapy), external beam radiotherapy, plaque radiotherapy, enucleation and, more recently, stereotactic radiotherapy.

10.5
Treatment Options and Results

10.5.1
External Beam Radiation Therapy

10.5.1.1
Techniques

External beam radiotherapy has been used for decades for effective palliation of ocular metastases in all subsites of the eye. Techniques vary slightly according to the intraocular or orbital location. General principles, however, emphasize respecting normal tissue tolerance of sensitive surrounding ocular structures when fashioning the treatment field. Lens-sparing techniques include right-angled wedged fields (BRADY et al. 1982), direct lateral field posterior to the lens, i.e., anterior margin at the outer canthus (BRADY et al. 1982; CHU et al. 1977; NYLEN et al. 1994), oblique lateral field with lens shielding (CHU et al. 1977; MAOR et al. 1977), and anterior field with lens block (CHU et al. 1977). Field sizes typically range from 3+3 cm to 5+5 cm. Radiation energies used in the past have included cobalt-60, megavoltage 4–15 MV photons, or 4- to 16-MeV electrons, depending upon the depth of the target volume.

The most commonly accepted doses are in the range of 30–40 Gy in 2- to 3-Gy fractions over 2–4 weeks. Some groups (CHU et al. 1977; MAOR et al. 1977; ROSSET et al. 1998) have described a significant dose–response relationship. ROSSET et al. (1998) found improved tumor response and visual acuity for doses higher than 35.5 Gy. CHU et al. (1977) recommended the biologic equivalent dose of 40 Gy in 15 fractions over 3 weeks for best results. MAOR et al. (1977) found doses below 30 Gy in 10 fractions to be inferior with regard to tumor control. Other studies failed to find any effect of dose on outcome (RUDOLER et al. 1997b).

Stereotactic radiotherapy is a specialized technique, which delivers highly focused external beam radiation to small immobilized targets, generally in single or hypofractionated high doses. Surrounding structures outside the three-dimensional target volume receive little or nothing of the radiation dose. While this technique has been widely used in the setting of intracranial malignancy and benign diseases such as arteriovenous malformations and acoustic neuromas, its application to the treatment of solitary, unilateral choroidal metastases is much more recent. In the only published study (BELLMANN et al. 2000) in which this technique was applied, patients received doses ranging from 30 Gy in 10 fractions to 12–20 Gy in a single fraction. With a short median follow-up time of 26 weeks, no tumor growth was observed in any of the ten patients treated; tumor regressed in five of the ten, and visual acuity remained stable or improved in eight patients. No side effects were observed. Additional study of the efficacy and efficiency of this technique in comparison with conventional external beam radiation is indicated. However, selected patients with excellent performance status, no other sites of systemic disease, and a good overall long-term prognosis may benefit from such an approach.

10.5.1.2
Results

Radiotherapy for ocular metastases is purely palliative, the relevant endpoints being restoration and preservation of vision, tumor control, and globe preservation. Overall survival is not affected by this treatment, as patients with ocular and orbital metastases generally have a poor prognosis with a median survival in the range of 9 months. Results of radiotherapy reported in the literature are compiled and referenced in Table 10.3. To summarize, the overall response rate for this tumor is generally in the range of 80–85%. Vision is improved in 33–89% of cases, depending upon the report. Globe preservation is 98–100%.

RUDOLER et al. (1997b) defined preradiotherapy prognostic factors to predict the group of patients with posterior uveal metastases who would be most likely to benefit from radiotherapy. Patients younger than 55 years of age, with tumors smaller than 15 mm and preradiotherapy visual acuity better than 20/60, were statistically significantly more likely to achieve and maintain the highest level of functional vision. The authors therefore recommend early intervention for all patients with symptomatic uveal lesions, unless there is superseding rapid systemic deterioration.

10.5.1.3
Sequelae

Vision loss, blindness, and intractable pain requiring enucleation can be psychosocially devastating to patients with a short expected life span. Therefore, palliative treatment of ocular metastases should not diminish patients' quality of life by causing ocular complications leading to vision loss or acute symptoms necessitating enucleation. Acute and late effects of radiotherapy

Table 10.3. Results of external beam radiotherapy for uveal metastases

Reference	No. of eyes treated	Overall response (%)	Vision improvement (%)	Globe preservation (%)
JAEGER et al. (1971)	21	33	33	NR
ORENSTEIN et al. (1972)	7	86	43	NR
THATCHER and THOMAS (1975)	57	80	80	100
CHU et al. (1977)	57	63	63	NR
MAOR et al. (1977)	62	NR	89	NR
REDDY et al. (1981)	10	80	70	NR
MEWIS and YOUNG (1982)	52	NR	26.9	NR
BRADY et al. (1982)	93	88.9	NR	NR
RATANATHARATHORN et al. (1991)	17	NR	71.5	NR
NYLEN et al. (1994)	21	82	81	NR
RUDOLER et al. (1997b)	233	83	57	98
Rosset et al. (1998)	78	82	62	99

to sensitive eye structures must be balanced against the overall efficacy of treatment.

The most common and most extensively documented complication of radiation to the eye is cataract formation (BRAY et al. 1991; CHAO et al. 1995; DEEG et al. 1984; MERRIAM and FOCHT 1957; RUDOLER et al. 1997a; SAGERMAN 1993). Other possible sequelae of radiation include radiation retinopathy, optic neuropathy, exposure keratopathy (or dry eye syndrome), neovascularization, and narrow-angle glaucoma (BROWN et al. 1982; PARSONS et al. 1994; VIEBAHN et al. 1991; WARA et al. 1979; ZAMBER and KINYOUN 1992).

RUDOLER et al. (1997a) analyzed 233 eyes that had received external beam radiotherapy for uveal metastases with standard doses of 30.0–40.0 Gy in 2.0- to 3.0-Gy fractions. Only 12% of eyes developed one or more significant radiation complication. These included cataracts (16 eyes), radiation retinopathy (6 eyes), optic neuropathy (5 eyes), exposure keratopathy (5 eyes), and neovascularization of the iris (4 eyes). Two eyes developed acute narrow-angle glaucoma, and one of these required enucleation. Univariate analysis failed to show any predisposition to complications based on biologic effective radiation dose, energy type, or concurrent systemic therapy. Interestingly, there was no difference in the incidence of complications, including cataract formation, between patients treated with lens-sparing techniques and those who received treatment to the whole globe. The authors concluded that the known benefits of vision and globe preservation after palliative external beam radiation therapy outweigh the very small risk that radiation-induced complications will be manifest during the patients' short expected life span.

10.5.2
Plaque Radiotherapy

Brachytherapy utilizing a radioactive plaque applied directly to a solitary lesion can be an excellent treatment choice in selected patients. Potential candidates for plaque placement include patients who have a solitary choroidal, ciliary body or iris lesion and controlled systemic disease, and are medically fit enough to undergo an operative procedure (SHIELDS et al. 1997a). Patients who have failed external beam treatment may also benefit from this approach, in lieu of enucleation. Tumor thickness and location in relation to the optic disc and foveola are also important in determining an individual patient's eligibility for plaque placement. Iodine-125 is the most common radioactive source in use today, with lead or gold shields used to protect deep structures. The typical dose is 40 Gy over 2–4 days (SHIELDS et al. 1997a).

SHIELDS et al. (1997a) have reported the results of plaque radiotherapy for choroidal metastases. Thirty-six patients with uveal metastases were treated as described above. It is noteworthy that one fourth of the patients had failed on other methods of treatment previously. Complete tumor response was seen in 94% of patients. Vision improved or remained stable in 58%, and complications were seen in only 8%. The authors conclude that plaque radiotherapy can be a highly effective treatment in selected patients with refractory disease or solitary uveal metastases.

10.5.3
Systemic Therapy

Chemotherapy and/or hormonal therapy are often used in patients with systemic or recurrent disease, and will also concurrently act on an eye lesion. The specific choice of chemotherapy or hormonal therapy is determined by the underlying primary disease. Definitive response rates of ocular metastases to systemic therapy alone are not well documented in the literature, but are thought to mirror response rates of metastatic disease elsewhere in the body (NELSON et al. 1983). However, in one report, MEWIS and YOUNG (1982) describe studying a subgroup of patients with choroidal metastases from breast cancer whose ocular disease was observed during systemic therapy. Vision remained stable in 71.4%, and improved by two lines or more on the Snellen chart in 7.1%. In the reported experience of BRADY et al. (1982), about 50% of observed lesions remained stable while the patients are receiving chemotherapy. Systemic therapy is often given concurrently with local radiotherapy to the eye, with no increased risk of complications (RUDOLER et al. 1997a).

10.5.4
Observation

Close follow-up, in the absence of active treatment, may be appropriate in selected patients with clinically inactive ocular tumors, or in patients with very poor performance status and rapid deterioration. The risk of this approach is that growth of the metastatic deposit(s) may cause vision loss or angle-closure glaucoma with resultant significant pain, requiring enucleation.

10.6
Conclusions

In summary, ocular and orbital metastases are relatively common, usually occur in the setting of advanced disease, and can result in blindness or pain, or possibly lead to enucleation. Treatment with external beam radiotherapy, plaque radiotherapy, and/or systemic therapy can effectively and safely prevent

these outcomes, which impact negatively on patients' quality of life. The best palliative responses are seen in patients with smaller tumors and only limited visual impairment prior to treatment. Therefore, oncologists and ophthalmologists should be aggressive in diagnosing ocular and orbital metastases. Early intervention is indicated for all patients with symptomatic lesions, unless rapid systemic deterioration supervenes.

References

Bellmann C, Fuss M, Holz FG et al (2000) Stereotactic radiation therapy for malignant choroidal tumors. Ophthalmology 107:358–365

Bloch RS, Gartner S (1971) The incidence of ocular metastatic carcinoma. Arch Ophthal 85:673–675

Brady LW, Shields JA, Augsburger JJ et al (1982) Malignant intraocular tumors. Cancer 49:578–585

Bray LC, Carey PJ, Proctor SJ et al (1991) Ocular complications of bone marrow transplantation. Br J Ophthal 75:611–614

Brown GC, Shields JA, Sanborn G et al (1982) Radiation retinopathy. Ophthalmology 89:1494–1501

Chao CKS, Lin H, Devineni VR et al (1995) Radiation therapy for primary orbital lymphoma. Int J Radiat Oncol Biol Phys 31:929–934

Chu FCH, Huh SH, Nisce LZ et al (1977) Radiation therapy of choroid metastasis from breast cancer. Int J Radiat Oncol Biol Phys 2:273–279

Deeg HJ, Flournoy N, Sullivan KM et al (1984) Cataracts after total body irradiation and marrow transplantation: a sparing effect of dose fractionation. Int J Radiat Oncol Biol Phys 10:957–964

Eliassi-Rad B, Albert DM, Green WR (1996) Frequency of ocular metastases in patients dying of cancer in eye bank populations. Br J Ophthalmol 80:125–128

Ferry AP, Font RL (1974) Carcinoma metastatic to the eye and orbit. A clinicopathologic study of 227 cases. Arch Ophthalmol 92:276–286

Jaeger EA, Frayer WC, Southard ME et al (1971) Effect of radiation therapy on metastatic choroidal tumors. Trans Am Acad Ophthalmol Otol 75:94–101

Kiratli H, Shields CL, Shields JA et al (1996) Metastatic tumours to the conjunctiva: report of 10 cases. Br J Ophthalmol 80:5–8

Maor M, Chan RC, Young SE (1977) Radiotherapy of choroidal metastases. Breast cancer as primary site. Cancer 40:2081–2086

McCormick B, Harrison LB (1993) Radiation therapy for orbital metastases. In: Alberti WE, Sagerman RH (eds) (1993) Radiotherapy of intraocular and orbital tumors, 1st edn. (Medical radiology – diagnostic imaging and radiation oncology) Springer, Berlin Heidelberg New York, pp 187–189

Merriam GR, Focht EF (1957) A clinical study of radiation cataracts and the relationship to dose. AJR Am J Roentgenol 77:759–785

Mewis L, Young SE (1982) Breast carcinoma metastatic to the choroid. Analysis of 67 patients. Ophthalmology 89:147–151

Nelson CC, Hertzberg BS, Klintworth GK (1983) A histopathologic study of 716 unselected eyes in patients with cancer at the time of death. Am J Ophthalmol 95:788–793

Nylen U, Kock E, Lax I et al (1994) Standardized precision radiotherapy in choroidal metastases. Acta Oncol 33:65–68

Orenstein MM, Anderson DP, Stein JJ (1972) Choroid metastasis. Cancer 29:1101–1107

Parsons JT, Bova FJ, Fitzgerald CR et al (1994) Radiation retinopathy after external-beam irradiation: analysis of time-dose factors. Int J Radiat Oncol Biol Phys 30:765–773

Ratanatharathorn V, Powers WE, Grimm J et al (1991) Eye metastasis from carcinoma of the breast: diagnosis, radiation treatment and results. Cancer Treat Rev 18:261–276

Reddy S, Saxena VS, Hendrickson F et al (1981) Malignant metastatic disease of the eye: management of an uncommon complication. Cancer 47:810–812

Rosset A, Zografos L, Coucke P et al (1998) Radiotherapy of choroidal metastases. Radiother Oncol 46:263–268

Rudoler SB, Corn BW, Shields CL et al (1997a) External beam irradiation for choroid metastases: identification of factors predisposing to long-term sequelae. Int J Radiat Oncol Biol Phys 38:251–256

Rudoler SB, Shields CL, Corn BW et al (1997b) Functional vision is improved in the majority of patients treated with external beam radiotherapy for choroid metastases: a multivariate analysis of 188 patients. J Clin Oncol 15:1244–1251

Sagerman RH (1993) Radiation-induced cataracts: simple but difficult to quantify. Int J Radiat Oncol Biol Phys 26:713–714

Shields JA, Shields CL (1992) Intraocular tumors: a text and atlas. Saunders, Philadelphia

Shields JA, Shields CL (1999) Atlas of intraocular tumors. Lippincott / Williams and Wilkins, Philadelphia, pp 152–164

Shields JA, Shields CL, Kiratli H et al (1995) Metastatic tumors to the iris in 40 patients. Am J Ophthalmology 119:422–430

Shields CL, Shields JA, DePotter P et al (1997a) Plaque radiotherapy in the management of uveal metastasis. Arch Ophthalmol 115:203–209

Shields CL, Shields JA, Gross NE et al (1997b) Survey of 520 eyes with uveal metastases. Ophthalmology 104:1265–1276

Shields JA, Shields CL, Singh AD (2000) Metastatic neoplasms in the optic disc (the 1999 Bjerrum Lecture, part 2). Arch Ophthalmol 118:217–224

Shields JA, Shields CL, Brotman HK et al (2001) Cancer metastatic to the orbit (the 2000 Robert M. Curts Lecture). Ophthal Plast Reconstr Surg 7:343–354

Sobottka B, Kreissig I (1999) Ultrasonography of metastases and melanomas of the choroid. Curr Opin Ophthalmol 10:164–167

Stephens RF, Shields JA (1979) Diagnosis and management of cancer metastatic to the uvea: a study of 70 cases. Ophthalmology 86:1336–1349

Thatcher N, Thomas PRM (1975) Choroidal metastases from breast carcinoma: a survey of 42 patients and the use of radiation therapy. Clin Radiol 26:549–553

Viebahn M, Barricks ME, Osterloh MD (1991) Synergism between diabetic and radiation retinopathy: case report and review. Br J Ophthalmol 75:629–632

Wara WM, Irvine AR, Neger RE et al (1979) Radiation retinopathy. Int J Radiat Oncol Biol Phys 5:81–83

Wiegel T, Kreusel KM, Bornfeld N et al (1998) Frequency of asymptomatic choroidal metastasis in patients with disseminated breast cancer: results of a prospective screening program. Br J Ophthalmol 82:1159–1161

Zamber RW, Kinyoun JL (1992) Radiation retinopathy. West J Med 157:530–533

11 Diagnosis and Management of Retinoblastoma

Winfried E. Alberti and Robert H. Sagerman

CONTENTS

11.1
General Aspects

Although retinoblastoma accounts for only 1 % of all childhood malignancies, it has been studied intensively because of its genetic features, the association with chromosomal deletions, and the known predisposition of children with retinoblastoma to develop other nonocular malignant tumors.

This chapter discusses the clinical features, diagnosis, and treatment of retinoblastoma. It is based partly upon the published experiences from New York City, Essen, and Utrecht, and partly upon the authors' experience.

11.2
Introduction

Retinoblastoma was described as early as 1597 by PETRUS PAWINUS, Professor of Anatomy at the University of Leiden. In 1809, JAMES WARDRUP called the tumor "fungus haematodes" and advocated enucleation of the eye as a life-saving measure. Enucleation became possible with the development of chloroform anesthesia in the middle of the nineteenth century. In 1864, RUDOLF VIRCHOW identified the tumor and named it "glioma of the retina," considering the tumor to be of glial origin. FLEXNER (1891) and WINTERSTEINER (1894) described the classical rosettes which are apparent in many retinoblastomas and named the tumor "neuroepithelioma" because of the close resemblance of the tumor cells to the rods and cones. In 1922, VERHOEFF proposed the term "retinoblastoma," indicating its origin from primitive retinoblasts. This term is now generally accepted. Investigations by KYRITSIS et al. (1984) using immunofluorescence to search for the presence of a neuronal marker, neuron-specific enolase, and a glial marker in retinoblastoma cells support the notion that retinoblastoma originates from a primitive neuroectodermal cell.

11.3
Incidence

Retinoblastoma is the most common tumor of the eye in children. The worldwide incidence of retinoblastoma is remarkably constant, ranging from 1 in 15 000 to 1 in 30 000 live births (MACKLIN 1960; DEVESA 1975; SCHIPPER 1980; SHIELDS and

W. E. ALBERTI, MD
Professor, Radiologische Klinik, Abteilung für Strahlentherapie und Radiooncologie, Universitäts-Klinikum, Hamburg-Eppendorf, Martinistrasse 52, 20246 Hamburg, Germany
R. H. SAGERMAN, MD, FACR
Professor in the Department of Radiation Oncology at the State University of New York, Upstate Medical University, 750 East Adams Street, Syracuse, NY 13210, USA

AUGSBURGER 1981; AMERICAN CANCER SOCIETY 1983; WINTHER et al. 1988). An increase in the last generation has been attributed to the better life expectancy of patients with the germinal mutation, allowing them to mature and bear children, and to more complete and accurate registration of new cases.

Retinoblastoma shows no predilection for sex or race. The tumor occurs bilaterally in 25%–30% of all cases. Bilateral disease is diagnosed earlier than unilateral disease. In the Essen series of 580 patients, the tumor was detected at a median age of 11 months in bilateral cases and 20 months in unilateral cases. About 47.8% of the unilateral (97/203) cases presented within the first 2 years of life, whereas 315 of the 377 bilateral cases (83.6%) were diagnosed within the same interval. Only 28 tumors were detected after the fifth year. Eight patients were older than 10 years when diagnosed (HEINRICH 1989).

Children born to parents successfully treated for retinoblastoma should be examined in the first few days after birth; if no tumors are seen, examination under general anesthesia should occur at 1-month intervals for the first 6 months, every 2 months to 1 year of age, and at 3-month intervals for the next 2 years.

11.4
Heredity

Retinoblastoma occurs in hereditary and non-hereditary forms. Nearly 10% of affected children appear as familial cases. Seven percent of unilateral and 22% of bilateral cases have a family history of retinoblastoma (HOPPING et al. 1985a).

Approximately 90% of all cases have no family history of retinoblastoma. In these cases, the gene may be acquired by a new mutation. About 80% of these sporadic cases have a somatic mutation, which means that family members are not at increased risk of retinoblastoma. The remaining 20% of the sporadic cases have a germinal mutation and can pass the disease to their children.

The hereditary and nonhereditary types of retinoblastoma present distinctive characteristics. The nonhereditary type accounts for approximately 60% of all cases (Knudson 1971). These children have unilateral and unifocal disease, i.e., one focus in one eye. In the other 40% of cases (including patients with new germinal mutations) either a positive family history of retinoblastoma exists or both eyes are affected. About 12% of children with unilateral disease have a positive family history and these cases belong to the heredi-

tary category (VOGEL 1979). The genetic form of the disease shows an autosomal dominant inheritance pattern with high penetrance of about 80%. In approximately 5% of patients, a deletion of the long arm of chromosome 13 has been observed (SPARKES et al. 1983). These children can suffer from multiple congenital abnormalities such as growth retardation, motor and mental retardation, and craniofacial dysmorphism and have a high incidence of secondary neoplasms (HOWARD 1982; MOTEGI et al. 1983).

KNUDSEN (1971) proposed that at least two independent events were necessary for a retinal cell to develop into retinoblastoma. In the hereditary form, the first mutation is germinal and is followed by the second occurring in the somatic retinal cell. This hypothesis accounts for the multicentricity and earlier development of hereditary retinoblastoma in one or both eyes, as well as the older age of patients with unilateral, non hereditary disease, in whom two events must take place in a single retinal cell. Genetic counseling is essential if there is a positive family history or hereditable disease.

11.5
Clinical Features

11.5.1
Local Tumor Growth Pattern and Related Disorders

Retinoblastomas show characteristics caused by the tumor itself and by the surrounding tissues. Fragments of the tumor can break free and cause vitreous seeding. These spheroids are rarely greater than 1 mm (FOLKMANN 1974), but may settle on parts of the retina or uveal tract and grow as separate tumor foci. They may localize around the primary tumor focus or disseminate throughout the vitreous and into the anterior chamber. Most eyes with diffuse vitreous seeding cannot be salvaged because radiation therapy and chemotherapy are less effective.

Retinoblastomas may grow in two ways. Endophytic retinoblastoma grows from the inner surface of the retina into the vitreous. As the tumor becomes larger, there is a tendency to produce seeding into the vitreous cavity (Fig. 11.1). Exophytic tumors grow from the retina into the sub retinal space, frequently causing an extensive retinal detachment.

There is a third, rarer type of growth: retinoblastoma diffusely growing over the entire retina without exophytic or endophytic signs. Schipper

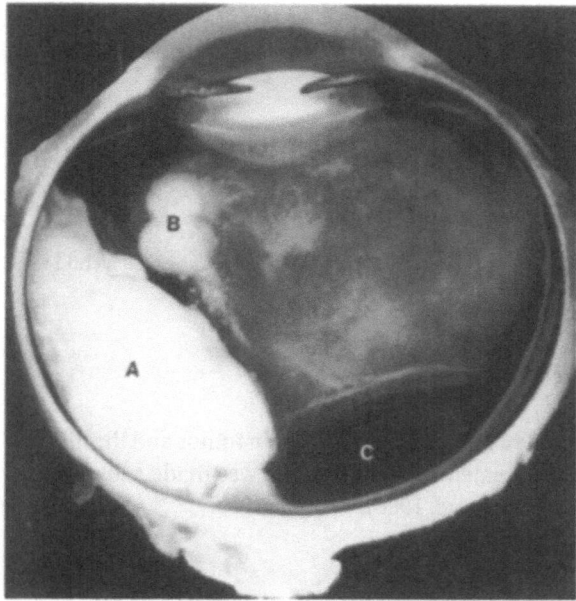

Fig. 11.1. Cross-section of an eye with retinoblastoma. *A*, tumor; *B*, seeding; *C*, retinal detachment caused by fixation. (ALBERTI et al. 1987; by courtesy of Dr. E.P. MESSMER, Zürich)

(personal communication, 1992) has seen two such cases, which were diagnosed at the age of 4–5 years.

Extraocular extension of retinoblastoma is rare and is seen particularly due to late diagnosis in countries where medical care is underdeveloped. Invasion of the optic nerve is more common in advanced lesions, especially in those arising close to the disk. Survival is excellent for retinoblastoma confined to the retina but the prognosis worsens when optic nerve, scleral, and deep choroidal invasion is present.

11.5.2
Distant Metastases

Intracranial involvement usually occurs via direct spread along the optic nerve or subarachnoid space, via choroidal invasion along the emissary vessels, or by direct extension through the sclera (CARBAJAL 1959). Advanced disease follows these routes to the orbit, skull, brain or via lymphatics. Hematogenous metastases can be found in bone, liver, lung, and other sites (CARBAJAL 1959; STANNARD et al. 1979). In the Essen series, most metastases were seen within 5 years after diagnosis of retinoblastoma (HEINRICH 1989). Fortyone patients (7%) developed metastases; among these were 33/377 (8.7%) with bilateral and 8/203 (3.7%) with unilateral disease. The median in-

terval between diagnosis of retinoblastoma and metastases was 7 months in unilateral and 24 months in bilateral disease. Two-thirds of all metastases and all of those in patients with unilateral retinoblastoma were present within 2 years after diagnosis. The median latency to metastasis was 5.5 months in patients in whom the optic nerve was involved, compared with 11 months for those without involvement at the cut end of the nerve. Eleven of 16 metastases occurring within 1 year after diagnosis were associated with invasion of the optic nerve whereas in ten patients with metastases within the fourth year, no invasion of the optic nerve could be diagnosed. In the literature, the mean interval between diagnosis of retinoblastoma and occurrence of distant metastases has been reported as 5.5 months (CARBAJAL 1959), 23 months (MERRIAM 1950), and 12 months (MCKAY et al. 1984). The prognosis of children with metastatic disease is dismal and most die within 12 months (MERRIAM 1950; CARBAJAL 1959; MCKAY et al. 1984). Thirty-three of 41 patients (80%) with metastases in the Essen series died due to intracranial tumor progression. Only a few patients have been reported as having had a long period of survival after treatment for metastatic disease (STANNARD et al. 1979; FREEMAN et al. 1980; JUDISCH et al. 1980).

Occasionally, late distant metastases can be difficult to distinguish histologically from second nonocular malignancies, even with immunohistochemical study (DONOSO et al. 1981).

11.5.3
Spontaneous Regression

Spontaneous regression of retinoblastoma was first reported by KNIEPER (1911). The regressed tumors resemble retinoblastoma controlled by radiotherapy, presenting a calcified mass surrounded by translucent tissue and a chorioretinal scar. The terms „retinoma" (GALLIE et al. 1982) and "retinocytoma" (MARGO et al. 1983) have been proposed for this apparently benign process whose pathogenesis is unclear. Clinically, spontaneous regression occurs in two forms: large regressed retinoblastoma may produce ocular phthisis causing a blind eye and requiring enucleation, while visual acuity may not be impaired when there are small regressed lesions. These retinomas are frequently detected when apparently normal parents of children with retinoblastoma are examined.

BONIUK and ZIMMERMAN (1962) reported 14 such patients; unilateral disease with a phthisic eye was present in six cases, while in eight bilateral cas-

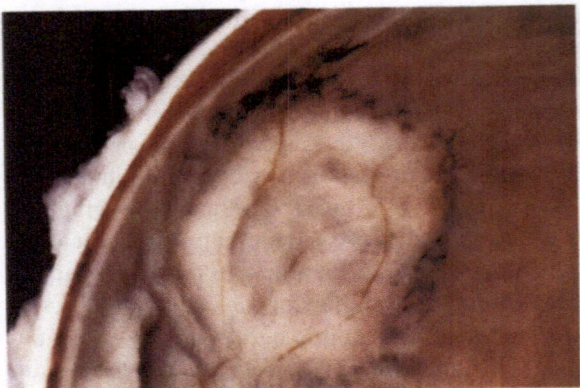

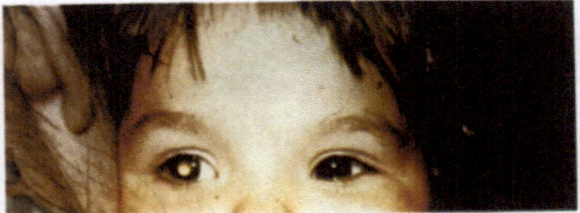

Fig. 11.3. Unilateralleukocoria (cat's eye reflex) in a child with retinoblastoma

Fig. 11.2. Low-power photomicrograph of a retinoma diagnosed 43.5 years after enucleation of the blind fellow eye. The patient developed small cell lung cancer at age 55. (MESSMER et al. 1987; by courtesy of Dr. E.P. MESSMER, Zürich)

es, spontaneous regression was observed in one eye and a viable tumor in the other. KHODADOUST et al. (1977) reviewed 50 cases with spontaneous regression; 43 were bilateral with regression in both eyes and seven were unilateral.

In 580 patients with retinoblastoma treated between 1959 and 1985 in Essen, the incidence of spontaneous regression was about 1 % (HAVERS et al. 1986), which corresponds to the findings of other authors (REESE 1976; GALLIE et al. 1982). In one of these patients, a retinoma was diagnosed in one eye (Fig. 11.2) when the diagnosis of bilateral retinoblastoma was established in his son. This 47-year-old man had undergone enucleation of the blind fellow eye when 3.5 years old. He developed small cell lung cancer at age 55 and died from extensive metastatic disease. Neuroectodermal cells were noted in the area of the scar at autopsy (MESSMER et al. 1987).

Because retinoma may be a benign manifestation of the retinoblastoma gene (CONOLLY et al. 1983), it carries the same significance for genetic Gounseling as retinoblastoma. This is also true if retinoma is considered a spontaneous regression of a developed tumor.

11.5.4
Trilateral Retinoblastoma

Bilateral retinoblastoma may be associated with ectopic intracranial retinoblastoma in the pineal gland and suprasellar region (JAKOBIEC et al. 1977), and such cases have been termed "trilateral retinoblastoma" (BADER et al. 1980). In Essen, two patients with trilateral retinoblastoma were observed. Histologic examination re-

vealed a neuroectodermal brain tumor and the diagnosis of bilateral retinoblastoma was made subsequently (HAVERS et al. 1986).

11.5.5
Presenting Symptoms

The signs and symptoms of retinoblastoma are related to its size and location. The most frequent sign is leukocoria, or cat's eye reflex, in one or both eyes (Fig. 11.3). Leukocoria is a white pupillary reflex caused by a rentrolental mass due to tumor or retinal detachment, visible through the pupil. Leukocoria has been reported in 44% (HÖPPING et al. 1985b), 56% (ELLSWORTH 1977), and 76% (LENNOX et al. 1975) of patients.

Strabismus is the next most frequent sign. Strabismus arises when the tumor is located in the macular or paramacular area of the retina, causing loss of central vision. Unfortunately, strabismus seldom leads to early diagnosis because it is so common. Other disorders such as an inflamed painful eye, caused by uveitis, endophthalmitis, or hypopyon, or glaucoma, rubeosis, phthisis, and decreased vision are less common presenting signs of the tumor.

11.6
Diagnosis

The diagnosis can be established clinically by binocular indirect ophthalmoscopy under general anesthesia with fully dilated pupils. Bilateral fundus examination with 3600 scleral depression is essential to exclude tumors at the ora serrata which cannot be otherwise detected. Multiple white or pink tumors in one or both eyes are highly suggestive of retinoblastoma. The presence of calcification strongly suggests retinoblastoma although other conditions, such as Coats' disease, angiomatosis retinae, retinal astrocytoma, and nematode endophthalmitis may produce intraocular calcium deposits.

Generally, clinical diagnosis is possible with high accuracy by ophthalmoscopy and B-scan ultrasonography. Attention should be paid to a family history of the disease. Occasionally, a parent may have had an enucleation during childhood but not know why it was done. The parents and siblings should also be examined ophthalmoscopically. A retinoma may be discovered in parents without a family history of retinoblastoma, indicating the hereditary nature of this disease. Biopsy of the tumor should be avoided when retinoblastoma is suspected. If the diagnosis is in doubt, enucleation of a blind eye is reasonable.

Modern diagnostic imaging methods include two-dimensional B-scan ultrasonography, fluorescein angiography, brain and orbital computed tomography (CT) (Fig. 11.4), and magnetic resonance imaging (see chapters 1, 22, 23, 28 this volume).

Laboratory tests may be helpful for diagnosis or follow-up of retinoblastoma. A paracentesis of aqueous from eyes containing retinoblastoma shows significant elevation of lactate dehydrogenase (LDH) in 93% of cases (ABRAMSON et al. 1979a). This test seems to be safe as long as the tumor is not located in the anterior chamber. FELDBERG et al. (1977) reported that elevated aqueous to plasma LDH and phosphoglucose isomerase ratios are helpful in differentiating retinoblastoma from pseudoretinoblastoma. In cases with suspected *Toxocara canis* infections the enzyme-linked immunosorbent assay (ELISA) has a high degree of specificity (90%) and sensitivity (levels of 1 to 64) (CYPRESS et al. 1978). POLLARD et al. (1979) reported toxocariasis to be the cause of 15 (37%) of 41 cases of diagnosed retinal diseases. It should be taken into account that 5% of the population have elevated antibody levels to *Toxocara;* therefore 5% of patients with retinoblastoma may also have positive ELISA tests

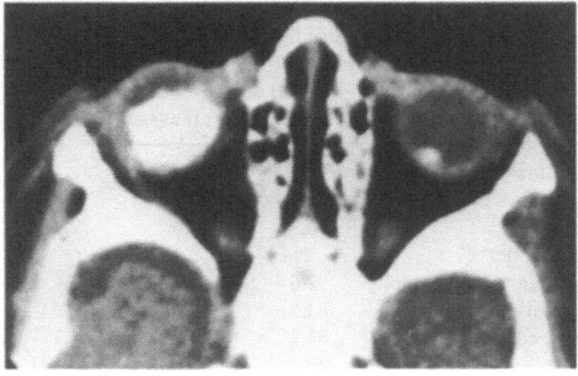

Fig. 11.4. Orbital CT of a patient with bilateral retinoblastoma. (ALBERTI et al. 1987)

for toxocariasis. Bone marrow aspiration and lumbar puncture should be performed in cases with proven extraocular tumor invasion to search for metastases (PRATT et al. 1989).

The lesions simulating retinoblastoma most closely are Coats' disease, persistent hyperplastic primary vitreous, retinal dysplasia, retinopathy of prematurity, and *Toxocara canis* toxocariasis (SHIELDS and AUGSBURGER 1981).

11.7
Staging

Each eye should be evaluated individually to determine the size of the tumor(s) and the extent of involvement. This evaluation allows the team of ocular, radiation, and pediatric oncologists to decide whether conservative treatment can preserve vision or whether enucleation is necessary.

Several staging systems have been published which classify disease within the globe (REESE and ELLSWORTH 1963; HÖPPING 1983; DE SUTTER et al. 1987a) or beyond the globe (PRATT 1972) (Table 11.1) or have the aim of predicting survival (DE SUTTER et al. 1987b). The REESE-ELLSWORTH classification was introduced to predict visual prognosis, i.e., the likelihood of tumor control and preservation of vision, in eyes treated by external beam irradiation (Table 11.2).

The advent of modern irradiation equipment and techniques, and of improved ophthalmologic treatments such as cryo- and photocoagulation, has improved the outcome for patients with small lesions anterior to the equator (IIIa) or the ora serrata (IVb), and for those with slight vitreous seedings (Vb). The need for revision of groups IIIa, IVb, and Vb has been recognized by several authors.

HÖPPING (1983) developed a new prognostic classification. He divided affected eyes into five categories according to the likelihood of preservation of vision after conservative treatment, based upon tumor parameters including size and location, the presence or absence of retinal detachment (partial or complete), and vitreous seeding (localized or diffuse). The use of retinal detachment (IIIb, IVa, Vc), location close to or overlapping the disk (IIIa, IVb), and the distinction between localized (IIIc, IVa) and diffuse vitreous seeding (Vb) allows a more accurate prediction of preservation of vision.

The staging system of DE SUTTER et al. (1987a) is based upon a computer-assisted analysis of the Essen data from 1958 to 1986. It utilized the number of tumors,

Table 12.1. Clinical staging of unilateral and bilateral retinoblastoma. (PRATT 1972)

Stage I: disease confined to the retina
A. Unifocal or multifocal disease of one quadrant or less
B. Unifocal or multifocal disease of two quadrants or less
C. Unifocal or multifocal disease of more than 50% of the retinal surface

Stage II: disease confined to the globe
A. Unifocal or multifocal disease with vitreous seeding
B. Unifocal or multifocal disease with extension to optic nerve head
C. Unifocal or multifocal disease with extension to choroid
D. Unifocal or multifocal disease with extension to choroid and optic nerve head
E. Unifocal or multifocal disease with extension to emissaries, ora serrata, iris, or anterior chamber

Stage III: extraocular extension of disease – regional
A. Extension beyond cut end of optic nerve
B. Extension through sclera into orbital contents
C. Extension to choroid and beyond cut end of optic nerve (including subarachnoid extension)
D. Extension through sclera into orbital contents and beyond cut end of optic nerve (including subarachnoid extension)

Stage IV: distant metastases
A. Extension via optic nerve to brain
B. Blood-borne metastases to soft tissues, bone
C. Bone marrow metastases

Table 12.2. Reese-Ellsworth classification for retinoblastoma. (REESE and ELLSWORTH 1963; cure rates according to ELLSWORTH 1968)

Group I
Very favorable (95% cure)
a) Solitary tumor, less than 4 dd[a] in size, at or behind the equator
b) Multiple tumors, none more than 4 dd in size, all at or behind the equator

Group II
Favorable (83% cure)
a) Solitary lesion 4–10 dd in size, at or behind the equator
b) Multiple tumors, 4–10 dd in size, behind the equator

Group III
Doubtful (76% cure)
a) Any lesion anterior to the equator
b) Solitary tumors larger than 10 dd behind the equator

Group IV
Unfavorable (71 % cure)
a) Multiple tumors, some larger than 10 dd
b) Any lesion extending anteriorly to the ora serrata

Group V
Very unfavorable (35% cure)
a) Massive tumors involving more than half the retina
b) Vitreous seeding

[a]dd, optic disk diameter = 1.6 mm

site, size, vitreous seeding, and retinal detachment to calculate failure rate scores for each parameter; these range from 0 to 29 points and are divided into four groups.

Despite its disadvantages, the REESE-ELLSWORTH classification remains the most commonly used system for comparing results from different centers. It must be emphasized that this classification should not be used to predict patients' survival.

11.8
Prognosis

Survival for 5 years after diagnosis depends largely on the risk for developing distant metastases. Although the risk for distant metastases is difficult to estimate clinically, it correlates significantly with invasion into other ocular structures (Table 11.3) (DE SUTTER et al. 1987b). The metastatic risk is 3% for noninvasive tumors, 20% with optic nerve invasion but a clean cut end as against 40% when the margin is involved, 40% with choroidal invasion, and 67% with orbital involvement. There is no relationship

between grade or age and metastasis. Among patients with retinoblastoma limited to the retina, 5-year survival drops from 92.2% to 33.7% in those with tumors invading the optic nerve at the plane of transection.

These findings are in agreement with data published by STANNARD et al. (1979) and REDLER and

Table 12.3. Correlation of survival with histopathologic characteristics in 590 patients enucleated between 1959 and 1986, Eye Clinic University of Essen. (Modified from DE SUTTER et al. 1987b)

Site of involvement	No. of eyes	5-year survival (%)	P value (Savage test)
Retina only	414	92.2	0.9
Vitreous body	101	92.1	0.8
Choroid	85	80.3	0.0
Optic nerve			
Prelaminar	86	92.6	0.5
Postlaminar	30	82.9	0.0
Cut end	23	33.7	0.0
Iris	10	90	0.06
Sclera	16	78.7	0.0
Extraocular	5	60	0.0

ELLSWORTH (1973) regarding invasion of the choroid and by ROOTMAN et al. (1976) and STANNARD et al. (1979) for invasion of the optic nerve. In the Essen series, undifferentiated histology (MESSMER 1989) and large tumor size (DE SUTTER et al. 1987b) did not correlated with poor risk, in contrast to the findings of RUBIN et al. (1985).

Patients with orbital extension, i.e., with tumor cells outside the sclera after enucleation, are at increased risk for metastasis to the central nervous system or bone marrow (MCKAY et al. 1984). External beam therapy to the orbit is indicated to prevent orbital recurrence but most of these patients die owing to distant metastases. Therefore, many centers add intrathecal and systemic chemotherapy although its effectiveness in improving survival has been hard to document.

Patients with hereditary retinoblastoma are at increased risk of developing a second nonocular cancer during the rest of their lives. Therefore, long-term survival is worse for bilateral than for unilateral disease (10-year survival: 88% vs 97%; HÖPPING et al. 1985a).

11.9
Treatment

11.9.1
General

The management of retinoblastoma continues to evolve clearly indicating the need for conjoint efforts involving ophthalmological, radiotherapeutic and pediatric oncologists, as well as imaging specialists and physicists. In addition to the time tested modalities of enucleation, external beam irradiation, laser photocoagulation and cryotherapy, plaque brachytherapy, thermotherapy and chemotherapy, individually and especially in a 'combined modality program', along with advances in surgical techniques, have contributed to the goal of 'cure with presevation of form and function'. The technical advantages of proton beam irradiation, so far utilized mostly for choroidal melanoma, are limited to those few institutions which have both ophthalmological and radiotherapeutic expertise and the machinery.

The choice of therapy depends upon the size, location and number of lesions, whether vision can be preserved or not, and the potential late effects of each treatment modality. In most circumstances where ne useful vision can be expected, attempts at preservation of the globe may carry more risks than benefits and should not be attempted (SHIELDS CL and SHIELDS JA, 1999).

11.9.2
Surgical Treatment Modalities

11.9.2.1
Enucleation

Because most children with unilateral disease have far-advanced tumors, enucleation of the affected eye is the treatment of choice. Bilateral enucleaion is rarely indicated as there will be no sight. Usually, the more severely affected eye will not have vision and is enucleated while the remaining eye is irradiated. When tumor is advanced in both eyes and there is little to indicate which eye will do better, bilateral irradiation should be performed and bilateral vision may be preserved; enucleation can always be performed when an eye fares badly. Similarly, bilateral irradiation is indicated when there is bilateral vision in earlier stage disease, even though the disease may be more advanced in one of the eyes. Enucleation is appropriate when there is invasion of the optic nerve, choroid, anterior chamber and orbit, secondary glaucoma, pars plana seeding, failure of conservative treatments, and when there is persistent vitreous hemorrhage in which the cours of the disease cannot be assessed (SHIELDS CL and SHIELDS JA, 1999).

If enucleation is necessary, attention should be paid to removing a long segment of the optic nerve (>10mm). In patients with invasion of the choroid or optic nerve, or with orbital recurrence, exenteration is not indicated; postenucleation irradiation yields better results (ABRAMSON and ELLSWORTH 1980).

11.9.2.2
Cryotherapy

Cryotherapy for retinoblastoma, first reported in 1967 (LINCOFF et al. 1967), is used as a primary treatment or for selected tumor recurrences.

The cryotherapy probe is placed on the sclera over the tumor. Lesions with a diameter less than 6 mm, less than 3 mm thick, and located at the ora serrata, which are not treatable with light coagulation, can be destroyed by transscleral cryotherapy. If eyes with multiple tumors are to be irradiated with external beam therapy, cryotherapy may be useful in treating tumors at the ora serrata before or during the course of radiotherapy because most irradiation techniques do not provide the full tumor dose anterior to the equator. Eighty-five percent of new tumors developing after external beam irradiation, and 90% of tumors with a poor response to irradiation, have been cured by cryotherapy (ABRAMSON et al. 1982a). These authors emphasized that this modality is most effective in tumors not larger than 3-4dd (optic disk diameter = 1.6 mm). Between 20% and 30% of the tumors required more than one treatment.

11.9.2.3
Light Coagulation

Light coagulation, developed and first used for retinoblastoma by MEYER-SCHWICKERATH (MEYER-SCHWICKERATH and HELFERICH 1958; MEYER-SCHWICKERATH 1961; HÖPPING and MEYER-

SCHWICKERATH 1964), is a valuable therapeutic tool for primary or recurrent lesions of less than 4 dd. Whereas the main indication for cryotherapy is a tumor in the anterior retina, light coagulation is suitable for tumors at the posterior pole. The principle of this method is to ‚ring‘ the tumor(s) with two or three rows of coagulation, occluding the nutritional retinal vessels (Fig. 11.5). Because the resultant chorioretinal scar is much larger than the tumor itself, light coagulation is contraindicated for tumors close to the macula or optic disk. Even in small, single, centrally located lesions, external beam therapy should be performed to avoid central scotoma. In hereditary disease, the whole retina is at risk due to multicentric tumor origin. Under certain circumstances it may be justified to use local treatment modalities such as coagulation therapy instead of external beam therapy which includes

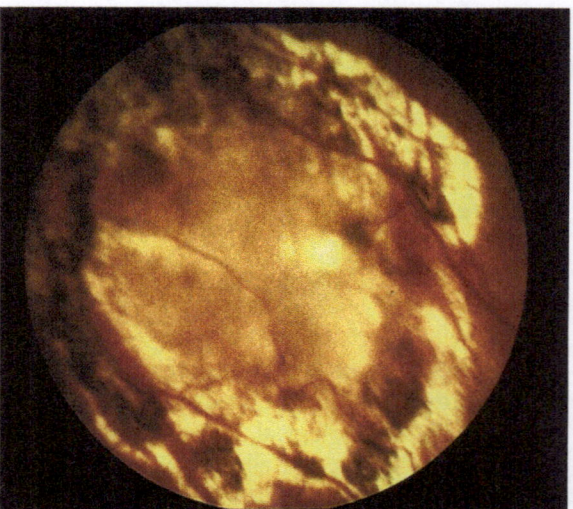

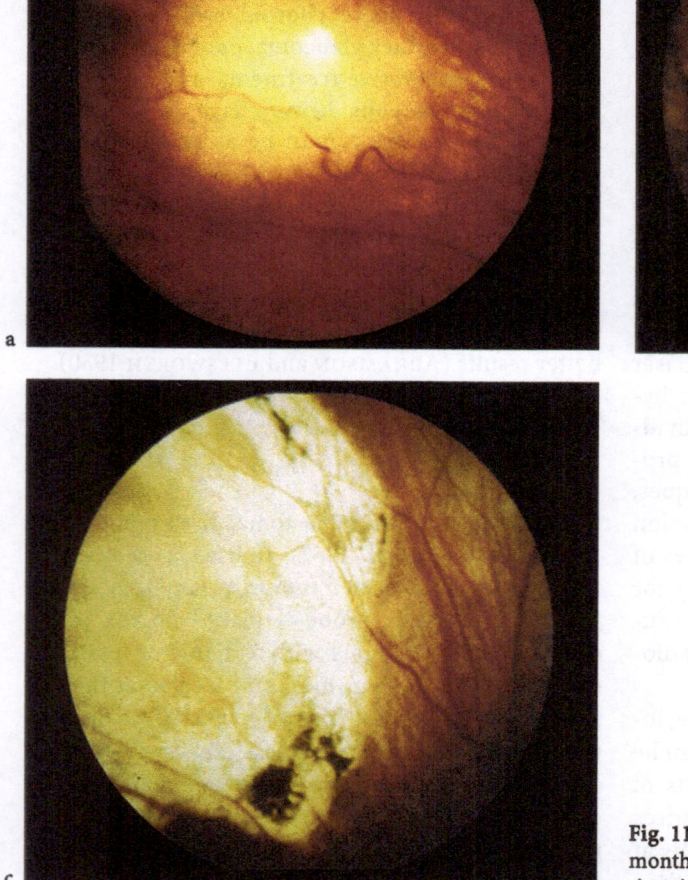

Fig. 11.5. a Retinoblastoma in the peripheral fundus. b Two months after photocoagulation. c Scar after 1 year. The patient is free of recurrence at 5 years. (LOMMATZSCH 1989)

the entire retina in order to avoid the potential hazard of ionizing radiation (HÖPPING and BUNKE-SCHMIDT 1985).

11.9.3
Radiation Treatment

11.9.3.1
Radioactive Plaque Therapy

ABRAMSON et al. (1983) reported on the use of 81 cobalt plaques in 71 eyes in 64 patients with advanced retinoblastoma. Of the 64 patients, 60 had already failed prior treatment with external beam therapy, photocoagulation, cryotherapy, or a combination of these. The fellow (contralateral) eye had been enucleated in 60 of 63 patients with bilateral disease. More than half (45/81) of the tumors were larger than 10 mm in base diameter. Forty-four of the 71 eyes (62%) could be preserved. In 21 of the 27 enucleated eyes, the reason for enucleation was continued tumor growth. Two eyes were lost to complications and four were lost to a combination of tumor growth and treatment- or tumor-related complications.

STANNARD et al. (1987) published their findings on the effects of ^{125}I plaque irradiation of 19 tumors in 14 eyes (seven untreated eyes and seven eyes with recurrence after external beam therapy). Local control was achieved in 63% (12/19). Local control was better in the untreated group (nine of ten tumors) than in the previously treated group (three of nine tumors).

MESSMER et al. (1990) reported on ten patients with hereditary disease treated primarily with plaques. Ruthenium plaques were used in six cases and cobalt plaques in four. A dose of 40 Gy at the apex of the tumor was delivered in 70% of the cases. Additional coagulation therapy was performed in five cases. All eyes were preserved with useful vision. In contrast to ABRAMSON et al. (1983), MESSMER et al. treated only group I-III patients, who have a good prognosis for tumor control with preservation of vision.

Regression patterns in 30 patients receiving 31 ^{60}CO plaques were studied by Buys et al. (1983). Type I, II and III radiation regression patterns appeared to be identical to those seen after external beam therapy (Fig. 11.6a-c). Nine patients had a radiation regression pattern that did not fall into any of these three categories. In these patients, the tumor completely disappeared, no calcification was found, and a flat scar was left. The authors labeled this regression type IV (Fig. 11.6d). Type IV regression has been described by STALLARD (1968) and by ROSENGREN and TENGROTH (1963).

STALLARD (1966) reported successful treatment of 63 of 69 eyes with retinoblastoma by means of cobalt plaques; approximately 40 Gy was delivered at the tumor apex. Experience with ^{106}Ru/ ^{106}Rh applicators, introduced by Lommatzsch in 1966, has been gained in retinoblastoma not exceeding a height of 5 mm; LOMMATZSCH (1978) reported tumor destruction in 28 of 33 cases (84%) (Fig. 11.7).

At present, most centers have replaced ^{60}CO plaques with ^{125}I or ^{106}Ru/^{106}Rh plaques, resulting in less radiation damage to uninvolved intraocular and orbital structures (see also chapters 4, 5, 6, 25, 26 this volume).

Indications for a radioactive plaque are:
1. Unifocal, unilateral retinoblastoma less than 12 mm in diameter and 3-7 mm thick (CHAR 1989).
2. Recurrent, localized lesions following external beam therapy, not suitable for treatment with cryotherapy or light coagulation.
3. As part of a combined modality program.

SHIELDS et al. (2001) reported 208 tumors in 141 patients treated with plaque brachytherapy, 148 (71%) recurrent after failing one or more prior therapies. Kaplan-Meier estimated tumor control was 83% at one year and 79% at five years. The authors concluded that plaque brachytherapy "was particularly useful for photocoagulation, thermotherapy and cryotherapy".

11.9.3.2
External Beam Therapy

External beam therapy (EBRT) has been successfully employed since 1903 (HILGARTNER 1903). The introduction of megavoltage radiation and improved techniques allowed treatment to be optimized. EBRT should be performed for bilateral disease and is most frequently used for the treatment of the second eye after the one with the more advanced tumor has been enucleated. It is the treatment of choice if the second eye has a tumor close to the fovea or optic disk, if there are several tumors, or if advanced vitreous seeding is present. Eyes with large tumors in which successful coagulation therapy is not possible are also candidates for irradiation. Today, chemoreduction, thermochemotherapy and plaque brachytherapy and other combined-modality programs are employed, in an effort to avoid late complications after EBRT.

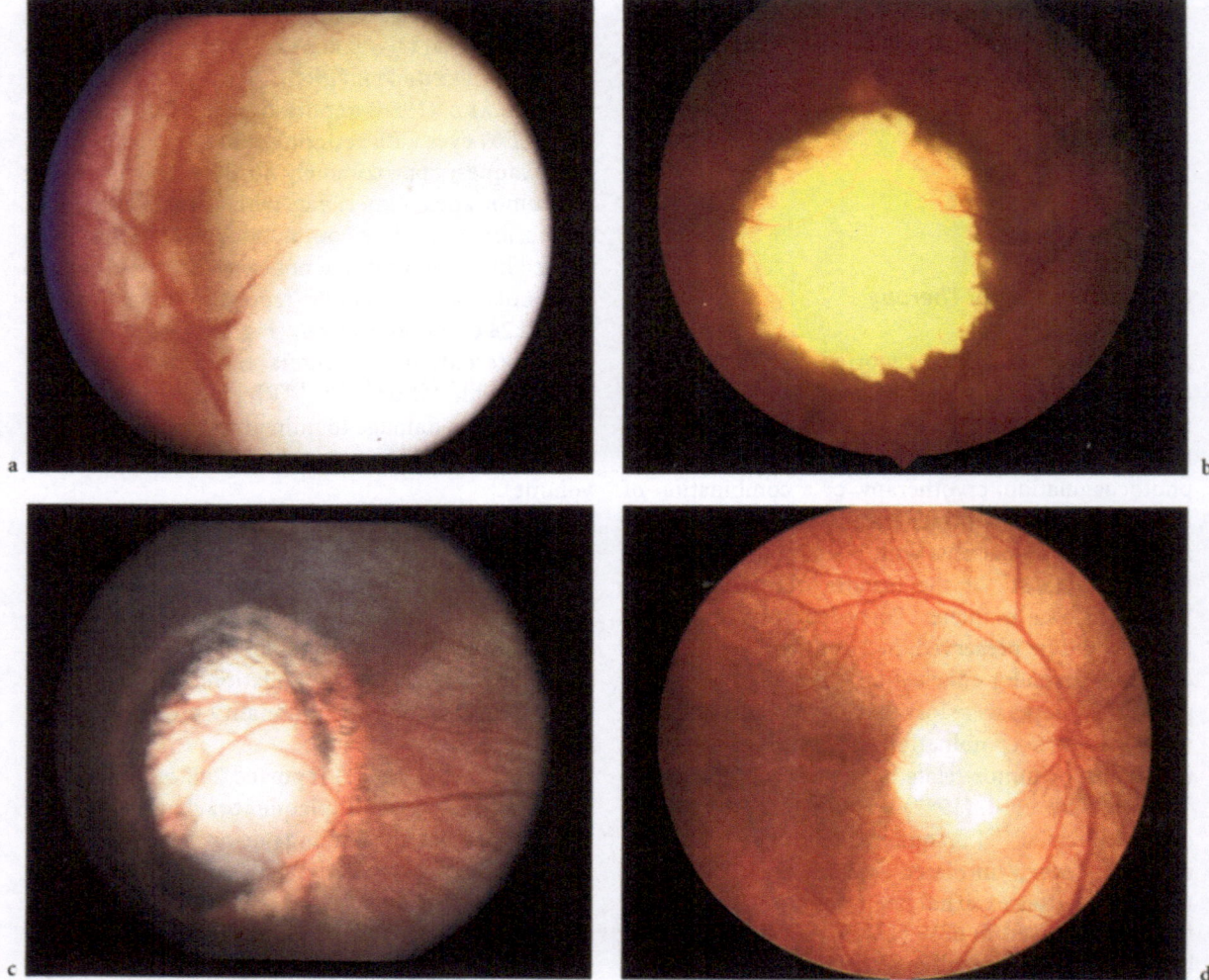

Fig. 11.6. a Unilateral, sporadic retinoblastoma OD in a 7 month old girl before irradiation. **b** Type I regression pattern is seen 4 months after external beam irradiation. **c** Type 2 regression pattern is seen OS in this 8 month old boy with familial, bilateral retinoblastoma after ^{125}I plaque therapy. **d** Type 3 regression pattern is seen in this 6 month old boy with unilateral, sporadic retinoblastoma after ^{125}I plaque therapy. (Courtesy of Dres. SHIELDS, Wills Eye Hospital, Philadelphia)

In far-advanced, bilateral cases, it is sometimes difficult to determine in which eye some vision is present and can be preserved. In this case, both eyes should be irradiated (ABRAMSON et al. 1981a; SCHIPPER et al. 1985; ALBERTI et al. 1987; DONALDSON and EGBERT 1989). Bilateral irradiation is indicated in the unusual situation of bilateral, early group retinoblastoma, with good prospects of preserving binocular vision (Fig. 11.8).

If there is active disease after EBRT, coagulation treatment can usually control the residual foci. A second or third course of irradiation is seldom successful, as demonstrated by Abramson et al. (1982c). Of 104 re-treated eyes receiving total irradiation doses of 54–165 Gy (average 84 Gy), only 14 could be preserved. Of the 90 eyes in which treatment failed,

60 (67%) were enucleated because of tumor regrowth, 22 (24%) because of radiation complications, and 6 because of tumor growth and complications. Twelve of the 14 eyes that were salvaged belonged to groups I, II, or III. Nine of these eyes were cured and maintained useful vision after an observation period of 3–3 years (average 11 years). It was striking that in this series, 23% of the survivors developed a second nonocular cancer. This supports the findings of SAGERMAN et al. (1969) and ALBERTI et al. (1987) that there is a dose–effect relationship and those of DRAPER et al. (1986) and ALBERTI et al. (1987) that chemotherapy increases the risk of non-ocular malignancies. In addition, more radiation injury can be expected in eyes treated with a second course and a higher total dose.

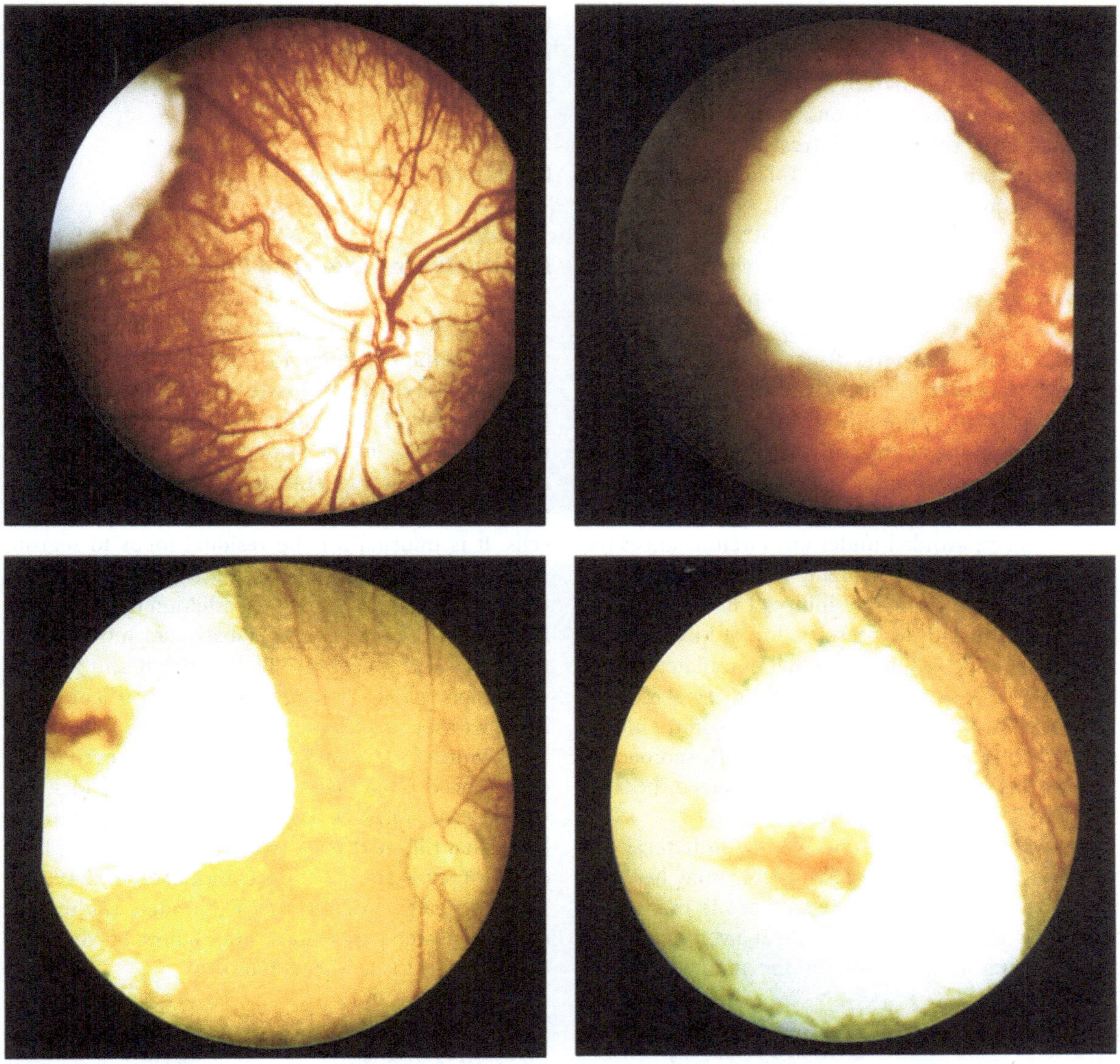

Fig. 11.7. a,b Retinoblastoma with calcification in the midperiphery, nasally of the optic disk, before treatment. **c,d** Appearance 5 years after ^{106}Ru/^{106}Rh plaque treatment (500 Gy at the base and 40 Gy at the summit of the tumor). Flat scar with a devitalized remnant in the center. (LOMMATZSCH 1989)

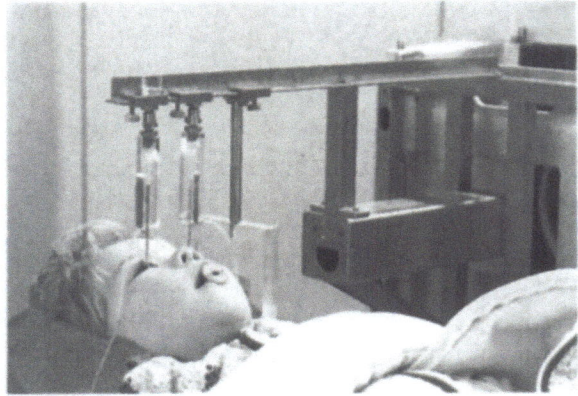

Fig. 11.8. Bilateral irradiation of a child with bilateral retinoblastoma with the Schipper technique

EBRT is also indicated for unilateral disease that is not treatable by focal methods (cryotherapy, light coagulation, plaque therapy) and in which useful vision can be expected (ABRAMSON et al. 1982c). These authors recommend treating patients with unilateral tumors in groups I–III conservatively, without primary enucleation. Of 39 such eyes, 34 were preserved. Another argument for nonsurgical treatment is that 10–20% of patients with unilateral involvement will eventually develop retinoblastoma in the second eye (CARLSON et al. 1979). This is true especially when unilateral disease is diagnosed at an early age (less than 12 months) and more than one tumor is present. If the initially affected eye were to be enucleated, the chance of retaining useful vision might be compromised.

However, many ophthalmologists feel that irradiation should be avoided under any circumstances because of the hazards of ionizing radiation. This must be weighed against the possibility of useful vision in the treated eye and the preservation of binocular vision. It should be kept in mind that in unilateral, nonhereditary disease the incidence of radiation-induced nonocular cancer is low. If the size of the tumor in unilateral disease allows for treatment with radioactive plaques this modality should be preferred, because uninvolved tissues will receive a lower dose.

Generally, eyes with group IV or V unilateral disease should be enucleated. Exceptions may be when a positive family history exists, there is more than one tumor, the diagnosis is made at a very early age, or the tumor is not close to the macula or disk

(ABRAMSON et al. 1982b). Irradiation techniques are reviewed in Chapter 24 (this volume).

11.9.4
Results After Therapy

11.9.4.1
Preservation of Vision and Eye(s)

The response to irradiation may be quite different in various retinoblastoma foci within the same eye. Three typical regression patterns have been described (ELLSWORTH 1969). Type I is characterized by dramatic shrinkage of the tumor, resulting in a "cottage cheese" remnant (Fig. 11.9). It is suggested that tumors with such regression patterns consist of differentiated cells. It is unusual for the residual focus to regrow. Type II regression shows only a slight or moderate reduction in size at the end of radiation therapy and a little, if any, change during subsequent months. The tumor has the appearance of like "fish flesh." Type III regression, which occurs in more than 50% of cases, contains aspects of both type I and type II. Types II and III must be followed carefully, because even for an experienced ophthalmologist it is difficult to judge whether the tumor is active or not. It is important to know that different tumors in the same eye can have different regression patterns (ABRAMSON et al. 1981c). This correlates with the histopathologic findings in eyes enucleated primarily or after failure of conservative treatment (MESSMER 1989).

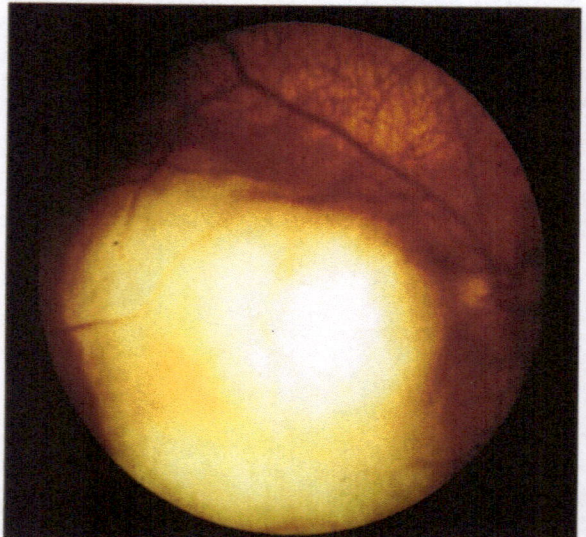 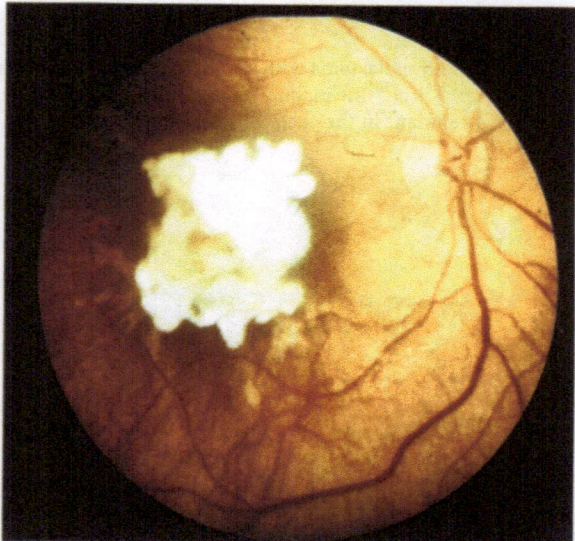

Fig. 11.9. a Retinoblastoma covering the macula, close to the optic disk. **b** Type I regression pattern with a cottage cheese appearance 1 year after 45 Gy. (LOMMATZSCH 1989)

Preservation of the eye with useful vision is one of the main goals in the treatment for retinoblastoma. In Table 11.4 results from different centers are compared, tumor control being demonstrated in more than 80% of eyes affected by group I to group IV disease. Excluding group V eyes, in which only poor results can be expected, 86% (284 of 332) of the eyes were preserved. Many eyes received concurrent or subsequent cryotherapy, photocoagulation, or plaque therapy for residual or recurrent disease or because of the appearance of new tumors in previously uninvolved retina. The percentages of patients receiving additional coagulation therapy in various series were 25% (ABRAMSON 1985, New York), 54% (SCHIPPER et al. 1985, Utrecht), and 74% (ALBERTI et al. 1987, Essen). It should be noted that the reason for the use of coagulation therapy was not always irradiation failure; many eyes were treated because of the uncertainty of tumor control after irradiation and others because close follow-up examination was not possible since the patient in question had come from another country.

Total doses of between 35 and 50 Gy delivered with different fractionation schemes are usual in most centers. If general anesthesia is induced, single doses of 2.5-3.5 Gy are used to reduce the number of sessions (WEISS et al. 1975; SCHIPPER et al. 1985; ALBERTI et al. 1987). Others do not consider general anesthesia necessary (CASSADY et al. 1969; FREEMAN et al. 1980; HAYE et al. 1986; AMENDOLA et al. 1990) and treat children soon after they have been fed, with or without sedation.

Conclusions can be drawn from the analysis of 127 eyes treated with megavoltage irradiation between 1974 and 1988 in Essen (MESSMER et al. 1990).

Tumors with group V disease and those with total retinal detachment, were not included in this study. Eyes were irradiated (74 with a lateral field, 53 with the Schipper technique) with total doses of about 40 or 50 Gy. Weekly fractionation changed over the years: 1974-1976: 4-5 times 2-2.5 Gy; 1977-1983: 3 times 3.3 Gy; 1984-1988: 4 times 2.5 Gy. Eyes treated with radiation doses of 50 Gy developed significantly fewer new and recurrent tumors than those treated with about 40 Gy (22% vs 49%, $P=0.037$). Eyes treated with 50 Gy had significantly larger tumors (>10 D) than those treated with 40 Gy ($P=0.0003$).

On the basis of their experience, MESSMER et al. (1990) recommended a dose of 50 Gy (20 fractions, 5 weeks). However, it must be emphasized that single doses of more than 2.0 Gy may be critical for structures such as the optic nerve and retina if total doses of 50 Gy are delivered. Total doses of 50-60 Gy with conventional fractionation, as recommended by DONALDSON and EGBERT (1989), may be better tolerated by the ocular structures, especially in patients receiving additional treatment such as coagulation, plaque therapy, and/or chemotherapy.

There is an inherent conflict between the need to treat the anterior retina and the desire to spare the lens and the anterior chamber, which is only partially resolved by accuracy in the application of the particular technique chosen. With almost all techniques, underdosage results in a higher incidence of new tumors anterior to the equator (MESSMER et al. 1990).

An important question is whether the delay in enucleation after several attempts to save the remaining eye might increase the risk of metastatic

Table 11.4. Results of irradiation for retinoblastoma (± coagulation ± plaque therapy)

Reese-Ellsworth group	New York ABRAMSON et al. 1981a,b[a] 1955-1980[d]		Paris HAYE et al. 1986[b] 1963-1977[d] 1971-1988[d]		Utrecht SCHIPPER 1992[c] (personal communication)		Essen ALBERTI et al. 1987 1973-1984[d]		All centers	
I	34/37[e]	92%	17/170	100%	32/320	100%	12/120	100%	95/980	97%
II	15/18	83%	29/38	76%	14/14	100%	25/27	93%	83/97	86%
III	16/19	84%	20/24	83%	20/25	80%	17/22	77%	73/90	81%
IV	12/13	92%	4/5	80%	20/28	71%	39/51	76%	75/97	77%
V	7/51	14%	3/10	30%	9/32	28%	4/17	23%	23/90	25%
	84/138	61%	73/94	78%	95/131	73%	97/129	75%	347/472	73.5%

[a] Series with 40% group V
[b] Including 15 eyes treated with cobalt 60 plaques
[c] Including 22 eyes treated with hyperthermia
[d] Period of treatment
[e] Eyes saved/total

disease. HEINRICH (1989) found that survival in patients in whom retinoblastoma was confined to the retina, i.e., without any histological risk factors, was the same as in those in whom the eye had been enucleated primarily or secondarily soon after failure of the primary treatment. However, 5-year survival was significantly worse in patients whose eyes were enucleated after a long interval and when they were showing choroidal invasion than in patients who underwent earlier enucleation with a similar grade of invasion (52% vs 92%). Patients with other risk factors were excluded from this analysis.

It can be concluded that a low incidence of cataract formation correlates with a higher incidence of new tumors anteriorly in the retina when a temporal approach is used. However, this is not true for the highly accurate beam technique developed by SCHIPPER (1983) and used in several centers (SCHIPPER et al. 1985; ALBERTI et al. 1987; HARNETT et al. 1987). Fortunately, most of the failures in the underdosaged area can be managed successfully with coagulation therapy and occasionally with plaque therapy. In the Essen series, the remaining eye in two patients had to be enucleated owing to failure anteriorly, in an area not included in the treatment volume with a lateral field (ALBERTI et al. 1987). As in the series of SCHIPPER et al. (1985), only one of the 54 irradiated eyes developed a new tumor within the area receiving a full radiation dose.

11.9.4.2
Recurrent and New Tumors

Because of the multicentric origin of hereditary retinoblastoma, most authorities agree that the entire retina is at risk and should be treated. This is best achieved with EBRT or with a multistage combined modality program.

The incidence of multifocality is high, ranging from 75% to 84% (ELLSWORTH 1969; SCHIPPER 1980; DE SUTTER et al. 1987b). The mean number of tumors spread over the two retinas is four to six (STALLARD 1955; KITCHIN 1976; DE SUTTER et al. 1987b). As demonstrated by HÖPPING and BUNKE-SCHMIDT (1985), small foci up to a diameter of 4 D and elevated by 4 D can be treated successfully by primary photocoagulation and/or cryotherapy. Tumors too close to the fovea or optic disk, pedunculated tumors with a small base, and those with massive vitreous seeding and retinal detachment should not be treated primarily by coagulation therapy.

The occurrence of new and recurrent tumor foci following local treatment (coagulation and plaque

therapy) and EBRT was analyzed in 200 patients treated in Essen since 1960 (MESSMER et al. 1990). The study comprised 229 eyes from 200 patients with multifocal disease, including 196 bilateral and four familial unilateral cases. Primary local treatment was performed in 102 eyes, including 69 with light coagulation, 27 with cryocoagulation, and 10 with plaque therapy. The remaining 127 eyes received EBRT, 81% of them with doses of 40-50 Gy. The two treatment groups were comparable for age and tumor size. Patients with retinal detachment, diffuse vitreous seeding, and tumors larger than one-half the size of the retina were excluded from the study. The risk for developing new tumors was calculated using life-table methods. During a 5-year follow-up, the risk was 20% in eyes treated with local methods and 27% following treatment with EBRT (difference not significant). The risk was age related: 11% in children older than 12 months and 35% in those younger than 6 months ($P=0.0009$). The median latency between the start of treatment and the appearance of a new tumor was 4 months with local treatment and 9 months with EBRT ($P=0.02$). New tumors were equally distributed anterior and posterior to the equator (16/16) in locally treated patients, whereas after EBRT most of the tumors arose in the anterior retina (40 vs 9 posteriorly; $P=0.003$). In the local treatment group, 2 eyes required additional irradiation and both were preserved. In the irradiation group, 2 eyes with new tumors received a second course of irradiation, and 1 had to be enucleated.

The rate of recurrent tumor calculated with the life-table method was 26% after local treatment and 28% after EBRT. There was no significant difference between photo- and cryocoagulation. Five of the ten patients with plaque therapy required additional coagulation therapy. The incidence of recurrence showed no age-related variation; all recurrences were documented within 24 months in the local treatment group and within 54 months in the EBRT group. In both treatment groups, most recurrences were posterior to the equator (63% and 65%). Recurrent tumors could be controlled by additional conservative methods in all eyes in the locally treated group, while 10 eyes had to be enucleated in the EBRT group and 6 eyes required a second course of EBRT (no longer performed). If new and recurrent tumors are combined, the incidence in the two groups was 35% and 44%, respectively (difference not significant). Because of the difference in latency of new and recurrent tumors following local treatment modalities and EBRT, follow-up visits should be adapted to the mode of treatment received.

11.9.4.3
Complications (see also Chapter 27 this volume)

As the survival of patients treated for retinoblastoma in specialized centers is 90%, treatment-related late complications and, especially, the hazard of second malignancies, are important. Therefore, each case should be evaluated with the aim of preserving the eye with useful vision while avoiding complications. The most frequent reason for secondary enucleation is residual or recurrent disease not controlled by irradiation or any other treatment. New tumors arising in formerly uninvolved retina can usually be managed successfully with coagulation and occasionally with plaque therapy. Thus, most eyes with a favorable prognosis (stages I–III) can be preserved (ABRAMSON et al. 1981b; HÖPPING et al. 1985b; HAYE et al. 1986; SCHIPPER et al. 1985).

HOWARD (1966) reported a clinicopathologic evaluation of 100 globes enucleated for retinoblastoma, 21 of which had been irradiated. The usual radiation therapy schedule at this time was 36 Gy given in 11 fractions over 3 1/2 weeks. Microscopic examination of the enucleated eyes showed pathologic changes such as synechial closure of the angles, atrophy, thickening, and hyaline degeneration of the retinal vessels, and sclerosis and shrinkage of the choroidal vessels. These changes were present in 10 of 14 eyes (71%) which had received two courses of irradiation (average total dose 84 Gy), and in 1 of the 7 eyes receiving one course (average dose 37.5 Gy). The pathologic changes were significantly more frequent and severe in the eyes treated with 80 Gy than in those treated with 36 Gy. Similar results were obtained in minipig eyes irradiated with total doses of 40, 50, 60, and 70 Gy in 16–28 fractions over 4–7 weeks (ALBERTI et al. 1990). Today, radiation-induced cataracts no longer pose the technical challenge that they did the past; but visual rehabilitation is difficult in young children.

Radiation-induced cataracts can arise at low doses. The latent period between irradiation and cataract formation decreases as the dose increases and is related to the extent of the germinative zone of the lens epithelium included in the volume of irradiation. If the total dose is delivered through an anterior field, radiation cataract of varying degree can be expected in almost all patients (MCFAUL and BEDFORD 1970). Posterior lens cataracts of varying severity were observed in 25 of 38 eyes irradiated for retinoblastoma with a temporal approach (EGBERT et al. 1978). The dose to the retina ranged from 35 to 60 Gy, but the dose to the lens is difficult to assess in this report. SCHIPPER et al. (1985) reported 39 children

with retinoblastoma (73 affected eyes) treated with a precise megavoltage irradiation technique (SCHIPPER 1983). Forty-five gray was given to the retina in 15 fractions delivered in 3 sessions per week. Eighteen eyes developed a clinically detectable cataract; in 5 of these the lens was aspirated. Cataracts developed exclusively in those lenses where more than 1 mm of the posterior lens was included in the treatment field. The likelihood and the degree of cataract formation were related only to the dose absorbed by the germinative zone of the lens epithelium. The minimum cataractogenic dose found in this series was 8 Gy in 15 fractions. These cataracts did not impair vision. When the dose to the germinative zone of the lens epithelium was increased from 8 to 25 Gy the severity of the cataract also increased.

The most significant long-term complications that occur after irradiation of retinoblastoma are optic nerve damage and radiation retinopathy.

Radiation retinopathy was first described by STALLARD (1933) following radon seed implantation for treatment of retinoblastoma. It is characterized by microaneurysms of the capillaries, 'cotton-wool spots,' and vitreous hemorrhages. Chronic changes include retinal detachment and optic nerve atrophy with blindness. Retinopathy usually occurs within 1 year after radiotherapy, but a longer latency of 3–5 years is not uncommon (ELLSWORTH 1969; EGBERT et al. 1978; ALBERTI 1991).

Data on the threshold dose producing retinal damage vary. ELLSWORTH (1977) showed that some vascular damage occurred in 10% of children with retinoblastoma treated with 35 Gy, in 66% treated with 45 Gy, and in 100% treated with 80 Gy (3-Gy fractions were used in each case). SCHIPPER et al. (1985) reported a series of 54 patients with retinoblastoma treated with 45 Gy (15 fractions/5 weeks). They observed retinal vascular damage in three patients 8, 8, and 24 months after irradiation; all three eyes retained useful vision.

Vitreous hemorrhages can occur as a result of advanced retinopathy or from leaks in the retinal vessels supporting a shrinking tumor. Intensive photocoagulation increases the risk of vascular damage (EGBERT et al. 1978).

Histologically, the affected retinal vessels have thickened hyalinized walls, and the lumen may be partly or completely obliterated (HOWARD 1966; EGBERT et al. 1980). In addition, narrowing of central retinal and ciliary arteries has been observed (EGBERT et al. 1980).

Radiation optic neuropathy (RON) can arise after high-dose irradiation or plaque therapy for retinoblastoma. The exact pathogenesis of delayed radion-ecrosis of the optic nerve is unknown. Most authors believe that retinal vascular damage causes subsequent optic neuropathy. The clinical characteristics of RON have been described by several authors (for a review see ALBERTI 1991). Latency periods from the completion of radiotherapy until the onset of RON vary from several months to several years.

In the series of EGBERT et al. (1978), 1 of 28 children irradiated for bilateral retinoblastoma with a midplane dose of 47 Gy in 5 weeks received an additional 49 Gy in 5 weeks for recurrent disease in one eye. Vision later decreased to light perception only in each eye, in one after 16 and in the other afer 17 years. It was assumed that this patient had suffered an ischemic insult to the optic nerves as a result of late radiation damage.

ABRAMSON et al. (1982a) noted a 24.4% incidence of enucleation (22/104) for radiation complications after second or third courses of EBRT for retinoblastoma with total doses ranging from 54 to 165 Gy. Seventy patients received chemotherapy as well. In 90 patients, the eye was lost because of progressive tumor, enucleation, or death. Tumor control was achieved in 14 eyes, all but 2 belonging to Reese-Ellsworth groups I, II, or III at the time of the second course of irradiation. The main reason so few eyes were lost to irradiation complication is that the majority were lost to uncontrolled disease. Had more of the tumors been controlled, the majority of eyes might well have been lost to complications. These observations point to the significance of fractionation in the development of radiation retinopathy and RON. The risk for developing severe ocular complications is rather low in children with retinoblastoma treated with megavoltage irradiation wth up to 40–50 Gy using a careful technique.

Growth retardation of the irradiated bony structures resulting in facial malformation was a significant side effect in the past due to the high bone absorption of orthovoltage irradiation (REESE et al. 1949). With megavoltage irradiation, and doses in the range of 35–50 Gy in 3 1/2–5 weeks, this complication is now less frequent and less severe (SCHIPPER 1980).

11.9.5
Combined modality programs including chemotherapy, thermotherapy, plaque brachytherapy

The late effects of EBRT, cataract formation, dry eye, alteration of normal bone growth and, especially, the estimated incidence of second nonocular cancers in long-term survivors of hereditary retinoblastoma of

51% at 50 years after diagnosis have spurred on the search for alternative treatment methods (ABRAMSON 1999). Chemotherapy today may be classified as neoadjuvant chemotherapy, chemoreduction; chemo-irradiation, and chemothermotherapy (FINGER et al. 1999).

In 1953, KUPPER reported a response of intraocular retinoblastoma when nitrogen mustard was given concomitantly with irradiation. In the same year, REESE et al. (1955) introduced the alkylating agent triethylenemelamine (TEM) for retinoblastoma; this was given orally, intramuscularly, intravenously, and intra-arterially.

As detailed by SCHIPPER and ALBERTI (1985), a large number of patients with bilateral involvement treated at the Harkness Institute of Ophthalmology, Columbia-Presbyterian Medical Center, New York between 1953 and 1966 received TEM as an adjunct to irradiation. Thereafter, TEM was replaced by cyclophosphamide and vincristine, given to patients with advanced group V tumors (ELLSWORTH 1978). Patients receiving a second course of radiotherapy (ABRAMSON et al. 1982c) and those considered to be at risk for developing metastatic disease after enucleation (REESE 1976; ELLSWORTH 1978) were also given chemotherapy. Although chemotherapy was given in this institution to about two thirds of nearly 800 patients between 1953 and 1981, there has been no report describing the effect of chemotherapy on local control, survival, or carcinogenic risk. CASSADY et al. (1969) could not demonstrate any better tumor control in patients treated with adjunctive TEM given intramuscularly or by carotid artery injection than in those who received irradiation alone.

From 1963 to 1977, TEM was also frequently used concurrently with electron beam or ^{60}Co plaque irradiation at the Institut Curie in Paris (HAYE et al. 1986).

In 1977, the Children's Cancer Study Group initiated a randomized study in group V disease comparing enucleation with enucleation followed by chemotherapy for 57 weeks (cyclophosphamide and vincristine every 3 weeks) (ABRAMSON 1985). Although this study was closed in 1980 because of insufficient patient accrual, survival in the group with additional chemotherapy (n=41) was worse (87.6%) than in patients who had undergone enucleation alone (95%; n=47, P=0.368). Seven patients relapsed within 1 year after diagnosis. Two each of the orbital and systemic relapses were in the chemotherapy and control groups (WHITE 1983).

Adjuvant chemotherapy was given in patients considered to be at risk for metastatic disease at St. Jude Children's Hospital (HOWARTH et al. 1980).

From 1970 to 1977, patients were staged according to the results of histologic examination of the globe and clinical evaluation for metastatic disease. Of 42 patients, 38 (90.5%) received vincristine and cyclophosphamide for 1 year. Patients with CNS tumor extension also received intrathecal methotrexate and cranial or craniospinal irradiation. Thirty-nine of the 42 children survived for 6–90 months (median 42 months) from the start of treatment. When the use of chemotherapy is considered, the possibility of potentiating the risk of second malignancies in these young patients should always be borne in mind (DRAPER et al. 1986; SCHIPPER and ALBERTI 1985).

If histologic evaluation of the enucleated eye reveals that the tumor(s) involve(s) other structures than the retina, prognosis for life may be impaired. This is especially true when such involvement takes the form of significant choroidal invasion, postlaminar or cut-end involvement of the optic nerve, or scleral or extraocular extension of the disease (McKAY et al. 1984, DeSUTTER et al. 1987, HUNGERFORD 1993). Patients with these findings are at risk for local recurrences in the orbit, CNS disease or dissemination.

Because of the poor prognosis, aggressive treatment including radiation therapy of the orbit and chemotherapy is advocated, sometimes combined with cranial or craniospinal irradiation (CSI) (KINGSTON and HUNGERFORD 1992) or intrathecal chemotherapy (GRZESKOWIAK-MELANOWSKA et al. 1997). If intrathecal chemotherapy is given, no cranial irradiation or CSI should be delivered (KINGSTON et al., 2000).

In the past, most patients died of orbital recurrence, in most cases due to CNS disease or disseminated retinoblastoma (HUNGERFORD et al. 1987). Only one of ten children with orbital recurrences was cured by excisional biopsy of the recurrent tumor followed by radical orbital radiotherapy and systemic chemotherapy. The other nine patients died from disseminated disease. At the time of diagnosis, extraorbital spread had been ruled out in all patients. GOBLE et al. (1990), at the same institution, reported another four children with orbital recurrence treated by excisional biopsy, radiotherapy and chemotherapy. These patients received a radiation dose of 34–50 Gy at 4–6 weeks and systemic chemotherapy with vincristine, cyclophosphamide, cisplatinum, etoposide (OPEC protocol) and intrathecal methotrexate. They remained disease free for 8 months to 3 years. The authors suggest that orbital exenteration is unlikely to achieve surgical clearance of all recurrent tumor and recommend simple excision of the orbital mass.

PRADHAM et al. (1997) treated 28 patients (28 eyes) with EBRT to the orbit for locally advanced disease, usually after enucleation (24 eyes). Nineteen patients also had chemotherapy. One patient presented with an orbital recurrence after enucleation. Ten patients had involvement of the optic nerve to the cut margin. Local control was maintained in 71% of patients (20 orbits) within a mean follow-up period of 22.6 months.

During the last few years chemotherapy in combination with focal methods such as coagulation and plaque therapy has been used by several investigators (SHIELDS et al. 1996 and 1999, KINGSTON et al. 1996, GREENWALD and STRAUSS 1997, LEVY et al. 1998).

GALLIE et al. (1996) used chemotherapy to treat 40 eyes (in 31 patients) which would otherwise have been treated with EBRT. Because of vitreous seeds, large size, multifocality, ora serrata involvement, proximity to the macula or optic nerve, and previous radio- and/or chemotherapy, these tumors were not suitable for focal or radioactive plaque therapy. The chemotherapy protocol included vincristine-teniposide for 8 and additional carboplatin for 22 eyes, combined with cyclosporine. Chemotherapy was administered for 3–12 months and followed by laser therapy and cryotherapy. After a median follow-up of 2.8 years the actuarial relapse-free rate was 89% in patients without prior treatment (28 eyes) and 67% in patients treated after relapse since previous treatment (12 eyes). For eyes with vitreous seeds the relapse-free rate was 88%.

GREENWALD and STRAUSS (1996) treated six patients (11 eyes) with chemotherapy alone (carboplatin and etoposide) with 6–7 monthly cycles. Twelve of 33 small tumors were treated with coagulation therapy. All 8 larger tumors (>10 mm) underwent dramatic regression with chemotherapy alone. Six larger tumors remained without further growth for 7–21 months after chemotherapy. Eight of the 11 eyes were salvaged, including 5 of the 8 with larger tumors and all 4 of those with diffuse vitreous seeding, 3 of which were irradiated. These eyes appear to have been salvaged 16, 19, 26 and 40 months after treatment.

MURPHREE et al. (1996) reported 38 eyes with group 1 through 5b tumors that were treated with thermochemotherapy (carboplatin followed by diode laser thermotherapy). All 24 eyes with group 1 and 2 tumors were treated successfully and 2 of the 4 eyes with group 3 tumors and all 10 eyes with diffuse vitreous seeding (group 5b) were treated unsuccessfully. Chemoreduction (carboplatin, etoposide and vincristine for 3 cycles) plus sequential aggressive local therapy (SALT) was the primary treatment in

17 eyes and was successful in all 10 eyes with group 1 through 4 tumors and unsuccessful in all 7 eyes with extensive retinal detachment. Treatment in group 5b tumors consisted of 2 cycles each of chemotherapy before and after EBRT (45 Gy to the whole eye). All 18 eyes with diffuse vitreous seedings failed.

Ishu et al. (1996) reported successful treatment with ranimustine and carboplatin for recurrent intraocular retinoblastoma with vitreous seeding. The child has been treated primarily by photocoagulation and EBR with a total dose of 60 Gy 6 years before. Following 5 cycles, the patient has remained free of recurrence for more than 4 years.

Kingston et al. (1996) treated 14 patients in whom bilateral disease with group 5a (16 eyes) and group 5b tumors (12 eyes) was diagnosed. The children were each given 2 courses of chemotherapy (vincristine, etoposide, carboplatin) before (14 children) and after (7 children) whole-eye irradiation (40–44 Gy in 20–22 fractions). Four eyes had to be enucleated, primarily because of severe disease. After 2 courses of chemotherapy tumors decreased in thickness by more than 50%. Serous retinal detachment also resolved in all patients. Six eyes required enucleation, in 2 patients after glaucoma and in 4 patients for recurrent disease (2 each with group 5a and 5b tumors, respectively). Of the 20 eyes of the surviving children (excluding eyes enucleated primarily), 14 (70%) could be salvaged. Of the surviving children, 5 had a visual acuity of 1/60 or better, but many others required low vision aids. The median follow-up time for the 14 children was 60 months. The chemotherapy was well tolerated. The authors concluded that chemotherapy plus radiotherapy was successful in salvaging most eyes with R-E group 5 retinoblastoma. However, ocular complications were frequent and visual acuity was often poor.

The largest series treated by chemotherapy with subsequent thermotherapy was published by Shields et al. (1999). The effectiveness of chemotherapy (vincristine, etoposide, and carboplatin) followed by focal methods, such as cryotherapy, laser photocoagulation, thermotherapy or plaque radiotherapy, had been demonstrated in 20 patients with 54 retinoblastomas in 31 eyes in a previous publication (Shields et al. 1996). All 10 eyes with diffuse vitreous seeding treated with EBRT after failure of chemoreduction, could be salvaged. Shields et al. (1999) reported 188 retinoblastomas in 80 eyes of 58 patients who were treated with thermotherapy. Under general anesthesia, thermotherapy was delivered using infrared radiation (810 nm), either transpupillary or transscleral. The transpupillary method in-

volved infrared radiation delivered through an operating microscope or an indirect ophthalmoscope. Thermotherapy with the transscleral method was delivered via scleral depression and indirect ophthalmoscopy.

Tumors that were close to the optic disc and fovea and large in size (>6 m) were treated with the operating microscope (72 cases), whereas smaller ones or those situated peripheral to the macula were treated with the indirect ophthalmoscope (109 cases). One hundred eight foci (57.4%) were healed after chemoreduction. Tumors 3.0 mm or less across the base and 3.0 mm or less in thickness were treated with infrared radiation alone, and larger tumors and those with vitreous seeds with chemoreduction before thermotherapy.

Complications of thermotherapy in the 80 eyes included focal iris atrophy in 29 eyes (36%), peripheral focal lens opacity in 19 eyes (24%), retinal fraction in 4 eyes (5%) and sector optic disc atrophy in 10 eyes (12%).

After a mean follow-up of 12 months (median 10 months; maximum 45 months) local control was obtained in 85.6% (161/188) of the retinoblastomas. The authors state that about one third of their patients with retinoblastoma are selected for chemoreduction; the other two thirds are treated with nonchemotherapy methods (Shields et al. 1997). They use chemoreduction if a tumor is 4 mm or greater with subsequent thermotherapy after reduction. Tumors less than 3–4 mm across the base are treated initially with thermotherapy alone. However, the decision is often complicated by the many variables of the child and the tumors.

It seems at present that chemoreduction with carboplatin, vincristine and etoposide or teniposide, followed by focal methods such as cryotherapy, laser thermotherapy or radioactive plaque treatment can control more than the half of RE group 5 tumors. Chemoreduction and focal methods are more successful than EBR alone for the treatment of large tumors, tumors adjacent to the optic nerve and fovea and those with diffuse vitreous seeding. More eyes can be salvaged with useful vision, and EBR, with its late effects, can be avoided.

So far, it is not known whether adjuvant chemotherapy reduces the risk of micrometastases in patients with adverse histologic risk factors. However, Kingston et al. 2000, reported that only 1 of 55 children with adverse histological features treated with adjuvant platinum-based chemotherapy (1986–1997) died from metastatic disease, whereas 14 of 22 (63%) children with adverse histologic features not so treated (1970–1985) developed metastatic disease and had died at a median follow-up of 5 years.

Trilateral retinoblastoma is usually fatal despite aggressive treatments (KINGSTON et al. 1985). Only 2 of 20 patients with pinealoblastoma survived for 4 years with aggressive chemotherapy (BLACH et al. 1994). However, SHIELDS CL et al. (1999, 2001) report no cases of pinealoblastoma in 147 children treated with chemoreduction.

Authorities agree that chemotherapy has a part to play in the management of metastatic retinoblastoma. Metastases can occur in the brain or spinal cord, or systemically (DUNKEL et al. 2000). CNS and systemic dissemination have a poor prognosis, although there have been a few reported cases of long-term or prolonged survival in patients with metastatic disease following chemotherapy (JUDISCH et al. 1980; CHAN et al. 1997; PETERSEN et al. 1987; SANDRI et al 1998).

Some institutions have pushed the boundaries further, employing high-dose chemotherapy with stem cell rescue (NAMOUMI et al. 1997).

11.9.6
Treatment-related Nonocular Malignancies

The occurrence of second malignant neoplasms in survivors of retinoblastoma has been reported by many authors (REESE et al. 1949; FORREST 1961; SOLOWAY 1966; SAGERMAN et al. 1969; JENSEN and MILLER 1971; SHAH et al. 1974; ABRAMSON et al. 1976, 1984; MEADOWS et al. 1980; MEADOWS 1988; SCHLIENGER et al. 1985; DRAPER et al. 1986; ALBERTI et al. 1987; KOTEN et al. 1988; SMITH et al. 1989; JENKINSON et al. 2000). ABRAMSON et al. (1984) reported that more than 98% of patients who developed second nonocular tumors had bilateral disease. These tumors have frequently been attributed to the irradiation. However, one-third to one-half of these patients develop tumors outside the irradiation field (ABRAMSON et al. 1984; SCHLIENGER et al. 1985; DRAPER et al. 1986; ALBERTI et al. 1987; SMITH et al. 1989) or without having received irradiation (JENSEN and MILLER 1971; SCHIMKE et al. 1974; LENNOX et al. 1975; ABRAMSON et al. 1979b; ALBERTI et al 1987).

The majority of second malignant tumors are osteosarcoma and soft tissue sarcoma. Modern molecular genetic techniques have demonstrated similar deletions of DNA sequences in retinoblastoma, osteosarcoma, and possibly other mesenchymal tumors at the retinoblastoma locus (band q14 on chromosome 13). The genetic link between these tumors

is probably responsible for the high risk in patients with hereditary retinoblastoma, making it difficult to quantify the role of radiation or chemotherapy in the induction of nonocular cancer.

SAGERMAN et al. (1969) described a dose–response relationship demonstrating an increased risk of second malignant tumors with increasing radiation dose. This was confirmed by ALBERTI et al. (1987), who demonstrated a 47.5% incidence at 16 years for second tumors within the field in patients treated with 55 Gy or more and a 5% incidence in those treated with lesser doses ($P=0.0006$) (Fig 11.10). ABRAMSON et al. (1984) studied 688 survivors of hereditary retinoblastoma and concluded that a second or third course of betatron irradiation did not increase the incidence of second cancer; the role of chemotherapy was not analyzed. Whereas two thirds of the second malignancies occurred in the irradiated volume in the series of SAGERMAN et al. (1969), only one third occurred in this region in the series of ABRAMSON et al. (1984), in which no irradiation was given.

DRAPER et al. (1986) reported 882 patients with retinoblastoma, 90 of whom received cyclophosphamide. They found that the addition of chemotherapy significantly increased the risk of secondary malignancies both within and outside the irradiation field.

The cumulative risk at 10, 20, and 30 years was 6%, 19%, and 38%, respectively, in the study of SMITH et al. (1989), and 20%, 50%, and 90% in the series of ABRAMSON et al. (1984). DRAPER et al. (1986) reported a cumulative risk of 4.3% at 12 years and 8.4% at 18 years. KOTEN et al. (1988) reported an 11% incidence at 35 years in heritable disease.

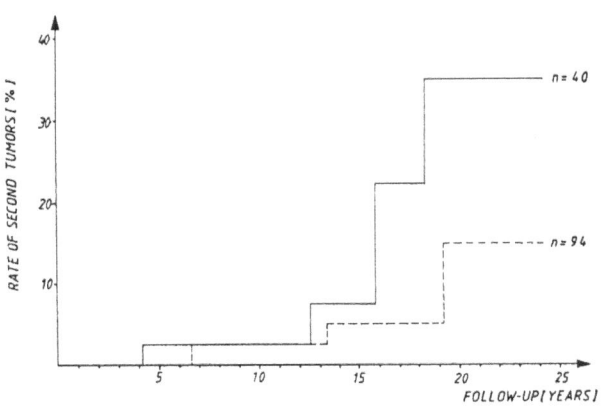

Fig. 11.10. Risk of nonocular malignancy in bilateral retinoblastoma patients treated in Essen from 1959 to 1973. Comparison of patients treated with 55 Gy or more *(solid line)* or less than 55 Gy *(broken line)* ($P = 0.006$, Wilcoxon-Breslow). (ALBERTI et al. 1987)

Two hundred fifteen cases of bilateral retinoblastoma were registered at the Department of Ophthalmic Pathology at the Armed Forces Institute of Pathology (AFIP), Washington, D.C. (ROARTY et al. 1988). Eighty-seven patients died of retinoblastoma, and second tumors developed in 24 patients. The median follow-up was 7.2 years (range 0-49.1 years). The latency period from the time of enucleation to diagnosis of the second tumor ranged from 1.4 to 44.3 years (median 12.2 years). The cumulative incidence of second neoplasms calculated using the life-table method was 4.4% after 10 years, 18.3% after 20 years, and 26.1% after 30 years. Thirteen of 20 tumors in the group of 137 patients treated with irradiation developed in the treatment field, while seven developed outside the field. In the group of 78 patients not treated with radiation, second tumors developed in 4. These data are in agreement with the studies of SCHLIENGER et al. (1985), DRAPER et al. (1986), LUEDER et al. (1986), DER KINDEREN et al. (1987), and ALBERTI et al. (1987), in all of which a significantly lower rate of second tumors was observed than was reported by ABRAMSON et al. (1984). It may be that the last-named group was more successful in obtaining long-term follow-up data on patients with a second tumor than on patients who did not have a second tumor. On the other hand, additional chemotherapy has been given in more than two thirds of the patients reported by ABRAMSON et al. (1984). Chemotherapy was demonstrated by SCHIPPER and ALBERTI (1985) to increase the risk of second nonocular cancers. In the series of SCHLIENGER et al. (1985), 230 patients with retinoblastoma (162 bilateral, 68 unilateral) were irradiated between 1943 and 1972. Fifty-seven of 130 patients treated between 1963 and 1972 received TEM intra-arterially. Four of 94 survivors with bilateral disease with a minimum follow-up of 10 years developed osteosarcoma either within (2) or outside (2) the radiation field. Six additional patients developed other sarcomas (3) within or other tumors (3) outside the field.

WINTHER et al. (1988) investigated the risk of nonocular cancer among survivors of retinoblastoma treated in Denmark between 1943 and 1984. All patients were treated with either radiotherapy or surgery, and chemotherapy was not administered. Among 150 surviving patients, 3 cases of new primary malignancy were observed. No second tumors occurred within the field of irradiation among 47 patients treated with X-rays. Parents not having retinoblastoma themselves were not at increased risk for nonocular cancer. The overall risk for a new primary cancer was 4.2% in both groups, including hereditary and nonhereditary cases. In the subgroup of genetic retinoblastoma the risk was 15.4% and in the group of nonhereditary disease, 1.7%.

In a retrospective study, 194 patients with bilateral retinoblastoma treated in Essen between 1940 and 1973 were divided into three groups according to the treatment received (HILLE 1989). The groups were comparable with respect to age at diagnosis, radiation beam quality, type of chemotherapy, and duration of follow-up. Using multivariate (Cox model) and univariate analyses (Kaplan-Meier), the influences of additional chemotherapy and radiation dose on the incidence and location of second nonocular cancer were investigated. The first group comprised 86 patients treated with radiotherapy alone, the second, 48 patients receiving irradiation and chemotherapy, and the third, 60 patients treated by surgery alone (enucleation and/or photo- and cryocoagulation). Patients in groups 1 and 2 (134) received orthovoltage irradiation (300 kV) and 48 received additional single-agent chemotherapy with alkylating drugs, mostly cyclophosphamide but in some cases busulfan. Second nonocular cancer sdeveloped in 15 of 134 irradiated patients (11.2%) after a median latency of 13.5 years (range 4--20 years). Eleven tumors developed within or close to the irradiation field (ipsilateral orbit, maxilla, nose, temporal bone, base of the skull), while 4 developed outside the field. Osteosarcoma was the most frequent tumor within (5/11) and outside the field (2/4). Soft tissue sarcoma occurred exclusively within the field (5). Only 1 of the 60 patients treated surgically developed an osteosarcoma (of the femur), and this was first observed 16 years after treatment. The rate of second tumors was 8.1% (7/86) in group 1, 16.7% (8/48) in group 2, and 1.7% in group 3 (1/60) (Fig. 11.11). The

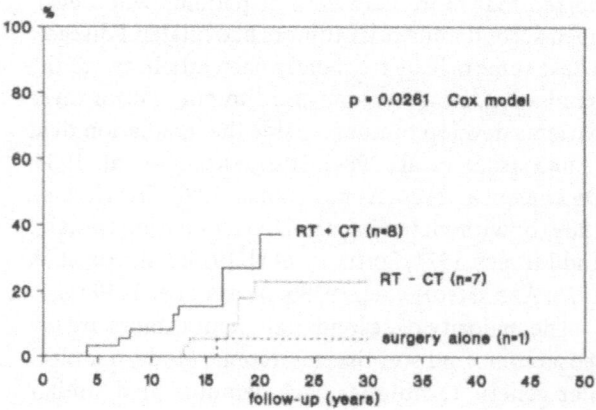

Fig. 11.11. Risk of nonocular malignancies in bilateral retinoblastoma patients treated in Essen from 1940 to 1973 with radiotherapy alone *(RT)* (*n* = 48) vs chemo- and radiotherapy *(CT + RT)* (*n* = 86) vs surgery alone (*n* = 60). (HILLE 1989)

median follow-up intervals were 190 months (range: 2–512) in the radiotherapy group and 145 months (range: 8–270) in the combined modality group. The incidence of second tumors was significantly higher in group 2 than in group 1 ($P=0.01$, Wilcoxon-Breslow). This is in agreement with data published by DRAPER et al. (1986), who found a significantly higher incidence for tumors within and outside the radiation field. In the Essen series, second tumors within the field occurred significantly more frequently in patients with additional chemotherapy than in those receiving radiotherapy alone ($P=0.02$, Cox model). This could not be demonstrated for tumors outside the field, probably because of the small numbers in our series.

The risk for second tumors after 20 years was calculated in a multivariate analysis: the rate was 21% in group 1 vs 38% in group 2 ($P=0.02$). When tumors within the radiation field were considered the difference between the two groups was also significant: 13% vs 28% ($P=0.004$, Wilcoxon-Breslow). For tumors outside the radiation field, the incidence of second nonocular cancer after 20 years was 9% after radiotherapy alone, compared with 14.5% with additional chemotherapy ($P=0.564$). Patients treated with surgery alone had a 4.4% risk of second tumors after 20 years.

Recent analyses indicate a statistically significant increase in the incidence of second cancers only in the 961 patients with hereditary retinoblastoma among 1,604 retinoblastoma patients surviving for at least 1 year after diagnosis (190 cancers developed vs 6.3 expected in the general population; relative risk 30, 95% confidence interval 26–47). The cumulative incidence of a second cancer was 51% (±6.2%) at 50 years for hereditary retinoblastoma, as against 5.0% (±3.0%) for nonhereditary retinoblastoma. All 114 sarcomas developed among the hereditary group, and there was a stepwise increase at all dose categories above 5 Gy, rising to 10.7-fold at 60 Gy or greater. An underlying genetic predisposition, enhanced by irradiation, indicates that these patients should be followed up throughout their lifetimes (ABRAMSON 1999; WONG et al. 1997).

In the future, more patients with retinoblastoma will die from secondary cancer than from metastatic disease. Careful treatment planning, sophisticated radiation techniques, limitation of the radiation dose, and the employment of combined-modality programs, utilizing plaque brachytherapy and omitting EBT when possible, should reduce the risk of second tumors.

References

Abramson D (1999) Second nonocular cancers in retinoblastoma: A unified hypothesis. (The Franceschetti lecture) Ophthalmic Genet 20:193–204

Abramson DH (1985) Treatment of retinoblastoma. In: Blodi FC (ed) Retinoblastoma. Churchill Livingstone, New York, pp 63–93

Abramson DH, Ellsworth RM (1980) The surgical management of retinoblastoma. Ophthalmic Surg 11:596–598

Abramson DH, Ellsworth RM, Zimmerman LE (1976) Nonocular cancer in retinoblastoma survivors. Trans Am Acad Ophthalmol Otolaryngol 81:454–457

Abramson DH, Piro P A, Ellsworth RM et al. (1979a) Lactate dehydrogenase levels and isoenzyme patterns: measurements in the aqueous humor and serum of retinoblastoma patients. Arch Ophthalmol 97:870–872

Abramson DH, Ronner HJ, Ellsworth RM (1979b) Second tumors in nonirradiated bilateral retinoblastoma. Am J Ophthalmol 87:624–627

Abramson DH, Ellsworth RM, Tretter P et al. (1981a) Simultaneous bilateral irradiation for advanced bilateral retinoblastoma. Arch Ophthalmol 99: 1763–1766

Abramson DH, Ellsworth RM, Tretter P et al. (1981b) Treatment of bilateral groups I through III retinoblastoma with bilateral radiation. Arch Ophthalmol 99:1761–1762

Abramson DH, Jereb B, Ellsworth RM (1981c) External beam radiation for retinoblastoma. Bull NY Acad Med 57:787–803

Abramson DH, Ellsworth RM, Rozakis GW (1982a) Cryotherapy for retinoblastoma. Arch Ophthalmol 100:1253–1256

Abramson DH, Marks RF, Ellsworth M et al. (1982b) The management of unilateral retinoblastoma without primary enucleation. Arch Ophthalmol 100:1249–1252

Abramson DH, Ellsworth RM, Rosenblatt M et al. (1982c) Retreatment of retinoblastoma with external beam irradiation. Arch Ophthalmol 100:1257–1260

Abramson DH, Ellsworth RM, Haik B (1983) Cobalt plaques in advanced retinoblastoma. Retina 3:12–15

Abramson DH, Ellsworth RM, Kitchin FD et al. (1984) Second nonocular tumors in retinoblastoma survivors. Are they radiation-induced? Ophthalmology 91:1351–1355

Alberti W (1991) Effects of radiation on the eye and ocular adnexa. In: Scherer E, Streffer C, Trott KR (eds) Radiopathology of organs and tissues. Springer, Berlin Heidelberg New York, pp 269–282

Alberti W, Halama J, Wannenmacher M (1987) Tumoren im Kopfbereich. Tumoren des Auges und der Orbita. In: Scherer E (ed) Strahlentherapie. Radiologische Onkologie. Springer, Berlin Heidelberg New York, pp 412–453

Alberti W, EI-Hifnawi S, Foerster MH, Bornfeld N (1990) Late effects after fractionated external beam therapy of minipig eyes in the retina and optic nerve. Int J Radiat Oncol Biol Phys 19: 158–159

Amendola BE, Lamm FR, Markoe AM et al. (1990) Radiotherapy of retinoblastoma. Cancer 66:21–26

American Cancer Society, New York (1983) Cancer facts and figures.

Amoaku WM, Willshaw HE, Parkes SE et al (1996) Trilateral retinoblastoma: a report of five patients. Cancer 78:858–863

Bader IL, Miller RW, Meadows AT et al. (1980) Trilateral retinoblastoma. Lancet 11:583–583

Blach LE, McCormick B, Abramson DH et al (1994) Trilateral retinoblastoma .– incidence and outcome: a decade of experience. Int J Radiat Oncol Biol Phys 29:729–733

Boniuk M, Zimmerman LE (1962) Spontaneous regression of retinoblastoma. Int Ophthalmol Clin 2:525–542

Buys RJ, Abramson DH, Ellsworth RM et al. (1983) Radiation regression patterns after cobalt plaque insertion for retinoblastoma. Arch Ophthalmol 101: 1206–1208

Carbajal UM (1959) Metastasis in retinoblastoma. Am J Ophthalmol 48:47–60

Carlson EA, Letson MD, Ramsay NKC et al. (1979) Factors for improved genetic counseling for retinoblastoma based on a survey of 55 families. Am J Ophthalmol 87:449–459

Cassady JR, Sagerman RH, Tretter P et al. (1969) Radiation therapy in retinoblastoma. Radiology 93:405–409

Chan HS, DeBoer G, Thiessen JJ et al (1996) Combining cyclosporin with chemotherapy controls intraocular retinoblastoma without requiring radiation. Clin Cancer Res 2:1499–1508

Char DH (1989) Clinical ocular oncology. Churchill Livingstone, New York, pp 179–230

Connolly MJ, Payne RH, Johnson G et al. (1983) Familial, EsD-linked, retinoblastoma with reduced penetrance and variable expressivity. Hum Genet 65:122–124

Cypress RH, Karol MH, Zidian JL et al. (1978) Larva specific antibodies in patients with visceral larva migrans. Am J Trop Med Hyg 27:492–498

der Kinderen DJ, Koten IW, Wolterbeek R et al. (1987) Nonocular cancer in hereditary retinoblastoma survivors and relatives. Ophthalmic Paediatr Genet 8:23–25

de Sutter E, Havers W, Hopping W et al. (1987a) The prognosis of retinoblastoma in terms of globe saving treatment. A computer assisted study. Part I. Ophthalmic Paediatr Genet 8:77–84

de Sutter E, Havers W, Hopping W et al. (1987b) The prognosis of retinoblastoma in terms of survival. A computer assisted study. Part II. Ophthalmic Paediatr Genet 8:85–88

Devesa SS (1975) The incidence of retinoblastoma. Trans Am Ophthalmol Soc 67:263–265

Donaldson SS, Egbert PR (1989) Retinoblastoma. In: Pizzo PA, Poplack DG (eds) Principles and practice of pediatric oncology. JB Lippincott, Philadelphia, pp 555–569

Donoso LA, Feldberg NT, Shields JA et al. (1981) Immunodiagnosis of late, recurrent retinoblastoma. Retina 1:107–112

Draper GI, Sanders BM, Kingston IE (1986) Second primary neoplasms in patients with retinoblastoma. Br J Cancer 53:661–671

Dunkel IJ, Aledo A, Kernan NA et al (2000) Successful treatment of metastatic retinoblastoma. Cancer 89:2117–2121

Egbert PR, Donaldson SS, Moazed K et al. (1978) Visual results and ocular complications following radiotherapy for retinoblastoma. Arch Ophthalmol 96:1826–1830

Egbert PR, Fajardo LF, Donaldson SS et al. (1980) Posterior ocular abnormalities after irradiation for retinoblastoma: a histopathological study. Br J Ophthalmol 64:660–665

Ellsworth RM (1968) Treatment of retinoblastoma. Am J Ophthalmol 66:49–51

Ellsworth RM (1969) The practical management of retinoblastoma. Trans Am Ophthalmol Soc 67: 462–534

Ellsworth RM (1977) Retinoblastoma. Mod Probl Ophthalmol 18:94–100

Ellsworth RM (1978) Current management of retinoblastoma. In: Jakobiec FA (ed) Ocular and adnexal tumors. Aesculapius, Birmingham, pp 128–136

Feldberg NT, McFall R, Shields JA (1977) Aqueous humor enzyme patterns in retinoblastoma. Invest Ophthalmol Yis Sci 16:1039–1046

Ferris FL, Chew EY (1996) A new era for the treatment of retinoblastoma. Arch Ophthalmol 114:1412

Finger PT, Czechonska G, Demirci H et al (1999) Chemotherapy for retinoblastoma: a current topic. Drugs 58:983–996

Flexner S (1891) A peculiar glioma (neuro epithelioma?) of the retina. Bull Hopkins Hosp 2:115–119

Folkmann J (1974) Tumor angiogensis factor. Cancer Res 34:2109–2113

Forrest AW (1961) Tumors following radiation about the eye. Trans Am Acad Ophthalmol Otolaryngol 65:694–717

Freeman CR, Esseltine DL, Whitehead YM et al. (1980) Retinoblastoma: the case for radiotherapy and for adjuvant chemotherapy. Cancer 46:1913–1918

Gallie BL, Budning A, DeBoer G et al. (1996) Chemotherapy with focal therapy can cure intraocular retinoblastoma without radiotherapy. Arch Ophthalmol 114:1321–1328

Gallie BL, Ellsworth RM, Abramson DH et al. (1982) Retinoma: spontaneous regression of retinoblastoma or benign manifestation of the mutation? Br J Cancer 45:513–554

Goble RR, McKenzie J, Kingston JE et al (1990) Orbital recurrence of retinoblastoma successfully treated by combined therapy. Br J Ophthalmol 74:97–98

Greenwald MJ, Strauss LC (1995) Treatment of intraocular retinoblastoma with carboplatin and etoposide chemotherapy. Ophthalmology 103:1989–997

Harnett AN, Hungerford IL, Lambert GD et al. (1987) Improved external beam radiotherapy for the treatment of retinoblastoma. Br J Radiol 60:753–760

Havers W, Alberti W, Messmer EP et al. (1986) Retinoblastoma. Monogr Paediatr vol 18. Karger, Basel, pp 342–358

Haye C, Desjardins L, Schlienger P et al (1987) Treatment of bilateral retinoblastoma stage V at the Curie Foundation. Ophthalmic Paediatr Genet 8:73–76

Haye C, Schlienger P, Calle R et al. (1986) Traitement conservateur des tumeurs de la retine a l'Institut Curie. Bull Cancer (Paris) 73:260–270

Heinrich T (1989) Das Metastasierungsrisiko beim Retinoblastom. Eine Prognoseklassifikation auf dem Boden einer multivariaten Analyse potentieller Einflußfaktoren. Dissertation, University of Essen

Hilgartner HL (1903) Report of a case of double glioma treated by x-rays. Tex Med J 18:322

Hille P (1989) Spätergebnisse der Strahlentherapie bilateraler Retinoblastome unter besonderer Berücksichtigung maligner Zweitneoplasien. Essen 1940–1973. Dissertation, University of Essen

Hopping W (1983) The new Essen prognosis classification for conservative sightsaving treatment of retinoblastoma. In: Lommatzsch PK, Blodi FC (eds) Intraocular tumors. Akademie, Berlin, pp 497505

Höpping W, Bunke-Schmidt A (1985) Light coagulation and cryotherapy. In: Blodi FC (ed) Retinoblastoma. Churchill Livingstone, New York, pp 95–110

Höpping W, Meyer-Schwickerath G (1964) Light coagulation treatment in retinoblastoma. In: Boniuk M (ed) Ocular and adnexal tumors. New and controversial aspects. C.Y. Mosby, St. Louis, pp 192–196

Höpping W, Havers W, Alberti W et al. (1985a) Klinische Gesichtspunkte des Retinoblastoms. In: Hammerstein W, Lisch W (eds) Ophthalmologische Genetik. Ferdinand Enke, Stuttgart, pp 324–338

Höpping W, Alberti W, Havers W et al. (1985b) Das Retinoblastom. In: Lund DE, Waubke TN (eds) Die Augenerkrankungen im Kindesalter. Enke, Stuttgart, pp 199–217

Howard GM (1966) Ocular effects of radiation and photocoagulation. Arch Ophthalmol 76:7–10

Howard RO (1982) Chromosome errors in retinoblastoma. Birth Defects 18:703–727

Howarth C, Meyer D, Hustu 0 et al. (1980) Stage-related combined modality treatment of retinoblastoma. Cancer 45:851–858

Jakobiec FA, Tso MOM, Zimmerman LE et al. (1977) Retinoblastoma and intracranial malignancy. Cancer 39:2048–2058

Ishii E, Matsuzaki A, Ohnishi Y et al (1996) Successful treatment with ranimustine and carboplatin for recurrent intraocular retinoblastoma with vitreous seeding. Am J Clin Oncol 19:562–565

Jenkinson HC, Hawkins MM, Draper GJ, Kingston JE (2000) The risk of second primary tumors in 3-year survivors of retinoblastoma in Britain. Medical and Pediatric Oncology 35:206

Jensen RD, Miller RW (1971) Retinoblastoma: epidemiology characteristics. N Engl J Med 285: 307–311

Judisch GF, Apple DI, Fratkin ill (1980) A survivor 12 years after treatment for metastatic disease. Arch Ophthalmol 98:711–713

Khodadoust AA, Roozitalab HM, Smith RE et al. (1977) Spontaneous regression of retinoblastoma. Surv Ophthalmol 21:468–478

Kingston JE, Hungerford JL, Madreperla SA et al (1996) Results of combined chemotherapy and radiotherapy for advanced intraocular retinoblastoma. Arch Ophthalmol 114:1339–1343

Kingston JE, Hungerford JL, Stiller CA, Plowman PN (2000) Improved survival of children with advanced retinoblastoma – the role of adjuvant chemotherapy. Medical and Pediatric Oncology 35:179

Kingston JE, Plowman PN, Hungerford JL (1985) Ectopic intracranial retinoblastoma in childhood. Br J Ophthalmol 69:742–748

Kitchin FD (1976) Genetics of retinoblastoma. In: Reese AB (ed) Tumors in the eye. Harper and Row, Hagerstown, pp 125–132

Knieper C (1911) Ein Fall von doppelseitigem Glioma retinae mit Enucleation des einen und nunmehr fast 11-jahriger Atrophie des anderen Auges. A.v. Graefes Arch Klin Ophthalmol 78:310–330

Knudson JR (1971) Mutation and cancer: statistically study of retinoblastoma. Proc Natl Acad Sci USA 68:820–823

Koten JW, der Kinderen DJ, Otter WD (1988) Editorial reply. N Engl J Med 318:581–582

Kupfer C (1953) Retinoblastoma treated by intravenous nitrogen mustard. Am J Ophthalmol 36:1721–1724

Kyritsis AP, Tsokos M, Triche TI et al. (1984) Retinoblastomaorigin from a primitive neuroectodermal cell? Nature 307:471–473

Lennox EL, Draper GJ, Sanders BM (1975) Retinoblastoma: a study of natural history and prognosis of 268 cases. Br Med J 3:731–734

Levy C, Doz F, Quintana E et al (1998) Role of chemotherapy alone or in combination with hyperthermia in the primary treatment of intraocular retinoblastoma: preliminary results. Br J Ophthal 82:1154–1158

Lincoff H, McLean J, Long R (1967) The cryosurgical treatment of intraocular tumors. Am J Ophthalmol 63:389–399

Lommatzsch PK (1978) Experience with beta-irradiation (IO6Ru/1O6Rh) of patients suffering from retinoblastoma (report on 33 patients). Jpn J Ophthalmol 22:424–430

Lommatzsch PK (1989) Intraokulare Tumoren. Enke, Stuttgart

Lueder GT, Goyal R (1996) Visual function after laser hyperthermia and chemotherapy for macular retinoblastoma. Am J Ophthalmol 121:582–584

Lueder GT, Judisch GF, O'Gorman TW (1986) Second nonocular tumors in survivors of heritable retinoblastoma. Arch Ophthalmol104:372–3

Macklin MT (1960) A study of retinoblastoma in Ohio. Am J Hum Genet 12:1–43

Margo CE, Hidayat A, Kopelman I et al. (1983) Retinocytoma: a benign variant of retinoblastoma. Arch Ophthalmol 101:1519–1531

McFaul FA, Bedford MA (1970) Ocular complications after therapeutic irradiation. Br J Ophthalmol 54: 237–247

McKay CI, Abramson DH, Ellsworth RM (1984) Metastatic patterns of retinoblastoma. Arch Ophthalmol 102:391–396

Meadows AT (1988) Risk factors for second malignant neoplasms. Report from the Late Effects Study Group. Bull Cancer (Paris) 75:125–130

Meadows AT, Strong LC, Li FP et al. (1980) Bone sarcoma as a second malignant neoplasm in children: influence of radiation and genetic predisposition. Cancer 46:2603–2606

Merriam GR (1950) Retinoblastoma: analysis of 17 autopsies. Arch Ophthalmol 44:71–108

Messmer EP (1989) Die Histopathologie des Retinoblastoms unter besonderer Berücksichtigung des Differenzierungsverhaltens. Thesis, University of Essen

Messmer EP, Richter HJ, Hopping W et al. (1987) Nichtokularer, maligner Zweittumor nach Spontanheilung eines Retinoblastoms. Klin Monatsbl Augenheilkd 19:299–303

Messmer EP, Sauerwein W, Heinrich T et al. (1990) New and recurrent tumor foci following local treatment as well as external beam radiation in eyes of patients with hereditary retinoblastoma. Graefes Arch Clin Exp Ophthalmol 228:426–431

Meyer-Schwickerath G (1961) The preservation of vision by treatment of intraocular tumors with light coagulation. Arch Ophthalmol 66:458–466

Meyer-Schwickerath G, Helferich E (1958) Zur Therapie des Retinoblastoms. Klin Monatsbl Augenheilkd 132:806–817

Motegi T, Kaga M, Yanagawa Y et al. (1983) A recognizable pattern of the midface of retinoblastoma patients with interstitial deletion of 13q. Hum Genet 64:160–162

Murphree AL, Villablanca JG, Deegan WF et al (1996) Chemotherapy plus local treatment in the management of intraocular retinoblastoma. Arch Ophth 114:1348–1356

Murray TG, Roth DB, O'Brian JM et al (1966) Local carboplatin and radiation therapy in the treatment of murine transgenetic retinoblastoma. 4:385–386

Namouni F, Doz F, Tanguy ML et al (1997) High dose chemotherapy with carboplatin, etoposide and cyclophosphamide followed by a haematopoietic stem cell rescue in patients with high risk retinoblastoma: a SFOP and SFGM study. Eur J Cancer 33:2368–2375

Pollard ZF, Jarrett WH, Hagler WS et al. (1979) ELISA for diagnosis of ocular toxocariasis. Am J Ophthalmol 86:743–749

Pradhan DG, Sandridge AL, Mullaney P et al (1997) Radiation therapy for retinoblastoma: aretrospective review of 120 patients. Int J Radiat Oncol Biol Phys 39:3–3

Pratt CB (1972) Management of malignant solid tumors in children. Pediatr Clin North Am 19:1141–1155

Pratt CB, Meyer D, Chenaille P et al. (1989) The use of bone marrow aspirations and lumbar punctures at the time of diagnosis of retinoblastoma. J Clin Oncol 7:140–143

Redler LD, Ellsworth RM (1973) Prognostic importance of choroidal invasion in retinoblastoma. Arch Ophthalmol 90:294–296

Reese AB (1976) Retinoblastoma and other neuroectodermal tumors of the retina. In: Haverstraw MD (ed) Tumors of the eye, 3rd edn. Harper & Row, New York, pp 89–133

Reese AB, Ellsworth RM (1963) The evaluation and current concept of retinoblastoma therapy. Am Acad Ophthalmol Otolaryngol 67:164–172

Reese AB, Merriam GR, Martin HE (1949) Treatment of bilateral retinoblastoma by irradiation and surgery. Am J Ophthalmol 32:175–190

Reese AB, Hyman G, Merriam GR et al. (1955) Treatment of retinoblastoma by radiation and triethylene melamine. Arch Ophthalmol 53:505–513

Roarty ID, McLean IW, Zimmerman LE (1988) Incidence of second neoplasms in patients and their parents. Cancer 95: 1583–1587

Rootman J, Hofbauer J, Ellsworth RM et al. (1976) Invasion of the optic nerve by retinoblastoma: a clinicopathologic study. Can J Ophthalmol 11:106–114

Rosengren BH, Tengroth B (1963) A modified cobalt 60 applicator for the treatment of retinoblastoma. Acta Radiol Oncol Radiat Phys BioI 1:310–314

Rubin CM, Robinson LL, Camaron JD et al. (1985) Intraocular retinoblastoma group V: an analysis of prognostic factors. J Clin Oncol 3:680–685

Sagerman RH, Cassady JR, Tretter P et al. (1969) Radiation induced neoplasia following external beam therapy for children with retinoblastoma. AJR 105:529–535

Sandri A, Besenzon L, Acquaviva A et al (1998) Eight drugs in one day chemotherapy in a nonfamilial bilateral retinoblastoma with recurrent cerebrospinal fluid metastases. Pediatr Hematol Oncol 15:557–561

Schimke RN, Kowman IT, Cowan GAB (1974) Retinoblastoma and osteogenic sarcoma in siblings. Cancer 34:2077–2079

Schipper J (1980) Retinoblastoma. A medical and experimental study. Thesis, Utrecht

Schipper J (1983) An accurate and simple method for megavolt age radiation therapy of retinoblastoma. Radiother Oncol1:31–41

Schipper J, Alberti W (1985) Second non ocular cancer in retinoblastoma survivors. Letter to the editor. Ophthalmology 92:60A–62A

Schipper J, Tan KEWP, van Peperzeel A (1985) Treatment of retinoblastoma by precision megavoltage radiation therapy. Radiother Oncol 3:117–132

Schlienger P, Calle R, Haye C et al. (1985) Sarcomes osseux et tumeurs malignes de la retine. Bull Cancer (Paris) 72:16–24

Shah IC, Arlen M, Miller T (1974) Osteogenic sarcoma developing after radiotherapy for retinoblastoma. Am Surg 40:485–490

Shields CL, Shields JA (1999) Recent developments in the management of retinoblastoma. J Pediatr Ophthalmol Strabismus 36:8–18

Shields CL, DePotter P, Himelstein BP et al (1996) Chemoreduction in the initial management of intraocular retinoblastoma. Arch Ophthalmol 114:1330–1338

Shields CL, Shields JA, Needle M et al (1997) Combined chemoreduction and adjuvant treatment for intraocular retinoblastoma. Ophth 1997:2101–2111

Shields CL, Santos MC, Diniz W et al (1999) Thermotherapy for retinoblastoma. Arch Ophthalmol 117: 885–893

Shields CL, Shields JA, Cater J et al (2001) Plaque radiotherapy for retinoblastoma. Ophthalmology 108:2116–2121

Shields CL, Meadows AT, Shields JA et al (2001) Chemo-reduction for retinoblastoma may prevent intracranial neuroblastic malignancy (trilateral retinoblastoma). Arch Ophth 119:1269–1272

Shields JA, Augsburger JJ (1981) Current approaches to the diagnosis and management of retinoblastoma. Surv OphthalmoI25:347–353

Smith LM, Donaldson SS, Egbert PR et al. (1989) Aggressive management of second primary tumors in survivors of hereditary retinoblastoma. Int J Radiat Oncol BioI Phys 17:499–505

Soloway HB (1966) Radiation-induced neoplasms following curative therapy of retinoblastoma. J Am Soc Cancer 19:1984–1988

Sparkes RS, Murphree AL, Lingua RW et al. (1983) Gene for hereditary retinoblastoma assigned to human chromosome 13 by linkage to esterase D. Science 219:971–973

Stallard HB (1933) Radient energy as (a) a pathogenic (b) a therapeutic agent in ophthalmic disorders. Br J Ophthalmol, Monograph Supplement 6

Stallard HB (1955) Multiple islands of retinoblastoma. Br J Ophthalmol 39:241–243

Stallard HB (1966) The treatment of retinoblastoma. Ophthalmologica 151:214–230

Stallard HB (1968) The treatment of retinoblastoma. Mod Probl Ophthalmol 7:149–173

Stannard C, Lipper S, Sealy R et al. (1979) Retinoblastoma: correlation of invasion of the optic nerve and choroid with prognosis and metastases. Br J Ophthalmol 63:560–570

Stannard C, Sealy R, Shackleton D et al. (1987) The use of iodine-125 plaques in the treatment of retinoblastoma Ophthalmic Paediatr Genet 8:89–93

Verhoeff FH (1922) Primary intraneural tumors (gliomas) of the optic nerve. Arch Ophthalmol 51:120

Virchow R (1864) Die krankhaften Geschwiilste, vol 2. Hirschwald, Berlin

Vogel F (1979) Genetics of retinoblastoma. Hum Genet 52:1–54

Weiss DR, Cassady JR, Petersen R (1975) Retinoblastoma: a modification in radiation therapy technique. Radiology 114:705–708

Wintersteiner H (1894) Über Bau, Wachstum und Genese des Glioma Retinae. Wien Klin Wochenschr 7:493

Winther J, Olsen JH, de Nully Brown P (1988) Risk of nonocular cancer among retinoblastoma patients and their parents. Cancer 62:1458–1462

Wong FL, Boice JD, Abramson DH (1997) Cancer incidence after retinoblastoma. JAMA 278:1262–1267

12 Heat Treatment of Choroidal Melanomas

J. A. Oosterhuis, J. E. E. Keunen, H. G. Journée-de Korver

CONTENTS

12.1 Introduction

The therapeutic effect of heat on tumors was recognized more than a century ago, when it was noted that attacks of high fever, as in erysipelas, could reduce the size of malignant tumors. Today, heat in three temperature ranges is used to treat choroidal melanomas. These three temperature ranges (hyperthermia, meaning a tumor temperature of 42–44°C; thermotherapy, with a tumor temperature of 45–65°C; and photocoagulation and diathermy, requiring a tumor temperature of over 65°C) are discussed separately.

J.A. Oosterhuis, MD
Prinsenweg 57, 2242 EB Wassenaar, The Netherlands
J.E.E. Keunen, MD
Department of Ophthalmology, Leiden University Medical Center, P.O. Box 9600, 2300 RC Leiden, The Netherlands
H.G. Journée-de Korver, PhD
Department of Ophthalmology, Leiden University Medical Center, P.O. Box 9600, 2300 RC Leiden, The Netherlands

12.2 Hyperthermia

Hyperthermia is used in the treatment of human tumors because it has a synergistic effect when combined with radiotherapy or cytostatic drug therapy. The effect is optimal when both treatments are given simultaneously. Well-oxygenated tumor cells are more sensitive to radiation than hypoxic cells, and the opposite applies for hyperthermia. Many choroidal melanomas have areas of hypoxia or even of spontaneous necrosis. Hyperthermia is not effective as a sole therapy, because in this range of temperatures cell damage is largely reversible. At best, hyperthermia alone causes a temporary retardation of tumor growth.

Brachytherapy of choroidal melanomas is complicated by macular radiation vasculopathy with impairment of visual acuity in 42% of patients because the macular capillaries are highly susceptible to radiation (Gündüz et al. 1999). The combination of brachytherapy and hyperthermia allows the dose of radiation to be reduced without interfering with its therapeutic effect.

Hyperthermia was introduced into ophthalmic oncology in 1982. Episcleral applicators are used in three hyperthermia techniques: microwave, localized current field and ferromagnetic thermoseeds; a fourth hyperthermia technique provides transscleral heat by high-intensity ultrasound produced by a transducer.

In hyperthermia treatment of choroidal melanomas most experience has been gathered with *microwave thermoradiotherapy*, and this is the form of hyperthermia that has also yielded the best treatment results. After brachytherapy with iodine-125 (^{125}I) or palladium-103 (^{103}Pd) seeds, heat is produced by electromagnetic induction by means of an applicator containing a disc-shaped microwave antenna connected to a power source. Finger (1997) reported treatment results obtained in 48 patients with uveal melanoma with an average follow-up of 5 years. The tumor apex was heated to at least 42°C for

45 min. The episcleral temperature, which ranged from 46.6° to 52.5°C, was well tolerated by the sclera. The mean radiotherapy dose at the apex was 52.6 Gy, i.e., about half the dose commonly used for brachytherapy as sole treatment. Tumor control was obtained in all but 3 eyes (93.8%), which were enucleated, as were 4 eyes with neovascular glaucoma. In 33 (69%) of the patients visual acuity remained within 3 lines of the pretreatment value or improved. The most striking heat-induced side effect was choroidal infarction, which was observed in 15 (32%) of the patients and which led to scar formation in and around the treatment area.

In *localized current field hyperthermia* an episcleral applicator is provided with a radiofrequency electrode; a second, larger, electrode is placed on the patient's cheek. The tumor is heated by the current between the two electrodes, which is greatest next to the smaller electrode. The tumor is almost uniformly heated as the temperature gradient is only 0.23°C mm^{-1}. Twenty-five patients with mainly large (T3) choroidal melanomas were treated by localized current field hyperthermia at a tumor temperature of 43–45°C for 45 min and with 73.3 Gy ^{125}I brachytherapy at the tumor apex. The average follow-up was 2.5 years (PETROVICH et al. 1996). Twenty patients (80%) showed permanent tumor regression. Sixty percent of the patients had a visual acuity of 20/50 or better before treatment, but only 20% had it at the last examination. Mild transient complications developed in 6 (24%) patients and cataract in 5 (20%) patients.

Ferromagnetic hyperthermia is generated by ferromagnetic thermoseeds, which are placed in an electromagnetic field. The seeds maintain the desired temperature in a self-regulated manner, depending on the rate of the ferromagnetic element. There are no electrical connections to a power source. An applicator temperature of 54°C for 60 min caused chorioretinal scarring but was well tolerated by the sclera (MURRAY et al. 1997). In experimental retinoblastomas tumor control after heating for 20 min was 33% at 48°C and 100% at 54°C. After treatment at the latter temperature, 25% of the eyes were lost owing to treatment complications (MURRAY et al. 1996).

Ultrasonically induced transscleral hyperthermia is produced by a transducer providing high-intensity ultrasound. Ultrasonic energy can easily be focused and localized in the tumor, where it induces selective heating based on the high acoustic absorption coefficient of choroidal melanomas. The rate of tumor necrosis in experimental melanomas is related to the increase in temperature (BRAAKMAN et al. 1989). For clinical treatment, ultrasonic hyperther-

mia has been combined with cobalt-60 (^{60}Co) brachytherapy (COLEMAN et al. 1997). Tumor temperatures estimated in experimental models to be 43–45°C were maintained for 30 min. Complications in a 5-year follow-up study of 11 patients treated with ultrasonic thermoradiotherapy were tumor regrowth, choroidal effusion with vitreous hemorrhage, subretinal hemorrhages, radiation retinopathy, and cataract, each in 1 patient.

Microwave thermoradiotherapy is the only technique that has provided well-documented, favorable results based on 10 years' experience of treating choroidal melanomas. Hyperthermia as an adjuvant to brachytherapy makes it possible to reduce the radiation dose by about 50% without interfering with its therapeutic effect. However, this treatment modality is not used on a large scale.

12.3
Thermotherapy

Temperatures of 45–65°C have been designated thermotherapy, because heat in this temperature range exerts an irreversible cytotoxic effect. Thermotherapy of intraocular tumors (melanomas, retinoblastomas and hemangiomas) is carried out as transpupillary thermotherapy (TTT), meaning that an infrared laser beam is directed at the surface of the tumor through the pupil. This treatment modality has gained worldwide acceptance since its introduction by OOSTERHUIS et al. in 1995.

12.3.1
Histopathologic Results of Experimental Thermotherapy

For TTT a near-infrared laser is used at 810 nm, a wavelength that provides an optimal depth of penetration of heat into tissue. Penetration is also promoted by the use of a large radiation beam, up to 3.5 mm in diameter, and a long exposure time, generally 1 min (JOURNÉE-DE KORVER et al. 1992).

Tumor cell destruction by thermotherapy is predominantly caused by a direct effect of heat, which causes necrosis of the nuclei of the tumor cells, as revealed by electron microscopy. Shutdown of the circulation in the tumor contributes to the cell damage by causing mitochondrial breakdown, but it is not the primary cause of necrosis (JOURNÉE-DE KORVER et al. 1995). Histopathologic examination of hamster and human choroidal melanomas after thermotherapy shows a continuous field of tumor necrosis up to 6 mm deep in hamster melanomas and 3.9 mm in human choroidal melanomas (Fig. 12.1) (JOURNÉE-DE KORVER et al. 1992). All blood vessels in the necrotic part of the tumor are occluded, which explains why there are only a few hemorrhages present or none at all. There is a sharp demarcation between the necrotic and the viable parts of the tumor, as revealed by fluorescein angiography (Fig. 12.2). This is due to the rather steep decrease in temperature in the tumor: about 5°C per millimeter of tumor tissue. Treated and non-treated parts of the tumor are separated by a small (0.5–0.7 mm) transitional zone, which contains small hemorrhages, because heating is sufficient to damage the vessel walls but not to cause thrombosis. The anterior segment of the eye and the ocular media are normal (JOURNÉE-DE KORVER et al. 1997).

12.3.2
Technique of Transpupillary Thermotherapy (TTT)

TTT for the treatment of choroidal melanomas is performed as an outpatient procedure and thus can be repeated if necessary. Prior to treatment mydriatic eyedrops and parabulbar anesthesia are administered. TTT is performed with an 810-nm diode laser attached to a slit-lamp for monitoring the laser beam, which is delivered through a contact lens. Treatment is started with a relatively low energy level

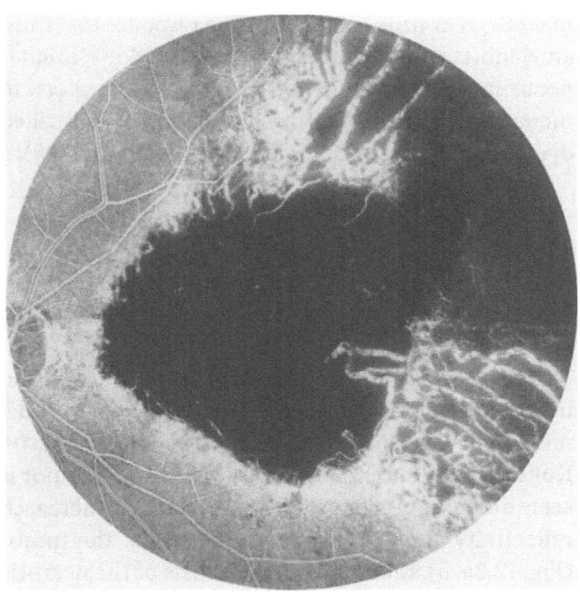

Fig. 12.2. Fluorescein angiogram after TTT of a marginal recurrence of a choroidal melanoma after [106]Ru plaque treatment. The TTT-treated area in and around the macula is almost completely nonfluorescent and is sharply demarcated from the surrounding area with normal background fluorescence. The border of the brachytherapy-treated area shows a wide marginal zone of choriocapillaris atrophy with perfusion of the large choroidal vessels. (Reproduced from OOSTERHUIS et al. 1998; copyrighted 1998, American Medical Association)

that has little or no visible effect after 1 min. The energy level is then increased stepwise until a gray or slightly white discoloration of the tumor develops in the last 15–20 s of the 1-min exposure. This discoloration is a good indicator of the energy level to be used. Energy levels that produce a white photocoagulation effect in the first 30 s of TTT should be avoided, because increased reflection and scatter reduce the rate of transmission of light into the tumor and hence the depth of tumor necrosis. The entire surface of the tumor should be confluently covered by overlapping applications extending 1–1.5 mm into the normal choroid. Several days after TTT the tumor becomes white, a sign of tumor necrosis.

The absence of pigmentation in amelanotic melanomas allows for increased penetration of infrared radiation into tissue, but also for a lower volume uptake of radiation. Therefore, amelanotic melanomas require treatment at a higher energy level than pigmented melanomas. The mean energy required for TTT of amelanotic melanomas has been found to be 15% higher than that needed for pigmented melanomas, and the reduction in thickness was 33% greater in the amelanotic tumors than in pigmented melano-

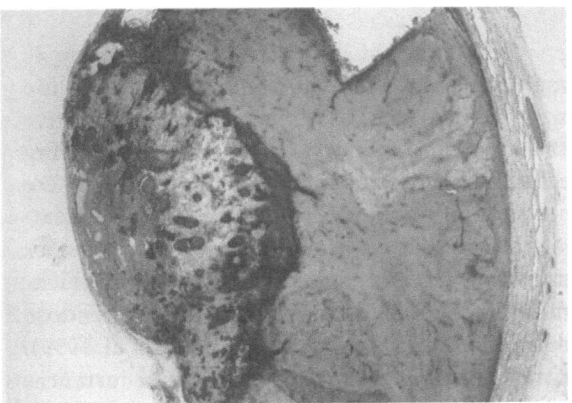

Fig. 12.1. Histopathological examination of a human choroidal melanoma after experimental TTT shows necrosis to a depth of 3.9 mm, with a sharp demarcation between the viable and the necrotic parts of the tumor. In the necrotic part all vessels are occluded, which explains the absence of hemorrhages. (Reproduced from JOURNÉE-DE KORVER et al. 1992, with kind permission of the copyright holder, Kluwer Academic Publishers)

mas (OOSTERHUIS et al. 1998). The response to TTT in amelanotic melanomas can be improved by simultaneous intravenous injection of indocyanine green to increase the uptake of infrared radiation, for so-called dye-enhanced thermotherapy (SHIELDS et al. 1998).

12.3.3
Heat Damage After TTT of Choroidal Melanomas

TTT-induced tumor necrosis and vascular occlusion in the heat-damaged part of the human choroidal melanoma develop within 3 days (JOURNÉE-DE KORVER et al. 1997). The necrotic part of the tumor is seen on B-scan echography as a zone of increased reflectivity about 3 mm from the top of the tumor (Fig. 12.3a, b). Clearance of the debris of the necrotic tumor takes 3–4 months; the reduction in tumor thickness is evident on ultrasonography (Fig. 12.3c). At this stage, additional TTT can be performed to flatten the tumor further by inducing necrosis in another layer of the tumor, the "cheese slice procedure" (Fig. 12.3d). Tumor regression may be associated with loss of pigment in the tumor progressing over years. In one study, intraretinal pigment proliferation was found in one third of the patients 1 year and longer after TTT (ROBERTSON et al. 1999).

The conduction of heat from the tumor into the retina causes atrophy of the retina in the treated area. Patients develop dense scotomas, including nerve fiber bundle defects, which reflect the disturbance of the overlying retina (ROBERTSON et al. 1999).

Signs of inflammation in the posterior segment of the eye are surprisingly mild; a transient increase in subretinal fluid after TTT is a common finding; it resolves within several weeks. Incidentally the amount of fluid over the tumor is very large; in these cases TTT may cause a hole in the atrophic retina, resulting in retinal detachment.

TTT is remarkably well tolerated by the ocular media. The absorption of laser radiation on its way thorough clear ocular media is about 5%, too low to cause side effects (JOURNÉE-DE KORVER et al. 1997). TTT does not have a cataractogenous effect, as established by fluorophotometric examination of the lens before and 1–7 years after TTT (WEENINK et al. 1998). The anterior chamber and vitreous humor are free of any significant inflammation; they sometimes show a slight flare and some cells. GODFREY et al. (1999) mentioned vitritis over the tumor area. A study of endothelial cells of the cornea did not reveal any differences before and after TTT (ROBERTSON et al. 1999). There are no signs of iritis, except when the radiation beam accidentally touches the pupillary margin, which causes focal iris atrophy and a posterior synechia, sometimes associated with a local, white, nonprogressive cataract.

12.3.4
Exclusion Criteria for TTT

TTT is not indicated as the sole treatment for choroidal melanomas when the tumors are more than 4 mm in thickness, and TTT combined with [106]Ru plaque radiotherapy is not indicated for tumors more than 8 mm in thickness.

TTT is not feasible when opacities preclude a clear view of the tumor. In one study, a tumor that could not be treated adequately because of cataract showed viable tumor cells on histopathologic examination (DIAZ et al. 1998). TTT is not technically possible when the pupil cannot be dilated sufficiently or when the tumor is located in the distant periphery and not visible in its full extension with the wide field contact lens. TTT is not indicated when subretinal fluid measures more than 3 mm in elevation (SHIELDS et al. 1998).

12.3.5
TTT Combined with Brachytherapy: "Sandwich Therapy"

The combination of TTT and brachytherapy is termed "sandwich therapy." The two treatments are complementary, with TTT being maximally effective at the top of the tumor and brachytherapy being effective at the base of the tumor (Fig. 12.4). There are several advantages of combining the two treatments. It makes it possible to treat tumors thicker than 5 mm, which is generally the maximum thickness for [106]Ru brachytherapy, and to use a lower dose of radiation in brachytherapy (KEUNEN et al. 1999). Insufficient melanoma regression and recurrences after combined treatment can be retreated with TTT alone.

OOSTERHUIS et al. (1998) reported on 50 eyes of patients with choroidal melanomas treated with TTT and [106]Ru brachytherapy. The tumors were up to 8.0 mm in thickness and 5.8–15 mm in diameter. Most tumors were treated with a laser spot size of 3.0 or 3.5 mm, but tumors close to the fovea or optic disc

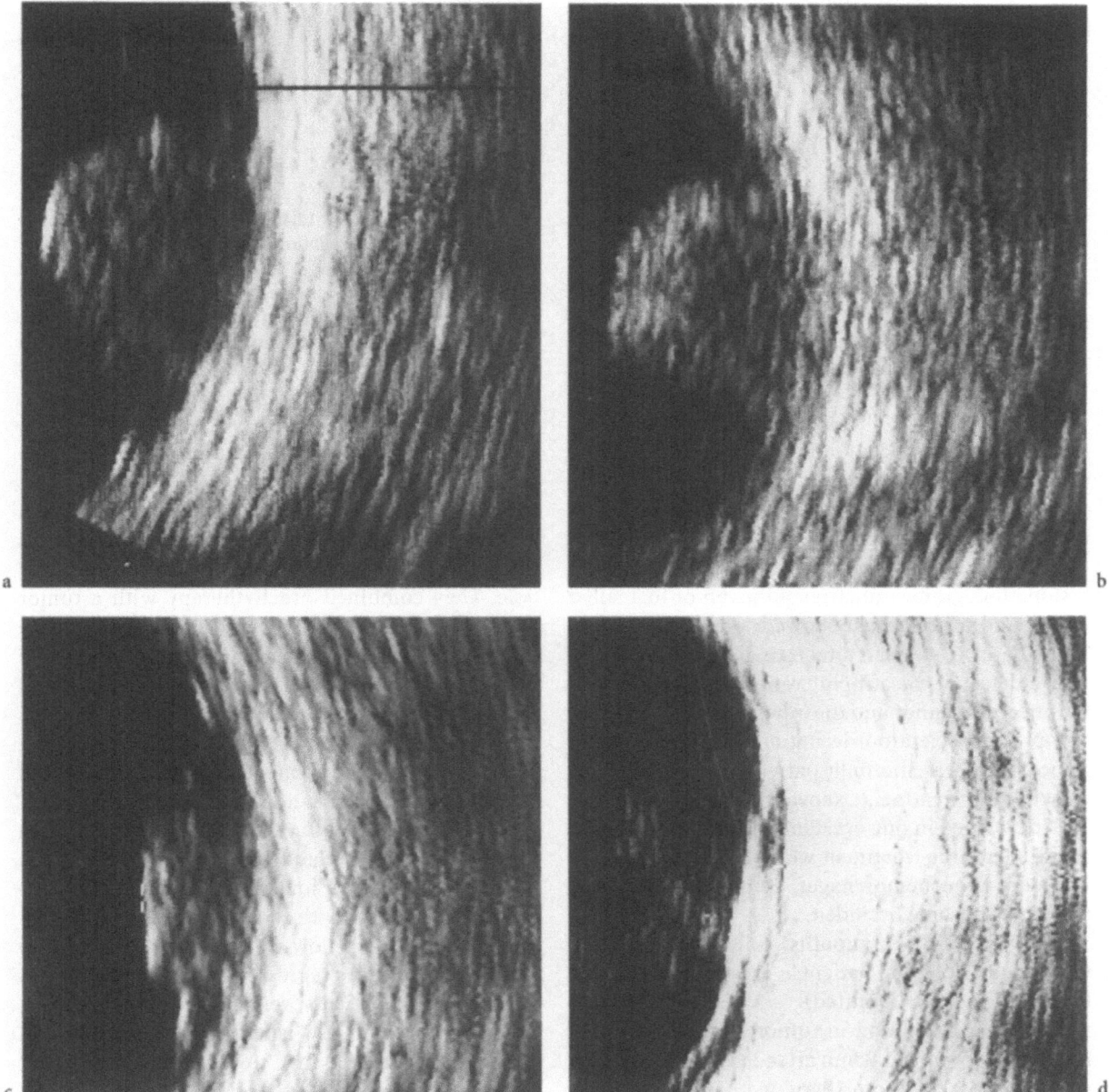

Fig. 12.3. a B-Scan echogram of a choroidal melanoma before treatment shows uniform reflectivity of the tumor. **b** The echogram 1 week after TTT shows increased reflectivity about 3 mm from the top of the tumor, which is indicative of tumor necrosis. **c** Two months after TTT the zone of increased reflectivity has disappeared on the echogram, associated with flattening of the top of the tumor. **d** Seven months after the second TTT, which was performed 4 months after the first TTT, echographic examination showed compete flattening of the tumor. (Reproduced from OOSTERHUIS et al. 1995; copyrighted 1995, American Medical Association)

were treated with a spot size of 2 or 2.5 mm. Because of the variations in spot size, the energy output of the laser is given in watts per square centimeter on the target area. Depending on the amount of pigmentation, energy levels ranged from 6.0 to 13.0 W/cm^2; in 54% of the patients an energy level of 8.0–9.5 W/cm^2 was used, corresponding to 565 and 670 mW laser output-energy for a spot size of 3 mm. The number of applications ranged from 5 to 15, depending on the diameter of the tumor. The follow-up was 20.5 (6–49) months.

All but one tumor exhibited a reduction in thickness at a mean follow-up period of 20.5 (6–49) months. The tumors flattened completely in 41 (82%) eyes. Flattening of large tumors required two to three thermotherapy treatments. The mean de-

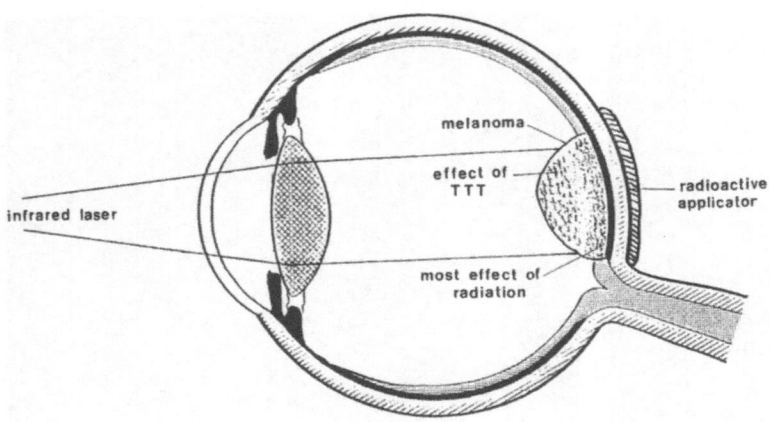

Fig. 12.4. Schematic drawing of "sandwich therapy," where TTT is more effective at the top of the tumor and brachytherapy at its base. (Reproduced from Journée-de Korver et al. 1997, by kind permission of the BMJ Publishing Group)

crease in thickness 3 months after the first TTT in melanomas more than 5 mm thick was 3.0 mm (1.3–4.5 mm); in melanomas 5 mm thick or less it was 2.3 mm (0.7–4.5 mm).

Three eyes were enucleated after TTT. In one eye, histopathologic examination of the tumor that failed to respond to treatment showed total cell necrosis. The other two eyes had total retinal detachment, one with a defect of the atrophic retina overlying the totally necrotic tumor and the other with tumor necrosis up to the sclera bordering on a vital part of the tumor. This was the only patient with tumor outgrowth after treatment. Neovascular glaucoma after TTT developed in one eye. Fine retinal hemorrhages at the site of the treatment were common, but there were no large hemorrhages. Retinal arteries and veins may become occluded.

The 5-year (60–92 months) follow-up results in this group of 50 patients are also favorable (Bartlema et al. submitted).

The mean reduction in tumor thickness was 1.9 mm after 3 months, 3.2 mm after 2 years, and 3.3 mm after 5 years. The tumor flattened completely in 31 patients (62%) within 1 year, in 39 patients (78%) within 2 years, and in 45 patients (90%) within 5 years. Complete flattening required one session in 32 eyes (71%), 2 sessions in 11 eyes (25%), and 3 sessions in 2 eyes (4%). Eight of the 15 retreatments were performed along the central margin of the previously treated area. Five rather thick or amelanotic tumors failed to flatten completely. Tumor recurrence was only observed in 2 (4%) patients, 41 and 51 months after TTT. Five eyes (10%) were enucleated. Radiation retinopathy was observed in 29 patients (58%). It caused a considerable visual loss, as visual acuity was 20/60 or better in 41 patients (82%) before treatment, but remained at this level in only 30 patients (60%) after 6 months, in 15 patients (30%) after 1 year, and in 9 patients (18%) after 5 years.

Schneider et al. (1999) performed sandwich therapy in 11 patients with choroidal melanomas thicker than 5 mm or with tumors near the posterior pole. They combined brachytherapy with a tumor apex dose of 100 Gy [106]Ru with TTT with a spot size of 1.5–3 mm and an exposure time of 30–60 s. Three months after treatment, the mean tumor thickness had decreased from 4.9 to 1.0 mm; in half the patients the tumor had flattened completely. Mean visual acuity, 1 year after treatment, was 0.5 (0.3–0.8) in 8 patients whose tumors did not involve the macula.

Seregard and Landau (2001) performed TTT as an adjunct to [106]Ru plaque treatment in 11 patients with juxtapapillary or juxtafoveal choroidal melanoma and 14 patients with recurrent growth at the tumor margin. The follow-up was 6–29 (median 20) months. The tumors regressed completely in 18 and partially in 11 patients, remained unchanged in 6, and progressed in 2. Visual acuity remained unchanged or improved in 17 (63%) of these patients. Two eyes were enucleated.

12.3.6
TTT As Sole Treatment

Results of TTT as the only treatment of small choroidal melanomas have been published by Keunen et al. (1997), Shields et al. (1998); Robertson et al. (1999); Godfrey et al. (1999), and Schneider et al. (1999). In these studies the maximum tumor thickness ranged from 2.2 mm (Schneider et al. 1999) to 4 mm (Shields et al. 1998). Laser treatment was usually performed with applications of 60 s and a spot size of 2.5–3.0 mm. Smaller spots were used for tumors near the macula or optic disc. The number of treatment sessions ranged from only one treatment for rather flat melanomas (SCHNEIDER et al. 1999), through one plus a single retreatment in 21% (GODFREY et al. 1999) and 35% (ROBERTSON et al. 1999), to a mean of three (range 1–6) sessions per tumor to ensure complete tumor control (SHIELDS et al. 1998). The mean follow-up period after TTT was rather short, ranging from14 to18.5 months.

The treatment was successful, with a reduction in tumor thickness to a flat scar, in 90–94% of the tumors in all studies. Failures included eyes with amelanotic melanomas that showed little or no response to thermotherapy. Recurrences were observed in 1 of 20 patients (ROBERTSON et al. 1999) and in 2 of 100 patients (SHIELDS et al. 1998); however, later data on 256 patients showed a 22% tumor recurrence after 3 years of follow-up (SHIELDS et al. 2001). Treatment results in juxtapupillary melanomas were less favorable, as KEUNEN et al. (1997) observed tumor recurrence after TTT of juxtapapillary melanomas in 4 of 5 patients with a follow-up of 2–6 years.

The visual acuity after TTT was the same (within one line) or better than the pretreatment visual acuity in 58 (58%) eyes of 100 patients (SHIELDS et al. 1998). Vision improved when subretinal fluid was resorbed. These results are favorable because in 25 eyes treatment through the foveola was the main reason for visual loss. ROBERTSON et al. (1999) found that visual acuity remained within one line after treatment in 15 (75%) of 20 patients. GODFREY et al. (1999) observed this outcome in 6 (47%) of 14 eyes. Proximity of the tumor to the fovea or the optic disc was the main reason for visual loss.

12.3.7
Complications

Fine superficial hemorrhages are commonly observed after TTT, but large hemorrhages rarely develop. Retinal traction folds and epiretinal membranes, an important cause of loss of visual acuity, developed after TTT in 25% (ROBERTSON et al. 1999) and 20% (SHIELDS et al. 1998) of patients; half of these patients had macular tumors.

Branch retinal artery occlusion has been reported in 12% (SHIELDS et al. 1998) and in 50% (ROBERTSON et al. 1999) of patients, and branch retinal vein occlusion in 23% (SHIELDS et al. 1998) and 30% (ROBERTSON et al. 1999) of patients. New vessel formation in the retina occurred secondary to branch retinal vein occlusion in 6% of patients (SHIELDS et al. 1998). TTT retreatment may promote occlusion of retinal vessels, as branch artery occlusion developed in 6 of

7 TTT-retreated patients but in only 4 of 13 patients treated only once (ROBERTSON et al. 1999). In all 20 patients, TTT-induced retinal atrophy was associated with dense scotomas that corresponded with the area of treatment. In all but 1 patient retinal atrophy was combined with wedge-shaped nerve fiber bundle defects (ROBERTSON et al. 1999). Occasional findings were macular edema, cystoid macular edema, and optic disc edema.

12.3.8
Comments on TTT

Good tumor reduction has been obtained with TTT combined with brachytherapy in melanomas up to 8 mm thick with a mean follow-up of 21 months. TTT as sole treatment yielded good tumor control in tumors up to 4 mm thick with a follow-up of 14–18.5 months. In all papers but one, the follow-up period after TTT has been rather short, so that the final evaluation of TTT in the treatment of choroidal melanoma has to await more results of long-term investigations.

Visual acuity is better after TTT as sole treatment than after TTT combined with brachytherapy. This is probably because in TTT the infrared radiation beam can be focused on the treatment area, resulting in a sharp demarcation between the heat-treated and the non-heat-treated area. In contrast, in brachytherapy the radiation cannot be focused; this can result in radiation maculopathy with a loss of central vision in almost half the patients (GÜNDÜZ et al. 1999).

Is TTT as sole treatment a safe technique or does it need to be combined with brachytherapy for adequate treatment of intrasclerally located tumor cells? This is a dilemma (KEUNEN et al. 1999). Intra- and episcleral melanoma cells were found in 55.7% and 8.2%, respectively, on histopathologic examination of eyes with choroidal melanomas (COLLABORATIVE OCULAR MELANOMA STUDY GROUP 1998). Even small melanomas already showed scleral ingrowth in 17 (81%) of 21 enucleated eyes (KAKEBEEKE-KEMME et al. 1985). It is, therefore, imperative that during heat treatment the scleral temperature increases to a level sufficient to destroy these tumor cells. Surviving intra- and episcleral melanoma cells are a source of tumor recurrences, which are associated with a two- to three-fold increase in the rate of metastasis (KARLSSON et al. 1990; SEREGARD et al. 1997; GRAGOUDAS 1997). The consequences of insufficient penetration of heat into the sclera are evident from the results of xenon arc photocoagulation of choroidal melanomas, in which eyes enucleated after treatment showed scleral invasion in 55% and extraocular extension of the tumor in 35% (DE LAEY et al. 1986). However, even with TTT, which causes tumor necrosis to a depth of 3.9 mm in human choroidal melanomas, viable tumor cells have been observed in the inner layers of the sclera of an eye, very close to the tumor, which was necrotic up to the sclera (JOURNÉE-DE KORVER et al. 1997). These cells may have survived because the increase in temperature in the sclera is lower than that in the tumor, as the production of heat by absorption of infrared radiation is considerably less in the nonpigmented sclera than in the pigmented tumor. This was also observed in a study of transscleral infrared laser thermotherapy of experimental melanomas covered by sclera, where a tumor temperature of 60°C was associated with a scleral surface temperature of only 45°C (REM et al. 1998). This may explain the recurrence rate of 22% at 3 years' follow-up after TTT as the sole treatment for choroidal melanomas, as opposed to a 2% recurrence rate at 5 years' follow-up after "sandwich treatment (BARTLEMA et al. submitted; SHIELDS et al. 2001).

The conduction of heat into the sclera may be promoted by performing TTT on tumors already flattened by previous TTT. For this reason, SHIELDS et al. (1998) treated melanomas with three TTT sessions on average. Unfortunately, sensitive clinical techniques are not available to evaluate the destructive effect of TTT on intrascleral and episcleral tumor cells and to detect early extrascleral recurrences. To avoid the risk of insufficient treatment of the sclera, the combination of TTT and brachytherapy should be considered for the treatment of small choroidal melanomas, despite the increased risk of loss of visual acuity.

TTT is now performed in many oncologic eye centers, but it may be many years before we know whether the effect of TTT as sole treatment is sufficient to destroy intra- and episclerally located tumor cells. Recurrences may develop rather late and have been observed on average 2.5 years after treatment with argon laser photocoagulation and 6 years after xenon arc photocoagulation of choroidal melanomas (SHIELDS et al. 1990). At present, one has to choose between "sandwich" treatment, which may be the safest modality, and TTT as sole treatment, which has a better visual prognosis, for the treatment of patients with small choroidal melanomas.

TTT is not restricted to the treatment of choroidal melanomas and can also be used to treat retinoblastomas (SHIELDS et al. 1999) and circumscribed chor-

oidal hemangiomas (RAPIZZI et al. 1999; GARCIA-ARUMI et al. 2000; OTHMANE et al. 1999).

12.4
Photocoagulation and Diathermy

Photocoagulation is performed with xenon or laser irradiation. Long-term results of two series of patients have shown good tumor regression in 59–65% of patients (DE LAEY et al. 1986). Enucleation was performed in 33–50% of patients because of incomplete tumor response, recurrences, or complications. Treatment was restricted to small tumors not exceeding 3 mm in thickness, and multiple treatments were required because the heat-induced tumor necrosis was rather superficial, only extending to a depth of 0.5–1.0 mm. In the only recent study, photocoagulation was not recommended as treatment for small posterior choroidal melanomas (EIDE 1999). At present, photocoagulation is only indicated for supplemental treatment of tumor recurrences or for residual tumor following treatment with other modalities. It can be used to make a barrier of coagulation scars around the tumor prior to TTT, to lower the risk of retinal detachment after treatment.

Diathermy was used by Weve to treat 21 patients with choroidal melanomas between 1935 and 1953. There were no recurrences during a follow-up of 1–15 years. Three eyes were enucleated because of complications; viable tumor cells were found to be present in two of them (MELCHERS [thesis] 1953). The destructive effect of diathermy on a tumor can be attributed partly to the occlusion of feeder vessels at the base of the tumor. DAVIDORF et al. (1970) obtained good results with diathermy in four slightly elevated melanomas; however, the surface of the sclera was shrunken and heavily burned. This may explain why, despite the favorable results, diathermy is not generally accepted as a treatment modality for choroidal melanomas.

Photocoagulation as treatment for choroidal melanomas has largely been replaced by TTT. Diathermy is of only historical interest.

References

Bartlema YM, Oosterhuis JA, Journée-de Korver HG, Tjho-Heslinga RE, Keunen JEE (2001) Treatment of choroidal melanoma with brachytherapy and transpupillary thermotherapy: 5 year follow-up. (submitted for publication)

Braakman R, van der Valk JL, van Delft JL et al (1989) The effects of ultrasonically induced hyperthermia on experimental tumors in the rabbit eye. Invest Ophthalmol Vis Sci 30:835–844

Coleman DJ, Silverman RH, Ursea R et al (1997) Ultrasonically induced hyperthermia for adjunctive treatment of intraocular malignant melanoma. Retina 17:109–117

Collaborative Ocular Melanoma Study Group (1998) Histopathologic characteristics of uveal melanomas in eyes enucleated, from the collaborative ocular melanoma study. (COMS report no 6) Am J Ophthalmol 125:745–766

Davidorf FH, Gordon H, Newman GH et al (1970) Conservative management of malignant melanoma. Arch Ophthalmol 83:273–280

Diaz CE, Capone A, Grossniklaus HE (1998) Clinicopathologic findings in recurrent choroidal melanoma after transpupillary thermotherapy. Ophthalmology 105:1419–1424

Eide N (1999) Primary laser photocoagulation of "small" choroidal melanomas. Acta Ophthalmol Scand 77:351–354

Finger PT (1997) Microwave thermoradiotherapy for uveal melanoma, results of a 10 year study. Ophthalmology 104:1794–1803

Garcia-Arumi J (2000) Transpupillary thermotherapy for circumscribed choroidal hemangiomas. Ophthalmology 107:351–357

Godfrey DG, Waldron RG, Capone A (1999) Transpupillary thermotherapy for small choroidal melanoma. Am J Ophthalmol 128:88–93

Gragoudas ES (1997) Long term results after proton irradiation of uveal melanomas. Graefes Arch Clin Exp Ophthalmol 235:265–267

Gündüz K, Shields CL, Shields JA et al (1999) Radiation retinopathy following plaque radiotherapy for posterior uveal melanoma. Arch Ophthalmol 117:609–614

Journée-de Korver JG, Oosterhuis JA, Kakebeeke-Kemme HM et al (1992) Transpupillary thermotherapy (TTT) by infrared irradiation of choroidal melanoma. Doc Ophthalmol 82:185–191

Journée-de Korver JG, Oosterhuis JA, Vrensen GFJM (1995) Light and electron microscopic findings on experimental melanomas after hyperthermia at 50°C. Melanoma Res 5:393–402

Journée-de Korver JG, Oosterhuis JA, de Wolff-Rouendaal D et al (1997) Histopathological findings in human choroidal melanomas after transpupillary thermotherapy. Br J Ophthalmol 81:234–239

Kakebeeke-Kemme HM, Oosterhuis JA, de Wolff-Rouendaal D (1985) Five year follow-up study of choroidal and ciliary body melanomas after enucleation. In: Oosterhuis JA (ed) Ophthalmic tumours, 1st edn. Junk, Dordrecht, pp 9–26

Karlsson UL, Augsburger JJ et al (1990) Recurrence of posterior uveal melanoma after ^{60}Co episcleral plaque therapy. Ophthalmology 96:382–388

Keunen JEE, Bleeker JC, Journée de Korver JG et al (1997) Juxtapapillary melanomas and transpupillary thermotherapy. Invest Ophthalmol Vis Sci 38 [Suppl]:S720

Keunen JEE, Journée-de Korver JG, Oosterhuis JA (1999) Transpupillary thermotherapy of choroidal melanoma with or without brachytherapy: a dilemma. Br J Ophthalmol 83:1212–1213

Laey JJ de, Hanssens M, Ryckaert S (1986) Photocoagulation of malignant melanomas of the choroid, a reappraisal. Bull Soc Belge Ophthalmol 213:9–18

Melchers MJ (1953) Diathermy treatment of intraocular tumours. Thesis, University of Utrecht

Murray TG, O'Brien JM, Steeves RA et al (1996) Radiation therapy and ferromagnetic hyperthermia in the treatment of murine transgenic retinoblastoma. Arch Ophthalmol 114:1376–1381

Murray TG, Steeves RA, Gentry G et al (1997) Ferromagnetic hyperthermia: functional and histopathologic effects on normal rabbit ocular tissue. Int J Hyperthermia 13:423–436

Oosterhuis JA, Journée-de Korver HG, Kakebeeke-Kemme HM, Bleeker JC (1995) Transpupillary thermotherapy in choroidal melanomas. Arch Ophthalmol 113:315–321

Oosterhuis JA, Journée-de Korver HG, Keunen JJE (1998) Transpupillary thermotherapy. Results in 50 patients with choroidal melanoma. Arch Ophthalmol 116:157–162

Othmane IS, Shields CL, Shields JA et al (1999) Circumscribed choroidal hemangioma managed by transpupillary thermotherapy. Arch Ophthalmol 117:136–137

Petrovich Z, Pike M, Astrahan MA et al (1996) Episcleral plaque thermoradiotherapy of posterior uveal melanomas. Am J Clin Oncol 19:207–221

Rapizzi E, Grizzard S, Capone A (1999) Transpupillary thermotherapy in the management of circumscribed choroidal hemangioma. Am J Ophthalmol 127:481–482

Rem AI, Journée-de Korver JG, Oosterhuis JA, et al (1998) Feasibility of Nd:YAG (1064 nm) for transscleral thermotherapy of intraocular tumors. Invest Ophthalmol Vis Sci 39:289

Robertson DM, Buettner H, Bennett SR (1999) Transpupillary thermotherapy as primary treatment for small choroidal melanomas. Arch Ophthalmol 117:1512–1519

Schneider H, Fischer K, Fietkau R et al (1999) Transpupilläre Thermotherapie des malignen Aderhautmelanoms. Klin Monatsbl Augenheilkd 214:90–95

Seregard S, Landau I (2001) Transpupillary thermotherapy as an adjunct to ruthenium plaque radiotherapy for choroidal melanoma. Acta Ophthalamol Scand 79:19–22

Seregard S, Trampe E, Lax I et al (1997) Results following episcleral ruthenium plaque radiotherapy for posterior uveal melanoma. Acta Ophthalmol Scand 75:11–16

Shields CL, Shields JA, Cater J et al (1998) Transpupillary thermotherapy for choroidal melanoma. Ophthalmology 105:581–590

Shields CL, Santos MCM, Diniz W et al (1999) Thermotherapy for retinoblastoma. Arch Ophthalmol 117:885–893

Shields CL, Shields JA, Perez N, Singh AD, Cater J (2001) Primary transpupillary thermotherapy for choroidal melanoma in 256 consecutive cases: outcomes and limitations. International Congress on Ocular Oncology, Amsterdam, 17–21 June 2001, p 174 (ISBN 9-0901-4923-6)

Shields JA, Glazer LC, Mieler WF et al (1990) Comparison of xenon and argon laser photocoagulation in the treatment of choroidal melanomas. Am J Ophthalmol 1009:647–655

Weenink AC, van Best JA, Oosterhuis JA et al (1998) Lens transmission by fluorophotometry after brachytherapy and thermotherapy of choroidal melanoma. Ophthalmic Res 30:402–406

13 Orbital Rhabdomyosarcoma

R. H. SAGERMAN

CONTENTS

13.1
Incidence, Age, Sex, Race

Rhabdomyosarcoma (RMS) accounts for 4–8% of malignancies in children under 15 years old (CRIST et al. 1990). RMS is the most common orbital malignancy in children and was the primary site in 65 of 686 (9.47%) patients reported in the Intergroup RMS studies I and II (CRIST et al. 1990). KNOWLES et al. (1978) gathered data from four major reviews (ASHTON and MORGAN 1965; FRAYER and ENTERLINE 1959; JONES et al. 1965; PORTERFIELD and ZIMMERMAN 1962); of 161 patients, 64 (40%) were 0–5 years old, 57 (35%) were 6–10 years, 28 (17%) were 11–15 years, 7 (4%) were 16–20 years, 3 (2%) were 21–25 years, and 2 (1%) were older than 25. The average age was approximately 8 years in each of the four reviews, and the median age was 6 years in the Intergroup RMS study. RMS is rare in the newborn and not common before 1 year. The oldest patient reported was 78 years of age (KASSEL et al. 1965). Its occurrence during pregnancy has been reported (OLURIN 1969).

The male-to-female ratio has varied in the reported series. KNOWLES et al. (1978) reported 99 males vs 64 females, and SAGERMAN et al. (1974), 18 boys and 13 girls, but girls outnumbered boys (53% vs 47%) in the Intergroup RMS report (WHARAM et al. 1987). The Intergroup RMS study gathered 132 patients under the age of 21 years, of whom 84% were white, 13% black, and 3% other. In a compilation of 306 patients from four cooperative groups there were 186 from North America and 120 from Europe; 51% were boys; and the median age was 6.8 years (OBERLIN et al. 2001).

13.2
Epidemiology and Pathology

Although sometimes associated with trauma, there is no direct evidence of a causal relationship. LI and FRAUMENI (1969) reported an elevated incidence of cancer in the family and of sibling involvement by RMS. An oncogenetic relationship between congenital defects and RMS has been reported by MILLER (1968). In contrast to epidemiologic studies, however, these relationships are not usually seen in individual institutional reports (SAGERMAN et al. 1974).

All histologic types of RMS, embryonal, alveolar, pleomorphic, and botryoid, have been reported in the orbit, but the embryonal type is the most frequent, accounting for 84% in the Intergroup RMS report (WHARAM et al. 1987). PORTERFIELD and ZIMMERMAN (1962) considered the alveolar and pleomorphic types to be less controllable, and this belief is supported by experience at other body sites (GEHAN et al. 1981); however, there are insufficient data to know whether this holds true in the orbit.

More extensive pathological descriptions, with histologic illustrations, are found in KNOWLES et al. (1978). However, it is important to note that the majority of these tumors are not encapsulated or well defined (Fig. 13.1), putting the orbital contents at risk. This is illustrated by ASHTON and MORGAN (1965): 25 of 28 patients treated initially by excision later required exenteration and/or irradiation, and orbital recurrence was frequent even after exenteration (JONES et al. 1965).

R.H. SAGERMAN, MD, FACR
Department of Radiation Oncology, SUNY Upstate Medical University, 750 E. Adams Street, Syracuse, NY 13210, USA

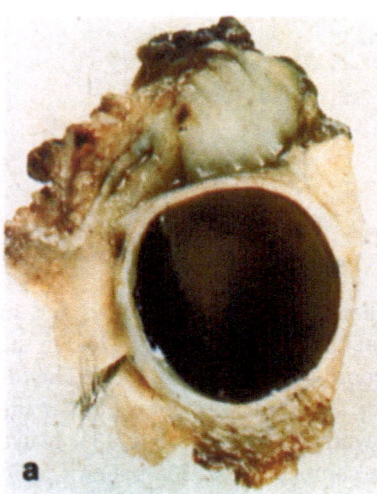
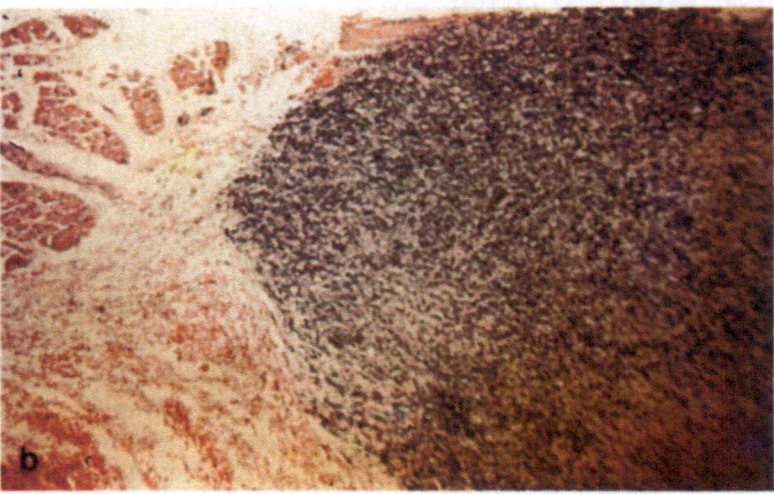

Fig. 13.1. a Exenteration specimen showing an unencapsulated tumor extending into the surrounding soft tissues. **b** Histologic appearance of a typical RMS without a capsule, showing tumor cells infiltrating the muscle

13.3
Clinical Presentation

Rapidly progressing exophthalmos is the most common presentation. A palpable mass was noted in only 25% of 62 patients by JONES et al. (1965). There may also be conjunctival involvement and edema. Judging from displacement of the globe, FRAYER and ENTERLINE (1950) and SAGERMAN et al. (1968) reported the superior nasal segment of the orbit to be the most common site of origin. This can now be demonstrated more accurately with computed tomography and magnetic resonance imaging.

The clinical differential diagnosis includes hemangioma, lymphangioma, dermoid, leukemia, neuroblastoma, pseudotumor, hyperthyroidism, and inflammatory diseases. Hemangiomas may grow rapidly during infancy, but there is often an obvious cutaneous lesion to suggest the diagnosis. Lymphangiomas usually progress slowly. Dermoids are usually found in the superotemporal quadrant, with a bony defect seen on radiographic study. Hematologic studies should indicate the diagnosis of leukemia, which often shows bilateral involvement, and the child will be sick. The child is also usually sick, and the diagno-

sis known, when neuroblastoma metastasizes to the orbit(s). Far advanced retinoblastoma that has broken out of the globe can mimic RMS, but this is rare in medically advanced societies (JONES et al. 1966; PORTERFIELD and ZIMMERMAN 1962).

13.4
Clinical Evaluation

Spatial limits within the bony orbit force displacement of the globe in response to an enlarging intraorbital mass, and the location of the mass can be reasonably well deduced from the direction of displacement. This leads to a change in appearance. The earliest changes may not be noticed (Fig. 13.2a, b), but the rapid growth of RMS usually makes itself known to the parents in days to weeks (Fig. 13.2c). At this time the child does not complain, seems healthy, and in the absence of a high index of suspicion this rare tumor is not suspected. Various conservative measures may be undertaken, but ophthalmological consultation is soon requested when there has been no response (Fig. 13.2d).

Fig. 13.2a, b. An asymptomatic girl when diagnosed with rhabdomyosarcoma (RMS) at the age of 6 years and 10 months; her mother had noted a reddish mass in the medial right conjunctiva. This did not respond to antibiotic therapy given for a concomitant upper respiratory infection. A biopsy was obtained, but a histologic diagnosis could not be established. **c** Rapid enlargement of the mass suggested the clinical diagnosis of RMS at examination 2 weeks later. **d** Four days later, there was a marked increase in swelling of the orbital tissues and the mass had now extended beyond the limbus and the midline. The histologic diagnosis of embryonal RMS was later established from a second biopsy obtained at this time. A pearly red mass was present in the nasal orbit. Radiotherapy began the next day: 60 Gy was delivered through shaped anterior (46 Gy at 2 Gy/day at Dmax) and anterior oblique fields (14 Gy). **e** Appearance 10 weeks after completion of radiotherapy. Note the loss of eyelashes and eyebrow and the resolving skin reaction, which is most marked at the biopsy site where bolus had been used. **f** Late effects (conjunctival telangiectasis, only partial regrowth of eyelashes) are demonstrated 1 year after radiotherapy. Note also the slight residual increase in tissue at the medial canthus. **g** There has been no change in the clinical or CT appearance at the medial canthus 8 years after radiotherapy. A progressive cataract began 14 months after therapy; cataract surgery was accomplished ▷▷

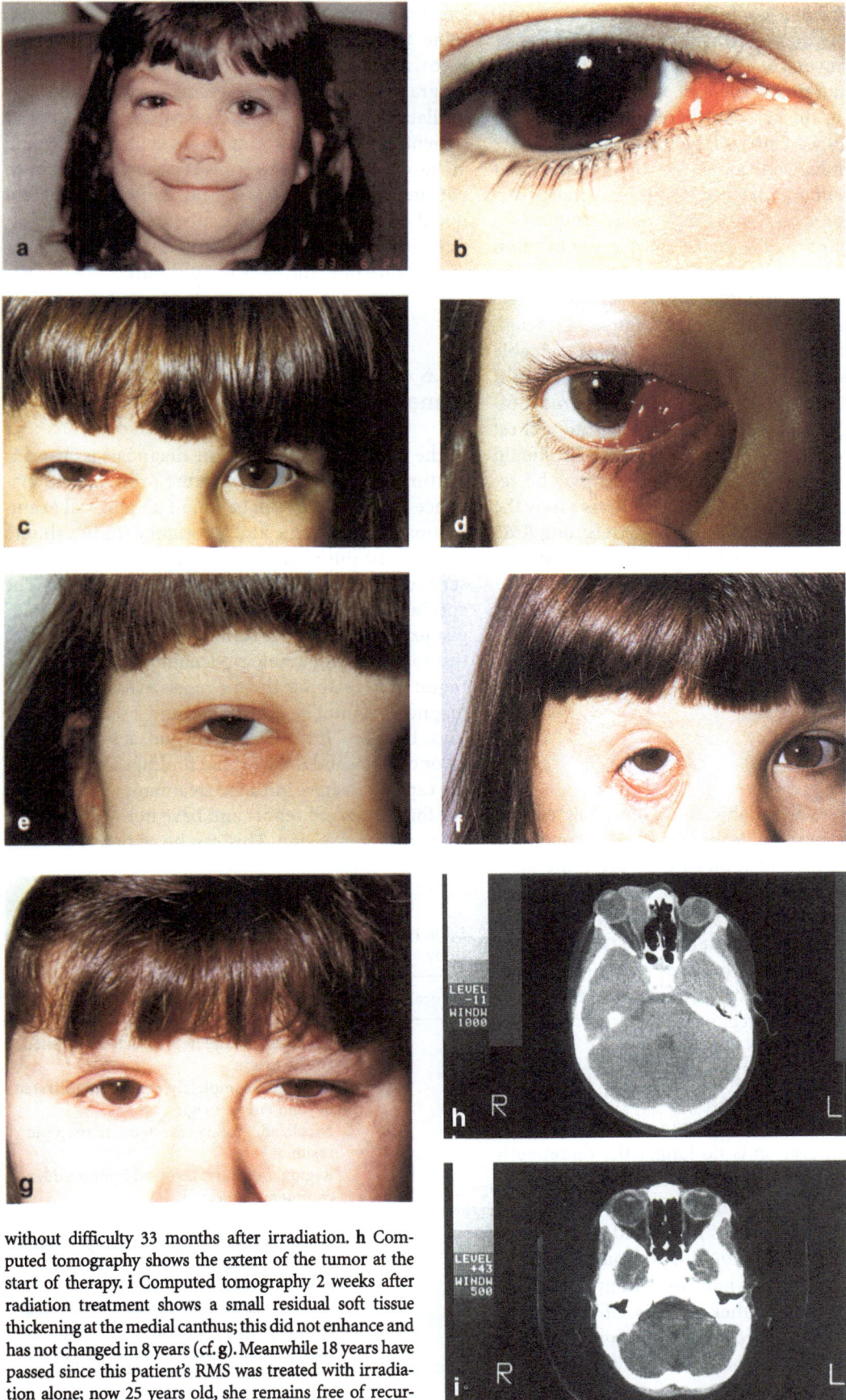

without difficulty 33 months after irradiation. **h** Computed tomography shows the extent of the tumor at the start of therapy. **i** Computed tomography 2 weeks after radiation treatment shows a small residual soft tissue thickening at the medial canthus; this did not enhance and has not changed in 8 years (cf. **g**). Meanwhile 18 years have passed since this patient's RMS was treated with irradiation alone; now 25 years old, she remains free of recurrence or development of a secondary malignancy

Only rarely will a careful history uncover a familial cancer, genetic abnormality, or abnormality of pregnancy, delivery, or childhood. Physical examination will be unremarkable except for the unilateral abnormality of the eye, and there will be no significant adenopathy. Acuity will be unchanged.

Contrast-enhanced computed tomography and magnetic resonance imaging have replaced all previous radiographic and ultrasonographic studies (see Chap. 22). They will document the size and location of the lesion and its extensions, the location of the globe and the lens, and invasion or erosion of bone and involvement of the paranasal sinuses. Although not often performed in the absence of palpable nodes, metastatic adenopathy may be discovered if these studies include the neck. Metastases most often involve the lungs, bones, and liver, and a chest film, blood count, and chemical liver profile should be obtained. More extensive evaluation may be required in special circumstances, but this is rarely the case: only 5 of 132 registrants in the Intergroup RMS study had disseminated disease at diagnosis (WHARAM et al. 1987).

Biopsy must be obtained quickly and evaluated promptly to establish the diagnosis.

13.5
Staging

After clinical, radiographic, and laboratory evaluation, each patient should be classified (staged) according to the bulk of tumor in the orbit, the presence or absence of bone destruction or paranasal sinus involvement, the presence of regional lymph node metastases or of distant metastases to lung, bone, liver, or the central nervous system, and histopathologic type. The most commonly used staging system is that employed by the Intergroup RMS study (Table 13.1).

This system was designed for the surgical treatment of RMS at any body site and is of limited value for orbital primaries because resection is rarely complete, exenteration is no longer the therapeutic mainstay, and lymph node metastases and distant metastases are uncommon at initial evaluation. Indeed, WHARAM et al. (1987) reported 132 patients gathered from participating institutions from 1972 to June 1983, only 5 of whom were in group IV and were excluded from further analysis. Of the remaining 127 patient, 6% were classed in group I, 24% in group II, and 70% in group III; only 7 patients had

exenteration at presentation. It is difficult to determine the stage for the 161 patients gathered by KNOWLES et al. (1978), and neither computed tomography nor magnetic resonance imaging was available at that time. In a similar time frame, the 31 patients irradiated by SAGERMAN et al. (1974) would all have been group III because only biopsy had been performed and there were no clinically apparent nodal or distant metastases, albeit after a less rigorous metastatic survey, as demonstrated by the later appearance of metastases in 10 children.

13.6
Management, Results

In the usual situation, once the diagnosis is suspected, tumor will be confined to the orbit and no evidence of metastases will be found on physical examination. Radiographic and laboratory studies should be initiated but should not delay the biopsy necessary to establish the histopathologic diagnosis. The specimen must be evaluated promptly by a pathologist experienced in the tumors of children and with the special histopathologic techniques that may be required to establish the diagnosis. On occasion, the diagnosis cannot be established and a second biopsy must be taken. If the clinical diagnosis is strongly in favor of RMS, and if the orbital findings are progressing rapidly, we have initiated treatment without waiting for the second report and have not yet had cause to regret the decision. This can be of practical value

Table 13.1. Staging system employed by the Intergroup RMS study

Clinical	Group	Definition
I	A	Localized, completely resected, confined to site of origin
	B	Localized, completely resected, infiltrated beyond site of origin
II	A	Localized, grossly resected, microscopic residual
	B	Regional disease, involved lymph nodes, completely resected
	C	Regional disease, involved lymph nodes, grossly resected with microscopic residual
III	A	Local or regional grossly visible disease after biopsy only
	B	Grossly visible disease after ≥50% resection of primary disease
IV		Distant metastases present at diagnosis

for radiotherapy and in limiting the chance for metastases. Clinical experience indicates that less than one-third of patients later developed metastases in the 1960s (SAGERMAN et al. 1974) and that, with better detection leading to a stage shift and the early introduction of chemotherapy, less than 5% of patients now develop metastases (WHARAM et al. 1987).

In the evaluation of treatment results, relapse-free survival at 2 or 3 years was sufficient to judge long-term results. In the series of JONES et al. (1965) and SAGERMAN et al. (1974), all recurrences and 25 out of 26 deaths occurred within 2 years of treatment. Among 202 patients with RMS of the head and neck treated with Intergroup RMS study I there were subsequent relapses in only 8% (6/75) of those without evidence of tumor at 2 years, and none among the patients with orbital primaries (SUTOW et al. 1982). In the present era of concomitant radiochemotherapy, all failures have occurred within 4 years (DONALDSON et al. 2001; WHARAM et al. 1987, 1997).

13.6.1
Management – Surgery

Orbital RMS was treated surgically for many years. Indeed, the surgical controversy centered about the extent of resection, with some authors favoring local excision and others immediate exenteration (ASHTON and MORGAN 1965; JONES et al. 1965). Limited resection was often followed by local recurrence owing to tumor cell infiltration beyond the obvious mass. Survival was poor; about 20% of tumors were controlled because they were small, localized, and resected in toto, or because exenteration had been accomplished. The best survival results were reported by JONES et al. (1965), who outlined the pressures brought to bear upon the physician by the family's desire to avoid mutilation. They concluded that exenteration cured "about half" of these patients. Indeed, 16 of 23 patients survived after exenteration alone. Of the total of 30 patients living and well, 3 were treated by excision alone and 11 received radiotherapy in addition to surgery. Given the selection factors that applied at that time, it is not surprising that 11 of 28 patients in whom irradiation was given survived but 17 died.

With rare exceptions, surgery is now restricted to biopsy in the primary management of orbital RMS. Enucleation, exenteration for special problems and treatment-related complications, cataract surgery, and plastic surgical repair are necessary aids within overall patient management.

13.6.2
Management – Irradiation

The role of irradiation in the primary management of orbital RMS before 1960 was summarized by LEDERMAN (1956), who indicated that these tumors were highly radiosensitive but rarely radiocurable because of prompt recurrence. This belief continued to be expressed in the 1970s and reflected the effects of the low dose and the small field size employed to avoid radiation damage, although several case reports and small series suggested that more conventional tumor doses to cover the entire volume at risk could sterilize these lesions and lead to long-term survival (CASSADY et al. 1968; LANDERS 1968; LEDERMAN 1956; SAGERMAN et al. 1968).

By 1968, SAGERMAN et al. were able to report long-term survival in all five patients irradiated after biopsy and local tumor control in seven of nine patients irradiated after surgery, with six of the seven surviving.

The first large series of children treated by primary radiation therapy was reported in 1972 by SAGERMAN et al. At a minimum tumor dose of $\geq$60 Gy, local tumor control was achieved in all 15 children. Two of four children with paranasal sinus extension were free of recurrence at 58 and 91 months. The limitations of metastatic involvement in this series are noted by the development of metastases in 6 of the 15 patients. Three developed distant metastases (two of lung, one of bone) and three, cervical adenopathy as the first manifestation of the failure of orbital irradiation. Although the neck nodes were controlled in the two patients who were treated adequately, only one, in whom no further metastases appeared, was a long-term survivor after surgery, radiotherapy, and chemotherapy.

Thirty-one consecutive patients treated by radiotherapy after biopsy were reported in 1974 by SAGERMAN et al. Local tumor control was achieved in 28 (90%). All 3 recurrences appeared within 10 months, and 2 of the 3 children were alive after exenteration and VAC chemotherapy (vincristine, actinomycin D, cyclophosphamide). Metastases developed in 10 patients and 9 died (the 1 survivor is noted above), again demonstrating the limitations of evaluation and of chemotherapy for metastatic RMS in the years 1963–1971. Although responses to chemotherapy were observed, it was not possible to establish a survival benefit for chemotherapy in these series. Nonetheless, chemotherapy was demonstrated to improve survival for RMS at other primary sites (DONALDSON et al. 1973; HEYN et al. 1974).

13.6.3
Management – Irradiation plus Chemotherapy

In 1979, ABRAMSON et al. reviewed the Columbia Presbyterian Medical Center experience with 58 nonrandomized patients, 25 of whom were treated with irradiation alone while 33 received chemotherapy in addition. After a mean follow-up of 5.2 years (6 months to 14 years), 75% were alive and local control was achieved in 91%. Three of four patients treated with radiochemotherapy following recurrence after exenteration were alive. Overall survival for 46 patients followed for 3 years was 70%, and all deaths but 1 occurred within 3 years. No difference could be demonstrated at 3 years (26 vs 20) or 5 years (23 vs 20) between patients treated with irradiation and those receiving irradiation plus chemotherapy. Three-year survival was approximately 50% for patients with abnormal tomograms whether they received chemotherapy or not, but increased from 67% (4/6 patients) to 91% (10/11 patients) for those with normal tomograms when chemotherapy was added. ABRAMSON et al. concluded that radiotherapy or radiochemotherapy had replaced exenteration as the treatment of choice and was of greatest benefit when disease was limited to the orbit.

Chemotherapy alone was employed as the primary therapy for RMS, with the goal of avoiding the deleterious effects of irradiation (VOUTE et al. 1981). It is not clear whether all or only some of the 11 patients also received irradiation and what dose was given, but 2 died of intracranial extension. Several additional patients were treated with initial chemotherapy at the Institut Gustave Roussy, Villejuif, France; it is my recollection that maintenance of a complete response was infrequent and that tumor regrowth led to the institution of irradiation within a period of months (SAGERMAN, notes of 1974, 1975, 1978). More recently, the results of the SIOP suggest that about 40% of patients with localized orbital rhabdomyosarcoma can be treated successfully without the use of irradiation (OBERLIN et al. 2001; ROUSSEAU et al. 1994).

The Intergroup RMS study began patient accrual in 1972 and has gathered the largest group of these patients. Their reports have provided detailed analyses of the many aspects of this disease, including orbital RMS. All children were treated according to protocols that required histologic proof and complete resection when possible, and were chemotherapy based. After surgical staging, the need for radiotherapy was tested in group I (histologically complete resection); few orbital RMS patients fell into this category, and such patients no longer receive immediate postoperative irradiation (WHARAM et al. 1997). Various chemotherapy regimens were tested in all other groups. Chemotherapy was given for 6 weeks before the start of irradiation in groups III and IV. The primary site received 50–60 Gy with conventional fractionation from supervoltage equipment, except for children under 3 years old, who received ≤40 Gy (MAURER et al. 1988). WHARAM et al. (1987) reported 132 patients with orbital RMS among a total of 1,461 cases registered from November 1972 to June 1983. Those with tumor confined to the eyelid or orbit (127) were analyzed. Ninety-four percent had histologic residual (20%) or gross (74%) tumor and received 30–64 Gy (50% received 45–55 Gy) in addition to one of several chemotherapeutic regimens (MAURER et al. 1988). The 3-year Kaplan-Meier survival estimate was 93%. There were 10 failures of primary chemoradiotherapy: 4 of the patients concerned were alive after salvage therapy. Two patients died of sepsis and 1 of leukemia, for 9 deaths in total. Relapse rates by clinical group were 1 out of 6 (16%), 2 out of 32 (16%), and 7 out of 89 (8%) for groups I, II, and III, respectively. Seven relapses were confined to the orbit (four were salvaged) and three were in regional nodes, but there were no distant metastases. Risk of relapse was not related to dose between 30–64 Gy or to histologic type. However, 3 of 5 children under 12 months relapsed and 9 of 10 failures occurred in girls.

Although local tumor control hovers at about 90%, more accurate staging and the development of effective chemotherapeutic regimens has decreased the incidence of later appearance of extraocular metastases from 30% to 2% (DONALDSON et al. 2001).

OBERLIN et al. (2001) reported overall results and differences in treatment strategy between the Intergroup RMS (IRS, 186 patients, 93% of whom received irradiation), the German Collaborative Soft Tissue Sarcoma Group (CSW, 28 of 40 patients irradiated), the Italian Cooperative Soft Tissue Sarcoma Group (ICG, 28 of 37 patients irradiated), and the International Society of Pediatric Oncology Sarcoma Committee (SIOP, 16 of 43 patients irradiated after failure of primary chemotherapy). The rate of local relapse varied from 5% (IRS) through 30% (CSW) and 35% (ICG) to 36% (SIOP; $P<0.001$ for IRS vs the other 3 groups). Event-free survival rates were 86% (IRS), 70% (CSW), 64% (ICG), and 58% (SIOP; $P<0.001$). Event-free survival was 86% with initial radiotherapy vs 53% without radiotherapy ($P<0.001$). Nevertheless, there was no significant difference in 10-year overall survival among the groups or with vs without initial radiotherapy, suggesting that irradiation after local relapse can be controlled in a significant proportion of these patients.

The techniques for orbital irradiation are varied; some are illustrated in Chap. 24. Proton beam therapy offers a unique approach to "painting" the tumor volume, and 3D conformal techniques and intensity-modulated radiation therapy provide better normal tissue sparing than conventional external beam irradiation (HUG et al. 2000). The physician is cautioned to choose the technique that best covers the tumor and spares sensitive structures as much as possible for each patient, recognizing that it is mandatory to achieve control at the primary tumor site and that visual and cosmetic changes may be rectified by newer surgical techniques. DONALDSON et al. (2001) report no significant difference in local/regional control, failure-free survival and overall survival for stages 1–3, group III rhabdomyosarcoma including the orbit, with hyperfractionated irradiation (59.4 Gy in 54 b.i.d. fractions) vs conventional irradiation (50.4 Gy in 28, 1.8-Gy fractions in the Intergroup RMS Study IV given with chemotherapy (DONALDSON et al. 2001).

13.6.4
Late Effects

Orbital RMS was present in 56 patients registered in the Intergroup RMS study I between 1972 and 1978 (HEYN et al. 1986). The overall survival was 86% (48/56), and the survival rate was 85% (33/39 in group III). Late effects were evaluated by questionnaire in the 50 who survived longer than 3 years. Forty patients underwent gross complete (15) or partial (25) resection and 10, biopsy only; there were 7 infectious complications related to surgery. Decreased vision was reported in 33 of 37 patients; it ranged from blurred vision to complete loss and was associated with cataracts. Cataracts appeared at all doses, and somewhat earlier at higher doses. Other functional problems included keratoconjunctivitis (10), photophobia (13), conjunctivitis (12), and dryness of the globe (4). Structural changes included cataracts (36/40, 90%), corneal changes (10), retinal changes (3), enophthalmos (10), stenosis of the lacrimal duct (7), facial asymmetry (19), and bony hypoplasia of the orbit. Defects in dentition were recorded in 3 children, and 61% (27/44) showed a downward deviation of >20% in height vs age percentile. Secondary surgery was performed in 17 children, in 9 cases for removal of a cataract. Plastic repair was accomplished for 3 children with ptosis and 1 with lacrimal

duct stenosis. Enucleation was done for a variety of reasons in 4 children (WEISS et al. 2001).

SAGERMAN et al. (1974) reported cataracts and bony hypoplasia in the vast majority of patients, but expected to find them in all patients if studied adequately. Changes were more profound the younger the child at the initiation of treatment. They noted dry eyes in those patients treated with the eyelids closed, which caused the loss of the "cornea-sparing" effects of the supervoltage beam, and in children undergoing subsequent ocular trauma or infection.

Although cataracts can be successfully removed, visual rehabilitation is a complicated matter and decreased tears may interfere with wearing a contact lens (see Chap. 21).

No second malignancies are known to have developed among the 31 children treated primarily by radiotherapy and with low-dose single-agent chemotherapy (SAGERMAN et al. 1974; R.M. Ellsworth, personal communication, 1992). HEYN et al. (1993) identified 22 second cancers among 1,770 patients with 9,877 patient-years of follow-up treated on the Intergroup RMS studies I and II. The orbit was the primary RMS site in 5. All received VAC-based chemotherapy, with Adriamycin in 2, in addition to 46.7–59 Gy. There were 2 acute nonlymphoblastic leukemias and 1 case each of leiomyosarcoma, adrenocortical carcinoma and fibrillary astrocytoma. Four patients died within 3 years of diagnosis of the second cancer; the patient with the leiomyosarcoma was alive with a 1-month follow-up.

13.7
Summary

Remarkable progress has been made in the management of orbital RMS in the last 39 years. Long-term survival improved from 25–67% to 85–90% with the replacement of surgery by irradiation, to which chemotherapy was then added. Staging is now more accurate. Tumor documentation by contrast-enhanced computed tomography and magnetic resonance imaging leads to more accurate radiotherapeutic treatment and can be exploited to reduce the volume of radiation and decrease late radiation effects (HUG et al. 2000). While the development of more effective chemotherapeutic agents and regimens may yet diminish or obviate the need for therapeutic surgery or irradiation, current protocols explore how to minimize the sequelae of treatment while improving tumor control.

References

Abramson DH, Ellsworth RM, Tretter P et al (1979) The treatment of orbital rhabdomyosarcoma with irradiation and chemotherapy. Ophthalmology 86:1330–1335

Ashton N, Morgan G (1965) Embryonal sarcoma and embryonal rhabdomyosarcoma of the orbit. J Clin Pathol 18:699–714

Cassady JR, Sagerman RH, Tretter P, Ellsworth RM (1968) Radiation therapy for rhabdomyosarcoma. Radiology 91:116–120

Crist WM, Garnsey L, Beltangady MS et al (1990) Prognosis in children with rhabdomyosarcoma: a report of the Intergroup Rhabdomyosarcoma Studies I and II. J Clin Oncol 8:443–452

Donaldson SS, Castro JR, Wilbur JR, Jesse RH (1973) Rhabdomyosarcoma of head and neck in children. Cancer 31:26–35

Donaldson SS, Meza JL, Breneman J et al (2001) Results from the IRS IV randomized trial of hyperfractionated radiotherapy in children with rhabdomyosarcoma. Int J Radiat Oncol Biol Phys 51:718–728

Frayer WC, Enterline HT (1959) Embryonal rhabdomyosarcoma of the orbit I children and young adults. Arch Ophthalmol 62:203–210

Gehan EA, Glover FN, Maurer HM et al (1981) Prognostic factors in children with rhabdomyosarcoma. Natl Cancer Inst Monogr 56:86–92

Heyn RM, Holland R, Newton WA et al (1974) The role of combined chemotherapy in the treatment of rhabdomyosarcoma in children. Cancer 34:2128–2142

Heyn R, Ragab A, Raney B et al (1986) Late effects of therapy in orbital rhabdomyosarcoma in children. A report from the Intergroup Rhabdomyosarcoma Study. Cancer 57:1738–1743

Heyn R, Haeberlen V, Newton WA, et al (1993) Second malignant neoplasms in children treated for rhabdomyosarcoma. J Clin Oncol 11:262–270

Hug EB, Adams J, Fitzek M et al. (2000) Fractionated, three-dimensional, planning-assisted proton-radiation therapy for orbital rhabdomyosarcoma: a novel technique. Int J Radiat Oncol Biol Phys 47:979–984

Jones IS, Reese AB, Krout J (1965) Orbital rhabdomyosarcoma: an analysis of sixty-two cases. Trans Am Ophthalmol Soc 63:223–255

Kassel SH, Copenhaver R, Arean VM (1965) Orbital rhabdomyosarcoma. Am J Ophthalmol 60:811–818

Knowles DM, Jakobiec FA, Potter GD et al (1978) The diagnosis and treatment of rhabdomyosarcoma of the orbit. In: Jakobiec FA (ed) Ocular and adnexal tumors. Aesculapius, Birmingham Ala, pp 708–734

Landers PH (1968) X-ray treatment of embryonal rhabdomyosarcoma of orbit. Case report of a 13-year survival without recurrence. Am J Ophthalmol 66:745–747

Lederman M (1956) Radiotherapy in the treatment of orbital tumors. Br J Ophthalmol 40:592–610

Li FP, Fraumeni JF (1969) Rhabdomyosarcoma in children: epidemiologic study and identification of a familial cancer syndrome. J Natl Cancer Inst 43:1365–1373

Maurer HM, Beltangady M, Gehan EA et al (1988) The Intergroup Rhabdomyosarcoma Study I. A final report. Cancer 61:209–220

Miller RW (1968) Relation between cancer and congenital defects: an epidemiologic evaluation. J Natl Cancer Inst 40:1079–1085

Oberlin O, Rey A, Anderson J et al (2001) Treatment of orbital rhabdomyosarcoma: survival and late effects of treatment – results of an international workshop. J Clin Oncol 19:197–204

Olurin O (1969) Orbital rhabdomyosarcoma in pregnancy. Cancer 24:1013–1016

Porterfield JF, Zimmerman LE (1962) Rhabdomyosarcoma of the orbit. A clinicopathologic study of 55 cases. Virchows Arch [A] 335:329–344

Raney RB, Anderson J, Kollath J et al (2000) Late effects of therapy in 94 patients with localized rhabdomyosarcoma of the orbit: report from the Intergroup Rhabdomyosarcoma Study (IRS)-III, 1984–1991. Med Pediatr Oncol 34:413–420

Rousseau P, Flamant F, Quintana E, et al (1994) Primary chemotherapy in rhabdomyosarcoma and other malignant mesenchymal tumours of the orbit: Results of the International Society of Paediatric Oncology MMT 84 Study. J Clin Oncol 12:516–521

Sagerman RH, Cassady JR, Tretter P (1968) Radiation therapy for rhabdomyosarcoma of the orbit. Trans Am Acad Ophthalmol Otolaryngol 72:849–854

Sagerman RH, Tretter P, Ellsworth RM (1974) Orbital rhabdomyosarcoma in children. Trans Am Acad Ophthalmol Otolaryngol 78:602–605

Sutow WW, Lindberg RD, Gehan EA et al. (1982) Three-year relapse-free survival rates in childhood rhabdomyosarcoma of the head and neck. Cancer 49:2217–2221

Voute PA, Vos A, de Kraker J, et al (1981) Rhabdomyosarcoma: chemotherapy and limited supplementary treatment program to avoid mutilation. Natl Cancer Inst Monogr 56:121–125

Wharam M, Beltangady M, Hays D et al (1987) Localized orbital rhabdomyosarcoma. An interim report of the Intergroup Rhabdomyosarcoma Study Committee. Ophthalmology 94:251–254

Wharam MD, Hanfelt JJ, Tefft MC, Johnston J, Ensign LG, Breneman J, Donaldson SS, Fryer C, Gehan EA, Raney RB, Maurer HM (1997) Radiation therapy for rhabdomyosarcoma: local failure risk for clinical group III patients on Intergroup Rhabdomyosarcoma Study II. Int J Radiat Oncol Biol Phys 38:797–804

14 Optic Pathway Glioma

R.H. Sagerman, G.F. Hatoum, S.S. Hahn

CONTENTS

14.1
Introduction

There is perhaps no other tumor of the eye or orbit whose treatment evokes as much controversy as that of the optic glioma. The reader is left thinking of a group of blind men describing an elephant while each touching a different part of the animal. Different specialists' preferred options range from no treatment, through partial excision, complete excision and radiation therapy to surgery plus radiotherapy, and now also include chemotherapy. The treatment selected is a direct reflection of the anatomical site of involvement, the symptoms and signs, the age of the patient, and the consequences of surgical extirpation of the lesion and of irradiation.

14.2
Anatomy and Histology

In 1988, Alvord and Lofton reviewed 623 cases of optic glioma that had been reported with information allowing actuarial analysis of several prognostic factors. The sites of involvement are shown in Table 14.1;

only the optic nerve was affected in 25% of cases, while in 75% the lesion also involved the chiasm. These tumors are often segregated into anterior lesions, which may extend to the chiasm, and posterior lesions. Complete or partial resection is feasible for anterior but not for posterior lesions, and anterior lesions have a better prognosis.

Optic nerve gliomas account for 1–5% of all intracranial gliomas. Histologically, they are usually reported as low-grade pilocytic astrocytoma, and occasionally as oligodendroglioma (Christiansen and Anderson 1952; Liss 1961; Rio-Hortega 1944). Russell and Rubinstein (1977) found only one case of malignant glioma in the literature; however, other malignant gliomas have been reported (Bataini 1991; Hoyt et al. 1973; Spoor et al. 1980). Pierce et al. (1990) reviewed nine reports of 171 patients, representing 82% of all patients, who had a biopsy for suspected optic chiasm glioma. One hundred and fifty-three (89%) were grade 1 or 2, eight were grade 3, four were not diagnostic, and there were three other tumors. Alvord and Lofton (1988) concluded that these gliomas have a wide but continuous range of growth rates and could not support the thesis that some of these lesions were hamartomas. Optic nerve gliomas may be the sole manifestation or part of the larger complex of von Recklinghausen's neurofibromatosis (Cohen and

R.H. Sagerman, MD, FACR; G.F. Hatoum, MD;
S.S. Hahn, MD
Department of Radiation Oncology, SUNY Upstate Medical University, 750 E. Adams Street, Syracuse, NY 13210, USA

Table 14.1. Sites of optic gliomas in 623 patients. (Modified from Alvord and Lofton 1988)

Tumor site	Total cases	Date of publication		
		<1960	1960–1979	>1980
Optic nerve	155	30	36	89
Optic chiasm	468			
Chiasm only	(229)	27	65	137
Plus hypothalamus	(180)	8	56	116
Plus hydrocephalus	(59)	7	8	44
Total cases	623	72	165	386

ROTHNER 1989). Several groups report an incidence of neurofibromatosis ranging from 14% to 50% (BATAINI et al. 1991; DANOFF et al. 1980; KOVALIC et al. 1990; PIERCE et al. 1990; RUSH et al. 1982; TENNY et al. 1982).

14.3
Clinical Presentation

Optic gliomas occur more often in children than in adults, 75% appearing within the first and 90% before the end of the second decade (FOWLER and MATSON 1957; TYM 1961). The age distribution for 623 patients, 386 (62%) of whom have been reported since 1980, is shown in Table 14.2; 59% were under 10 years and 82%, under 20 years old (ALVORD and LOFTON 1988).

Optic gliomas were found to be more frequent in girls than boys (62% vs 38%) and in the left than in the right eye (52% vs 41%, 7% bilateral) in the Armed Forces Institute of Pathology study of 63 patients (YANOFF et al 1978). In this study, proptosis was the first clinical sign in 50 patients, and tumor involved the orbit in 72%. Proptosis was directed laterally in 58% and axially in 21%.

The incidence of the several presenting signs and symptoms varies with the selection factors in the reported series. In the classic series of 36 patients of HOYT and BAGHDASSARIAN (1969), the presence of tumor in the anterior optic pathways was signaled by ophthalmic symptoms in 19: visual loss (8), proptosis (8), strabismus (2), and nystagmus (1). The incidental discovery of amblyopia and pallor of the optic disk led to the diagnosis in 7 patients. The tumor was discovered in the course of pediatric and radiologic investigation of nonocular problems in 9 children and as an incidental finding at autopsy in 1 adult. The diagnosis was established before the age of 5 years in 15 of the group of 19, but in the others were 10, 20, 26, and 40 years old before the diagnosis was made.

In a series of 56 patients (Table 14.3; CHUTORIAN et al. 1964), decreased visual acuity was the most common initial symptom (n=28); however, decreased vision was known to the patient or parents at the first neurologic examination in 11 cases, and testing detected diminished acuity of which the patient was unaware in 14 more. Thus, 53 (95%) of the 56 had decreased visual acuity at the time of diagnosis. In this series, exophthalmos, usually mild (<3 mm), was the initial symptom in 25 patients. Exophthalmos occurs with intraorbital optic glioma. Nys-

tagmus was the initial symptom in 8 patients, strabismus in 6, and increased intracranial pressure in 3. Changes in the optic nerve head were found in 55 patients; these took the form of simple optic atrophy in 33 and were more complex in 22. Although 12 patients had multiple café-au-lait spots, only 2 had other findings of neurofibromatosis and there was a family history of von Recklinghausen's disease in 4.

In contrast, series reported from radiation oncology centers, in which radiotherapy is given only for progressive signs and symptoms, report almost universal decreased visual acuity and restriction of visual fields, as well as frequent optic atrophy, endocrine abnormalities, hypothalamic symptoms, and even hydrocephalus (BATAINI et al. 1991; DANOFF et al. 1980; HORWICH and BLOOM 1985; PIERCE et al. 1990; WEISS et al. 1987). These patients have posteri-

Table 14.2. Ages of 623 patients with optic glioma. (Modified from ALVORD and LOFTON 1988)

Patients' ages (years)	Total cases	Date of publication		
		<1960	1960–1979	>1980
<10	370	40	98	232
10–19	140	18	33	89
20–29	36	4	7	25
30–39	5	6	12	
40–49	28	3	10	15
>49	23	2	11	10
Unknown	3			3
Total cases	623	72	165	386

Table 14.3. Symptoms and signs in 56 patients with optic glioma. (CHUTORIAN et al. 1964)

Presenting	Initial symptom	Presenting symptom	sign
Diminished visual acuity	28	39	53
Exophthalmos	25	27	29
Nystagmus	8	8	14
Strabismus	6	11	17
Field cut	1	1	12
Disk change			
Pallor			36
Pallor and blurring			11
Increased intracranial pressure	3	13	15
Enlarged head	1	1	4
Multiple café-au-lait spots		2	12
Paresis		3	4

orly located lesions not usually manageable by surgical extirpation, and a poorer prognosis (ALVORD and LOFTON 1988; JENKIN et al. 1993).

14.4
Diagnostic Studies

As suggested by the clinical presentation, a meticulous history, family history, and physical examination are needed. Ophthalmologic, endocrinologic, neurologic, and mental function details should be documented.

The most valuable radiographic studies are magnetic resonance imaging (MRI) and computed tomography (CT), which can document the size and location of the mass, infiltration of adjacent structures, and hydrocephalus and can usually distinguish glioma from meningioma of the optic nerve (BYRD et al. 1978; DANIELS et al. 1980; ST. LOUIS and HAIK 1993). Plain radiographic films, arteriography, and pneumoencephalography are rarely indicated. Radiographic determination of the diameter of the optic foramina is of value, but this is usually determined on CT. The normal optic foramen is 4.1–4.7 mm in diameter, and a diameter in excess of 6.5 mm is highly suggestive of glioma (SHIELDS 1989). Bone scan ultrasonography can show the enlarged optic nerve but does not allow evaluation of the optic canal. TAO et al. (1997) illustrated the importance of follow-up radiographic studies. The probability of at least a 50% radiographic response rose progressively from 18.1% through 38.2% to 45.9% at 2, 4, and 5 years, respectively.

14.5
Management

The management of optic nerve glioma is complicated by delays in diagnosis, patient age, location of the tumor, neurologic findings, visual acuity, loss of vision in an eye that has been enucleated or in which the optic nerve is resected, the late effects of irradiation, the uncertainty that tumor progression will occur, and the desire to maintain or improve vision. The seemingly widely diverging opinions regarding the management of optic nerve glioma are best resolved by choosing a plan after careful evaluation of the clinical situation. If there is clear evidence of tumor progression at the time of diagnosis, surgery

is indicated for lesions of the optic nerve and irradiation for tumors of the chiasm and posterior tracts. Lesions involving the optic chiasm, optic tracts, or the third ventricle are generally considered surgically unresectable (TENNY et al. 1982). Chemotherapy may be used for posterior lesions, especially in younger children (<5 years), in an attempt to avoid late sequelae from irradiation (JANSS et al. 1994).

When the history suggests a stable clinical state, when vision is good, or when tumor progression is uncertain, intervention should be delayed and the patient followed closely. Observation is also recommended when proptosis is moderate or severe, visual acuity is poor, the contralateral eye shows no field defect, and the tumor extends into the optic foramen or posterior to it. Complete removal should be accomplished if growth occurs posteriorly. Although about 5% of optic nerve gliomas are reported to recur in the chiasm following "complete" intraorbital excision, ALVORD and LOFTON (1988) found no reports of recurrence when the proximal end of the nerve was normal. Complete excision at the time of diagnosis is recommended when initial vision is poor, the tumor extends into the intracranial portion of the optic nerve, and there is a temporal field cut in the opposite eye.

When there is useful vision and the tumor involves the chiasm, and the opposite eye has a field defect, periodic observation is recommended until progression can be documented, at which time radiation therapy should be undertaken. When visual acuity is good, intervention should be postponed.

SHIELDS (1989) presents the following scenarios. If the tumor is confined to the intraorbital optic nerve, vision is good, and proptosis is mild and cosmetically acceptable, periodic evaluation is advised. Assessment of visual acuity, evaluation of the pupil, optic disk, and visual fields, and documentary photography are done at 6-month intervals. CT or MRI is repeated every 1–2 years, or sooner if suggested by clinical changes. Complete surgical removal through a lateral orbitotomy is recommended when acuity decreases, proptosis increases, and enlargement is seen on CT.

A histologic diagnosis was obtained in all seven patients with blinding optic nerve tumors or inflammation subjected to fine-needle aspiration biopsy under CT or bone scan ultrasound guidance (KENNERDELL et al. 1980). Although not without danger, a histologic diagnosis can be established with minimal invasion and might be valuable prior to irradiation when the clinical and radiographic findings are equivocal.

Radiotherapy reports present a selected group of patients with lesions of the chiasm and optic tracts who have neurologic involvement, endocrine deficits, and progressive disease. Nevertheless, they are universal in concluding that irradiation can arrest tumor progression in a majority of patients and improve visual acuity in some (DOSORETZ et al. 1980; FLICKENGER et al. 1988; HARTER et al. 1978; HORWICH and BLOOM 1985; MONTGOMERY et al. 1977; ROBERTSON and BREWIN 1980; WONG et al. 1987). BATAINI et al. (1991) reported an overall actuarial survival of 83.5% at both 5 and 10 years, and corresponding relapse-free survival rates of 89% and 82%, in their series of 57 patients, 21 of whom had involvement of the chiasm ± optic nerves ("group B") and 36 involvement of the chiasm with posterior extension ("group C"). The relapse-free survival rates found were 100% and 88% at 5 and 10 years, respectively, for group B and 82% and 72% for group C ($P<0.05$). Patients with neurologic signs fared worse than those without neurologic signs, overall survival at 5 and 10 years being 57% vs 92%, respectively ($P<0.02$).

BATAINI et al. (1991) reviewed 18 series involving a total of 234 patients with anterior chiasmal gliomas, 189 of which were irradiated. The failure rate after radiotherapy was 18.5% (35/189) and the mortality, 17.5% (41/234). There were 175 cases of posterior chiasmal gliomas in 15 series, 142 of which were irradiated: 50 of the 142 (35%) recurred after radiotherapy, and 44 of the 175 patients died (25%). The technical details given were not sufficient to determine the adequacy of tumor coverage.

A population-based study of 87 consecutive children with newly diagnosed optic nerve glioma at the University of Toronto hospital from 1958 to 1990 was reported by JENKIN et al. (1993). The 10-year survival, relapse-free survival, and freedom from second relapse rates were 84%, 68%, and 85%, respectively. Of the 27 patients who progressed or relapsed, 41% were free of a second relapse 10 years after the first relapse. Thirteen of the 14 patients suffering a second relapse died, and none survived 5 years. The 10-year survivals and 10-year relapse-free survivals were 95% vs 76% ($P=0.02$) and 80% vs 59% ($P=0.02$), respectively, for the 35 patients with anterior tumors involving the optic nerves or chiasm + optic nerves vs those with posterior spread beyond the chiasm. Primary irradiation and the presence of neurofibromatosis were favorable prognostic factors for first relapse. Primary irradiation was more effective in preventing relapse at 10 years than primary subtotal resection (75% vs 41%; $P=0.02$); however, salvage

therapy was somewhat successful, and neither factor significantly affected survival upon multivariate analysis.

In 1997, TAO et al. reported on 42 children with chiasmal gliomas. Eleven asymptomatic patients with neurofibromatosis were observed only. Two children less than 3 years old had surgery and chemotherapy to delay irradiation, and 29 with progressive disease were irradiated, with or without surgery or chemotherapy. With a median follow-up of 108 months the 10-year freedom from progression rate was 100% and the overall survival rate was 89% for the 29 irradiated patients. Vision stabilized or improved in 81% of the 26 evaluable irradiated patients.

A desire to avoid radiation morbidity has gradually changed the authors' practice for posterior optic gliomas; since 1977, the rate of surveillance has increased from 13% to 34% and that of primary resection alone from 4% to 38%, while the proportion treated with primary irradiation alone decreased from 57% to 17% and that treated with resection plus irradiation, from 26% to 10%. There has been no significant difference in survival or relapse-free survival at 10 years. These authors now resect gliomas involving the optic nerve when there is no or little vision in the affected eye, or when there is a history of tumor activity. Otherwise, children are followed carefully and primary irradiation is not used for tumors confined to the nerve. When tumor is limited to the optic nerves and chiasm, children with reasonable vision and no recent history of progression are followed; primary irradiation is given when visual defects are severe or progressive. In this series, the incidence of second malignant tumors was 5 out of 48 irradiated children versus none of 49 who were not irradiated; all second malignancies proved fatal (JENKIN et al. 1993). PIERCE et al. (1990) reported two patients developing second tumors; both tumors were gliomas and developed outside the radiation field in children with neurofibromatosis.

Although it has been difficult to establish significant differences in survival by virtue of location or treatment, the review of 623 reported cases by ALVORD and LOFTON (1988) led them to conclude that:

1. There is a broad range in growth rate from very slow to very rapid, despite the almost uniform histologic appearance of low-grade astrocytomas.
2. There is a gradient for death due to tumor: it is rare in the case if tumors limited to the optic nerve and increases progressively for gliomas of the chiasm, hypothalamus, and ventricle.

3. No reports of recurrence in the chiasm were found after resection of an optic nerve with a clean proximal margin.

4. Irradiation is more effective at doses above 45 Gy.

5. The increasing probability of death noted after the age of 20 years is marked in those older than 50 years, because half of these patients have malignant glioma.

6. The association with neurofibromatosis doubles the recurrence rate after complete excision of an intraorbital glioma but does not affect prognosis following irradiation of chiasmal gliomas.

A major concern in management of children with optic gliomas has been the avoidance of late radiation effects (JANSS et al. 1994). These can include basal ganglia calcification (8), cerebral atrophy (5), white matter degeneration (8), and the arterial stenosis of moyamoya syndrome (2), which were noted in the 24 irradiated children studied by PIERCE et al. (1990). In addition, 15 of the 18 patients evaluated showed growth hormone deficiency. Endocrinologic deficiency is thought to be more frequent and more severe when radiation therapy is given at an earlier age, but no correlation was found with tumor location, tumor dose, or neurofibromatosis. Of even greater potential significance is neuropsychological abnormality. After exclusion of patients with progressive disease, altered learning ability and decreased memory were found in 10 of 19 patients (PIERCE et al. 1990). Six of 16 patients had hydrocephalus at presentation in the series of WEISS et al. (1987). Five patients were mentally retarded, 1 following meningococcal meningitis; 4 of these 5 were less than 2 years old when irradiated. LLOYD (1973) reported that one-third of patients were retarded prior to therapy.

Visual acuity improved in 5 and stabilized in 7 of the 14 irradiated patients of WEISS et al. (1987); the corresponding figures in the series of PIERCE et al. (1990) were 7 out of 23 (35%) and 14 out of 23 (61%), respectively. In 53 evaluable patients, BATAINI et al. (1991) reported complete response in 8 (15%), partial response in 25 (46%), and no progression in 12 (22%); vision improved or stabilized in 93%.

When radiation therapy is indicated, we recommend carefully tailored fields designed with the aid of CT or MRI, treatment with megavoltage accelerators, and treatment of all fields daily at 1.8–2 Gy per fraction to give a tumor dose of 50.4 Gy (45 Gy minimum to 54 Gy maximum). This will prevent further deterioration in about 90% of cases, and vision will improve in perhaps 30%. Pretreatment mental and endocrinologic function should be documented and long-term post-treatment studies, including a search for second tumors, must be accomplished. Endocrine replacement must be provided as necessary.

Advances in radiotherapeutic techniques, such as 3D conformal therapy, intensity-modulated irradiation, and linac or gamma knife radiotherapy, may reduce the incidence and degree of adverse reactions by decreasing the volume of normal tissue treated. Of note in this regard is the mechanical advantage provided by proton beam therapy (FUSS et al. 1999).

14.6
Chemotherapy

PACKER et al. (1983, 1988) and ROSENSTOCK et al. (1985) reported on 24 children under the age of 5 years (mean age 1.6 years) with chiasmatic/hypothalamic gliomas treated with actinomycin D plus vincristine, without radiotherapy. They had been followed up for a median of 4.3 years (range 0.3–10 years) and all were still alive; 9 had developed clinical or radiographic progression at a median of 3 years after start of treatment, and 8 of these 9 children then received radiotherapy, which stabilized the disease. Fifteen (62.5%) remained free of progression and had received no other treatment. Tumor shrinkage was documented in 9 of the 24 patients but did not correlate with long-term outcome. Full-scale intelligence quotient was normal, with a mean of 103 (range 84–133) at a median of 3.5 years.

Six children, ranging in age from 1 year to 10 years, have been treated with combination chemotherapy for progressing optic glioma at the SUNY Upstate Medical University at Syracuse, New York since 1982 (R.L. DUBOWY, personal communication, 1992). Five cases involved the chiasm (one with hydrocephalus and one with diencephalic syndrome) and one child had bilateral optic nerve tumors. Two had neurofibromatosis and were not biopsied; grade 1 (3) or grade 2 (1) pilocytic astrocytoma was reported in four patients. Chemotherapy consisted of vincristine (1.5 mg/m^2 weekly for 8 weeks) and actinomycin D (1.5 μg/kg daily for 5 days during the first week); five cycles were given at 12-week intervals. Marked regression of the mass was noted in two patients (Fig. 14.1) and minimal regression in one; there was no radiographic change in two. There has been no tumor progression requiring irradiation, although operative relief was accomplished for hydrocephalus in one child when there was only a minimal

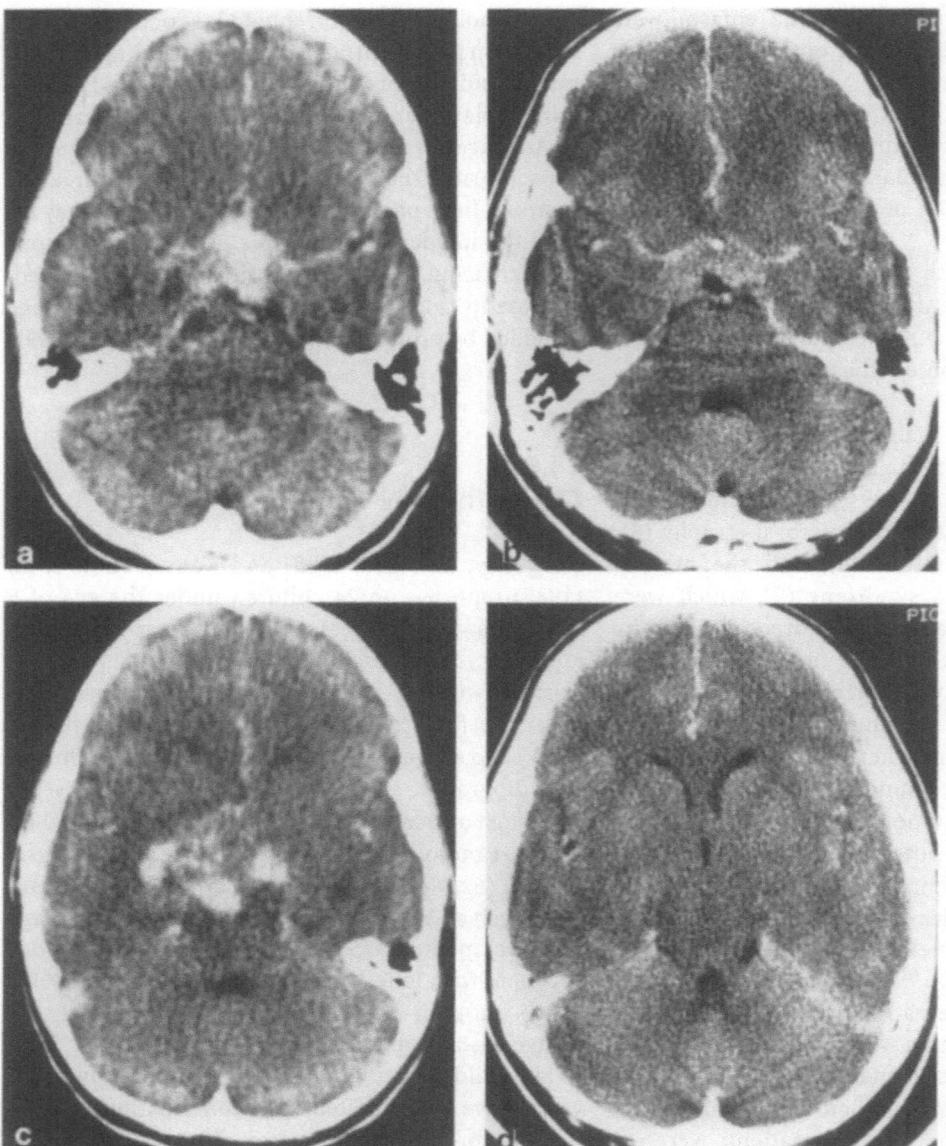

Fig. 14.1a–d. CT scan of a 10-year-old boy with neurofibromatosis and a large chiasmatic tumor treated with chemotherapy: **a** abnormal contrast enhancement before treatment; **b** minimal contrast enhancement 8 years after treatment; **c** abnormal, multinodular contrast enhancement before treatment; **d** normal appearance at this CT level 8 years after treatment. Regression was demonstrated at 8 months and there has been no further change in the CT appearance at 8 years. There has been no relapse during 9 years of observation but vision did not improve despite tumor regression

response after two cycles of chemotherapy. Vision has not improved in any of these children.

There were too few patients (five), and they have been treated too recently, to reach conclusions regarding the effectiveness of chemotherapy in the series of JENKIN et al. (1993). Similarly, ALVORD and LOFTON (1988) concluded that chemotherapy has been employed for too short a time and in too varied a population to be certain of its effects.

MAHONEY et al. (2000) presented the results of Pediatric Oncology Group (POG) studies 8935 and 8936,

which closed in 1994. POG 8936 was a phase II cooperative study designed to test the efficacy of single-agent chemotherapy with carboplatin as the primary treatment for children under 6 years of age. Fifty of the 51 patients enrolled were eligible for review; in 1 case the age threshold of 6 years had already been passed. All had progressive disease recognized from the symptoms or by neuroimaging Twenty-one had type 1 neurofibromatosis. Carboplatin, 560 mg/m^2, was given at 4-week intervals. Patients with stable disease after 3 months of therapy continued until disease progression was noted or for 18 months. Thirty-four of the 39 patients with stable disease or better completed 18 months of therapy. The proportion who achieved objective responses, defined as complete, partial, or minor response or stable disease, exceeded 30%. Twenty-one patients suffered disease progression, 15 during the chemotherapy and 6 after completing 18 months of chemotherapy. Six children died with progressive disease. The major toxicities were neutropenia and thrombocytopenia. The authors concluded that this regimen was safe and effective and that further studies, adding other chemotherapeutic agents, should be pursued.

14.7
Summary

Optic pathway gliomas are uncommon tumors of childhood, whose diagnosis is often delayed and which vary in the rate of progression. Their management is undergoing revision, and it will take years for mature data to be reported from the cooperative studies in progress. At present, careful follow-up is all that is necessary when the clinical picture is stable. Complete excision should be accomplished in the case of anterior lesions and irradiation for posterior lesions when tumor progression is demonstrated clinically or radiographically. Existing chemotherapy data indicate its usefulness, and chemotherapy should be the initial treatment in younger children with posterior lesions. Careful studies of vision, mentation, and endocrinologic function are necessary before and after treatment, and late effects must be recorded.

References

Alvord EC Jr, Lofton S (1988) Gliomas of the optic nerve or chiasm. Outcome of patients' age, tumor site, and treatment. J Neurosurg 68:85–98

Bataini JP, Delanian S, Ponvert D (1991) Chiasmal gliomas; results of irradiation management in 57 patients and review of literature. Int J Radiat Oncol Biol Phys 21:615–623

Byrd SE, Harwood-Nash DC, Fitz CR, Barry JF, Rogovitz DM (1978) Computed tomography of intraorbital optic nerve gliomas in children. Radiology 129:73–78

Christiansen E, Andersen SR (1952) Primary tumors of the optic nerve and chiasm. Acta Psychiatr Kbh 27:5

Chutorian AM, Schwartz JF, Evans RA, Carter S (1964) Optic gliomas in children. Neurology 14:83–93

Cohen BH, Rothner AD (1989) Incidence, types, and management of cancer in patients with neurofibromatosis. Oncology 3:23–30

Daniels DL, Haughton VM, Williams AL, Gager WE, Berns TF (1980) Computed tomography of the optic chiasm. Radiology 137:123–127

Danoff BF, Kramer S, Thompson N (1980) The radiotherapeutic management of optic nerve gliomas in children. Int J Radiat Oncol Biol Phys 6:45–50

Dosoretz DE, Blitzer PH, Wang CC, Linggood RM (1980) Management of glioma of the optic nerve and/or chiasm. An analysis of 20 cases. Cancer 45:1467–1471

Flickenger JC, Torres C, Deutsch M (1988) Management of low-grade gliomas of the optic nerve and chiasm. Cancer 61:635–642

Fowler FD, Mastson DD (1957) Gliomas of the optic pathways in childhood. J Neurosurg 14:515

Fuss M, Hug EB, Schaefer RA, Nevinny-Strickel M, Miller DW, Slater JM, Slater JD (1999) Proton radiation therapy (PRT) for pediatric optic pathway gliomas: comparison with 3D planned conventional photons and a standard photon technique. Int J Radiat Oncol Biol Phys 45:1117–1126

Harter DJ, Caderao JB, Leavens ME, Young SE (1978) Radiotherapy in the management of primary gliomas involving the intracranial optic nerves and chiasm. Int J Radiat Oncol Biol Phys 4:681–686

Horwich A, Bloom HJG (1985) Optic gliomas; radiation therapy and prognosis. Int J Radiat Oncol Phys 11:1067–1079

Hoyt WF, Baghdassarian SA (1969) Optic glioma of childhood. Natural history and rationale for conservative management. Br J Ophthalmol 53:793–798

Hoyt WF, Meshel LG, Lessel S et al (1973) Malignant optic glioma of adulthood. Brain 96:121–132

Janss AJ, Grundy R, Cnaan A et al (1994) Optic pathway and hypothalmic/chiasmatic gliomas in children younger than 5 years with a 6 year follow-up. Cancer 75:1051–1059

Jenkin D, Angyalfi S, Becker L et al (1993) Optic glioma in children. Surveillance, resection or irradiation. Int J Radiat Oncol Biol Phys 25:215–225

19. Kennerdell JS, Dubois PJ, Dekker A, Johnson BL (1980) CT guided fine needle aspiration biopsy of orbital optic nerve tumors. Ophthalmology 87:491–496

Kovalic JJ, Grigsby PW, Shepard MJ, Fineberg BB, Thomas PR (1990) Radiation therapy for gliomas of the optic nerve and chiasm. Int J Radiat Oncol Biol Phys 18:927–932

Liss L (1961) The oligodendrogliomas. A comparative study with tissue culture and silver carbonate techniques. J Neuropathol Exp Neurol 20:582

Lloyd LA (1973) Gliomas of the optic nerve and chiasm in childhood. Trans Am Ophthalmol Soc 71:488–535

Mahoney DH Jr, Cohen ME, Freidman HS, Kepner JL, Gemer L Langston JW, James HE, Duffner PK, Kun LE (2000) Carboplatin is effective therapy for young children with progressive optic pathway tumors: a Pediatric Oncology Group phase II study. Neurooncology 2:213–220

Montgomery AB, Griffin T, Parker RB, Gerdes AJ (1977) Optic nerve glioma: the role of radiation therapy. Cancer 40:2079–2080

Packer RJ, Savino PJ, Bilaniuk LT et al (1983) Chiasmatic gliomas of childhood. A reappraisal of natural history and effectiveness of cranial irradiation. Childs Brain 10:393–403

Packer RJ, Sutton LN, Bilaniuk LT et al (1988) Treatment of chiasmatic/hypothalamic gliomas of childhood with chemotherapy: an update. Ann Neurol 23:79–85

Pierce SM, Barnes PD, Loeffler, JS, McGinn C, Tarbell NJ (1990) Definitive radiation therapy in the management of symptomatic patients with optic glioma. Survival and long-term effects. Cancer 65:45–52

Rio-Hortega P del (1944) Contribucion al conocimente citologies de los tumores del nervio y guiasma opticos. Arch Histol B Aires 2:307

Robertson AG, Brewin TB (1980) Optic nerve glioma. Clin Radiol 31:471–474

Rosenstock JG, Packer RJ, Bilaniuk L, Bruce DA, Radcliffe J, Savino P (1985) Chiasmatic optic glioma treated with chemotherapy. A preliminary report. J Neurosurg 63:862–866

Rush JA, Young BR, Campbell RJ, MacCarty CS (1982) Optic glioma. Long-term follow-up of 85 histopathologically verified cases. Ophthalmology 89:1213–1219

Russell DS, Rubinstein LJ (1977) Pathology of tumors of the nervous system, 4th edn. Williams and Wilkins, Baltimore, pp 309–312

Saint Louis LA, Haik BG (1993) Imaging of diseases of the orbit. In: Alberti WE, Sagerman RH (eds) Radiotherapy of intraocular and orbital tumors, 1st edn, chap 30. Springer, Berlin Heidelberg New York, pp 273–282

Shields JA (1989) Diagnosis and management of orbital tumors. Saunders, Philadelphia

Spoor TC, Kennerdall JS, Martinez AJ et al (1980) Malignant gliomas of the optic nerve pathways. Am J Ophthalmol 89:284–292

Tao ML, Barnes PD, Billett AL et al (1997) Childhood optic chiasm gliomas: radiographic response following radiotherapy and long-term clinical outcome. Int J Radiat Oncol Biol Phys 39:579–587

Tenny RT, Laws ER Jr, Younge BR, Rush JA (1982) The neurosurgical management of optic glioma. Results in 104 patients. J Neurosurg 57:452–458

Tym R (1961) Piloid gliomas of the anterior optic pathways. Br J Surg 49:322–331

Weiss L, Sagerman RH, King GA, Chung CT, Dubowy RL (1987) Controversy in the management of optic nerve glioma. Cancer 59:1000–1004

Wong JYC, Uhl V, Wara WM, Sheline GF (1987) Optic gliomas. A reanalysis of the University of California, San Francisco experience. Cancer 60:1847–1855

Yanoff M, Davis RL, Zimmerman LE (1978) Juvenile pilocytic astrocytoma ("glioma") of optic nerve: clinicopathologic study of sixty-three cases. In: Jakobiec FA (ed) Ocular and adnexal tumors. Aesculapius, Birmingham, Ala, pp 685–707

15 Graves' Disease

S. S. Donaldson and I. R. McDougall

15.1
Introduction

The ophthalmopathy associated with thyroid disease most commonly accompanies hyperthyroidism and diffuse toxic goiter (Graves' disease). However, it can occur in euthyroid patients with Hashimoto's thyroiditis, in patients with myxedema who lack a history of thyrotoxicosis, and occasionally in patients without any recognized thyroid disease. Between 50% and 90% of patients with Graves' disease develop manifestations of ophthalmopathy (JACOBSON and GORMAN 1985; KRISS et al. 1983), although the symptoms may be minor and not progressive, and may not require treatment.

The disorder has been recognized for many years and is well characterized in the first patient described by Graves. Variable terms have been used for the problem, including malignant exophthalmos, thyrotropic exophthalmos, exophthalmic ophthalmoplegia, endocrine ophthalmopathy, dysthyroid ophthalmopathy, progressive exophthalmos and Graves' orbitopathy (JONES 1951). Currently the accepted term for it is Graves' ophthalmopathy, whether or not the patient has ever had Graves' hyperthyroidism.

S. S. DONALDSON, MD
Department of Radiation Oncology, Stanford University Medical Center, 300 Pasteur Drive, Stanford, CA 94305, USA
I. R. McDougall, MB, ChB, PhD
Stanford University Medical Center, 300 Pasteur Drive, Stanford, CA 94305, USA

15.2
Pathogenesis

The pathogenesis of Graves' disease has been widely studied and is known to be autoimmune. The ophthalmopathy is also considered to be an autoimmune disorder, but it remains unclear whether it has no relationship to Graves' disease and is causally related to antibodies interacting with orbital antigens, or is a complication of Graves' disease with shared antigenic determinants reacting between the thyroid gland and the orbital tissue (KRISS et al. 1987). There is a growing body of evidence supporting autoantibodies against TSH receptors in connective tissue of orbital muscles as a cause of the disorder (BAHN et al. 1998). The pathologic features include extraocular muscles that are enlarged, firm, rubbery, and resistant to passive stretching. The muscle volume may increase to 8–10 times the normal size, resulting in anterior displacement of the globe. The medial and inferior recti are the ones most frequently involved. The histologic features reveal an inflammatory cellular infiltrate of benign lymphocytes and associated edema. The inflammatory component may progress to one of fibrosis and scarring in the late stages of the disease. There is a strong association with cigarette smoking (PRUMMEL and WIERSINGA 1993). The relationship between induction or aggravation of eye disease and the treatment of hyperthyroidism continues to be controversial. BARTALENA et al. report that about 5% of patients treated with iodine-131 have longlasting exacerbation which merits treatment of the eyes (BARTALENA et al. 1998). Other experts do not confirm this (GORMAN 1995).

15.3
Clinical Characteristics

The clinical manifestations of Graves' ophthalmopathy are varied. Patients usually present with bilateral involvement, although unilateral ophthalmopathy may precede bilateral involvement. The symptoms can be symmetric or asymmetric, and the complex often appears to wax and wane and can undergo spontaneous remission. The ophthalmic symptoms include lacrimation, photophobia, burning, a sensation of tightness or pressure, diplopia, pain, and loss of vision. The clinical manifestations include periorbital edema, chemosis, proptosis, extraocular motor paresis, corneal irritation, and optic nerve dysfunction.

A comprehensive classification system adopted by the American Thyroid Association, the so-called NO SPECS classification (WERNER 1977), has become widely accepted and serves as a means of grading the severity of the disease, allowing assessment of its natural history and response to treatment. A modification of that system enabling an assessment of severity expressed as a useful ophthalmic index is shown in Table 15.1. Proptosis is measured using an exophthalmometer. Sight loss is measured by visual acuity. Drawbacks to this scoring system are that it does not differentiate acuity loss from other nonthyroid etiologies of sight loss, does not assess intraocular pressure, does not incorporate dependence upon corticosteroid medication, and assigns equal weight to all signs, which does not necessarily reflect their functional significance. Nevertheless it is widely accepted and serves as an excellent means of comparing pre- and posttreatment values in an individual patient while also allowing comparison between one individual and another. Other investigators have included the patient's subjective opinion about the natural history of the disorder and whether there is retraction of the lids.

15.4
Imaging Studies

Assessment of the orbit by ultrasound, computerized tomography (CT), or magnetic resonance imaging (MRI) is useful to confirm the diagnosis, and allows differentiation from other orbital disorders, such as pseudotumor and lymphoma. Of the three techniques, CT is the most commonly used to visualize the orbital contents and guide radiotherapy treatment planning, although comparative studies of the various techniques are not available. Orbital CT is not a requirement in all patients, but is recommended in any patient with symptoms/signs of ophthalmopathy who has no history of thyroid disease and for whom laboratory evidence of thyroid dysfunction or thyroid autoimmunity is lacking. In addition, imaging is essential in a patient presenting with unilateral ophthalmopathy. Patients with unilateral proptosis must be evaluated for primary orbital malignancy and orbital metastases, and must be differentiated from those with pseudotumor or lymphoma. MRI can determine whether there is acute inflammation, which helps some authorities determine whether to treat.

15.5
Indications for Radiotherapy

The first report of the effectiveness of orbital X-ray treatment in Graves' ophthalmopathy was in 1951 (JONES 1951). Since that time the use and techniques

Table 15.1. NO SPECS classification system and ophthalmic index[a]

Sign	Severity score		
	1	2	3
Soft tissue involvement	Slight conjunctival redness, chemosis, periorbital edema	Moderately severe conjunctival redness, chemosis, periorbital edema	Conjunctival redundancy, marked redness, periorbital edema
Proptosis	20–23 mm	>23–27 mm	>27 mm
Eye muscle involvement	Minimal limitation of movement, occasional diplopia	Moderate limitation of movement, frequent diplopia not in primary gaze	Severe limited movement, frequent symmetric diplopia in all gaze
Corneal involvement	Slight stippling	Marked stippling, corneal inflammation	Ulceration
Sight loss	20/25–20/40	20/45–20/100	20/>100

[a]Ophthalmic index = sum of scores for all five categories

of orbital radiation have evolved in such a way that today there are clear indications for the use of ionizing radiation in this "benign" condition. The rationale for the use of orbital radiotherapy is based on the premise that the ophthalmopathy is part of an autoimmune disorder and that the lymphocytes infiltrating the eye muscles have a role in the pathogenesis of the disease. Irradiation is used to ablate these lymphocytes. In contrast to the situation in most diseases or symptom complexes for which radiotherapy may be recommended, it is not necessary and not advisable to have histologic proof of a lymphocytic infiltrate in the eye muscle. However, it is important to elicit a history of thyroid dysfunction and thyroid status and also laboratory evidence of thyroid autoimmunity. When a patient presents with ophthalmopathy in a euthyroid state following radioiodine treatment or thyroidectomy while receiving oral replacement therapy, it is appropriate to focus management decisions on the eyes. Patients presenting with coexisting thyrotoxicosis or those who are euthyroid with antithyroid drug therapy require therapeutic decisions regarding thyroid dysfunction, as well as the ophthalmopathy. There is debate about the optimal type and timing of therapy. Treatment of the eyes does not influence the thyroid, but treatment of the thyroid can influence the ophthalmopathy.

The majority of patients with Graves' disease will develop some degree of ophthalmopathy; in some it can only be diagnosed by imaging. Most of these patients do not require orbital treatment, as mild ophthalmopathy can be appropriately managed symptomatically and spontaneous regressions are common.

Severe and progressive ophthalmopathy (generally an ophthalmopathy index score of 4 or greater) is an indication for considering treatment with corticosteroids or orbital irradiation. A previous trial of corticosteroids is not a prerequisite to radiotherapy. However, it is common for patients who have had an unsuccessful trial of corticosteroids, with either lack of response or intolerable side effects, to be referred for orbital irradiation. Once patients have become dependent on corticosteroid therapy, it is difficult to taper their corticosteroid medication. The tapering must be done very gradually over a long duration, which can cause iatrogenic Cushing's syndrome. Rapid tapering often results in a relapse of symptoms with the need for even higher corticosteroid dosage levels for temporary cessation of symptoms. A double-blind study comparing radiation with high-dose corticosteroids led to the conclusion that the former is the treatment of choice (PRUMMEL et al. 1993). BARTALENA et al. (1983) have evaluated the effect of orbital irradiation combined with systemic corticosteroids against that of systemic corticosteroids alone and found the combined therapy to be more effective.

Guidelines used in assessing candidates for radiotherapy are shown in Table 15.2, as are absolute contraindications to orbital irradiation. The goals of irradiation are to stop progression of the disease, eliminate functional disability, improve the appearance, and minimize side effects of treatment, including weaning from corticosteroids when patients are steroid dependent.

15.6
Techniques of Treatment

The use of external beam irradiation in the treatment of patients with Graves' ophthalmopathy involves:
1. History and physical examination
2. Setup and localization of the position of the orbit and retro-orbital tissues
3. Design and fabrication of custom beam-shaping blocks
4. Simulation of the individualized blocks
5. Treatment
6. Verification (portal) films
7. Follow-up

The history must be oriented toward the thyroid history and any intercurrent disease which might

Table 15.2. Guidelines on orbital irradiation

Indications

1. History of thyroid disease, laboratory evidence of thyroid autoimmunity or CT scan showing enlarged retro-orbital muscles
2. Confirmation of progression by detailed ophthalmologic examination
3. Absence of coexisting illness characterized by retinopathy
4. Functional disability

Contraindications

1. Stable disease, no evidence of progression
2. Cosmetic indications only, without functional handicap
3. Inability to give informed consent

Goals of treatment

1. Stop progression
2. Reduce/eliminate functional disability
3. Improve cosmetic appearance
4. Minimize undesirable side effects of treatment

influence the present illness, while the physical examination needs to include findings in the eye/orbit, thyroid gland, and nonthyroidal sites related to Graves' disease. Particular attention should be paid to the presence of pre-existing globe or orbital abnormalities, cataract, and retinopathy, in addition to aspects of the disease itself. A history of diabetes mellitus, hypertension, or other disease complex manifesting small vessel abnormalities should be noted. Extent of eye involvement should be addressed by examination, exophthalmometry, tonometry, retinoscopy, visual acuity and field examinations, and tests of extraocular motor function. Extent and severity of involvement should be agreed upon by all members of the treatment team: the radiation oncologist, ophthalmologist, and thyroidologist.

Megavoltage photon radiation as generated by a linear accelerator, with beam energies of 4–6 MV, is optimal. The use of cobalt-60 should be discouraged because of excess penumbra and scatter radiation. It is essential to keep the radiation dose to the anterior chamber of the eye and lens to an absolute minimum. Figure 15.1 demonstrates setup, simulation, and portal fields for a typical patient with Graves' disease. Ideally, the patient is stabilized in the treatment position by means of a face mask. The radiation field is localized by aligning the patient so that the central axis of the planned radiation beam will rest at the lateral fleshy canthus of each eye. A radiopaque marker such as a BB is placed to confirm this position. The cornea is marked by means of a contact lens containing a radiopaque marker.

The treatment field is then shaped using a beam-splitting technique so that the central axis of the ra-diation beam becomes the anterior border of the effective beam. The area anterior to the central axis can then be blocked by double-thickness lead blocks to minimize scatter radiation. The superior, inferior, and posterior field borders are designed to spare the brain, maxillary antrum, and pituitary, but shaped to include the entire muscular cone of the globe. In practice, using shaped Cerrobend fields, the collimator is approximately 4×8 cm while the actual treatment field size is approximately 4×4 cm. Figures 15.2–15.4 show several isodose curves using a 4×4 cm treatment field, but with modifications of the technique. When two opposing fields are used with the central axis of the beam placed at the midportion of the treatment field, as opposed to the anterior border of the treatment field, the entire orbit is well contained in the 90% isodose curve; however, the lens dose is approximately 15% of the treatment dose (Fig. 15.2). Angling the treatment beam 3° posteriorly serves to diminish the lens dose to approximately 10%, while the entire orbit is well covered (Fig. 15.3). The preferred technique is the beam-splitting technique (Fig. 15.4) (OLIVOTTO et al. 1985). The anterior border of the actual beam becomes the central axis, with its edge being 50% of the total dose. The orbits are well contained by the 90% isodose curve, while the lens dose is diminished to 4%.

As 95% of patients with Graves' ophthalmopathy have bilateral disease, it is advisable to treat both orbits simultaneously, even if one eye is less involved than the other. Use of a single lateral 4- to 6-MV photon field for unilateral disease results in approximately 60% of the dose to the opposite uninvolved eye. This radiation dose becomes problematic when

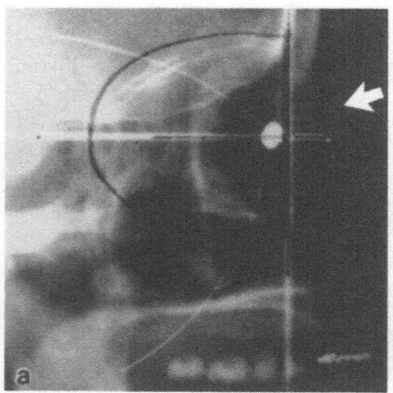 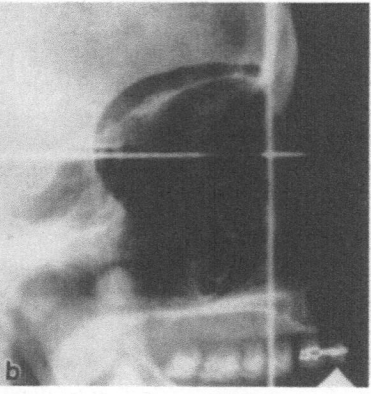 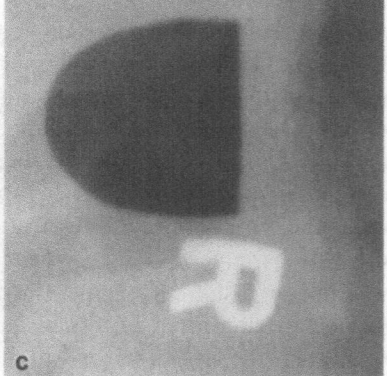

Fig. 15.1. A series of X-rays for a typical patient with Graves' ophthalmopathy, showing **a** setup, **b** simulation, and **c** portal film. The region within the D-shaped field is the treatment volume. The *arrow* points to the corneal marker. The radiopaque BBs are placed on the right and left lateral fleshy canthus. The *horizontal* and *vertical crossed lines* represent the central axis of the treatment field, with all structures anterior to the central axis shielded from radiation. The portal film verifies the accuracy of the setup and simulation film

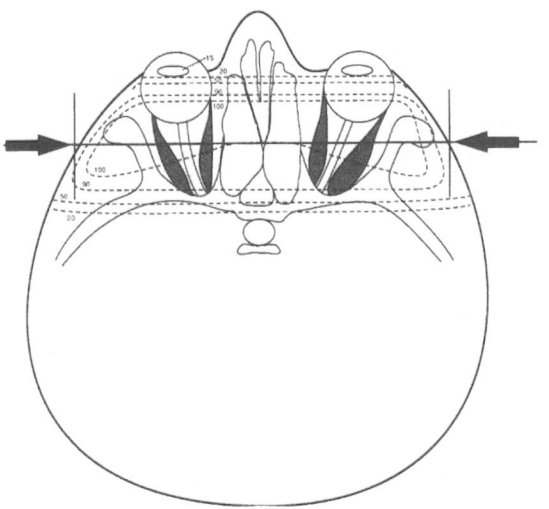

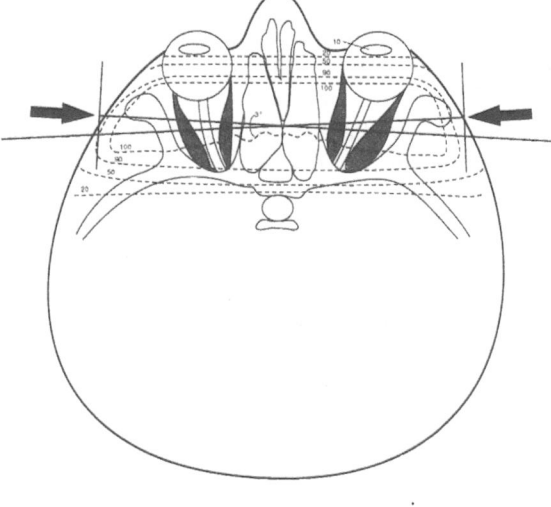

Fig. 15.2. Isodose curves using 6-MV photons from a linear accelerator with 4×4 cm opposed lateral fields with the central axis placed at the center of the treatment field. (Reproduced from ALBERTI and SAGERMAN 1993, chap 21, Fig. 21.2)

Fig. 15.3. Isodose curves using 6-MV photons from a linear accelerator with 4×4 cm lateral fields angled 3° posteriorly, with the central axis placed at the center of the treatment field. (Reproduced from ALBERTI and SAGERMAN 1993, chap 21, Fig. 21.3)

disease becomes apparent in the opposite, previously untreated, eye. Use of electron therapy has been suggested in theory (MARKOE et al. 1987). However, in practice a single lateral electron beam is unsatisfactory in terms of homogeneity of orbital dose. Using a single 20-MeV electron port results in a dose gradient of approximately 100% to 60% across the involved orbit, which is unacceptable. Furthermore, the lens dose is approximately 10%. Thus, it is advisable to treat the bilateral orbits with photons initially, to avoid subsequent problems.

Radiation doses used have generally been 20 Gy in 2 weeks, using 2-Gy fractions calculated to the midplane at the level of the central axis. Radiation doses of 30 Gy/3 weeks have not produced results superior to those seen with 20 Gy (PETERSEN et al. 1990).

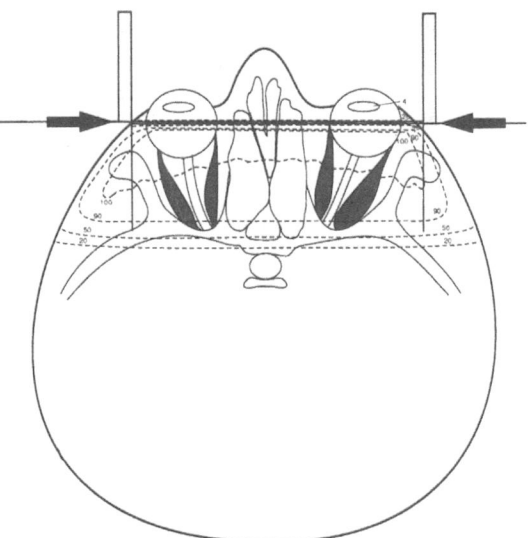

Fig. 15.4. Isodose curves using 6-MV photons from a linear accelerator with 4×8 cm opposed lateral fields with the central axis at the fleshy canthus, and the anterior border of the actual field, with the anterior half of the field blocked with lead, the beam-splitting technique. (Reproduced from ALBERTI and SAGERMAN 1993, chap 21, Fig. 21.4)

15.7
Results

Current results using orbital irradiation in the treatment of Graves' ophthalmopathy reveal that approximately two-thirds to three-fourths of irradiated patients have a good or excellent response to radiotherapy (BARTALENA et al. 1983; DONALDSON et al. 1973; KRISS et al. 1983, 1987; OLIVOTTO et al. 1985). However, as patient selection differs in different studies and prognostic factors vary, it is most useful to evaluate response as a function of each individual orbital sign and to predict response as a function of the degree of severity of the affliction prior to radiotherapy. Three hundred eleven patients undergoing orbital radiation from Stanford University Medical Center from 1968 to 1988 have recently been analyzed in consecutive series I, II, and III (PETERSEN et al. 1990). All patients were evaluated before and after therapy utilizing the ophthalmopathy index score shown in Table 15.1, and all patients had a minimum follow-up of 1 year. For the purposes of evaluating the effects of irradiation, the evaluation period was terminated at the time of any subsequent eye surgery. The demographic information regarding these 311 patients is shown in Table 15.3. All patients received photon radiation from a linear accelerator in 2-Gy daily fractions, although the total dose varied within the three consecutive series as shown.

The results of therapy in these 311 patients are shown in Table 15.4. The percentage of patients responding is shown for each of the specific signs, including soft tissue involvement, proptosis, eye muscle involvement, corneal involvement, and sight loss, as a function of the number of patients with involvement and the number of patients followed. Greater than 90% of patients presented with soft tissue involvement or eye muscle dysfunction. Nearly 75% had some degree of proptosis, and over 50% had some degree of sight loss prior to therapy. Scores for sight loss following treatment reflect non-thyroid-related conditions resulting in sight loss, such as pre-existing cataract, macular degeneration, and corneal injury. The best responses were seen in the categories of soft tissue involvement, corneal involvement, and sight loss; however, more than half the patients with proptosis and eye muscle dysfunction improved following treatment. An analysis of the prognostic factors related to each of the SPECS signs reveals that specific variables significantly influence outcome. They include age for soft tissue findings and sight loss, concurrent hyperthyroidism treatment for sight loss, an absent history of hyperthyroidism for extraocular muscle involvement, and gender for extraocular muscle involvement and proptosis (PETERSEN et al. 1990). Substantial improvements, even complete resolution of signs and symptoms, were often obtained following radiotherapy. Worsening after treatment was very rare.

Table 15.5 demonstrates that following radiotherapy approximately 30% of the patients required some form of eye surgery, usually to correct eye muscle or lid dysfunction. Subsequent surgery resulted in an excellent or a good response in greater than 80% of the patients. These surgical procedures are best undertaken when the inflammatory signs of ophthalmopathy have abated, which is usually a minimum of 6 months after treatment. Orbital decompression may be beneficial in severely affected individuals with threatening sight loss and in those with stable ophthalmopathy associated with proptosis. However, the early initiation of orbital radiotherapy has served to avoid decompression in the majority of patients.

Approximately 30% of patients were dependent upon corticosteroids at the time of radiotherapy, and approximately 75% of these were able to stop the medication. Patients rarely relapse after achieving an initial response to orbital irradiation. Most frequently their symptoms can be managed with low doses of corticosteroids gradually tapered off, such that additional radiotherapy or subsequent surgery is not necessary.

Table 15.3. Demographic information – 311 patients with Graves' ophthalmopathy

	Series		
	I	II	III
Number			
Total no.	156	69	86
Lost (n)	8	13	15
Followed (n)	148	56	71
Radiation dose (Gy)	20	30	20
Sex (% female)	66	69	72
Median age at onset (years)	52	51	55
Age <40 years (%)	12	19	8
Median pretreatment interval (months)	11	14	9
Median follow-up (months)	34	29	16
Prior thyroid status (%)			
Hyperthyroid	76	80	81
Hypothyroid	10	9	4
Hashimoto's thyroiditis	9	6	7
Prior X-ray therapy	2	0	0
Concurrent active hyperthyroidism (%)	9	23	26
Prior thyroid therapy			
Worse after ^{131}I treatment	33	19	37
Worse after thyroidectomy	4	6	0
Previous orbital decompression	5	0	2

15.8
Complications

No long-term complications have been reported among greater than 400 patients treated as described and followed up, some for 15–20 years. A small proportion of patients will experience mild exacerbation of the inflammatory symptoms of ophthalmopathy during the course of radiotherapy. Usually this is self-limiting, but occasionally corticosteroids are required for symptomatic relief. With irradiation as recommended there have been no radiation-induced

Table 15.4. Results of orbital irradiation in 311 patients[a]

Sign	Severity score	Worse			No response			Improved			Complete resolution		
		Series			Series			Series			Series		
		I	II	III	I	II	III	I	II	III	I	II	III
Soft tissue involvement	3				6		25	38	50	50	65	58	25
	2				2	13	18	32	56	45	67	32	45
	1	2	8	3	28	38	11				71	54	56
Proptosis	3				33	50	20	58	50	80	8		
	2	5	9	17	59	35	50	25	39	33	11	17	
	1	9	7	7	40	27	39				51	67	54
Eye muscle involvement	3				39	42	63	41	58	38	19		
	2	2		7	37	38	27	31	38	23	29	23	43
	1				37	57	29				63	43	71
Corneal involvement	3						100						
	2											100	100
	1	4			22	27	38				74	73	63
Sight loss	3					50	20	50	50	60	50		20
	2	4			16	25	33	36	38	44	44	38	22
	1	2	7	18	36	43	59				62	50	23

[a]Response is expressed as a percentage of those involved and followed for each sign

Table 15.5. Postirradiation therapy

	Series		
	I	II	III
Steroid therapy			
Taking prednisone during radiotherapy (%)	29	26	40
Weaned off prednisone (%)	80	76	68
Posttreatment eye surgery (%)	31	25	30

cataracts, although some patients have pre-existing senile cataracts prior to initiation of radiotherapy. In this experience no patient has developed any radiation-related retinopathy, nerve damage, or in-field radiation-induced malignancy.

Radiation retinopathy with subsequent blindness has been reported from one institution following an intended radiation dose of 20 Gy (KINYOUN and ORCUTT 1987). However, recalculation of treatment records revealed that a dosimetric error had been made and actually greater than 35 Gy/2 weeks in 3.5-Gy fractions had been given rather than the recommended 20 Gy/2 weeks (PARKER and WITHERS 1988). Large fraction sizes have been shown to be associated with irreversible visual complications.

If radiation therapy is to be administered in the course of treatment for this benign orbital condition, it is important that it be administered by a physician who has expertise in the technique and is familiar with the indications, and that it be given in a center where appropriate equipment is available.

References

Alberti WE, Sagerman RH (eds) (1993) Radiotherapy of intraocular and orbital tumors, 1st edn, chap 21. (Medical radiology – diagnostic imaging and radiation oncology) Springer, Berlin Heidelberg New York, pp 187–189

Bahn RS, Dutton CM, Naff N et al (1998) Thyrotropin receptor expression in Graves' orbital adipose/connective tissues: potential autoantigen in Graves' ophthalmopathy. J Clin Endocrinol Metab 83:998–1002

Bartalena L, Marcocci C, Chiovato L et al (1983) Orbital cobalt irradiation combined with systemic corticosteroids for Graves' ophthalmopathy: comparison with systemic corticosteroids alone. J Clin Endocrinol Metab 56:1139–1144

Bartalena L, Pinchera A, Martino E et al (1998) Relation between therapy for hyperthyroidism and the course of Graves' ophthalmopathy. N Engl J Med 338:73–78

Donaldson SS, Bagshaw MA, Kriss JP (1973) Supervoltage orbital radiotherapy for Graves' ophthalmopathy. J Clin Endocrinol Metab 37:276–285

Gorman CA (1995) Radioiodine therapy does not aggravate Graves' ophthalmopathy. J Clin Endocrinol Metab 80:340–342

Jacobson DH, Gorman CA (1985) Diagnosis and management of endocrine ophthalmopathy. Med Clin North Am 69:973–988

Jones A (1951) Orbital x-ray therapy of progressive exophthalmos. Br J Radiol 24:637–646

Kinyoun JL, Orcutt JC (1987) Radiation retinopathy. JAMA 258:610–611

Kriss JP, McDougall IR, Donaldson SS (1983) Graves' ophthalmopathy. In: Krieger DT, Bardin WC (eds) Current therapy in endocrinology 1983–1984. Becker/Mosby, Toronto, pp 104–109

Kriss JP, McDougall IR, Donaldson SS, Kraemer HC (1987) Non-thyroidal complications of Graves' disease: perspective on pathogenesis and treatment. In: Pinchera A, Ingbar S, Mckenzie J, Fenzi G (eds) Thyroid autoimmunity. Plenum, Pisa, pp 263–269

Markoe AM, Brady LW, Grant GD, Shields JA, Augsburger JJ (1987) Radiation therapy of ocular disease. In: Perez CA, Brady LW (eds) Principles and practice of radiation oncology. Lippincott, Philadelphia, pp 453–472

Marquez SD, Lum BL, McDougall R, Katkuri S, Levin PS, MacManus M, Donaldson SS (2001) Long-term results of irradiation for patients with progressive Graves' ophthalmology. Int J Radiat Oncol Biol Phys 53:766–774

Olivotto IA, Ludgate CM, Allen LH, Rootman J (1985) Supervoltage radiotherapy for Graves' ophthalmopathy: CCABC technique and results. Int J Radiat Oncol Biol Phys 11:2085–2090

Parker RG, Withers HR (1988) Radiation retinopathy. JAMA 259:43

Petersen IA, Donaldson SS, McDougall IR, Kriss JP (1990) Prognostic factors in the radiotherapy of Graves' ophthalmopathy. Int J Radiat Oncol Biol Phys 19:259–264

Prummel MF, Wiersinga WM (1993) Smoking and risk of Graves' disease. JAMA 269:518–519

Prummel MF, Mourits MP, Blank L et al (1993) Randomized double-blind trial of prednisone versus radiotherapy in Graves' ophthalmopathy. Lancet 342:949–954

Werner SC (1977) Modification of the classification of the eye changes of Graves' disease: recommendations of the Ad Hoc Committee of The American Thyroid Association. J Clin Endocrinol Metab 44:203–204

16 Management of Orbital Lymphoma

J.A. BOGART, R.H. SAGERMAN, C.T. CHUNG

Contents

16.1
Epidemiology

Non-Hodgkin's lymphoma (NHL) is the sixth most common cancer in the United States in both incidence and mortality. NHL may involve the conjunctiva (bulbar or palpebral), lacrimal gland, or posterior orbit either primarily or as a manifestation of systemic disease. Primary orbital lymphomas account for approximately 1% (FITZPATRICK and MACKO 1984) of all NHL, with an annual incidence of 1 case per million. Although uncommon, NHL is the most common malignancy of the orbit and accounted for 55% of malignant orbital tumors in a report from the Florida Cancer Registry (MARGO and MULLA 1998). The median age of patients at diagnosis is approaching 65 years, and the diagnosis is rare in children and adolescents (KENNERDELL et al. 1999). The incidence is equal in men and women. Orbital NHL appears to be becoming more

common, with a 155% rise in incidence noted between 1987 and 1993 in the Florida Registry (MARGO and MULLA 1998).

Hodgkin's disease (HD) of the orbit is an extremely rare entity. Involvement of the lacrimal gland(s) has been reported in association with widely disseminated HD (PATEL and ROOTMAN 1983; KRAMER et al. 1983) and may be detected by clinical evaluation or radiographic examination. However, orbital involvement in early-stage HD has not been reported in the literature, and a diagnosis of primary orbital HD should be viewed with suspicion and alternative diseases considered.

16.2
Presentation

Orbital NHL is not usually suspected at a patient's initial presentation, and the average duration of symptoms prior to diagnosis is approximately 4–6 months (KNOWLES et al. 1990). Presenting signs and symptoms are dependent on the location and extent of the lesion. In one study of 95 patients, the most common presentation was a painless mass; visual impairment was seen in 13%, conjunctival redness in 25%, pain in 12%, and acute orbital inflammation in 15% of the patients (POLITO et al. 1996). Posterior orbital lesions may produce headaches or orbital pain (KNOWLES and JAKOBIEC 1980). Proptosis is often present with posterior orbital tumors, and decreased ocular motility is seen with more advanced lesions.

Conjunctival lesions are usually salmon-colored, fleshy masses. Chemosis and secondary blurred vision may occur. Ptosis may be secondary to inflammatory change or direct tumor invasion. Patients with benign and malignant ocular adnexal lymphoid proliferations do not differ significantly with respect to age, sex, presenting complaints, duration of symptoms, or ophthalmic findings, although pain has

J.A. BOGART, MD
Department of Radiation Oncology, SUNY Upstate Medical University, 750 E. Adams Street, Syracuse, NY 13210, USA
R.H. SAGERMAN, MD, FACR
Department of Radiation Oncology, SUNY Upstate Medical University, 750 E. Adams Street, Syracuse, NY 13210, USA
C.T. CHUNG, MD, FACR
Department of Radiation Oncology, SUNY Upstate Medical University, 750 E. Adams Street, Syracuse, NY 13210, USA

been reported more frequently in association with benign lesions in some series (KNOWLES et al. 1990).

16.3
Pathology

The pathologic classification for NHL continues to evolve. Several systems have been proposed, including the classifications of RAPPAPORT (1966) and LUKES and COLLINS (1974), and that from the Kiel group (LENNERT et al. 1975). In 1982 the Working Formulation was developed; this classifies lymphomas into three prognostic groups (low, intermediate, and high grade) based on patient survival analyses (ANONYMOUS 1982). However, the grouping of several distinct diseases in the same category has been recognized as a major limitation of the Working Formulation. The Revised European-American Lymphoma (R.E.A.L.) classification was established in 1994 by hematopathologists from the United States, Europe, and Asia (HARRIS et al. 1994). This classification incorporates morphology, phenotype, cytogenetics and clinical features to define disease entities (KOEPPEN and VARDIMAN 1998). It has better interobserver reproducibility (85%) than other classifications, as demonstrated in the International Lymphoma Study (HARRIS et al. 1994). Major categories in the R.E.A.L. classification are: B-cell neoplasms, T/NK neoplasms, and HD. New clinical entities are described, including follicle center lymphoma, mantle cell lymphoma (MCL), and marginal zone B-cell lymphoma (MZBCL). Mucosa-associated lymphoid tissue (MALT) lymphoma, a subtype of MZBLC, correlates with small lymphocytic lymphoma in the Working Formulation and is commonly encountered in ocular adnexal lesions. A comparison of the R.E.A.L. classification and the Working Formulation is shown in Table 16.1.

The histologic distribution of NHL varies among series. In a prospective analysis of 117 ocular adnexal lymphoid proliferations, 27% were polyclonal lymphoid hyperplasia; 69% monoclonal B-cell lymphoma; 1% null cell lymphoma; and 3% histologically indeterminate (KNOWLES et al. 1990). Reports generally demonstrate low-grade lymphoma in 60–90% of cases (SAUERWEIN et al. 1997), and all 15 cases of stage I-E orbital lymphoma were diagnosed as low-grade MALT lymphoma in one series (GALIENI et al. 1997). Conversely, a comparison of MALT lymphoma with other subtypes from the Royal Victoria Eye and Ear Hospital and from the Moorfields Eye Hospital and St. Bartholomew's Hospital showed that a significantly higher proportion of patients with MALT lymphoma had early-stage disease (CAHILL et al. 1999; JENKINS et al. 2000).

A frequent difficulty encountered in the pathologic evaluation of ocular adnexal lymphoid proliferations, despite the utilization of histopathologic and immunophenotypic criteria, is the classification of lesions as either benign or malignant (KNOWLES and JAKOBIEC 1980). Some series have reported the development of malignant lymphoma in greater than one-third of patients initially diagnosed with lymphoid hyperplasia with long-term follow-up (KELETI et al. 1992; POLITO et al. 1996). Genotypic abnormalities may be found in lymphoid hyperplasia from patients who ultimately develop systemic lymphoma (SMITT and DONALDSON 1999). Increasing utilization of molecular biologic analysis, including the polymerase chain reaction (PCR), should improve the detection of malignant orbital lymphomas, but at present patients with lesions classified as lymphoid hyperplasia should be evaluated and followed for the possibility of developing malignant lymphoma.

16.4
Clinical Evaluation and Staging

A careful history should include evaluation for possible systemic symptoms (fever, malaise, drenching night sweats, weight loss) as well as local disease infiltration (sinus and nasal congestion, headache). A careful, complete physical examination should be performed, with particular attention given to both orbits, the remainder of the head and neck, peripheral lymph node stations, and abdominal organs. Laboratory examination should include a complete blood count, serum electrolytes, liver function tests, and serum LDH.

Imaging studies are essential in the evaluation of orbital lesions. Computed tomography (CT) and magnetic resonance imaging (MRI) findings have been utilized in an attempt to differentiate benign and malignant lesions, with mixed results. Lymphomatous lesions are more likely than reactive lesions to appear homogenous on CT, and bone destruction, while unusual with malignant lymphoma, does not occur with benign lesions (WESTACOTT et al. 1991). MRI signal characteristics are of limited value in the diagnosis of lymphoma. GUFLER et al.

Table 16.1. Comparison of the Working Formulation and the Revised European-American Lymphoma (*R.E.A.L.*) classification (Revised European American Classification)

Working Formulation	R.E.A.L. classification	
	B-Cell neoplasms	T-Cell neoplasms
Low grade		
Small lymphocytic consistent with CLL	B-cell CLL/PLL/SLL Marginal zone/MALT Mantle cell	T-cell CLL/PLL LGL ATL/L (chronic and smoldering types)
Plasmacytoid	Lymphoplasmacytic-immunocytoma Marginal zone/MALT B-cell CLL/PLL/SLL	
Follicular, predominantly small cleaved cell	Follicle center, follicular, grade I Mantle cell Marginal zone/MALT	
Follicular, mixed small cleaved and large cell	Follicle center, follicular, grade II Marginal zone/MALT	
Intermediate grade		
Follicular, large cell	Follicle center, follicular, grade III	
Diffuse, small cleaved cell	Mantle cell Follicle center, diffuse small cell Marginal zone/MALT	T-cell CLL/PLL LGL ATL/L Angioimmunoblastic Angiocentric
Diffuse, mixed small and large cell	Large B-cell lymphoma (rich in T-cells) Follicle center, diffuse small cell Lymphoplasmacytoid Marginal zone/MALT Mantle cell	Peripheral T-cell, unspecified ATL/L Angioimmunoblastic Angiocentric Intestinal T-cell lymphoma
Diffuse, large cell	Diffuse large B-cell lymphoma	Peripheral T-cell, unspecified ATL/L Angioimmunoblastic Angiocentric Intestinal T-cell lymphoma
High grade		
Large-cell immunoblastic<?4>	Diffuse large B-cell lymphoma	Peripheral T-cell, unspecified ATL/L Angioimmunoblastic Angiocentric Intestinal T-cell Anaplastic large cell
Lymphoblastic	Precursor B-lymphoblastic	Precursor T-lymphoblastic
Small noncleaved cell Burkitt's Non-Burkitt's	Burkitt's High-grade B-cell, Burkitt-like Diffuse large B-cell	Peripheral T-cell, unspecified

(1997) reported that 12 of 16 orbital lymphomas were hypointense (4 intermediate) on T1-weighted images and 12 of the 16 were hyperintense (3 intermediate, 1 hypointense) on T2-weighted images, but only 35% of lymphoid lesions were hyperintense on T2-weighted images in a study of 95 patients reported by Polito et al. (1996). At this time, imaging studies cannot replace the need for biopsy. We utilize imaging studies to help define the extent of the orbital lesion and to assist in radiotherapy treatment planning. Both thin-slice CT and MRI provide valuable information. The tests are complementary, and while MRI may provide better tissue characterization, CT may provide information on possible bone erosion, and the location of the tumor relative to bony landmarks may more easily be assessed for radiotherapy treatment planning. Both orbits should always be imaged, as bilateral disease may be seen in 5–20% of patients (McNally et al. 1987; Vogiatzis 1984).

Staging evaluation, including CT of the chest, abdomen, and pelvis, and a bone marrow biopsy should be obtained in patients with documented NHL. Lumbar puncture is generally not necessary, and metastasis to the central nervous system from primary orbital lymphoma is unusual. The Ann Arbor staging system should be utilized for the classification of NHL. Lesions confined to the orbit in patients without systemic symptoms are staged as 1 AE. Systemic disease has been reported in as many as 51% of patients with orbital lymphoma at presentation, but in most series disease is reported to have been limited to the orbit in 60–85% of patients (Bessell et al. 1987; Esik et al. 1996; Restrepo et al. 1998).

16.5
Treatment

Treatment options are dictated by histologic classification and disease stage. Radiotherapy is the mainstay of treatment for low-grade lesions (Working Formulation) confined to the orbit (stage 1 AE), although limited experience has been reported with surgery or systemic chemotherapy for these patients. The overall survival for this group of patients may be similar to that in the normal population (Table 16.2) (Bessell et al. 1987). There is less agreement regarding the prognosis and treatment of stage 1 E intermediate or high-grade lymphoma. Survival for these patients is lower than in patients with low-grade lesions in some but not all series (Table 16.2). Chemotherapy may have a role in the management of these patients. A recent prospective cooperative group trial randomized patients with stage I and II intermediate-grade NHL (i.e., diffuse large cell lym-

Table 16.2. Results of radiotherapy for primary orbital lymphoma (*CF* cataract formation, *LC* local control, *LD* lacrimal dysfunction, *IHG* intermediate or high grade, *KS* keratitis, *LG* low grade, *NS* not specified, *ON* optic neuropathy, *RN* retinopathy, *SS* sicca ayndrome)

Series	N	Dose (median)	LC	Complications/comments
Esik et al. (1996)	37	30 Gy	100%	11 CF; lens block not placed in all cases with CF; 1 enucleation (glaucoma)
Bessell et al. (1987)	115 (18 IHG)	30 Gy (LG) 40 Gy (IHG)	NS	8 CF 5 mild LD
Erkal et al. (1997)	14	40 Gy	87%	9 CF, 4 mild LD Single anterior Co-60 field
Reddy et al. (1988)	17	35 Gy	100%	3 patients developed systemic disease
Fitzpatrick and Macko (1984)	19	25–45 Gy	100%	No serious complications 37% developed systemic disease
Bolek et al. (1999)	20 6 (IHG)	25 Gy	95%	CF 7/21 without lens shielding; 0/17 with lens shielding Reduced disease free survival for high grade lesions
Letschert et al. (1991)	33	21–57 Gy	94%	2 ON, 3 RN, 18 KS, 10 SS Treatment delivered with closed eyelid and bolus; 20% developed systemic disease
Chao et al. (1995)	20	30 Gy	100%	7 CF, 3 mild LD
Austin-Seymour et al. (1985)	8	3165	NS	No significant complications Oblique wedge-pair technique
Kennerdell et al. (1999)	21	24 Gy	95%	32% transient chemosis No significant late complications
Vogiatzis (1984)	18	NS	NS	All patients with bilateral tumors developed systemic disease
Jereb et al. (1984)	18	24–37.5 Gy	100%	No cataract formation; low-vac lens shield used
Galieni et al. (1997)	15	30 Gy	93%	8/15 patients treated with primary surgery/chemotherapy
Barthold et al. (1986)	9	35.47 Gy	85%	2 patients with benign disease developed systemic lymphoma

phoma) to either eight cycles of cyclophosphamide, doxorubicin, vincristine, and prednisone (CHOP) or three cycles of CHOP combined with involved field radiotherapy (MILLER et al. 1998). A survival benefit was observed for patients receiving limited chemotherapy and radiotherapy, although it is not clear that these results can be extrapolated to the treatment of orbital lesions. Patients unable to receive chemotherapy may be treated with radiotherapy alone. Systemic "B" symptoms are unusual in patients presenting with localized orbital lymphoma and must prompt a careful search for the possibility of systemic disease. The International Prognostic Index, which accounts for age, disease stage, serum LDH and performance status, should be utilized to assess prognosis for patients with more advanced disease and intermediate- and high-grade lymphomas (SHIPP 1994).

Results recorded in the literature with radiotherapy alone for orbital lymphoma are shown in Table 16.2. Local tumor control in the irradiated orbit is excellent in most series, with few true in-field failures. Doses of 24–57 Gy have been employed without evidence of a clear dose response. Many series indicate that a 30-Gy dose delivered over 3 weeks is adequate for control of low-grade lesions, with good control reported with a dose as low as 24–25 Gy (BOLEK et al. 1999; KENNERDELL et al. 1999). Our experience at Upstate Medical University includes 25 patients with low-grade lymphoma treated with local external beam photon or electron beam irradiation. The median tumor dose was 30 Gy given in 2-Gy fractions. Of these patients, 13 received photon irradiation (255 kV to 6 MV peak energy) and 12, electron beam therapy (6–20 MeV). Local tumor control was obtained in all patients, and marked tumor regression was generally noted by the completion of therapy (Fig. 16.1). Two of 25 patients developed recurrent low-grade lymphoma in the contralateral orbit 19 and 46 months after their initial unilateral radiotherapy. Both patients were salvaged with orbital radiotherapy, although one subsequently developed systemic lymphoma. Two patients with low-grade lymphoma developed brain involvement 2–15 months after radiotherapy, and both have died; 1 additional patient relapsed systemically.

16.5.1
Radiotherapy Technique

The technical aspects of treatment for lymphomas of the orbit are critical owing to the high probability

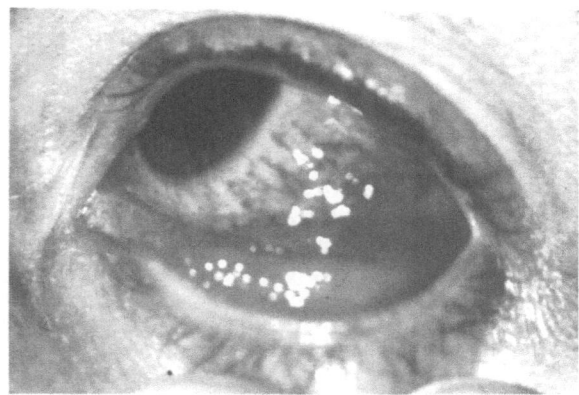

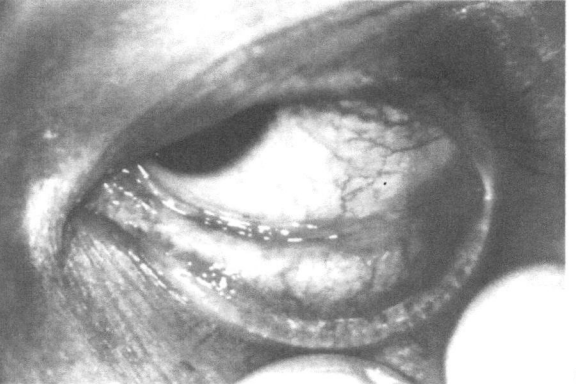

Fig 16.1. Well-differentiated lymphocytic conjunctival lymphoma **a** at diagnosis and **b** after completion of photon radiotherapy (30 Gy/3 weeks)

that tumor control will be countered by the severe consequences of a treatment-related complication. The impact of different treatment techniques and shielding methods on local tumor control is difficult to evaluate critically, given the paucity of in-field treatment failures with modest-dose radiotherapy. Several techniques employing electron or photon treatment appear equally efficacious. Thin-slice CT or MRI should be utilized routinely for radiotherapy treatment planning. We have generally irradiated the entire orbit and have most frequently used a 6 cm×6 cm field size with custom shielding. Placement of a "hanging" lens shield has not compromised tumor control when used with either treatment modality, although reports have shown a better dose distribution throughout the orbit with the use of an electron field than with a photon arrangement when an anterior lens shield is placed. We have generally treated with a direct anterior field, with the eyelids open and the patient looking directly forward at the lens shield (HARISIADIS et al. 1985; WILSON et al. 1992). The lens block hangs over the isocenter approximately 5 mm in front of the cornea (Fig. 16.2).

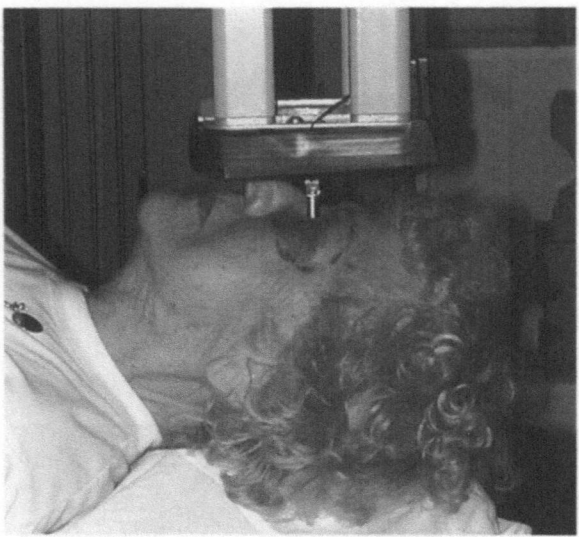

Fig. 16.2. Hanging lens block technique utilized with electron beam therapy

Other lens blocking techniques have been described, including a "low-vac lens" technique (Jereb et al. 1984) and use of an eye bar (Austin-Seymour et al. 1985). A tissue-equivalent bolus has occasionally been used in irradiation of superficial lesions with megavoltage quality photons, but care must be taken to preserve surface sparing of the uninvolved cornea. Electron beam therapy without bolus has been adequate to control superficial conjunctival lesions despite the concern about constriction of the isodose curves and a potentially reduced surface dose delivered by low-energy (i.e., 6–9 MeV) electrons with small fields. Deep lesions are treated with either an anterior and lateral wedged pair arrangement or with high-energy (16–20 MeV) electrons. Alternate photon field arrangements have been proposed to reduce target dose variation, including combined sagittal and transverse wedged pair beams, and an anterior wedged pair technique (Austin-Seymour et al. 1985). However, these techniques increase the complexity of the treatment without necessarily improving local tumor control.

16.5.2
Complications of Therapy

While tumor control has not correlated to radiation dose or treatment technique, serious sequelae may relate to these factors, given the abundance of radiosensitive structures in the region, including cornea, lens, lacrimal gland, retina, and optic nerve. The rate

of cataract formation varies from less than 10% (Bessell et al. 1987) to greater than 50% (Letschert et al. 1991). While the contribution of radiotherapy to cataract formation may be difficult to evaluate in this older population, the incidence of cataracts is reported to be reduced with lens shielding (Bolek et al. 1999; Esik et al. 1996). Mild conjunctival erythema is a commonly observed acute reaction during treatment, but late injury is uncommon. Although utilization of high-energy electrons in the treatment of deep (i.e., retroorbital) lesions may increase surface dose to the conjunctiva, the unblocked cornea, and the lacrimal apparatus (owing to loss of skin-sparing effect), we have not observed severe conjunctival reactions or dry eye in patients irradiated with electrons. The paucity of complications in our series may be secondary to the use of modest total doses with lens shielding. The solitary severe complication (corneal ulceration) in our series developed following 4 MV photon radiation to a total dose of 54 Gy, with a dose of 34 Gy delivered prior to placement of the lens (and cornea) shield (Fig. 16.3). Several field arrangements for photon beam irradiation have been utilized, including a direct anterior, anterior and lateral wedged pair and an oblique wedged pair. All have been employed without significant complications. However, use of complex set-ups, including multiple angled fields, may lessen daily reproducibility. An angled beam may the irradiate the conjunctiva and cornea tangentially and increase the complexity of lens shield placement. Meticulous care should be taken with any treatment plan, and physician visualization of the daily treatment is routine at our center.

Utilization of doses 40 Gy and higher appears to increase the risk of severe acute and late side effects (Table 16.2). Letschert et al. (1991) reported keratitis and reduced vision in more than half of 33 patients, and sicca syndrome in 30%, who had been irradiated with photons to a minimum dose of 40 Gy. Two optic nerve neuropathies and three retinopathies in five patients developed 12–60 months following doses of 4000–5700 cGy. Esik et al. (1996) reported 2 severe late complications (1 case of glaucoma requiring enucleation and 1 of severe dry eye) following irradiation of 22 patients to a median dose of 40 Gy, and Erkal et al. (1997) reported lacrimal disorders in 4 of 14 patients irradiated with single anterior field (cobalt-60) to 40 Gy in 2-Gy daily fractions.

Treatment techniques that eliminate the skin sparing effect of photons by placement of bolus or treating with a closed eyelid may also increase cor-

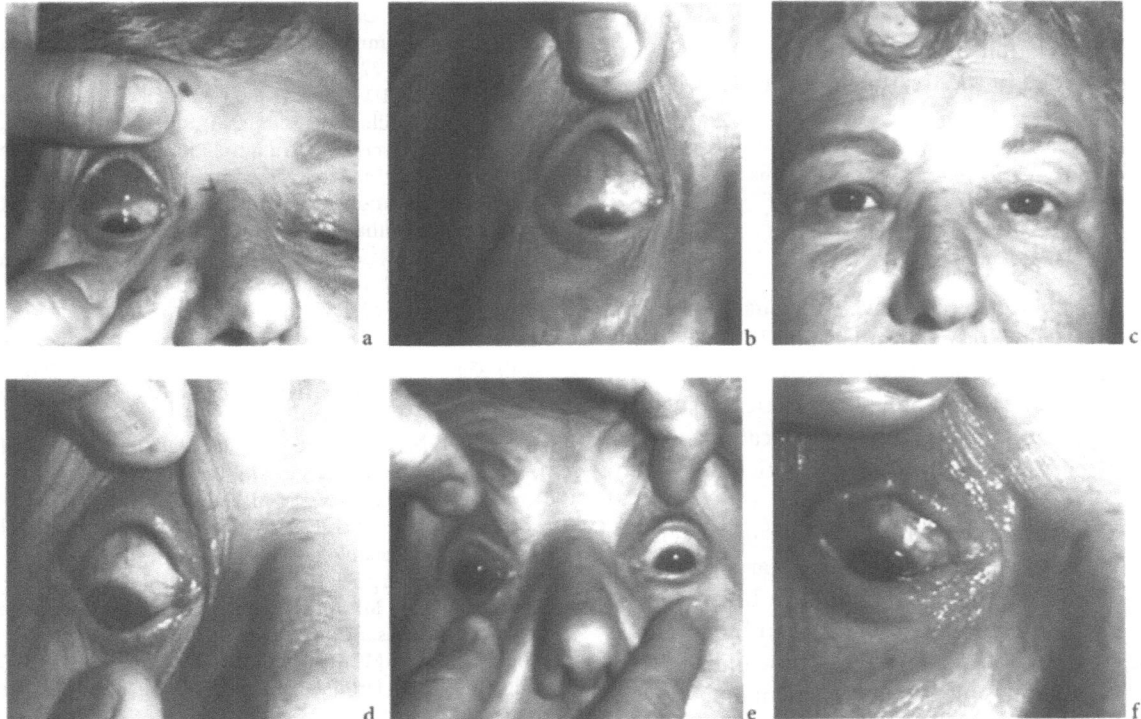

Fig. 16.3. a Lymphoma involving the superior bulbar conjunctiva at diagnosis. **b** Residual tumor following 3400 cGy (200 cGy/fx with 4 Mv photons using a direct anterior field). **c** Appearance after 5200 cGy total (additional 18 Gy/9 fx delivered after a 1-week treatment break). **d** Regression of tumor 3.5 months after completion of radiotherapy. **e** Corneal abrasion 10 months after radiotherapy. Abrasion occurred after trauma from a wind storm. **f** Appearance 1.5 years after radiotherapy. Vision reduced to light perception in right eye

neal reactions and complications for patients receiving modest radiotherapy doses. In the series described above (LETSCHERT et al. 1991), in which a high keratitis rate was reported, no lens shielding was employed and conjunctival lesions were irradiated using 5 MV photons with an additional 0.5-cm tissue-equivalent bolus placed over the closed eyelid.

16.6
Intraocular Lymphoma

Intraocular lymphoma is a distinct entity that is clinically more aggressive than orbital adnexal lymphoma. Although isolated intraocular lesions have been reported, there is a strong correlation with central nervous system (CNS) disease. Approximately 80% of patients with intraocular lymphoma will eventually develop CNS disease, and conversely, approximately 20% of patients with primary CNS lymphoma will have ocular involvement. The most common presentation is decreased vision and "floaters" associated with posterior uveitis (CHAR et al. 1988). Ul-

trasound findings may include vitreous debris, choroidal thickening, widening of the optic nerve, and retinal detachment (URSEA et al. 1997). Bilateral disease is present in approximately 90% of cases. Pathologic confirmation is obtained via vitreous biopsy for lesions initially confined to the globe, and the most common histology is large B-cell lymphoma (AKPEK et al. 1999; BARDENSTEIN 1998). The treatment for patients with CNS disease is generally combined systemic chemotherapy and cranial irradiation. Ocular radiotherapy alone has occasionally been utilized for lesions confined to the eye, but relapse may occur in the opposite eye or CNS (PETERSEN et al. 1993). Therefore, aggressive therapy including systemic and/or intrathecal chemotherapy is generally entertained in the treatment of these patients. Although occasional cases of long-term survival have been reported following ocular radiotherapy, the majority of patients will die from progressive CNS disease within 3 years of diagnosis (VON BELOW et al. 1989). Ocular radiotherapy doses have ranged from 20 to 60 Gy (CHAR et al. 1998; PETERSON et al. 1993; VON BELOW et al. 1989), and although symptomatic involvement is common there are too few cases of long-term control to evaluate for a dose–response relationship. Therapeutic advances are clearly needed in the treatment of this disease.

16.7
Conclusion

Orbital lymphoma is a relatively unusual tumor with an overall good prognosis. Lesions limited to the orbit are highly curable with localized orbital radiotherapy. Despite the abundance of critical structures in the orbit, the risk of severe complications may be minimized by the utilization of meticulous radiotherapy technique and by limiting the radiation dose. Overall survival in this group of patients is excellent, although patients remain at risk for the development of systemic lymphoma. In contrast to orbital adnexal lymphoma, intraocular lymphoma is an aggressive disease associated with a high frequency of CNS involvement. Survival remains poor despite combined modality therapy, and new strategies are needed to improve treatment results.

References

Akpek EK, Ahmed I, Hochberg FH, Soheilian M, Dryja TP, Jakobiec FA, Foster CS (1999) Intraocular-central nervous system lymphoma: clinical features, diagnosis, and outcomes. Ophthalmology 106:1805–1810

Anonymous (1982) National Cancer Institute sponsored study of classifications of non-Hodgkin's Lymphomas. Summary and description of a working formulation for clinical usage. Cancer 49:2112–2135

Austin-Seymour MM, Donaldson SS, Egbert PR, McDougall IR, Kriss JP (1985) Radiotherapy of lymphoid diseases of the orbit. Int J Radiat Oncol Biol Phys 11:371–379

Bardenstein DS (1998) Intraocular lymphoma. Cancer Control 5:317–325

Barthold HJ, Harvey A, Markoe AM, Brady LW, Augsburger JJ, Shields JA (1986) Treatment of orbital pseudotumors and lymphoma. Am J Clin Oncol 9:527–532

Bessell EM, Henk JM, Whitelocke RA, Wright JE (1987) Ocular morbidity after radiotherapy of orbital and conjunctival lymphoma. Eye 1:90–96

Bolek TW, Moyses HM, Marcus RB, Gorden L, Maiese RL, Almasri NM, Mendenhall NP (1999) Radiotherapy in the management of orbital lymphoma. Int J Radiat Biol Phys 44:31–36

Cahill M, Barnes C, Moriarty P, Daly P, Kennedy S (1999) Ocular adnexal lymphoma – comparison of MALT lymphoma with other histological types. Br J Ophthalmol 83:742–747

Chao CK, Lin HS, Devineni VR, Smith M (1995) Radiation therapy for primary orbital lymphoma. Int J Radiat Oncol Biol Phys 31:929–934

Char DH, Ljung BM, Deschenes J, Miller TR (1988) Intraocular lymphoma: immunological and cytological analysis. Br J Ophthalmol 72:905–911

Coupland SE, Foss HD, Assaf C, Auw-Haedrich C, Anastassiou G, Anagnostopoulos I, Hummel M, Karesh JW, Lee WR, Stein H (1999) T-cell and T/natural killer-cell lymphomas involving ocular and ocular adnexal tissues: a clinicopathologic immunohistochemical, and molecular study of seven cases. Ophthalmology 106:2109–2120

Erkal HS, Serin M, Sak SD, Cakmak A (1997) Radiation therapy for stage I primary orbital non-Hodgkin's lymphomas. Tumori 83:822–825

Esik O, Ikeda H, Mukai K, Kaneko A (1996) A retrospective analysis of different modalities for treatment of primary orbital non-Hodgkin's lymphomas. Radiother Oncol 38:13–18

Fitzpatrick PJ, Macko S (1984) Lymphoreticular tumors of the orbit. Int J Radiat Oncol Biol Phys 10:333–340

Galieni P, Polito E, Leccisotti A, Marotta G, Lasi S, Bigazzi C, Bucalossi A, Frezza G, Lauria F (1997) Localized orbital lymphoma. Haematologica 82:436–439

Gufler H, Laubenberger J, Gerling J, Nesbitt E, Kommerell G, Langer M (1997) MRI of lymphomas of the orbits and the paranasal sinuses. J Comput Assist Tomogr 21:887–891

Harisiadis L, Schell MC, Working KR, Justice T, Wessels BW, Ling CC (1985) Orbital irradiation using non-coplanar beams. Radiology 156:823–824

Harris NL, Jaffe ES, Stein H, Banks PM, Chan JK, Cleary ML, Delsol G, DeWolf-Peeters C, Falini B, Gatter KC (1994) A revised European-American classification of lymphoid neoplasms: a proposal from the International Lymphoma Study Group. Blood 84:1361–1392

Jenkins C, Rose GE, Bunce C, Wright JE, Cree IA, Plowman N, Lightman S, Moseley I, Norton A (2000) Histological features of ocular adnexal lymphoma (REAL classification) and their association with patient morbidity and survival. Br J Ophthalmol 84:907–913

Jenkins C, Rose GE, Bunce C, Wright JE, Cree IA, Plowman N, Lightman S, Moseley I, Norton A (2000) Histological features of ocular adnexal lymphoma (REAL classification) and their association with patient morbidity and survival. Br J Ophthalmol 84:907–913

Jereb B, Lee H, Jakobiec FA, Kutcher (1984) Radiation therapy of conjunctival and orbital lymphoid tumors. Int J Radiat Oncol Biol Phys 10:1013–1019

Keleti D, Flickinger JC, Hobson SR, Mittal BB (1992) Radiotherapy of lymphoproliferative diseases of the orbit. Surveillance of 65 cases. Am J Clin Oncol 15:422–427

Kennerdell JS, Flores NE, Hartsock RJ (1999) Low dose radiotherapy for lymphoid lesions of the orbit and ocular adnexa. Ophthal Plast Reconstr Surg 15:129–133

Knowles DM, Jakobiec FA (1980) Orbital lymphoid neoplasms: a clinicopathologic study of 60 patients. Cancer 46:576–589

Knowles DM, Jakobiec FA, McNally L, Burke JS (1990) Lymphoid hyperplasia and malignant lymphoma occurring in the ocular adnexa (orbit, conjunctiva, and eyelids): a prospective multiparametric analysis of 108 cases during 1977 to 1987. Hum Pathol 21:959–973

Koeppen H, Vardiman JW (1998) New entities, issues, and controversies in the classification of malignant lymphoma. Semin Oncol 25:421–434

Kramer EL, Sanger JJ, Benjamin DD, Tiu S (1983) Detection of lacrimal gland infiltration on routine bone scintigraphy. Clin Nucl Med 8:546–549

Lennert K, Mohri N, Stein H et al (1975) The histopathology of malignant lymphoma. Br J Haematol 31:193–203

Letschert JGJ, Gonzalez DG, Oskam J, Koornneef L, van Dijk JDP, Boukes R, Bras J, van Heerde P, Bartelink H (1991) Results of radiotherapy in patients with Stage I orbital non-Hodgkin's lymphoma. Radiother Oncol 22:36–44

Lukes RJ, Collins RD (1974) Immunologic characterization of human malignant lymphomas. Cancer 34:1488–1503

Margo CE, Mulla ZD (1998) Malignant tumors of the orbit. Analysis of the Florida Cancer Registry. Ophthalmology 105:185–190

McNally L, Jakobiec FA, Knowles DM (1987) Clinical, morphologic, immunophenotypic, and molecular genetic analysis of bilateral ocular adnexal lymphoid neoplasms in 17 patients. Am J Ophthalmol 103:555–568

Miller TP, Dahlberg S, Cassady JR, Adelstein DJ, Spier CM, Grogan TM, LeBlanc M, Carlin S, Chase E, Fisher RI (1998) Chemotherapy alone compared with chemotherapy plus radiotherapy for localized intermediate and high-grade non-Hodgkin's lymphoma. N Engl J Med 339:21–26

Nicolo M, Truini M, Sertoli M, Taubenberger JK, Zingirian M (1999) Follicular large-cell lymphoma of the orbit: a clinicopathologic, immunohistochemical and molecular genetic description of one case. Ophthalmology 237:606–610

Patel S, Rootman J (1983) Nodular sclerosing Hodgkin's disease of the orbit. Ophthalmology 90:1433–1436

Peterson K, Gordon KB, Heinemann MH, DeAngelis LM (1993) The clinical spectrum of ocular lymphoma. Cancer 72:843–849

Polito E, Galieni P, Leccisotti A (1996) Clinical and radiological presentation of 95 orbital lymphoid tumors. Graefes Arch Clin Exp Ophthalmol 234:504–509

Rappaport H (1966) Tumors of the hematopoietic system. Atlas of tumor pathology, section III. Armed Forces Institute of Pathology, Washington DC

Reddy EK, Bhatia P, Evans RG (1988) Primary orbital lymphomas. Int J Radiat Oncol Biol Phys 15:1239–1241

Restrepo A, Raez LE, Byrne GE, Johnson T, Ossi P, Benedetto P, Hamilton K, Whitcomb CC, Cassileth PA (1998) Is central nervous system prophylaxis necessary in ocular adnexal lymphoma. Crit Rev Oncog 9:269–273

Sauerwein W, Hoederath A, Sack H (1997) Radiotherapy of primary orbital lymphomas. Universitats-Strahlenklinik Essen, Deutschland. Front Radiat Ther Oncol 30:192–194

Shipp MA (1994) Prognostic factors in aggressive non-Hodgkin's lymphoma: who has "high-risk" disease? Blood 83:1165–1173

Smitt MC, Donaldson SS (1999) Radiation therapy for benign disease of the orbit. Semin Radiat Oncol 9:179–189

Ursea R, Heinemann MH, Silverman RH, DeAngelis LM, Daly SW, Coleman DJ (1997) Ophthalmic, ultrasonographic findings in primary central nervous system lymphoma with ocular involvement. Retina 17:118–123

Vogiatzis KV (1984) Lymphoid tumors of the orbit and ocular adnexa: a long-term follow-up. Ann Ophthalmol 16:1046–1055

Von Below H, Ruprecht KW, Volcker HE, Naumann GOH (1989) Oculocerebral non-Hodgkin lymphoma (sub-RPE): report on 16 patients. Proceedings of the International Symposium on Tumors of the Eye, Essen, Germany

Westacott S, Garner A, Moseley IF, Wright JE (1991) Orbital lymphoma vs. reactive lymphoid hyperplasia: an analysis of the use of computed tomography in differential diagnosis. Br J Ophthalmol 75:722–725

Wilson CM, Schreiber DP, Russell JD, Hitchcock P (1992) Electron beam versus photon beam radiation therapy for the treatment of orbital lymphoid tumors. Med Dosim 17:161–165

17 Tumors of the Eyelids and Their Treatment by Radiotherapy

P. J. FITZPATRICK

The eye altering alters all.
William Blake

CONTENTS

17.1
Introduction

To most of us sight is the most precious of the senses. Tumors of the eye and orbit can be life threatening, cause blindness and be disfiguring. In planning management, the threat to life is the primary issue to be faced with the best treatment aimed at cure or long-term control having priority. Fortunately we have two eyes and the loss of vision in one does not prevent a person from living a normal life. Disfigurement caused by tumors around the eye is more serious than in any other part of the body, and this, together with preservation, forms the secondary priority. Radiotherapy can produce a high cure rate with good cosmesis and preservation of vision but is in danger of becoming a lost medical art (FITZPATRICK 1995, SCHLIENGER et al. 1996).

Tumors of the eyelids are the commonest of all cancers encountered in ophthalmology. They frequently arise from actinically damaged skin or from preexisting lesions. Basal and squamous cell carcinomas are the most common, melanoma is the most

P. J. FITZPATRICK, MB, BS, FRCPC, FRCR
Retired Professor of Radiation Oncology, Princess Margaret Hospital and University of Toronto, ON, Canada; Dalhousie University, Physican-in-Chief NSCC, Halifax, NS, Canada

serious, and keratoacanthoma or its acute epithelial variant, the most puzzling. In addition, adenocarcinomas arise from the appendageal structures in the skin. Eyelid tumors rarely metastasize and have little effect on survival. Their importance lies in their special site, with the ability to penetrate all layers of the eyelid. These destructive lesions, involving the lid margin or lacrimal system, can produce severe functional disability and, in addition, can be very disfiguring. Because of the specialized function of the eyelids and the proximity to the eye, treatment presents many technical problems. Radiotherapy is an effective and cost-effective method of treatment but it is not the only treatment. Fortunately, there are alternatives in surgery, chemosurgery, cryotherapy, and electrodessication. Some cases are better treated by these methods. Others benefit from combined treatments, with the final results superior to those which can be obtained by any one method alone. The selection of optimal treatment is best made by a multidisciplinary oncologic team with decisions based on the probability of cure, cosmesis, function, and the relative comfort, time, and cost of treatment. The patient's wishes must also be considered. The parameters concerned in determining optimal treatment include the patient's general condition, age, complexion, occupation, the location of residence and whether the skin shows signs of damage or other lesions are present. Tumor factors to be considered include the site, size, degree of invasion, multifocal neoplasms, and previous treatment.

Some controversy exists as to whether surgery or radiotherapy is the best treatment for eyelid lesions. In general, radiotherapy is contraindicated when post-treatment complications may be significant. The eye is a radiosensitive organ but can usually be protected from radiation and so most contraindications relate to the possibility of the radiation scar becoming unstable or worsening with time. Accordingly, tumors developing in young people or those with severely actinically damaged skin, and those in fairskinned people who have an excessive exposure to sunlight, may be better treated by surgery. Surgery is also preferred for most tumors that recur following irradiation. Every patient's treatment should be individualized and if the aforementioned parameters are considered by a multidisciplinary team, a consensus can be reached as to optimal care.

The skin essentially consists of three main layers. The epidermis is a stratified squamous epithelium that covers a connective tissue dermis and an underlying fatty layer. Its thickness on the eyelids is about 0.06 mm and at this special site, its anatomic-functional and biologic characteristics give it the status of an organ. Tumors develop from the epidermis or from the glands situated along the lid margins. The eyelids are defined as the area within the orbital margin.

17.2
Radiotherapy

Most eyelid tumors are relatively superficial and readily treated with superficial and orthovoltage x-rays or the electron beam (LEDERMAN 1976, FITZPATRICK et al. 1984, AMDUR et al. 1992, DALY et al. 1984). The radiation time-dose relationships necessary to destroy tumors without producing necrosis of normal tissues is well established. A single dose of 21.5 Gy has a 99% probability of curing basal cell carcinoma or squamous cell carcinoma and a 3% chance of late skin damage (GOLDSCHMIDT 1975; JOHNS and CONNINGHAM 1969; STRANDQVIST 1944). The choice of dose, time, number of fractions, and technique varies with the clinical problem. Common schedules that have proven to be effective are shown in Table 17.1. In practice, about 20% of patients are treated with a single exposure of 20 Gy, one half with 35 Gy in five fractions, and the other 30% with higher doses because of the tumor size and the complexity of the case (Table 17.2). In general, the dose is increased and the treatment time is extended for large tumors. Basal and squamous cell carcinomas of the skin have similar radiosensitivities and most are radiocurable. The preferred dose-time schedule for most tumors up to 2 cm is 35 Gy in five daily fractions, and for 3-cm lesions the dose is 42.5 Gy in ten fractions in 12 days. Tumor doses are calculated at the skin surface and the minimum dose should be at least 90% of the maximum (GOLDSCHMIDT and SHERWIN 1983). The area to be irradiated includes the tumor with a margin of normal skin. This should be at least 0.5 cm for tumors up to 2 cm, 1 cm for lesions 2–5 cm in width,

and 2 cm or more for large tumors. Monoenergetic electrons have a defined depth of penetration but because of the electron build-up the maximum dose is below the surface and so a bolus of varying thickness must be used to increase the surface dose. The eye is a radiovulnerable organ and every attempt must be made to limit the radiation that it receives, especially to its anterior segment. For most patients treated with photon radiation, the dose to the eye can be reduced by the insertion of a 2-mm acrylic-coated lead equivalent shield into the conjunctival sac (Fig. 17.1). The percentage of radiation that is transmitted is low and only increases by a few percent owing to scatter. A similar technique can be used with the electron beam but because of secondary x-ray emission the dose to the eye is about 15% of the tumor dose (AMDUR et al. 1992)

Following irradiation, a series of changes occur in both the skin and the tumor. These vary in degree and are dependent on the patient's complexion, field size, and dose. A brisk erythema appears about the 4th day after a single exposure and 1–2 weeks after a 5-day course of treatment, and during the 2nd and 3rd weeks of protracted therapy. The erythema fades after 2–3 weeks with a dry desquamation. A hyperpigmented patch may be left, which fades over sever-

Table 17.1. Dose-time relationships used to treat basal and squamous cell carcinoma

Gy	Fractions	Days
20	1	1
22.5	1	1
35	5	5
40	5	7
42.5	10	12
45	10–15	12–19
50–60	20–30	26–38

Table 17.2. Use of radiotherapy in a series of 901 patients with basal or squamous cell carcinoma of the eyelids, treated between 1975 and 1984 (basal to squamous cell carcinoma ratio, 11.5 : 1)[a,b]

Gy	Pts.	%	Tx	Days
20	165	20	1	1
35	456	55	5	5
42.5	149	18	10	12
50–60	58	7	20–30	26–38
	828	100		

[a] T_1 < 2 cm: 576 (64%)

[b] 3-Year local control rate: 777/828 (94%)

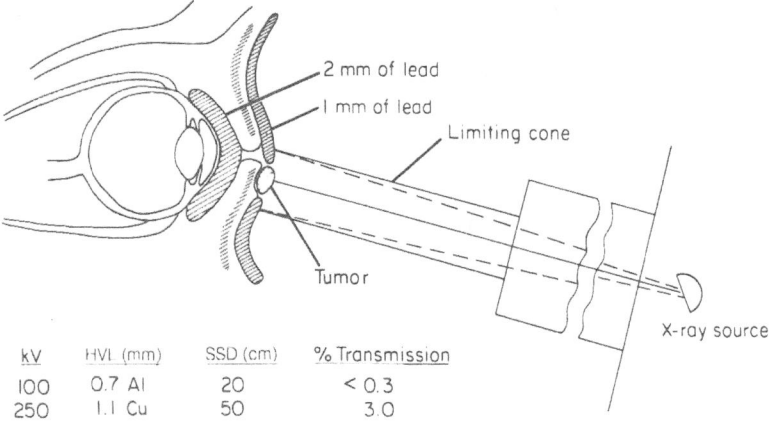

kV	HVL (mm)	SSD (cm)	% Transmission
100	0.7 Al	20	< 0.3
250	1.1 Cu	50	3.0

Fig. 17. 1. The radiovulnerable anterior segment of the eye is readily protected with a 2-mm lead shield

al weeks. In about half of patients, a moist reaction develops. Epilation of the lashes follows 3 Gy and is often permanent after 15 Gy. Most basal and squamous cell carcinomas start to regress following the first dose of radiation. This is not visible until the end of the 2nd week. At 1 month, the average tumor is flat with the surrounding eyelid and complete disappearance is usual within 8 weeks. Sometimes a ghost outline remains for several weeks before total disappearance. Any tumor detectable at 3 months is unlikely to be cured and further management should be considered. Melanomas and adenocarcinomas are slower in response and very variable in their behavior.

The radiation reactions require little care and the tissues are best left exposed to the air and kept dry. Cornstarch is used for this purpose, and if a moist desquamation develops it can be treated with 0.5% hydrocortisone or a 1% solution of aqueous gentian violet. This coagulates the serum and protects the healing tissues but is unsightly. Wet saline soaks help to remove the crusts but dressings are best avoided.

A late complication that may follow injury, usually actinic damage, months or years after treatment is tissue necrosis. This presents as a painful inflamed nonhealing ulcer. Most of these will heal if they are protected from further trauma and the healing can be hastened with the application of steroid and antibiotic creams. A persistent ulcer requires excision.

After radiotherapy patients are followed in order to assess the results of treatment and to detect the onset of other lesions. In general, patients are seen at 1 and 3 months following treatment in order to evaluate the response and advise on the care of reactions. Further visits are scheduled at 6 months and 1, 2, and 3 years when most patients are discharged from the clinic to the care of their family physician or ophthalmologist. Most recurrences occur within 2 years but 80% of patients will develop other skin neoplasms.

17.3
Basal Cell Carcinoma

Basal cell carcinoma, the most common tumor of the eyelids, arises from the basal layer of epidermis. It is so called because the tumor cells look like those ordinarily found in the basal layer of the epidermis but they do not mature and make keratin. Untreated, they burrow deeply, infiltrate vital areas, and cause hideous deformity. Commonly, they are known as rodent ulcers. All morphologic subtypes occur on the eyelid, including nodular, pigmented, morphea, superficial, and basisquamous cell types. These tumors do not metastasize. The average diameter is 19mm and the median duration of symptoms prior to diagnosis is 3.5 years. The relevant statistics on 829 patients seen between 1975 and 1984 are shown in Fig. 17.2. The preponderance of tumors arising from the inner canthal region is due to the specific referral of these patients for radiotherapy because of the site's special anatomy. Tumors arising from the upper lid or lateral canthal regions are most easy to excise and so these figures do not represent the true incidence of the site of origin. The median age was 61 years with a male to female incidence of 1.5 : 1, and 80%–90% of patients had other skin tumors.

The 3-year local control rate following radiotherapy in 720 patients was 94% and four (0.05%) had tumor-related deaths (Table 17.3). Figures 17.3 and 17.4 show the results of treatment in two cases.

BCC EYELIDS 1975 - 1984
829 PATIENTS

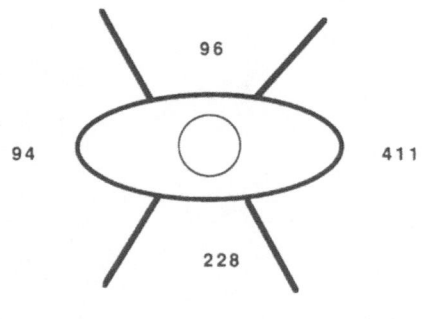

	Pts.	M:F	Years	Multiple Lesions %
Male	505	1.5:1	61 (29-97)	90
Female	324		57 (23-88)	80

Fig. 17.2. Clinical experience with basal cell carcinoma (BCC)

Table 17.3. Results of radiotherapy in 720 patients with basal cell carcinoma of the eyelids, treated between 1975 and 1984

	Pts.	%
3-Year local control	679	94
Metastases	0	0
Tumor-related deaths	4	0.05

Table 17.4. Results of radiotherapy in 58 patients with squamous cell carcinoma of the eyelids, treated between 1975 and 1984

	Pts.	%
3-Year local control	54	93
Metastases	2	3
Tumor-related deaths	1	2

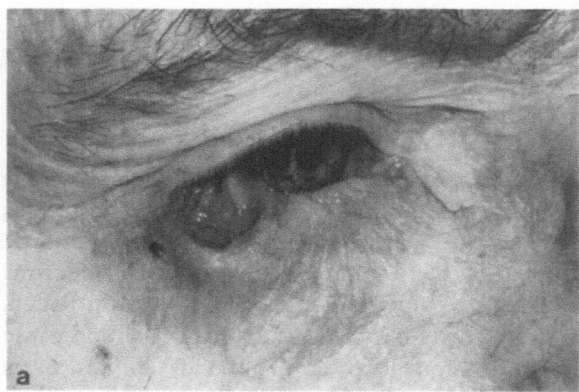
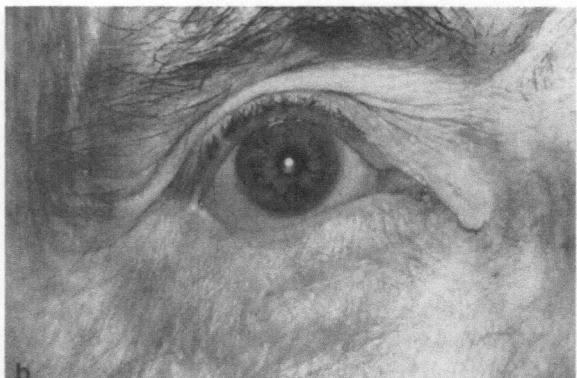

Fig. 17.3. Basal cell carcinoma of the lateral canthus **a** before and **b** 5 years after 42.5 Gy in ten exposures (125 kW, HVL 3.5 mm Al, 50 cm SSD)

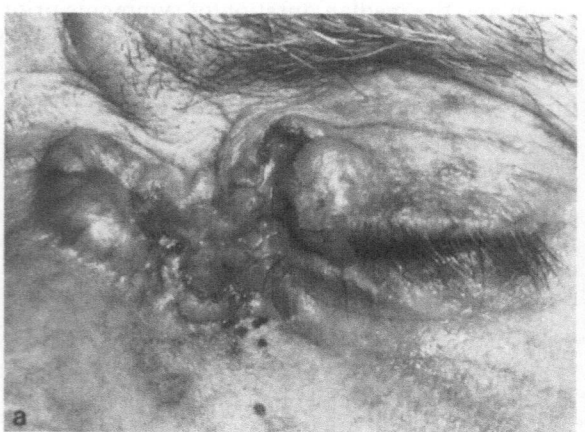
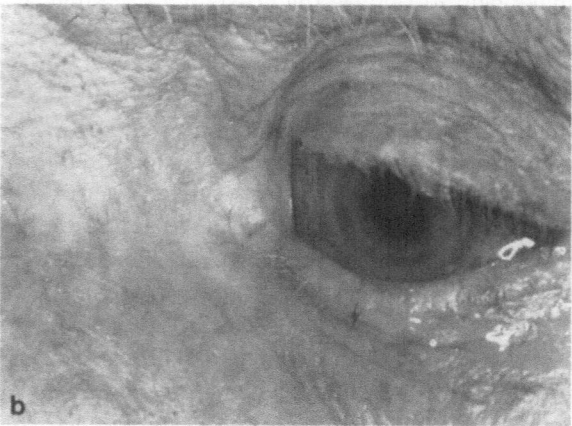

Fig. 17.4. Basal cell carcinoma of the inner canthus **a** before and **b** after treatment with 45 Gy in 15 exposures (250 kW, HVL 1.25 mm Cu, 50 cm SSD)

17.4
Squamous Cell Carcinoma

Most squamous cell carcinomas are well differentiated, produce keratin, and arise from actinically damaged skin. Typically, the tumors have firm, raised, rolled, everted edges; they have an average diameter of 19mm and a median history prior to diagnosis of 14 months. The relevant statistics for 72 patients seen between 1975 and 1984 are shown in Fig. 17.5. The median age was 67 and there was a male to female of 1.4 : 1 with 80% of patients having multiple lesions. The 3-year local control rate for 58 patients treated by radiotherapy was 93% (Table 17.4). Two (3%) tumors metastasized and one (2%) patient had a

tumor-related death. A typical case is shown in Fig. 17.6. Bowen's disease, or intraepithelial carcinoma in situ, is a radiosensitive lesion and control with excellent cosmetic results can be achieved with 25 Gy in five daily fractions.

17.5
Cosmesis and Function Following Radiotherapy

Cosmesis and function in patients with basal and squamous cell cancer were assessed in 115 patients at 1 and 5 years following radiotherapy by the patients themselves, a clinic nurse, a radiation oncologist, and an ophthalmologist (Fig. 17.7). The results show that all parties were more than satisfied with the treatment. On a scale of 1–10, the results were rated at 8 and confirm a previous report from our institute.

17.6
Complications Following Radiotherapy

In general there were few complications; they were mostly related to large tumors with extensive damage prior to radiotherapy. Our records, however, were not good enough to differentiate between prior damage and changes secondary to irradiation. In a previous report of 1166 cases of basal and squamous cell carcinoma treated by radiotherapy, signficant complications were reported in 112 (9.6%) patients but it was also not possible to differentiate between those

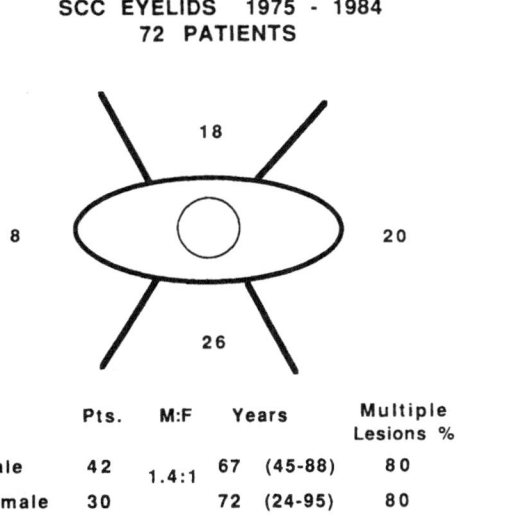

SCC EYELIDS 1975 - 1984
72 PATIENTS

	Pts.	M:F	Years	Multiple Lesions %
Male	42	1.4:1	67 (45-88)	80
Female	30		72 (24-95)	80

Fig. 17.5. Clinical experience with squamous cell carcinoma (SCC)

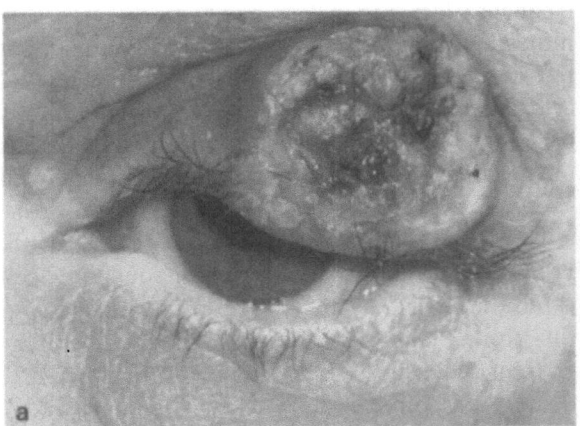
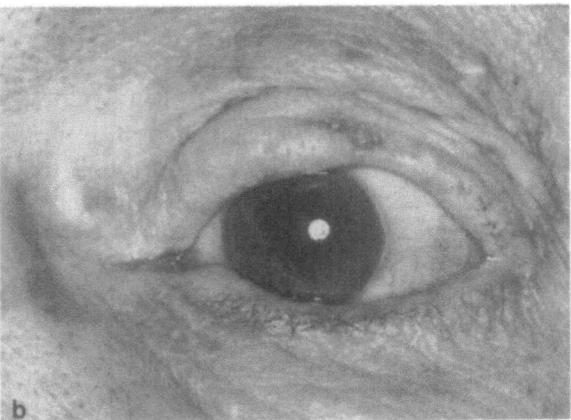

Fig. 17.6. Squamous cell carcinoma of the upper lid **a** before and **b** 6 years after treatment with 45 Gy in ten exposures (250 kW, HVL 1. 25 mm Cu, 50 cm SSD)

BCC/SCC EYELIDS
COSMESIS/FUNCTION AFTER RADIOTHERAPY

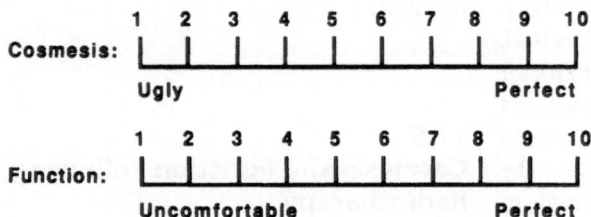

Pts.	Yrs.		Patient	Nurse	Radiation Oncologist	Ophthalmologist	Total
70	1.	Cosmesis	7	8	8	7	7.5
		Function	10	9.5	8	9	9.25
45	5.	Cosmesis	8	8	8	7	8.0
		Function	8	8	9	8	8.0
Total			8	8	8	7.5	8.0

Fig. 17.7. Assessment of cosmesis and function of eyelids following radiotherapy for basal (BCC) and squamous cell carcinoma (SCC)

due to the tumor and those due to the treatment (Table 17.5). Similar complication rates for 850 patients followed for 10–20 years were reported by SCHLIENGER et al. (1996).

17.7 Keratoacanthoma

The clinical course of keratoacanthoma is unpredictable. Many tumors will heal spontaneously if left alone or spurred on by a biopsy. Others will cause tremendous tissue destruction and may undergo malignant transformation with fatal results. To this group, we have given the name acute epithelioma and these tumors must not be underestimated. Between 1958 and 1988, 16 patients with a diagnosis of keratoacanthoma were seen with a median age of 70 and a male to female ratio of 2 : 1 (Table 17.6). Twelve lesions arose from the upper lid and four from the lower lid. Radiotherapy was used to treat all 16 lesions, with a median dose of 42.5 Gy in ten daily fractions. The 3-year control rate was 100%.

17.8 Acute Epithelioma

"Acute epithelioma" is the term that we use to describe an aggressive squamous cell carcinoma. It is

Table 17.5. Complications following radiotherapy [112/1166 (9.6%) patients affected][a]

Skin atrophy	64
Ectropion	36[b]
Entropion	6
Epiphora	27[b]
Keratinization conjunctiva	21
Keratitis	· 5
Cataract	11
Perforated globe	3
	173

[a] N.B. It was difficult to distinguish complications resulting from radiotherapy and those due to the tumor
[b] Often present before treatment

frequently larger than 2 cm and has a characteristic morphology with raised, rolled, and vascular but not everted edges. Commonly, there is a central crust covering a foul discharge on a papilliferous base. The biopsy is characteristically ambiguous but often that of a well-differentiated squamous cell carcinoma. Irrespective of the history, which is usually short, all tumors have a period of rapid growth. From a series of 125 patients with squamous cell carcinoma of the eyelid, 15 (12%) patients were in this group (Table 17.7). Ten (67%) had tumors larger than 2 cm, five (33%) developed regional metastases, and three (20%) had tumor-related deaths. The primary tumor was controlled by radiotherapy in 14 (93%) patients and the 3-year course-specific survival rate was 80%.

17.9
Melanoma

Nodular, superficial, and lentigo malignant melanomas occur on the eyelid. Between 1958 and 1988, 16 patients were registered (Fig. 17.8). Seven patients had nodular tumors and seven developed nodular tumors in an area of lentigo maligna while one patient had lentigo maligna alone. The median age was 69 with a male to female ratio of 0.7 : 1. Radiotherapy was used in the treatment of ten (62.5%) patients and was palliative in two, postoperative in one, and radical in seven (Table 17.8). Among the latter group, two patients had local recurrences after 3 and 7 years and one was lost to follow-up, while the other four had their disease controlled after 3–8 years. Three and four patients, respectively, received 45 Gy in ten fractions or 50 Gy in 10–15 fractions. Six (37%) patients died with distant metastatic disease. A case of lentigo maligna melanoma is shown in Fig. 17.9.

Table 17.6. Clinical experience with keratoacanthoma (16 patients seen between 1958 and 1988)

Sex	
Male	11
Female	5
M: F ratio	2:1
Age (years)	
Median	70
Range	44-91
Eyelid	
Upper	12
Lower	4
U: L ratio	3:1
Radiotherapy[a]	12
3-Year local control	12(100%)
Metastases	0
Deaths	0

[a] 42.5 Gy in ten daily fractions

Table 17.7. Clinical experience with the acute epithelioma variant of squamous cell carcinoma (15 patients seen between 1958 and 1982)

Sex	
Male	10
Female	5
M: F ratio	2:1
Age (years)	
Median	75
Range	49–84
Tumor size >2 cm	10(67%)
Positive nodes	5(33%)
Death	3(20%)
Local control	14(93%)
2nd Tx	15(100%)
3-Year CSS[a]	

[a] CSS, course-specific survival rate

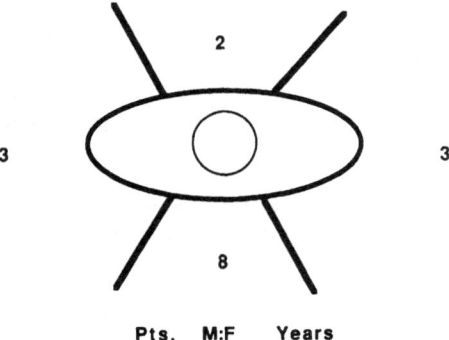

MELANOMA EYELIDS 1958 - 1988
16 PATIENTS

	Pts.	M:F	Years
Male	7	0.7:1	69 (23-83)
Female	9		

	Pts.	%
Lentigo maligna (LM)	1	
LM melanoma	7	
Nodular melanoma	7	
Dead with Metastases	6	37

Fig. 17.8. Clinical experience with melanoma on the eyelids

Table 17.8. Use of radiotherapy for melanoma of the eyelids (16 patients treated between 1958 and 1988)

Radiotherapy	10(62.5%)
Radical[a]	
45 Gy/10	3
50 Gy/10- 15	4
Palliative	2
Postoperative	1
Dead with metastases	6(37%)

[a] of the seven patients who underwent radical radiotherapy, four were alive and well after 3–8 years, two had local recurrences after 3 and 7 years, and one was lost to follow-up

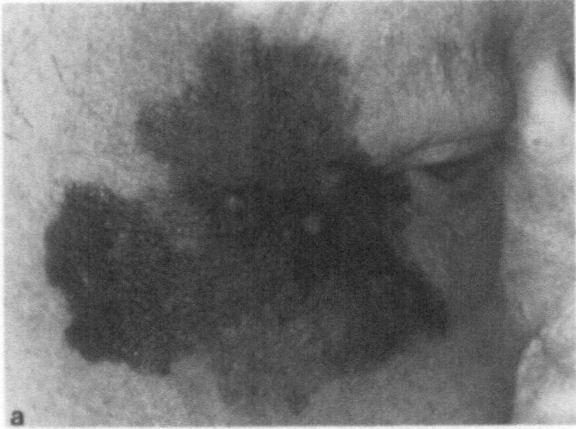

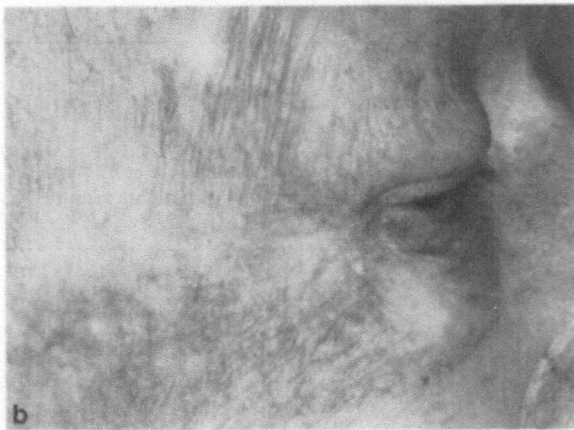

Fig. 17.9. A 69-year-old man with a lentigo maligna melanoma **a** before and **b** 5 years after treatment with 50 Gy delivered in 20 fractions in a month (100 kW, HLV 0.7 mm Al, 20 cm SSD)

17.10
Sebaceous Adenocarcinoma

Sebaceous adenocarcinomas arise from the ocular adnexae and most commonly from the meibomian glands. Between 1958 and 1988, 20 patients were registered with a median age of 68 and a male to female ratio of 0.6 : 1 (Table 17.9). Twelve tumors arose from the upper lid and eight from the lower. Fourteen (70%) patients had had previous surgery, with three having residual disease and six, recurrent disease; in five there was no evidence of tumor. Six were primary untreated cases and altogether seven patients received radiotherapy. Two patients receiving postoperative irradiation both had recurrences at the primary site, and of five tumors radically irradiated, two recurred locally while three remained controlled at 1, 3, and 6 years. Unfortu-

nately, the records were incomplete, with several patients being lost to follow-up, but two are known to have died of disease.

17.11
Conclusions

The treatment of eyelid tumors depends largely on the size and site of the tumor. Optimum treatment for every patient is most likely to be prescribed when there is close cooperation between the ophthalmic surgeon and the radiation oncologist. Some patients are best treated by surgery, others by radiotherapy, and some by combining both modalities. When irradiation is delivered carefully, it repudiates the sinister reputation that it has around the eye and orbit. The age and sex distributions of patients with basal and squamous cell carcinomas of the eyelid and their tumor size, tumor site, and treatment were similar to those in earlier reports from this institute. The increased incidence of both basal and squamous cell carcinomas of the inner canthus and lower lid is related to the referral pattern. It is more difficult to excise lesions at these sites because of the potential complications from scarring of the lid or damage to the lateral appendagea with consequent epiphora. About one-third of our patients were referred with residual or recurrent disease following surgical excision. Radiotherapy is just as effective in controlling these tumors as

Table 17.9. Clinical experience with sebaceous adenocarcinoma of the eyelids (20 patients seen between 1958 and 1988)

Sex	
Male	8
Female	12
M: F ratio	0.6:1
Age (years)	
Median	68
Range	35-92
Eyelid	
Upper	12
Lower	8
U: L ratio	1:0.6
Primary surgery	12(70%)
Radiotherapy	7(35%)
Postoperative	2[a]
Radical	5[b]

[a] Both tumors recurred at the primary site
[b] Two tumors recurred locally while in three cases there was no evidence of disease at 1, 3, and 6 years.

it is for untreated lesions. For tumors that recur following irradiation, surgical excision is preferred. Radiotherapy is given on an outpatient basis, takes only a few minutes a day, and allows patients to continue their normal occupation during treatment. The cost of treatment, including establishing the diagnosis by biopsy, is competitive with any other treatment; in these days of escalating medical costs and increased government surveillance this is an important consideration.

Basal and squamous cell carcinomas behave in a similar manner, the only difference being that 5% of the latter metastasize to the regional nodes. We use the same radiation dose for similar tumors, with the technique varied only according to the site and extent of the tumor. Acute epithelioma is an aggressive variant of squamous cell carcinoma of the skin which may arise as a result of malignant transformation in the pseudocancer or self-healing keratoacanthoma. In our experience, this type accounted for 12% of squamous cell carcinomas of the eyelids. We have postulated that these acute epitheliomas are virusinduced tumors and develop in actinicly damaged and immunologically suppressed skin. Fortunately, they are radiosensitive and radiocurable.

The place of radiotherapy in the treatment of melanoma of the eyelid is unclear but certainly some lesions are radiosensitive and radiocurable. This is especially so with lentigo maligna and lentigo maligna melanoma. Radiotherapy probably has a place in the treatment of sebaceous adenocarcinoma of the eyelids but from our experience it is not possible to draw conclusions or to make firm recommendations.

Acknowledgments. This chapter represents the combined efforts of many members of the staff of the Princess Margaret Hospital over many years.

References

Amdur RJ, Kalbaugh KJ, Ewald LM et al. (1992) Radiation therapy for skin cancer near the eye: kilovoltage x-rays versus electrons. Int J Rad Oncol Biol Phys 23:769–779

Daly NJ, LaFontan B, Combes PF (1984) Results of the treatment of 165 lid carcinomas by iridium wire implant. Int J Radiat Oncol Biol Phys 10:455–459

Fitzpatrick PJ (1995) Organ and functional perservation in the management of cancers of the eye and eyelid. Cancer Invest 13(1):66–74

Fitzpatrick PJ, Thompson GA, Easterbrook WM, Gallie BL, Payne DG (1984) Basal and squamous cell carcinoma of the eyelids and their treatment by radiotherapy. Int J Radiat Oncol Biol Phys 10:1319-1325

Goldschmidt H (1975) Dermatologic radiation therapy: current use of ionizing radiation in the United States and Canada. Arch Dermatol 111:1511-1517

Goldschmidt H, Sherwin W (1983) Office radiotherapy of cutaneous carcinomas, radiation techniques, dose schedules, and radiation protection. J Dermatol Surg Oncol 9: 1 January

Johns AE, Cunningham HR (1969) The physics of radiology, 3rd edn. Charles C. Thomas, Springfield, 111.

Lederman M (1976) Radiation treatment of cancer of the eyelids, Br J Ophthalmol 60:794-805

Schlienger P, Brunin F, Desjardins L et al. (1996) External radiotherapy for carcinoma of the eyelid: report of 850 cases treated. Int J Radiat Oncol Biol Phys 34:277-287

Strandqvist M (1944) Studien über die kumulative Wirkung der Roentgenstrahlen bei Fraktionierung. Acta Radiol [Suppl 55]

18 Conjunctival Tumors and Their Treatment by Radiotherapy

P. K. LOMMATZSCH and C. WERSCHNIK

P. K. LOMMATZSCH, MD
Private Eye Practice, Goldschmidtstrasse 30, 04103 Leipzig, Germany
C. WERSCHNIK, MD
Department of Ophthalmology, Martin Luther University of Halle-Wittenberg, Magdeburger Strasse 8, 06112 Halle, Germany

18.1
Introduction

The conjunctiva is often affected by neoplasms and by lesions that may simulate neoplasms, especially in elderly patients. This discussion of conjunctival tumors and their treatment by radiotherapy will follow the nomenclature, definition, and classification suggested by ZIMMERMAN and SOBIN (1980) in volume 24 of the World Health Organization International Classification of Tumors. Most of the conditions listed in this outline, such as pinguecula, corneal keloid, dermoid, dermolipoma, episcleral osseous choristoma, complex choristoma, benign epithelial tumors, and the inflammatory tumor-like lesions should not be treated by radiotherapy, and are mentioned briefly for systematic reasons only. However, lesions such as recurrent pterygium, malignant epithelial tumors, tumors and tumor-like lesions of the melanogenic system, and tumors and tumor-like lesions of the hematopoietic and lymphoid tissues are worthwhile targets for radiotherapy.

Radiation treatment can be employed alone or in combination with surgery. A pretreatment biopsy is indispensable.

18.2
Epithelial Tumors and Tumor-like Lesions

18.2.1
Surface Epithelial Lesions

18.2.1.1
Benign

Squamous Cell Papilloma. Various degrees of epithelial dysplasia exist; rarely, carcinoma may develop from a papilloma. Excision without radiotherapy is performed.

Keratotic Plaque. This leukoplakia is characterized by acanthosis, parakeratosis, and hyperkeratosis.

There is little or no potential for malignant change, and it is not an indication for radiotherapy.

Keratoacanthoma, pseudocarcinomatous hyperplasia, inverted follicular keratosis, and cysts are very rare conjunctival lesions with no significance for radiotherapy.

18.2.1.2
Precancerous

Actinic Keratosis (Senile Keratosis). This involves the bulbar and limbal conjunctiva and frequently develops in the epithelium overlying preexisting inflammatory lesions such as pinguecula or pterygium. The epithelium shows architectural disarray with acanthosis, keratosis, and parakeratosis. This lesion is the most common precursor of invasive squamous cell carcinoma.

Dysplasia. The epithelial changes in this lesion are similar to those of carcinoma in situ but typically do not involve the full thickness of the epithelial layer.

Xeroderma Pigmentosum. This is primarily a disease of the skin, but it is frequently marked by ocular complications (REESE 1976). The lesions are characterized by an abnormal reaction to light with development of various types of carcinoma. No effective treatment is known.

18.2.1.3
Malignant

Carcinoma in situ. Presently most clinicians use the term "conjunctival intraepithelial neoplasia" (CIN) for what was previously termed Bowen's disease, conjunctival dysplasia, conjunctival carcinoma in situ, dyskeratosis, or intraepithelial epithelioma. There is a moderate thickening of the conjunctival epithelium, mostly starting at the limbus. The tumor is characterized by large, oblong, hyperchromatic basaloid cells, which involve the full thickness of the epithelium. Mitotic activity is usually pronounced. Parakeratosis and hyperkeratosis are minimal, so that the affected tissue shows an opalescent rather than a leukoplakic appearance. This lesion frequently recurs but rarely changes into an invasive growth (Fig. 18.1). It may be treated successfully with a surface applicator (DAVID and CONSTABLE 1979).

Squamous Cell Carcinoma. This well-differentiated keratinizing tumor originates from the conjunctival epithelium, usually in the exposed interpalpebral

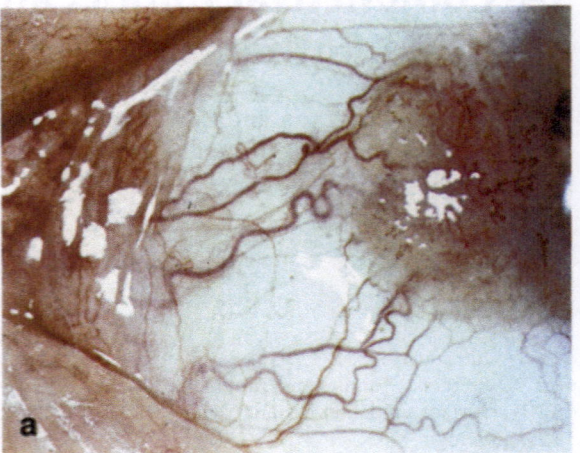
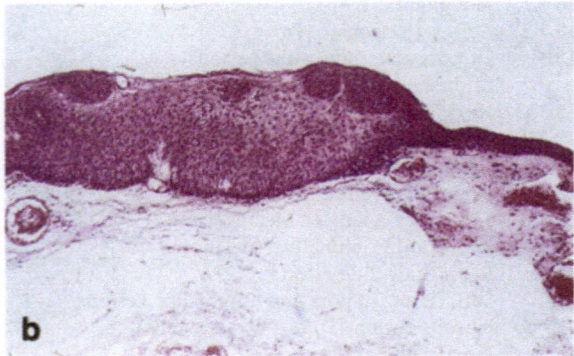
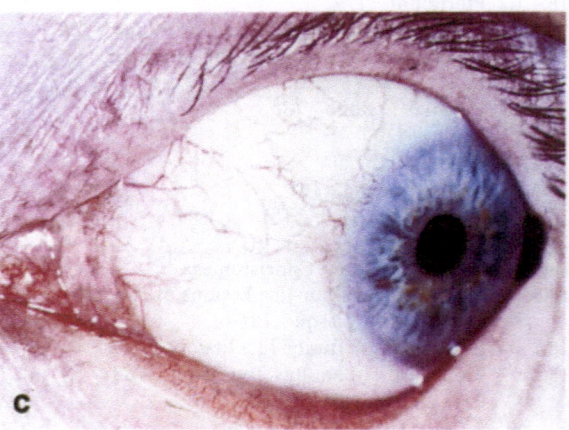

Fig. 18.1. a Small limbal tumor in a 45-year-old man. **b** Microscopic examination showed a carcinoma in situ with dyskeratosis, cellular atypia, some clumping of cells, and sharp demarcation against the underlying tissue. (Hematoxylineosin, ×75) **c** Two months after beta ray irradiation with 150 Gy: visual acuity 1.0

area. It tends to grow in an exophytic papillary fashion and is often only superficially invasive. It is impossible to distinguish this lesion from papilloma with certainty by slit-lamp examination. In both these lesions typical small loops of vessels are noted. Invasive squamous carcinoma has four common

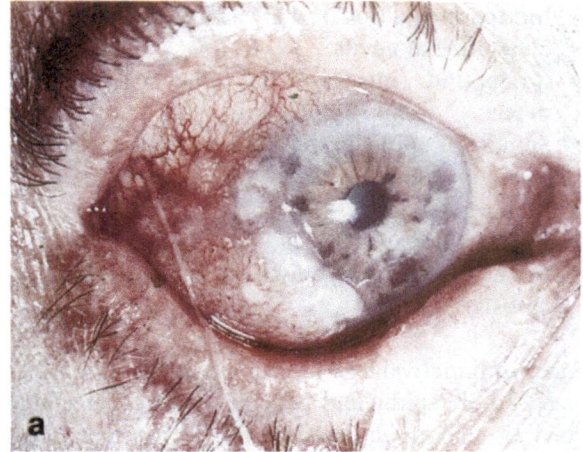

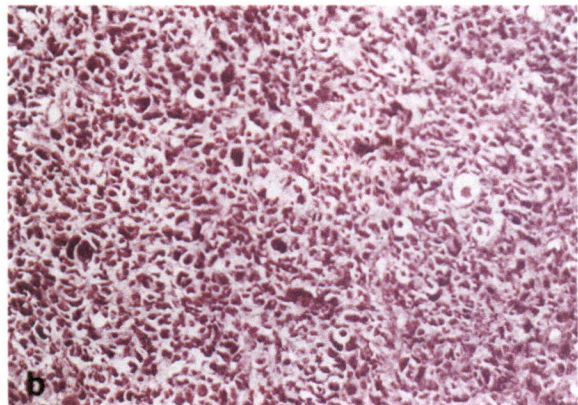

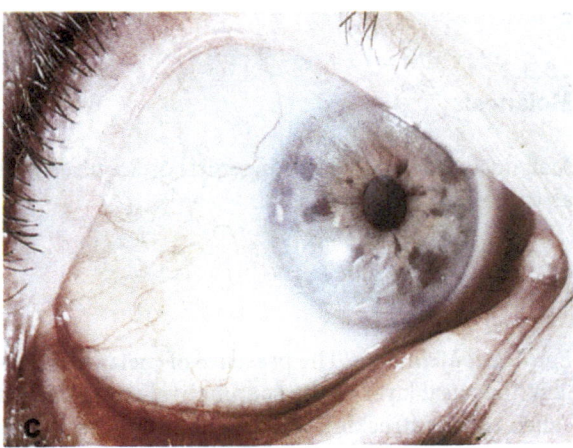

Fig. 18.2. a Squamous cell carcinoma in a 73-year-old man. **b** Microscopic appearance shows anaplasia and mitotic activity. **c** Three months after beta ray irradiation with 180 Gy: visual acuity 1.0

clinical presentations: as a gelatinous lesion with intrinsic vessels, a leukoplakic lesion, a vascular papilloma-like lesion, and pagetoid spread into the cornea (CHAR 1989). It may infiltrate into the eye or orbit, but rarely metastasizes. These tumors are typically seen in elderly people (Fig. 18.2).

Mucoepidermoid Carcinoma. This rare tumor contains an intimate admixture of mucus-secreting cells and squamous cells (BROWNSTEIN 1980). Extended follow-up after therapy is required because of the risk of late distant metastasis (HWANG et al. 2000).

Radiotherapy can be beneficial in all these different kinds of malignant epithelial conjunctival tumors.

The recurrence rate after surgical removal of squamous cell carcinoma in situ is 33% (PIZARELLO and JAKOBIEC 1978). A wide surgical margin should be included around the visible tumor mass, because invisible dysplastic cells can spread radially within the apparently healthy conjunctiva. Recurrence typically occurs within 2 years after excision; therefore, postoperative follow-up is essential.

Postoperative radiotherapy is effective in preventing recurrences of incompletely excised tumors. In addition, in those cases with deep corneal invasion, superficial local excision would be inadequate and irradiation is employed (ILIFF et al. 1975). There is no uniform method of treating malignant conjunctival tumors. A separate decision is needed in each case on which method of radiotherapy should be used.

LOMMATZSCH (1976) found beta ray irradiation with 150–180 Gy to the tumor surface to be effective when the thickness of the tumor did not exceed 5 mm. The tumors resolved in nine of ten patients with squamous cell carcinoma and in all four cases of carcinoma in situ; follow-up ranged from 1 to 8 years, with a median of 3.6 years. Only one patient had a recurrent tumor, after 5 years, which led to enucleation. In cases with very extended tumor growth involving almost the whole conjunctiva, radiotherapy with beta rays is the only treatment to salvage the eye and to destroy the tumor (LOMMATZSCH 1976). After termination of irradiation the tumors shrink slowly and finally disappear. Local irritation of the conjunctiva will accompany this process. Local scars in the conjunctiva at the site of the former tumor should not be considered a complication caused by beta ray irradiation.

For small lesions (less than 1 mm thick) and postoperative situations with minimal residual tumor, CEREZO et al. (1989) recommend a single fraction of 60 Gy surface dose or three fractions of 20 Gy. Gross lesions (more than 1 mm thick) are irradiated with four to seven fractions of 20 Gy at 1-week intervals to obtain a favorable protraction effect. In patients with a diagnosis of intraepithelial epithelioma their standard policy is to irradiate the entire conjunctiva and cornea prophylactically, with two or three fractions (40–60 Gy) given with the bidirectional applicator while the patient keeps his or her eyelids closed.

After this, any clinically apparent lesion is irradiated with the appropriate applicator to a total of 60–120 Gy according to its thickness.

The side-effects of any radiotherapy must always be considered. In our series one patient developed a local triangular opacity of the periphery of the lens without loss of visual acuity. One patient with a limbal intraepithelial carcinoma that grew around the cornea suffered from secondary glaucoma, and one patient had a partial symblepharon after tumor excision and beta ray irradiation.

To limit radiogenic side-effects other authors (ELKON and CONSTABLE 1979) recommend lower doses, 45 Gy after surgical removal or 70 Gy for primary treatment. Some authors recommend excision plus cryotherapy (double freeze-thaw technique), which leads to a recurrence rate of approximately 9% (FRAUNFELDER and WINGFIELD 1983; DUTTON et al. 1984). HABERLE et al. (1995) used brachytherapy with a ruthenium-106 applicator to treat recurrences of carcinoma in situ after complete tumor excision.

18.2.2
Adnexal Lesions

Adnexal tumors are typically encountered in the lacrimal caruncle. Most lesions of the caruncle are benign. Malignant tumors, such as squamous cell carcinoma of the conjunctiva, sebaceous gland carcinoma of the lid and conjunctival melanoma, involve the caruncle in less than 10% of cases (CHAR 1989).

The accessory lacrimal gland may be the site of:
- Pleomorphic adenoma (mixed tumor)
- Oxyphytic adenoma (oncocytoma)
- Other adenomas

The treatment for lesions of the sweat glands and sebaceous glands is local excision. In general there is no need for radiotherapy, but irradiation can control inadequately resected lesions.

18.3
Tumors and Tumor-like Lesions of the Melanogenic System

18.3.1
Nevi

Nevi of the conjunctiva are classified in a similar way to those of the skin, with only minor modifications:

- Intraepithelial (junctional) nevus
- Subepithelial nevus
- Compound (intraepithelial plus subepithelial) nevus
- Spindle or epithelioid cell nevus ("juvenile melanoma" or "Spitz nevus")
- Blue nevus
- Cellular blue nevus
- Nevus of Ota (congenital oculodermal melanocytosis)

Most conjunctival nevi are compound or subepithelial. Spindle/epithelioid cell, blue, and cellular blue nevi are seldom observed on the conjunctiva.

Subepithelial and compound nevi are typically elevated above the conjunctival surface. This tumefaction is often caused by solid and cystic epithelial inclusions. Most nevi that have been observed to grow are found on histologic examination to be entirely benign. Occasionally a nonpigmented nevus can become inflamed and vascularized so that it may be mistaken for an angiomatous tumor.

Nevi should not be treated with radiotherapy; the pigmented tissue does not regress even with a high dose, but telangiectasia and other complications may ensue. Nevi should be excised either for cosmetic reasons or when it is thought that malignant change has occurred.

18.3.2
Melanosis

Melanosis is classified as congenital or acquired and as epithelial or subepithelial.

18.3.2.1
Congenital Melanosis

Epithelial Melanosis. The presence of melanin mainly in the basal layer of the conjunctival epithelium is called ephelis (freckle), and it is of no significance as a precursor of malignant melanoma.

Subepithelial Melanosis. Subepithelial melanosis is not only a conjunctival abnormality; melanin-containing cells are also situated in the substantia propria and sclera. When only the eye is affected, this lesion is termed ocular melanosis. Sometimes the lesion is accompanied by ipsilateral melanosis of the deep cutaneous tissue of the periorbital skin, which is called oculodermal melanocytosis or nevus of Ota. Such lesions should not be treated, but only observed. They have a pronounced predisposition to the development of malignant melanoma, especially in the uveal tract of the afflicted side.

18.3.2.2
Primary Acquired Melanosis

Primary acquired melanosis occurs as an idiopathic melanotic pigmentation of the conjunctival epithelium. It begins in middle age and can involve any part of the conjunctiva. The evolution of primary acquired melanosis is unpredictable. It often progresses slowly, but may wax and wane (SPENCER and ZIMMERMAN 1985). Many patients are followed for many years without showing development of a malignant melanoma, but in some cases a malignant growth appears early in the course of this disorder. Treatment should not be given until a biopsy has been found to be positive.

18.3.2.3
Secondary Acquired Melanosis

Secondary acquired melanosis may occur following other pathologic processes, such as trauma, inflammation, cysts, papillomas, effects produced by epinephrine-containing drugs, ochronosis, and argyria. It can be observed in more heavily pigmented races and is never the precursor of malignant melanoma.

18.3.3
Malignant Conjunctival Melanoma

Malignant melanoma of the conjunctiva includes three major subtypes, those that are derived from preexisting nevi, those that are derived from acquired melanomas, and those that develop from previously normal conjunctiva (de novo).

Studies on the behavior of conjunctival melanoma (SPENCER and ZIMMERMAN 1985) are lacking in large series of well-documented cases of this relatively rare lesion. HENKIND (1978) stated that "much of what has been written about pigmented lesions of the conjunctiva is either anecdotal, speculative or controversial." We agree with JAKOBIEC (1981), ZIMMERMAN (1978) and FOLBERG et al. (1985) that the classification of cutaneous melanoma should not be used in the study of conjunctival melanoma.

The absence of stratification in the conjunctival substantia propria precludes use of the microstaging system of CLARK and FOLBERG (1979).

Tumor thickness seems to be the most important prognostic factor in conjunctival melanomas, but it remains impossible for the ophthalmologist to advise individual patients about their prognosis: the behavior of conjunctival melanoma, like that of primary acquired melanosis, remains unpredictable. Local excision followed by beta ray irradiation (^{90}Sr/^{90}Y) can be recommended as the treatment of choice (LOMMATZSCH 1978; LOMMATZSCH et al. 1990; STERKER and LOMMATZSCH 1993). STANNARD et al. (2000) used iodine-125 brachytherapy for melanomas of the palpebral conjunctiva.

The daily dose of ^{90}Sr/^{90}Y applied at the tumor surface is 10 Gy to a total dose of 150–200 Gy, depending on the thickness of the tumor. Regression of the irradiated tumor may take several weeks or months; this is a much longer time than that observed in squamous cell carcinoma of the conjunctiva. The first sign of regression will not appear for some weeks, and complete shrinkage with depigmentation will generally take more than 6 months. In some cases a small amount of pigment is left in the center of the radiogenic scar. This should not be regarded as an indication for further treatment (Figs. 18.3, 18.4).

18.3.3.1
Radiogenic Side-effects

In comparison with other tumors, melanoma requires the highest dose for cell destruction. It is, therefore, not surprising that undesirable side-effects occur in some patients, although in the case of beta rays the penetration depth of the electrons is very low.

The typical sector-shaped beta ray cataract will develop after some years, but does not impair visual acuity. Telangiectasia of the conjunctival vessels arises in most patients within the irradiated area and should not be regarded as a severe complication. In extended cases involving the cornea and parts of the limbus, we have observed corneal opacities and secondary glaucoma (LOMMATZSCH 1978). Our recent experience with conjunctival melanoma can be summarized as follows (LOMMATZSCH et al. 1990):

Eighty-one cases of conjunctival melanoma treated between 1960 and 1988 were studied to determine factors that might affect outcome in patients with such lesions. The therapeutic procedures performed were local excision (16), local excision followed by brachytherapy with ^{90}Sr/^{90}Y (32), local excision followed by liquid nitrogen (16), brachytherapy with ^{90}Sr/^{90}Y (12), local excision followed by external beam irradiation (3), and local excision followed by brachytherapy and cryotherapy (2). The median follow-up period was 5.5 years (range 1–26 years). Sixty-two patients (76.5%) showed complete regression

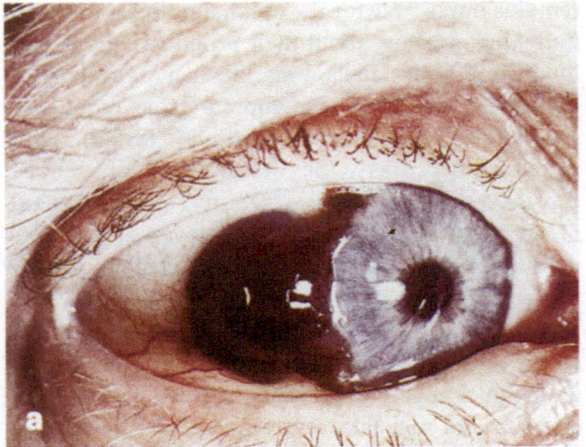

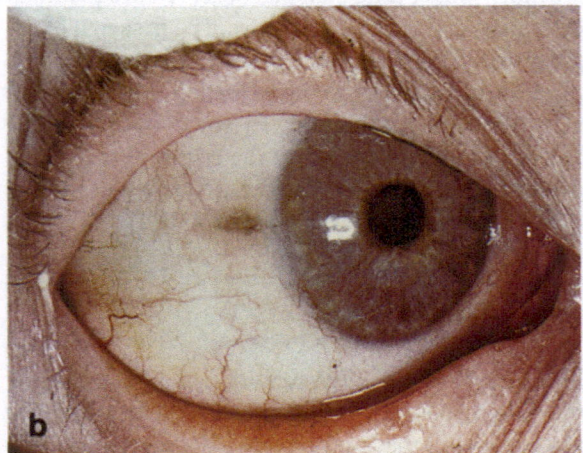

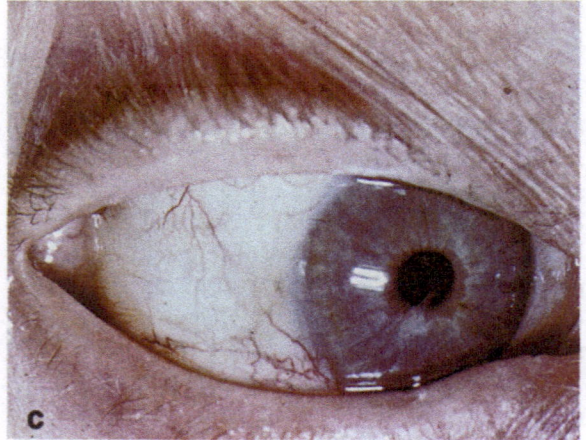

Fig. 18.3. a Conjunctival melanoma of an only eye in a 62-year-old woman. **b** Four years after beta ray irradiation with 150 Gy. **c** No recurrence 14 years after treatment: visual acuity 1.0

of the melanoma, 19 (23.5%) developed recurrences, and 15 (18.5%) died from metastases.

The melanoma had developed with almost equal frequencies from a preexisting nevus (25.9%), from primary acquired melanosis (25.9%), and de novo (30.9%). Small tumors of size pT1 and pT2 regressed more often than larger ones (pT3 and pT4): 80.6% vs 68.6%. The cumulative survival rate was 76% at 5 years and 60% at 10 years when all causes of death were taken into account, and 87.6% at 5 years and 76.3% at 10 years when only deaths caused by metastases were taken into account. The majority of deaths from metastases occurred within 5 years. The cumulative survival rate of 88.5% for patients with small tumors (T1) was significantly higher than that for patients with larger tumors (T2, T3, T4), which was only 65%, after 8 years. Local excision followed by beta ray irradiation (^{90}Sr/^{90}Y) or cryotherapy can be recommended as the treatment of choice. Locally applied mitomycin C is also used as an adjuvant in superficial melanoma or acquired melanosis with atypia (Werschnik and Lommatzsch 1998). A recent study including 85 patients with conjunctival melanoma with a mean follow-up of 13.8 years showed cumulative survival rates based on tumor-related death of 84.8% and 77.7% after 5 and 10 years, respectively. Age of patients (>55 years) and unfavorable tumor location (palpebral conjunctiva, fornix, caruncle, corneal stroma) were identified as risk factors for tumor-related death. Unfavorable tumor location, excision without adjuvant therapy and higher TNM grade were risk factors for recurrence (Werschnik and Lommatzsch 2001). Similar results are reported by Paridaens et al. (1994), De Wolff-Rouendaal (1990, 1999), and DePotter et al. (1993). Nevertheless, the behavior of conjunctival melanomas remains unpredictable.

18.4
Soft Tissue Tumors and Tumor-like Lesions

18.4.1
Fibrous Lesions

18.4.1.1
Pinguecula

Pinguecula is an elastoid degeneration of the collagen of the conjunctiva located nasally in the exposed bulbar conjunctiva; irradiation is not required.

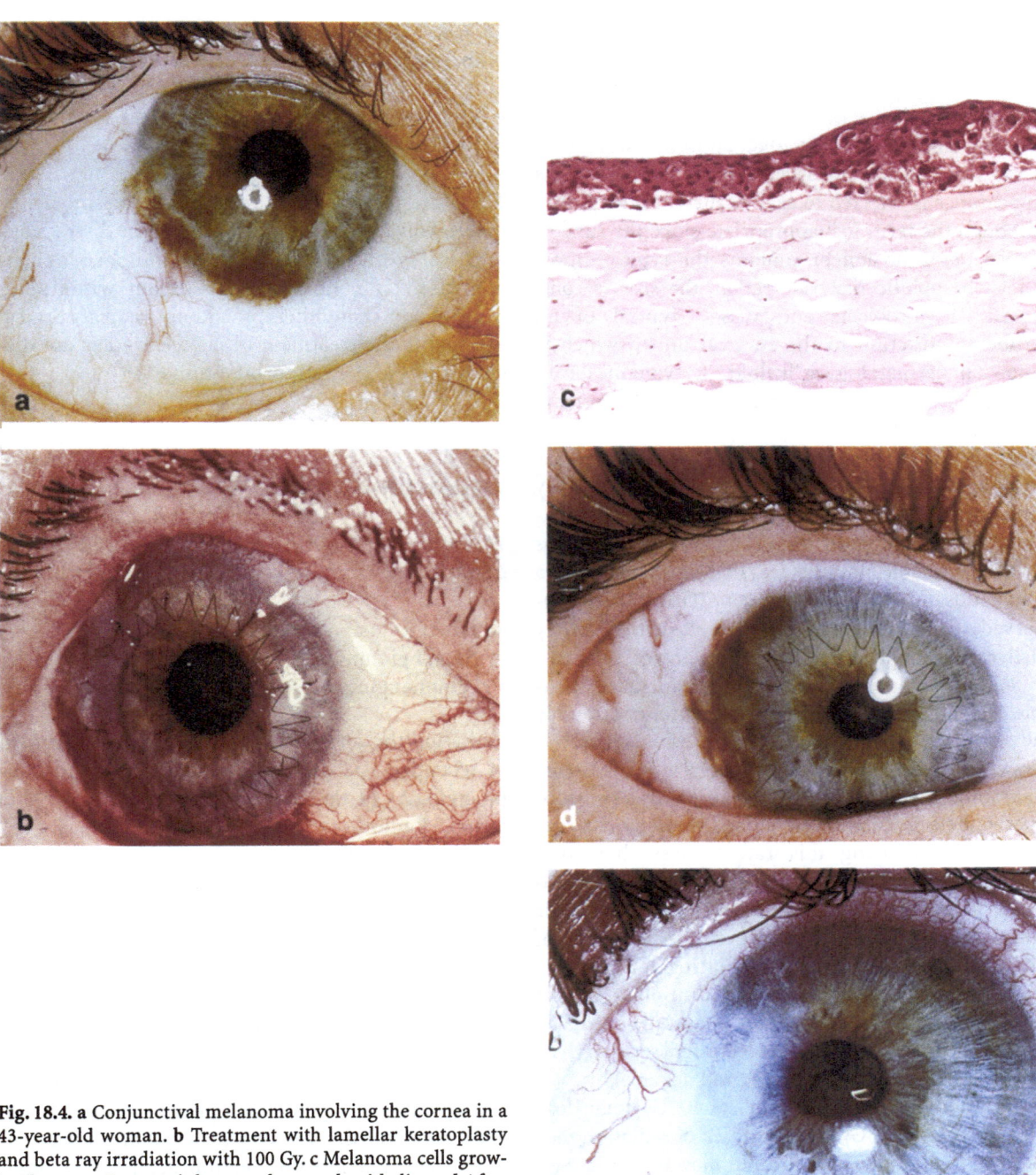

Fig. 18.4. a Conjunctival melanoma involving the cornea in a 43-year-old woman. **b** Treatment with lamellar keratoplasty and beta ray irradiation with 100 Gy. **c** Melanoma cells growing between Bowman's layer and corneal epithelium. **d** After 5 months there was a recurrence of the melanoma at the temporal corneal limbus, which was treated by cryotherapy. **e** 3 years after keratoplasty and beta ray irradiation

18.4.1.2
Pterygium

A pterygium arises at the nasal or temporal limbus, as a rule as an extension of a preexisting pinguecula. Pterygia are probably caused by prolonged solar exposure and are therefore also described as actinic degeneration of corneal and limbal conjunctiva.

The lesion is observed much more frequently in geographic areas with intense actinic stimulation.

The subepithelial limbal tissues, the periphery of Bowman's layer, and the superficial corneal stromal lamellae contain thickened, degenerated connective tissue in which the fibrous component is replaced by amorphous basophilic material, which is also called "elastotic" degeneration. Subsequently the overlying epithelium may undergo a variety of changes such as atrophy, acanthosis, or even dysplasia; it is difficult to exclude a very early carcinoma in situ. The therapy of choice is surgical removal of the pterygium (SUND-MACHER and MACKENSEN 1988). It is not unusual for a vascularized scar to develop postoperatively. This appearance is referred to as a "recurrent pterygium," although the term is inappropriate since the subepithelial tissue no longer contains the typical amorphous basophilic material; rather, the scar is composed of fibroblasts and vessels typical of an exuberant reaction to the surgical injury, which is known in dermatology as "keloid." To avoid the development of this so-called recurrent pterygium, brachytherapy with $^{90}Sr/^{90}Y$ is generally recommended. Immediately after surgical removal the treated area has to be irradiated with a maximum of 60 Gy in daily doses of 10 Gy (LOMMATZSCH et al. 1977). The irradiation field should cover the original lesion but be as small as possible. LEDERMAN (1972) recommended a single dose of 24 Gy after surgery. THIEL (1979) observed a decrease in the recurrence rate with 25–30 Gy delivered in single doses of 5+5 Gy per week.

Numerous surgical modifications, including simple excision, have been reported, but none is notably advantageous. Recurrence after excision alone has been reported to occur in 20–30% of patients (FARRELL and SMITH 1989). Use of adjuvant postoperative beta irradiation or topical thiotepa has succeeded in reducing this rate to less than 10% (HILGERS 1960; CAMERON 1972; KLEIS and PICO 1973; TARR and CONSTABLE 1980). On the other hand, beta irradiation to prevent recurrences of pterygia is a significant cause of iatrogenic disease.

TARR and CONSTABLE (1980) cautioned against beta ray treatment because they observed severe late complications such as scleral ulceration, sectorial lens opacities, ptosis, symblepharon, and iris atrophy 3–20 years after beta irradiation of 7.5–52 Gy total dose (mean 34.75±9.16 Gy). Lower doses of radiation may reduce the complication rate, but may also be less effective in preventing recurrences. A dose of 22 Gy after pterygium excision has been considered safe, even when repeated twice for subsequent recurrences.

18.4.2
Xanthomatous and Histiocytic Lesions

- Juvenile xanthogranuloma
- Fibrous histiocytoma (fibroxanthoma)

These rare lesions do not require radiotherapy.

18.4.3
Embryonal Mesenchymal and Muscular Lesions

- Embryonal sarcoma
- Rhabdomyosarcoma

These are primary tumors of orbital tissue, which may involve the conjunctiva. Sometimes the conjunctival involvement is the first symptom of a rhabdomyosarcoma. Combined treatment with radiotherapy and chemotherapy without radical surgical excision is the treatment of choice. Details are discussed in Chap. 13 on orbital tumors.

18.4.4
Vascular Lesions

18.4.4.1
Benign

- Telangiectasia
- Hemangioma
- Lymphangioma

Radiation therapy is not indicated in the treatment of telangiectasia. Isolated hemangiomas and lymphangiomas of the conjunctiva are extremely rare lesions. Radiotherapy may be required if local excision is impossible.

18.4.4.2
Malignant

Hemangiosarcoma (Kaposi's sarcoma) is the only known malignant vascular tumor of the conjunctiva. In the past, Kaposi's sarcoma was an uncommon disease that was usually limited to the skin on the legs of elderly patients. Ophthalmologists have recently become aware of this tumor which can affect the conjunctiva in patients suffering from acquired immunodeficiency syndrome (AIDS) (LOMMATZSCH 1999b; REICH et al. 1985). HOWARD et al. (1975) were the first to describe a case that responded satisfactorily to radiotherapy with 41 Gy. Later COOPER and FRIED (1988) reported on successful radiotherapy of an aggressive epidemic of Kaposi's sarcoma of the conjunctiva. Within 6 weeks after 30 Gy (94 kV, superficial X-ray machine) a pea-sized nodule under the left eyelid had disappeared completely, with no side-effects. KIROVA et al. (1998) successfully treated 362 patients with eyelid and conjunctival lesions using 20 Gy.

18.4.5
Neural Lesions

18.4.5.1
Benign

- Neurofibroma
- Neurofibromatosis
- Neurolemmoma (Schwannoma)

18.4.5.2
Malignant

- Malignant neurolemmoma (malignant Schwannoma)
- Others

We know of no experience of radiotherapy in these extremely rare tumors.

18.5
Hamartomas and Choristomas

These malformations are characterized by the formation of tissues that closely resemble skin with its associated dermal components. They are called dermoid tumors, dermolipoma, epibulbar osseous choristoma, or complex choristoma. There is no reason for radiotherapy. Local excision, if necessary, is the treatment of choice.

18.6
Tumors and Tumor-like Lesions of Hematopoietic or Lymphoid Tissue

Diagnostic procedures and classification of lymphoproliferative lesions according to the Revised European American Lymphoma Classification (R.E.A.L.) of 1994 have been discussed in detail by COUPLAND and STEIN (1999). The conjunctiva can be involved by many benign or malignant lymphoid lesions. They are typically apparent as a salmon-colored, subconjunctival infiltrate. Differentiation between benign and malignant lymphoid lesions can be very difficult, and often a distinction cannot be made at all (MORGAN and HARRY 1978).

Preexisting systemic lymphoma can be expected in approximately 10% of cases (CHAR 1989). All patients with conjunctival lymphoid lesions should undergo a general examination, including complete blood count, plasma protein electrophoresis, body computed tomography (CT), and bone marrow examination.

It is rare for any of these different tumors and tumor-like lesions of the hematopoietic or lymphoid tissue to be confined to the conjunctiva. Usually they involve the orbit and lids, and they are sometimes part of a generalized disease. In any case, all lymphatic tumors are highly radiosensitive. Radiotherapy is, then, an effective procedure either for local treatment or for local palliative treatment of patients with generalization of tumor cells (Fig. 18.5).

The extent of possible orbital involvement can be reliably shown by CT or ultrasound examination. Radiotherapy of the anterior part of the orbit, including the conjunctiva and lids, with protection of the eyeball, can be performed using high-energy electrons (for radiation technique, see Chap. 24). With 30–40 Gy, complete regression can be achieved in nearly all cases without serious side effects (LOMMATZSCH et al.

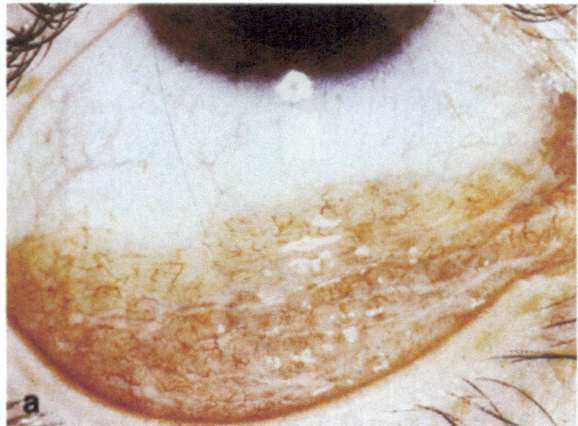

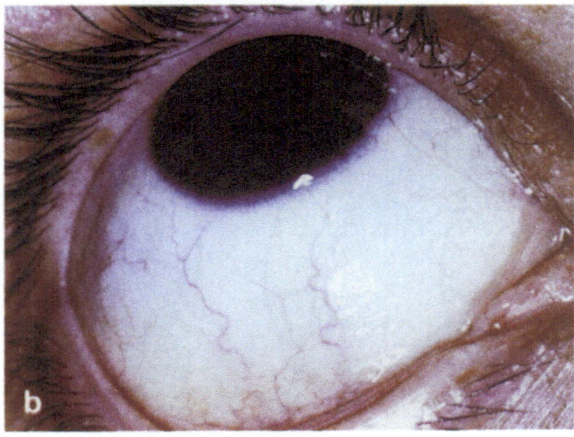

Fig. 18.5. a Reactive lymphoid hyperplasia in a 30-year-old woman. b Two years after radiotherapy (betatron, l6MeV, special eye tube with lens protection, 8 Gy)

1982). In benign lymphoid lesions that involve a diffuse area, low-dose irradiation with shielding of cornea and lens can be used successfully.

18.7
Inflammatory Tumor-like Lesions

• Chalazion
• "Hemangioma" of granulation tissue type (granuloma pyogenicum)
• Nodular fasciitis
• Amyloid and paramyloid deposits
• Vernal, ligneous, papillary, and other forms of conjunctivitis

These lesions should not be treated primarily with radiotherapy. In most cases corticosteroids are sufficient. Beta irradiation can be used in some tenacious cases of vernal conjunctivitis. High doses should not be delivered, because such side-effects as fibroplastic

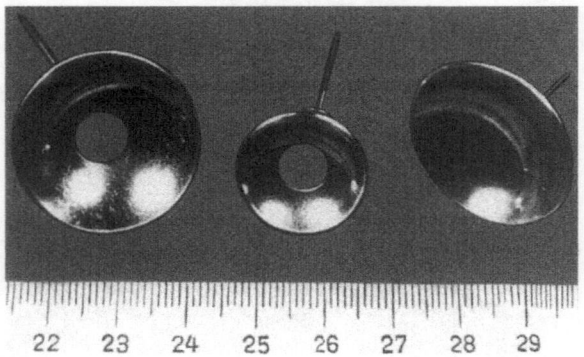

Fig. 18.6. Different kinds of concave ^{90}Sr/^{90}Y ophthalmic applicators (Isocommerz, Berlin-Buch, Germany)

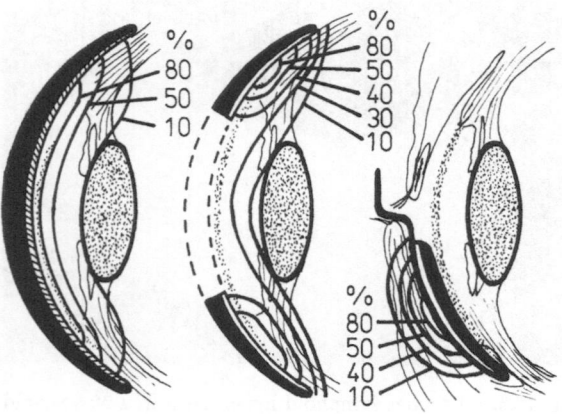

Fig. 18.7. Isodose curves of ^{90}Sr/^{90}Y eye applicators

scars and atrophy of the palpebral conjunctiva will later cause unpleasant complications.

18.8
Procedure of Beta Ray Treatment

Brachytherapy of conjunctival tumors can be performed with beta rays from radioactive strontium (^{90}Sr/^{90}Y) or ruthenium (^{106}Ru/^{106}Rh).

We use applicators of various shapes and sizes to cover the whole tumor as completely as possible. After local anesthesia of the conjunctiva, the applicator is placed directly .on the tumor. Depending on the applicator type, it is fixed with strings or supported by the doctor's hand during the radiation period of a few seconds per session. A lucite shield protects the radiotherapist against beta ray exposure.

In the case of melanoma the daily dose applied at the tumor surface should be 10 Gy until a total dose of 150 or 200 Gy has been delivered, depending on the thickness of the neoplasm. Epithelial tumors will regress after lower doses ranging between 100 and 150 Gy.

In patients with a localized tumor at the corneal limbus, we prefer a pestle-shaped applicator with a plane irradiation surface. For extended flat lesions of the conjunctiva we use concave applicators (Figs. 18.6–18.8). Irradiation times for the application of a single dose of 10 Gy may range from 40 s to 10 min, depending on the activity of the applicator. The tumors are irradiated with a single daily dose of 10 Gy to obtain a favorable protraction effect.

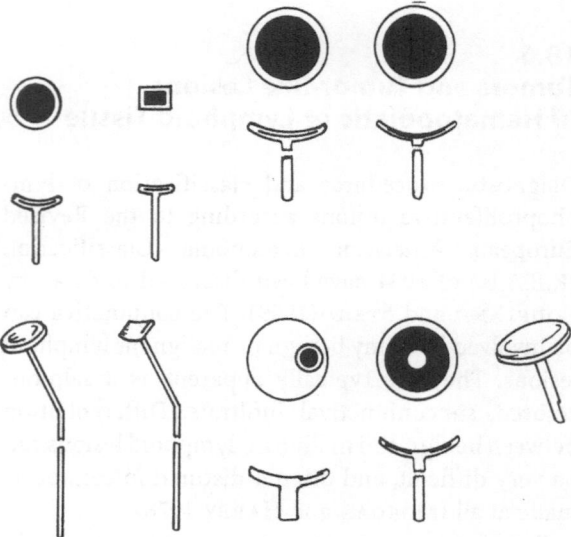

Fig. 18.8. ^{90}Sr/^{90}Y ophthalmic applicators (The Radiochemical Centre, Amersham, Bucks., UK)

References

Brownstein S (1980) Mucoepidermoid carcinoma of the conjunctiva with intraocular invasion. Ophthalmology 88:1226–1230

Cameron ME (1972) Preventable complications of pterygium excision with beta-irradiation. Br J Ophthalmol 56:52–56

Cerezo L, Otero J, Aragöu G, Polo E, de la Torre A, Valcárcel F, Magallön R (1989) Conjunctival intraepithelial and invasive squamous cell carcinoma treated with strontium-90. Radiother Oncol 17:191–197

Char DH (1989) Clinical ocular oncology. Churchill Livingstone, New York, pp 63–87

Clark WH, Folberg AM (1979) Tumor progression in primary human cutaneous malignant melanomas. In: Clark WH Jr (ed) Human malignant melanoma. Grune & Stratton, New York, pp 15–31

Cooper JS, Fried PR (1988) Treatment of aggressive epidemic Kaposi's sarcoma of the conjunctiva by radiotherapy. Arch Ophthalmol 106:20–21

Coupland SE, Stein H (1999) Lymphoproliferative Läsionen der okulären Adnexe. In: Lommatzsch PK (ed) Ophthalmologische Onkologie. Enke, Stuttgart, pp 107–123

David E, Constable WC (1979) The use of strontium-90 in the treatment of carcinoma in situ of the conjunctiva. Am J Ophthalmol 87:84–86

DePotter P, Shields CL, Shields JA (1993) Clinical predictive factors for development of recurrences and metastasis in conjunctival melanoma: a review of 68 cases. Br J Ophthalmol 77:624–630

De Wolff-Rouendaal D (1990) Conjunctival melanoma in the Netherlands: a clinico-pathological and follow-up study. Thesis, Leiden

De Wolff-Rouendaal D (1999) Konjunktivales Melanom. In: Lommatzsch PK (ed) Ophthalmologische Onkologie. Stuttgart, Enke, pp 88–95

Dutton JJ, Anderson RL, Tse DT (1984) Combined surgery and cryotherapy for scleral invasion of epithelial malignancies. Ophthalmic Surg 15:289–294

Elkon D, Constable WC (1979) The use of strontium-90 in the treatment of carcinoma in situ of the conjunctiva. Am J Ophthalmol 87:84–86

Farrell PLR, Smith RE (1989) Bacteria! corneoscleritis complicating pterygium excision. Am J Ophthalmol 107:515–517

Folberg R, McLean IW, Zimmerman LE (1985) Malignant melanoma of the conjunctiva. Hum Pathol 16:136–143

Fraunfelder ET, Wingfield D (1983) Management of intraepithelial conjunctival tumors and squamous cell carcinomas. Am J Ophthalmol 95:359–363

Haberle H, Pham DT, Scholman HJ, Wollensak J (1995) Ruthenium 105-applicator for radiation treatment of carcinoma in situ of the cornea and conjunctiva. Ophthalmologe 92:866–869

Henkind P (1978) Conjunctival melanocytic lesions: natural history. In: Jakobiec FA (ed) Ocular and adnexal tumors. Aesculapius, Birmingham, Ala, pp 572–582

Hilgers JM (1960) Prevention of recurrent pterygium by beta-radiation. Ophthalmologica 140:369–379

Howard GM, Jakobiec FA, De Voe A (1975) Kaposi's sarcoma of the conjunctiva. Am J Ophthalmol 79:420

Hwang IP, Jordan DR, Brownstein S, Gilberg SM, McEachren TM, Prokopetz R (2000) Mucoepidermoid carcinoma of the conjunctiva: a series of three cases. Ophthalmology 107:801–805

Iliff WJ, Marback R, Green WR (1975) Invasive squamous cell carcinoma of the conjunctiva. Arch Ophthalmol 93:119–122

Jakobiec FA (1981) Conjunctival melanoma: unfinished business. Arch Ophthalmol 98:1378–1384

Kirova YM, Belembaogo E, Frikha H, Haddad E, Calitchi E, Levy E, Piedbois P, Le Bourgeois JP (1998) Radiotherapy in the management of epidemic Kaposi's sarcoma: a retrospective study of 643 cases. Radiother Oncol 46:19–22

Kleis W, Pico G (1973) Thio-TEPA therapy to prevent postoperative pterygium occurrence and neovascularization. Am J Ophthalmol 76:371–374

Lederman M (1972) Radiotherapy. In: Sorsby A (ed) Modern ophthalmology, 2nd edn, vol 4. Butterworths, London, pp 887–900

Lommatzsch PK (1976) Beta-ray treatment of malignant epithelial tumors of the conjunctiva. Am J Ophthalmol [A] 1:198–206

Lommatzsch PK (1978) Beta-ray treatment of malignant epibulbar melanoma. Albrecht v Graefes Arch Klin Exp Ophthalmol 209:111–124

Lommatzsch PK (1999a) Tumoren der Bindehaut. Epitheliale Tumoren. In: Lommatzsch PK (ed) Ophthalmologische Onkologie. Enke, Stuttgart, pp 73–81

Lommatzsch PK (1999b) Tumoren der Bindehaut. Maligne Tumoren. In: Lommatzsch PK (ed) Ophthalmologische Onkologie. Enke, Stuttgart, pp 99–101

Lommatzsch PK, Fürst G, Vollmar R, Schmidt H (1977) Die therapeutische Anwendung von ionisierenden Strahlen in der Augenheilkunde. In: Velhagen K (ed) Der Augenarzt, 1st edn, vol 4. Thieme, Leipzig

Lommatzsch PK, Welker KE, Hüttner J, Bauke G (1982) Die Anwendung von hochenergetischen Elektronen bei der Behandlung von malignen Orbitatumoren. Klin Monatsbl Augenheilkd 180:198–202

Lommatzsch PK, Lommatzsch RE, Kirsch I, Fuhrmann P (1990) Therapeutic outcome of patients suffering from malignant melanomas of the conjunctiva. Br J Ophthalmol 74:615–619

Morgan G, Harry J (1978) Lymphocytic tumours of indeterminate nature. A 5-year follow-up of 98 conjunctival and orbital lesions. Br J Ophthalmol 62:381–383

Paridaens ADA, Minassian DC, McCartney ACE, Hungerford JL (1994) Prognostic factors in primary malignant melanoma of the conjunctiva: a clinicopathological study of 256 cases. Br J Ophthalmol 78:252–259

Pizarello LD, Jakobiec FA (1978) Bowen's disease of the conjunctiva: a misnomer. In: Jakobiec FA (ed) Ocular and adnexal tumors. Aesculapius, Birmingham, Ala, p 553

Reese AB (1976) Tumors of the eye, 3rd edn. Harper & Row, Hagerstown

Reich H, Hollwich F, Uthoff D (1985) Kaposi-Sarkom und AIDS. Klin Monatsbl Augenheilkd 187:1–8

Spencer WH, Zimmerman LE (1985) Conjunctiva. In: Spencer WH (ed) Ophthalmic pathology. An atlas and textbook, vol 1. Saunders, Philadelphia, pp 192–220

Stannard CE, Sealy GR, Hering ER, Pereira SB, Knowles R, Hill JC (2000) Malignant melanoma of the eyelid and palpebral conjunctiva treated with iodine-125 brachytherapy. Ophthalmology 107:951–958

Sterker I, Lommatzsch P (1993) Results of treatment in malignant epithelial conjunctival tumors. Ophthalmologe 90:62–65

Sundmacher R, Mackensen G (1988) Chirurgie der Konjunktiva und der Sklera. In: Mackensen G, Neubauer H (eds) Augenärztliche Operation, vol 1. Springer, Berlin Heidelberg New York, pp 333–382

Tarr KH, Constable IJ (1980) Late complications of pterygium treatment. Br J Ophthalmol 64:496–505

Thiel HJ (1979) Die Anwendung von Beta-Strahlern bei nichttumorösen Prozessen des vorderen Augenabschnittes. Ophthalmol Ges 76:283–288

Werschnik C, Lommatzsch PK (1998) Mitomycin C bei der Behandlung von Bindehautmelanomen und primär erworbenen Melanosen. Klin Monatsbl Augenheilkd 212:465–469

Werschnik C, Lommatzsch PK (2001) Long-term follow-up of patients with conjunctival melanoma. Am J Clin Oncol (in press) (presented in part by Lommatzsch PK at the International Congress for Ocular Oncology in Philadelphia 1999)

Zimmerman LE (1978) The histogenesis of conjunctival melanomas. In: Jakobiec FA (ed) Ocular and adnexal tumors. Aesculapius, Birmingham, Ala, pp 572–582

Zimmerman LE, Sobin LH (1980) International histological classification of tumours, vol 24: Histological typing of tumours of the eye and its adnexa. World Health Organization, Geneva

19 Epithelial Tumors of the Lacrimal Gland and Lacrimal Sac

R. H. Sagerman and M. Isaac

CONTENTS

19.1 Introduction

Tumors of the lacrimal gland are not common, and those of the nasolacrimal sac are rare. These two anatomic regions are affected by histologically different lesions and will be considered separately. Lymphoid tumors account for almost half of lacrimal gland malignancies and are reviewed in Chap. 17.

Treatment for tumors at both sites has been overwhelmingly surgical. We will review the limited radiotherapeutic experience, present our experience pointing to a potentially greater role for radiotherapy for lacrimal sac tumors, and refer the reader to Char (1989a, b), Font and Gamel (1978), Font et al. (1998), Forrest (1979), Henderson (1973), Reese (1976a, b), and Shields (1989) for more extensive discussions of differential diagnosis, histology, and surgery.

R.H. Sagerman, MD
SUNY Upstate Medical University, Department of Radiation Oncology, 750E. Adams Street, Syracuse, NY 13210, USA
M. Isaac, MD
SUNY Upstate Medical University, Department of Radiation Oncology, 750E. Adams Street, Syracuse, NY 13210, USA

19.2 Lacrimal Gland Tumors

19.2.1 Histology

Approximately 50% of lacrimal gland masses are epithelial, and about half of these are malignant. Recognizing the histologic similarity, Forrest (1954) and Zimmerman et al. (1962) applied the classification of salivary gland tumors (Foote and Frazell 1953) to lacrimal gland tumors. Font and Gamel (1978) were able to gather 265 cases whose distribution is shown in Table 19.1. Transformation from benign mixed tumor to malignant tumor has been reported (Perzin et al. 1980).

19.2.2 Clinical Presentation and Evaluation

Lacrimal gland tumors occur in adults, usually when they are between 20 and 70 years old (mean ~40 years), and are slightly more frequent in males (57% vs 43%). Pain has been found to be more frequent in malignant than in benign mixed tumors (31% vs 11%, respectively), and the latent period before diag-

Table 19.1. Reported lacrimal gland tumors. (*BMT* benign mixed tumor; Font and Gamel 1978)

Histopathologic diagnosis	No. of cases	Percentage of cases
BMT	136	51
Adenoid cystic carcinoma		
Arising de novo	70	27
Arising in BMT	9	3
Adenocarcinoma		
Arising de novo	19	7
Arising in BMT	25	9
Mucoepidermoid carcinoma	4	2
Miscellaneous carcinomas	2	1
Total	**265**	**100**

nosis to be longer for benign mixed tumors (FONT and GAMEL 1978). Bone destruction occurs with malignant but not benign tumors (CHAR 1989a). Magnetic resonance imaging (MRI) and thin-section computed tomography (CT) are valuable in documenting the primary lesion, its extensions, and resultant bone destruction or erosion (Fig. 19.1).

19.2.3
Management

Benign mixed tumors should be excised completely and without prior biopsy. The recurrence rate was 3% when the capsule was intact, but rose to 32% when biopsy preceded excision. The recurrence rate was 30% at 15 years, reflecting varying degrees of tumor removal, and malignant degeneration occurred in about 20% (FONT and GAMEL 1978). Recurrences were difficult to control, 70% recurring a second time within the next 15 years (FONT and GAMEL 1978). This suggests a poten-

tial role for irradiation, in an attempt to decrease recurrence when excision with an intact capsule has not been effected; this would be similar to its role in treatment for salivary gland tumors (GARDEN et al. 1995; MCNANEY et al. 1983; SAGERMAN 1984).

Treatment for malignant lesions has been unsatisfactory because few patients were suitable for local resection (WRIGHT 1982), because of extension to the central nervous system, and because distant metastases can appear even many years later. The 15-year survival was only 10% for adenoid cystic carcinoma (MARSH et al. 1981).

There are no large or prospective studies to document the role of irradiation. LEE et al. (1985) did not find radiotherapy to affect the course of adenoid cystic carcinoma. BRADA and HENK (1987) reported a median 10.4-year cause-specific survival in 33 patients irradiated following surgery. Tumor control was related to histology, extent of surgery, and radiation dose. All patients with adenocarcinoma, undif-

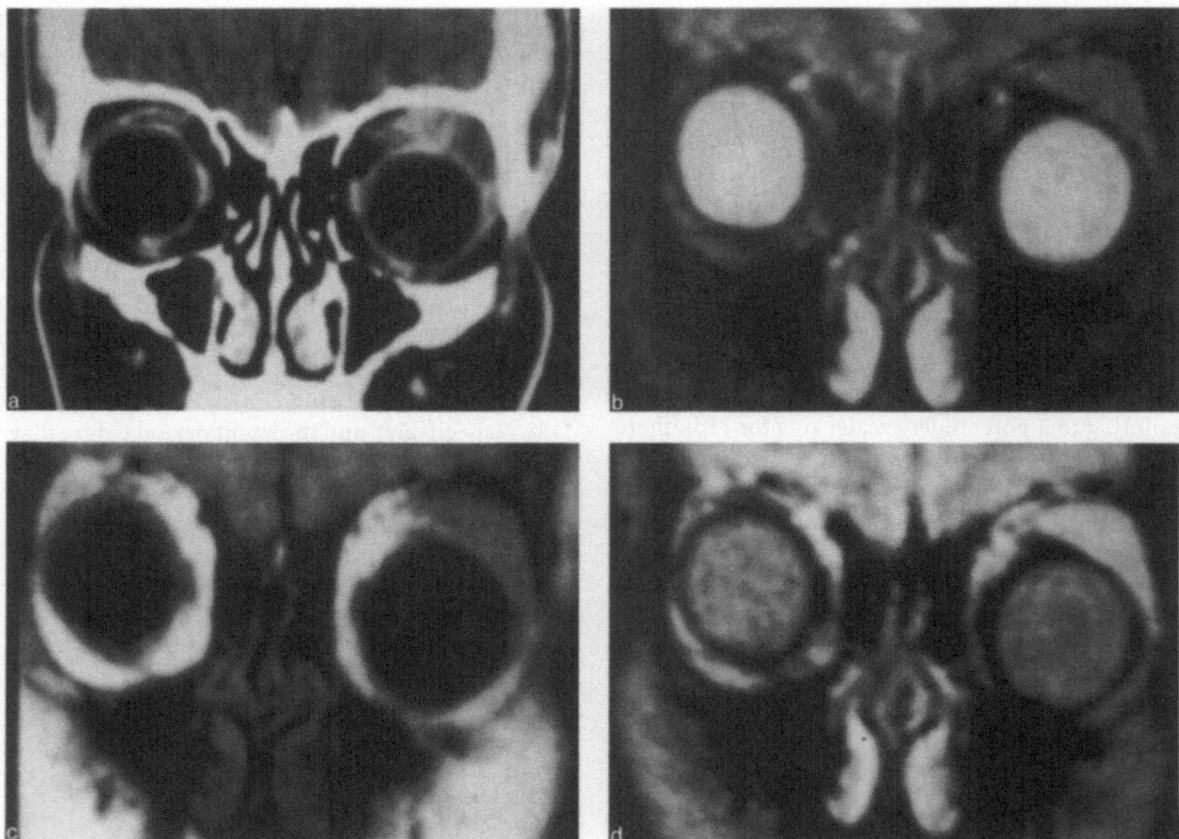

Fig. 19.1a–d. Mixed tumor of the lacrimal gland (courtesy of L. St. Louis). **a** Enhanced coronal CT scan. The left lacrimal gland is diffusely enlarged and causing downward proptosis. Enhancement is homogeneous but the gland is obscured by streak artifact from bone. **b–d** Coronal MRI spin-echo images: **b** T1 weighting (500/30), **c** spin density weighting (2000/30), and **d** T2 weighting (2000/90) show a homogeneous, diffusely enlarged lacrimal gland. Signal intensity is similar to that of gray matter in all sequences

ferentiated carcinoma, and malignant mixed tumor remained disease free following complete excision and adjuvant radiotherapy, but only 1 of 13 achieved local control if resection was incomplete. However, 7 of 13 patients with adenoid cystic carcinoma irradiated after incomplete resection were disease free. These authors used a beam-direction shell with a central block shielding the cornea, lens, and posterior retina, with the patient supine and receiving 60–65 Gy at 2 Gy daily or 50–55 Gy in 15–18 fractions of 3.1–3.3 Gy on alternate days. Visual deterioration attributed to irradiation occurred in 21% of patients who remained disease free.

19.3
Lacrimal Sac Tumors

19.3.1
Histology, Anatomy, Radiosensitivity

Tumors of the lacrimal sac were first reported in 1772. CHAR (1989b) estimated that some 300 cases had been reported. The majority of the 157 cases we found in the English-language literature were malignant, and 107 were of epithelial origin (Table 19.2). The most common lacrimal sac malignancies include squamous cell, transitional cell, and mucoepidermoid carcinoma, and melanoma. Involvement of the skin and conjunctiva is common, and bone destruction and extension into the sinuses may occur. The lymphatic drainage is to the submaxillary, deep parotid, preauricular, and upper cervical nodes.

The membranous lacrimal passages extend from the superior and inferior canaliculi to the lacrimal sac and through the nasolacrimal duct. Fear of radiation closing this passage has limited its use in treating tumors arising at this site. While stricture and obstruction may

Table 19.2. Reported nasolacrimal sac tumors

Authors	Year	No of tumors	Epithelial
DUKE-ELDER	1952	91	54
JONES	1956	6	3
SPAETH	1957	7	7
HARRY and ASHTON	1968	11	6
RYAN and FONT	1973	27	27
SCHENCK et al.	1973	10	6
Others[a]	1967–1978	5	4

[a]FLANAGAN and STOKES (1978), GRIFFITH (1967), MILDER and SMITH (1968), PAXTON et al. (1970)

follow irradiation, we believe this usually reflects the extent of tumor involvement, deep tumor extensions, and pre-existing damage. When the passages are patent at the initiation of therapy, they will usually remain patent, and the need for surgical repair or the placement of a stent has been rare in our experience with cancers arising in the skin, conjunctiva, sinuses, and orbit in which no shielding of the passages was employed (FITZPATRICK, Chap. 17 of this volume).

The radiation sensitivity of the membranous lacrimal tract was studied by dacroscintigraphy in 26 patients after irradiation, which was given for eyelid lesions in most cases (BRIZEL et al. 1975). Lid lesions received 5,200–5,400 R (air exposure with backscatter) divided into daily fractions over 3 weeks with a beam quality of 1–3 mm Al half-value layer. The entire orbit was treated with 20–40 Gy in 2–4 weeks, with megavoltage irradiation in 5 patients. Epiphora did not develop in any patient in whom it was not present originally. Severe epiphora with complete obstruction was present in 3 patients before irradiation; epiphora decreased in 2 of them after treatment. Three patients with mild to moderate epiphora before treatment had normal transit times and anatomy afterwards. Epiphora decreased in 4 of 6 patients after irradiation and did not increase in any patient. Similarly, 6 patients without epiphora maintained normal anatomy and tear transit time after irradiation.

19.3.2
Clinical Presentation and Evaluation

A high degree of suspicion is necessary to establish the diagnosis of a lacrimal sac tumor; initially, most patients are thought to have chronic dacryocystitis. Epiphora is a cardinal symptom, and bleeding may occur spontaneously or follow probing. A mass both above and below the medial canthal tendon is more suggestive of malignancy than inflammation.

In addition to history and physical examination, MRI and/or CT should be obtained. Dacryocystography can demonstrate the appearance, patency, and function of the drainage system (MILDER and DEMOREST 1954). Biopsy is required to establish the histologic diagnosis.

SPRATT (1940) identified three clinical stages, and JONES (1956) delineated four stages. In the earliest stage epiphora was present but the diagnosis was not suspected. The presence of a mass suggested the diagnosis in the intermediate stage(s) and extension beyond the sac made the diagnosis obvious in stage 3 or 4.

19.3.3
Management

Surgery remains the treatment of choice for malignant epithelial lacrimal sac tumors. The minimal procedure recommended includes removal of the upper and lower lacrimal canaliculi, lacrimal sac, nasolacrimal duct, bony lacrimal fossa, and surrounding ethmoid air cells (MILDER and WEIL 1983; SCHENCK et al. 1973). Dacryocystectomy is thought to be insufficient because these tumors have a propensity for diffuse mucosal involvement (PAXTON et al. 1970). Consequently, dacryocystectomy alone, without excision of the lacrimal canaliculi or nasolacrimal duct, carries the risk of an incomplete resection since there may be unsuspected involvement of these structures. Treatment should be individualized, and larger tumors may require exenteration (NAUGLE et al. 1994). RYAN and FONT (1973) cautioned against an overly aggressive surgical procedure in the elderly patient owing to their finding of a favorable prognosis for survival with lacrimal sac tumors.

When irradiation has been utilized, it has usually been given postoperatively after incomplete removal or when surgery has been rejected. Preoperative irradiation has been recommended by some authors (MILDER and WEIL 1983; SCHENCK et al. 1973).

Chemotherapy has not been studied adequately in this rare tumor (GOLDBERG 1998). Neoadjuvant intra-arterial chemotherapy has been given safely in 2 patients with extensive adenocystic carcinoma of the lacrimal gland, leading to downstaging prior to orbital exenteration, which was followed by orbital irradiation with long-term survival (MELDRUM et al. 1998).

It is difficult to draw any general conclusions on the results of treatment for epithelial malignancies of the lacrimal sac because of its rarity, the paucity of treatment details, and the short and incomplete follow-up in most cases. However, local recurrence is an acknowledged problem. A factor postulated to have a role in the development of local recurrence is the tendency for diffuse mucosal involvement, possibly secondary to multicentric foci of origin, or existence of a "field effect" (PAXTON et al. 1970). In addition, the true diagnosis is often established only after limited surgery undertaken for a "benign problem" (BOUZAS 1961; DUKE-ELDER 1952; SPRATT 1973). The 5-year local recurrence rate approximates 50% (RYAN and FONT 1973; SPAETH 1969). SPAETH (1969) reported that more than 50% of patients with recurrent primary epithelial carcinoma of the lacrimal sac died within 5 years.

Owing to the rarity of the disease and to incomplete follow-up, 5-year survival data are difficult to elucidate; however, the most favorable results quote 85% alive and well at 5 years postoperatively (FLANAGAN and STOKES 1978). Distant metastases appear most often in regional lymph nodes in the neck and in the lung (SCHENCK et al. 1973). In the literature reports, however, patients dying of tumor have usually died from uncontrolled local recurrence.

We have treated four patients with epithelial lacrimal sac malignancy with a definitive course of irradiation and have identified an important role for radiotherapy (SAGERMAN et al. 1991). There were two anaplastic carcinomas, one squamous cell carcinoma, and one mucoepidermoid carcinoma. Local tumor control was achieved in each patient. Two patients with anaplastic carcinoma developed metastatic cervical, but not preauricular or submaxillary, adenopathy, and the nodes were controlled with a second course of irradiation. The metastatic adenopathy appeared within 1 month in the patient with anaplastic carcinoma, and he died 26 months after starting radiotherapy, with widespread metastases but with tumor in the neck and primary site under control. Two patients died without recurrence at 11 and 17 years. The patient with mucoepidermoid carcinoma was lost to follow-up after 5 years of freedom from recurrence or metastasis.

The following case report illustrates several aspects that need consideration when irradiation is used. A 49-year-old white female patient presented with chronic dacryocystitis and epiphora OD, which did not resolve with antibiotic treatment. A 3-cm, round, elevated mass developed in the inner canthus, and the eye was displaced to the right (Fig. 19.2a). Vision and ocular motion were intact. There was no adenopathy. Computed tomography demonstrated a mass in the orbit without bone destruction (Fig. 19.3a). Biopsy revealed a mixed transitional cell and squamous cell carcinoma.

An operation was proposed but was unacceptable to the patient. She received 60 Gy in 30 fractions (fx) at 4 cm depth through an anterior 4-MV X-ray field with the cornea shielded. An electron boost of 6 Gy/2 fx was delivered to residual nodular disease. The tumor resolved 3 weeks after completion of irradiation (Figs. 19.2b, 19.3b).

A 4-cm mass developed below the right mandibular angle 8 months later. Biopsy revealed poorly differentiated carcinoma consistent with the original lesion. The uninvolved neck received 50 Gy, the nodal mass was boosted to 63.5 Gy, and the mass resolved.

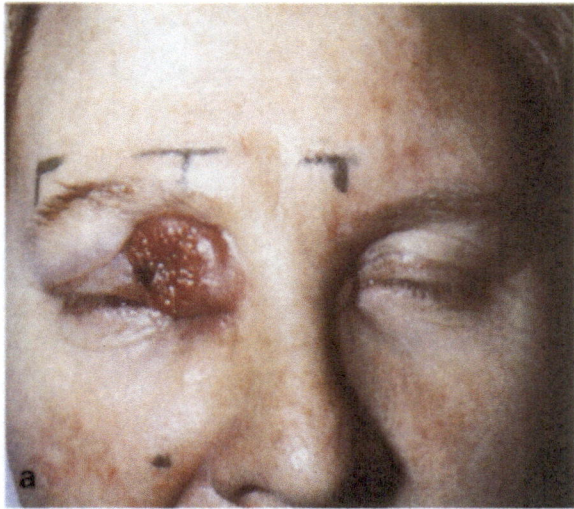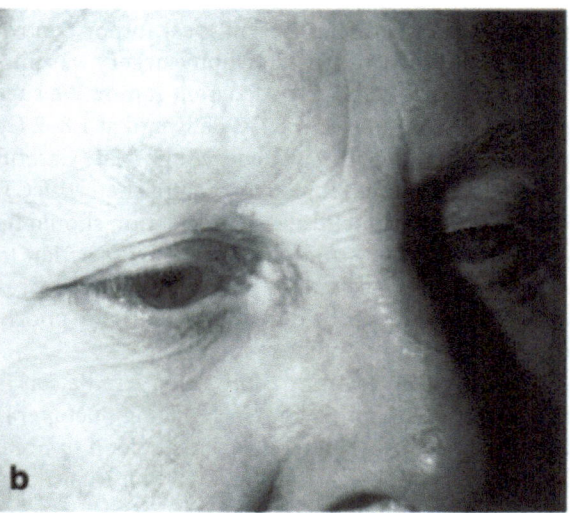

Fig. 19.2. a Medial canthal mass OD with ulceration and soft tissue swelling at the initiation of radiotherapy. The globe was pushed laterally. **b** Appearance 6 years after irradiation. Note mild hypopigmentation and telangiectasia. Lashes are present. The nasolacrimal system drained tears adequately and there was no overflow

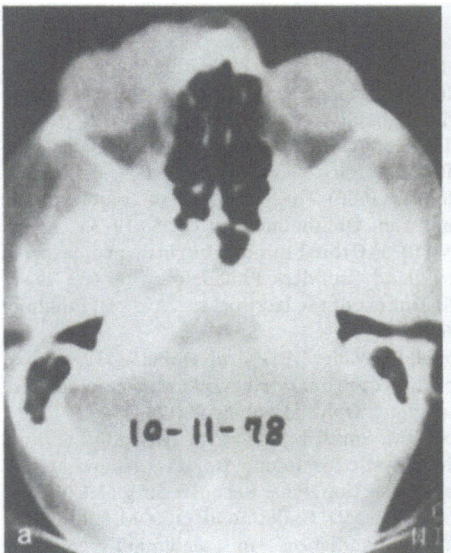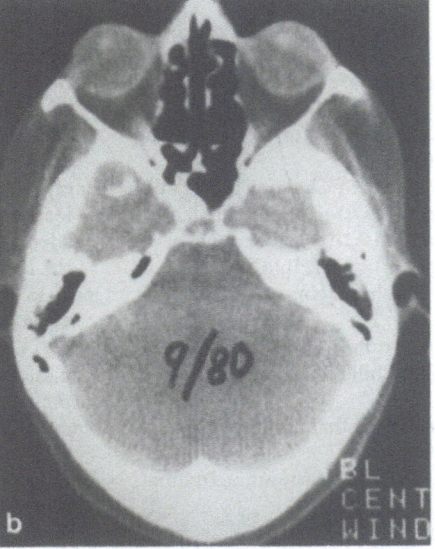

Fig. 19.3. a Pretreatment CT scan (10-11-78). Medical and posterior extension can be seen and there is clouding of the air spaces. **b** CT scan almost 2 years after therapy. The mass has resolved, the air spaces are aerated, and the small residual soft tissue density has been attributed to fibrosis, as there has been no further change in the ensuing 10 years

Blurred vision OD, with finger counting at 1 m and a positive afferent defect developed at 6 1/2 years. Acuity was 6/9 at 1 m OS. An old central retinal vein occlusion with secondary macular degeneration was seen ophthalmoscopically (Fig. 19.4). Photocoagulation was performed to prevent bleeding and further loss of vision.

This woman died 17 years after completing irradiation to the right eye, with no clinical or radiographic evidence of cancer and with no further change in vision.

19.4
Summary

We foresee a definite role for irradiation in the management of epithelial malignancies of the lacrimal sac when surgical extirpation cannot be accomplished and in the presence of locoregional tumor recurrence. Irradiation should be used postoperatively after incomplete resection or tumor spill. Preoperative irradiation and planned subtotal removal with postoperative irradiation do not seem worthwhile in view of the long-term local tumor control achieved in three patients in whom surgery was limited to biopsy or who had recurrent tumor. We suggest a tumor dose of 55–65 Gy, delivered at 1.8–2 Gy per fraction with megavoltage equipment. Careful treatment planning should be accomplished with CT, and beam quality, field size, and direction should be chosen to encompass the entire lesion with a view to sparing cornea, lens and retina. Elective nodal irradiation should be considered, especially for poorly differentiated carcinomas.

Similar considerations apply when irradiation is recommended in an attempt at reducing postoperative recurrence for epithelial lacrimal gland tumors. Primary radiation therapy has a proven role in the treatment of lymphoma of the orbit.

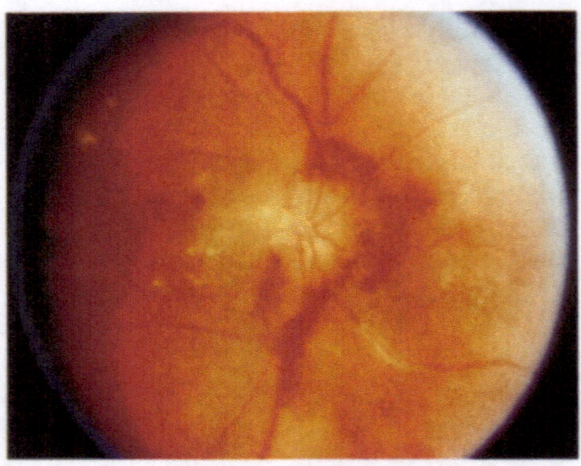

Fig. 19.4. Appearance of the retina 6 1/2 years after irradiation, demonstrating the central retinal vein occlusion. Analysis demonstrated the dose at the disk had been approximately 68 Gy/31 fractions at 2.2 Gy/fraction

References

Bouzas A (1961) Polyps of the lacrimal sac. Arch Ophthalmol 66:236–240

Brada M, Henk JM (1987) Radiotherapy for lacrimal gland tumors. Radiother Oncol 9:175–183

Brizel HE, Sheils WC, Brown M (1975) The effects of radiotherapy on the nasolacrimal system as evaluated by dacroscintigraphy. Radiology 116:373–381

Char DH (1989a) Lacrimal gland tumors. In: Char DH (ed) Clinical ocular oncology. Churchill Livingstone, New York, pp 305–318

Char DH (1989b) Lacrimal sac tumors. In: Char DH (ed) Clinical ocular oncology. Churchill Livingstone, New York, pp 319–322

Duke-Elder S (1952) Textbook of ophthalmology, vol V: The ocular adnexa. Mosby, St. Louis

Flanagan JC, Stokes DP (1978) Lacrimal sac tumors. Ophthalmology 85:1282–1287

Font RL, Gamel JW (1978) Epithelial tumors of the lacrimal gland: an analysis of 265 cases. In: Jakobiec FA (ed) Ocular and adnexal tumors. Aesculapius, Birmingham, Ala, pp 787–805

Font RL, Smith SL, Bryan RG (1998) Malignant epithelial tumors of the lacrimal gland: a clinicopathologic study of 21 cases. Arch Ophthalmol 116:613–616

Foote FW Jr, Frazell EL (1953) Tumors of the major salivary glands. Cancer 6:1065–1133

Forrest AW (1954) Epithelial lacrimal gland tumors: pathology as a guide to prognosis. Trans Am Acad Ophthalmol Otolaryngol 58:848–866

Forrest AW (1979) Lacrimal gland tumors. In: Jones IS, Jakobiec FA (eds) Disease of the orbit. Harper & Row, Hagerstown, Md, pp 355–370

Garden AS, Weber RS, Morrison WH et al (1995) The influence of positive margins and nerve invasion in adenoid cystic carcinoma of the head and neck treated with surgery and radiation. Int J Radiat Oncol Biol Phys 32:619–626

Goldberg RA (1998) Intra-arterial chemotherapy: a welcome new idea for the management of adenocystic carcinoma of the lacrimal gland. Arch Ophthalmol 116:372–373

Griffith BH (1967) Squamous cell carcinoma of the lacrimal sac. Plast Reconstr Surg 40:332–336

Harry J, Ashton N (1968) The pathology of tumors of the lacrimal sac. Trans Ophthalmol Soc UK 88:19–35

Henderson JW (1973) Orbital tumors: Intrinsic neoplasms of the lacrimal gland. Saunders, Philadelphia, pp 409–443

Jones IS (1956) Tumors of the lacrimal sac. Am J Ophthalmol 42:561–566

Lee DA, Campbell RJ, Waller RR, Ilstrup DM (1985) A clinicopathologic study of primary adenoid cystic carcinoma of the lacrimal gland. Ophthalmology 92:128–134

Marsh JL, Wise DM, Smith M, Schwartz H (1981) Lacrimal gland adenoid cystic carcinoma: intracranial and extracranial en bloc resection. Plast Reconstr Surg 68:577–585

McNaney E, McNeese MD, Guillamondegui OM et al (1983) Post-operative irradiation in malignant epithelial tumours of the parotid. Int J Radiat Oncol Biol Phys 9:1289–1295

Meldrum ML, Tse DT, Benedetto P (1998) Neoadjuvant intracarotid chemotherapy for treatment of advanced adenocystic carcinoma of the lacrimal gland. Arch Ophthalmol 116:315–321

Milder B, Demorest BH (1954) Dacryocystography. Arch Ophthalmol 51:180–195

Milder B, Smith ME (1968) Carcinoma of lacrimal sac. Am J Ophthalmol 65:782–784

Milder B, Weil BA (1983) The lacrimal system. Appleton-Century-Crofts, Norwalk, Conn, pp 145–149

Naugle T, Tepper DJ, Haik BG (1994) Adenoid cystic carcinoma of the lacrimal gland: a case report. Ophthalmic Plast Reconstr Surg 10:45–48

Paxton BR, Davidorf FH, Makley TA (1970) Carcinoma of lacrimal canaliculi and lacrimal sac. Arch Ophthalmol 84:749–753

Perzin KH, Jakobiec FA, Livolsi VA, Desjardins L (1980) Lacrimal gland malignant mixed tumors (carcinomas arising in benign mixed tumors): a clinico-pathologic study. Cancer 45:2593–2606

Reese AB (1976a) Epithelial tumors of the lid, conjunctiva, cornea, and lacrimal sac. In: Reese AB (ed) Tumors of the eye, 3rd edn. Harper & Row, Hagerstown, Md, pp 58–59

Reese AB (1976b) Tumors of the lacrimal gland. In: Reese AB (ed) Tumors of the eye, 3rd edn. Harper & Row, Hagerstown, Md, pp 399–431

Ryan SJ, Font RL (1973) Primary malignant neoplasms of the lacrimal sac. Am J Ophthalmol 76:73–88

Sagerman RH (1984) Salivary gland tumors. In: Gilbert HA (ed) Modern radiation oncology. Classic literature and current management, vol 2. Harper & Row, Philadelphia, pp 21–57

Sagerman RH, Fariss AK, Chung CT, King GA, You HS, Fries PD (1991) Epithelial malignancies of the nasolacrimal sac. Radiology 181:276

Schenck NL, Ogura JH, Pratt LL (1973) Cancer of the lacrimal sac. Ann Otol 82:153–161

Shields JA (1989) Diagnosis and management of orbital tumors. Saunders, Philadelphia, pp 259–274

Spaeth EB (1957) Carcinomas in the region of the lacrimal sac. Arch Ophthalmol 57:689–693

Spaeth EB (1969) A surgical technique for lacrimal sac malignancy. Trans Ophthalmol Soc UK 89:351–354

Spratt CN (1940) Carcinoma of the lacrimal sac. Arch Ophthalmol 24:1237–1243

Spratt CN (1973) Primary carcinoma of the lacrimal sac. Arch Ophthalmol 18:267–273

Wright JE (1982) Factors affecting the survival of patients with lacrimal gland tumors. Can J Ophthalmol 17:309

Zimmerman LE, Sanders TE, Ackerman LV (1962) Epithelial tumors of the lacrimal gland: prognostic and therapeutic significance of histologic types. Int Ophthalmol Clin 50: 337–367

20 Radiation-Related Orbital Injury: Clinical Manifestations and Considerations for Surgical Repair

R. A. WEISS, J. L. IWATA, R. S. GONNERING

CONTENTS

20.1 Overview

Deformity and contracture of ophthalmic soft tissues and the orbital bones which compose the orbital complex may be the result of mechanical, chemical, thermal, and/or radiation injury. While reconstruction is most commonly necessary following traumatic orbital injuries, iatrogenically induced deformities account for a large number of cases as well. Iatrogenic causes range from unavoidable surgically induced deformity resulting from excision of a primary orbital neoplasm or ocular tumor with orbital extension, to contracture resulting from secondary effects of radiation. Radiation-related injury may develop following radiation therapy directed to the globe, orbit, or nasopharynx. Secondary considerations which may exacerbate radiation-induced injury include poor fitting or excessively heavy pros-

R.A. WEISS, MD
Clinical Associate Professor in the Departments of Ophthalmology and Visual Science, and Neurosurgery, the University of Illinois at Chicago, Director of Oculoplastic and Reconstructive Surgery, and Ophthalmologic Oncology, Chicago Eye Institute and Advocate Illinois Masonic Medical Health Systems, 3982 North Milwaukee Avenue, Chicago, IL 60641, USA
J.L. IWATA, Pharm.D., DO
Clinical Instructor of Ophthalmology, Medical College of Wisconsin, Division of Oculoplastics, Eye Institute, 925 N. 87th Street, Milwaukee, Wisconsin 53226, USA
R.S. GONNERING, MD
Professor of Ophthalmology, Medical College of Wisconsin, Division of Oculoplastics, Clinical Professor of Ophthalmology, University of Wisconsin, Eye Institute, 925 N. 87th Street, Milwaukee, Wisconsin 53226, USA

theses in anophthalmic (no globe) patients with orbital volume deficiency, and normal aging changes which may lead to or contribute to socket deformity.

Radiation therapy is a proven therapeutic approach used individually or in consort with chemotherapy and/or surgical excision for a large number of ocular, orbital, and periorbital lesions, both benign and malignant. Radiation therapy is a particularly powerful tool; it often enables treatment of the primary pathologic process without permanently affecting vision, eyelid function, or cosmesis. However, when radiation therapy is a contributing factor to ophthalmic soft tissue contracture, the ophthalmic plastic surgeon is confronted with his/her most challenging reconstructive task. Unfortunately, cicatricial and atrophic changes in orbital soft tissues are very resistant to surgical correction. An especially difficult problem is mucous membrane contracture, which may develop from radiation-related cicatrization and loss of normal baseline lubrication of the eyelid and anterior globe surfaces. This lubrication derives from the goblet cells, main and accessory lacrimal glands, and the sebaceous glands. These glands, respectively, supply the mucinous, aqueous, and oily components of the tear film. Each of these tear film layers is required for normal lubricating and rewetting of the cornea, and the palpebral and bulbar conjunctival surfaces (LENP and HAMILL 1973; VANTLEY et al. 1977; LEMP 1989).

Surgical intervention may be necessary to repair radiation-related misdirection of the eye lashes and malposition of the eyelids to avoid conjunctival- corneal irritation and injury, and to allow smooth excursion of the lids. For the postradiation therapy anophthalmic patient, reconstruction may be necessary to enable the individual to wear and retain a prosthesis comfortably. The hardship of loss of an eye can be significantly compounded by the inability to wear a prosthesis in an attempt to maintain the semblance of a normal appearance. The inability of patients with irradiated sockets to retain their prostheses is usually related to secondary mal position of the lower eyelid, with canthal tendon laxity and contracture of the inner lamellar mucous membrane surface of their eyelids (Fig. 20.1).

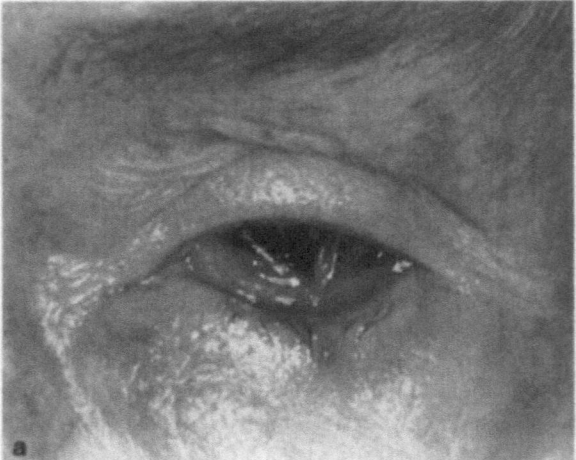

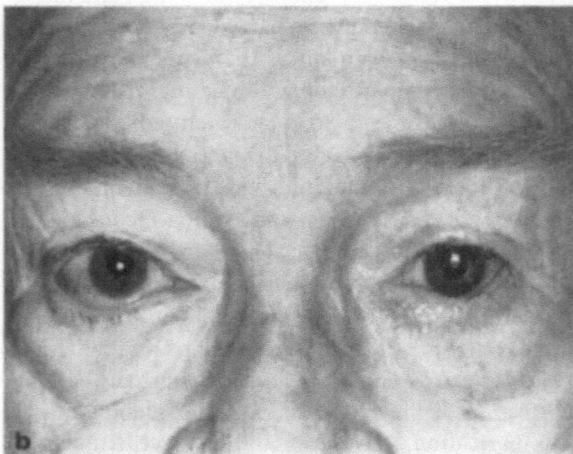

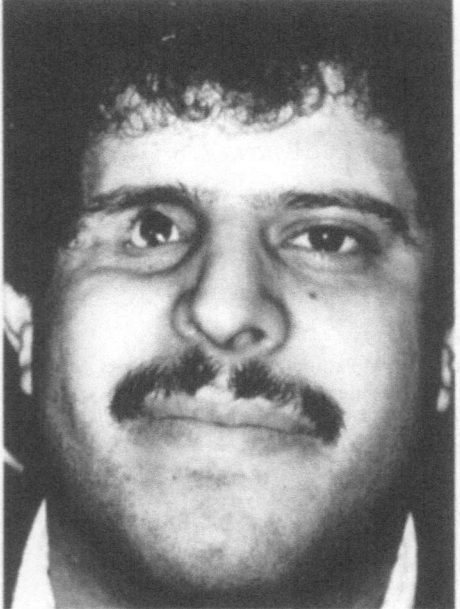

Fig. 20.2. Clinical photograph demonstrating significant contracture of the right orbito-maxillary complex with poor retention of a prosthesis and poor cosmesis

Fig. 20.1. a Clinical photograph of a patient unable to wear a prosthesis secondary to mucous membrane contracture of both fornices. b Clinical photograph of the same patient demonstrating ability to retain a prosthesis with improved cosmesis, following the first procedure of a two-staged socket reconstruction. The second stage, not shown in this photograph, involves rotation and repositioning of the inturned, misdirected eyelashes

The task of reconstructing the radiation-damaged socket becomes even more difficult when trying to rectify asymmetries in unilateral cases in which a normal contra-lateral orbitomaxillary complex is present (Fig. 20.2). Remarkably little information is available in the scientific literature regarding reconstruction of the irradiated orbit and socket. Presumably, this is because the ophthalmic plastic surgeon usually achieves very limited results in the vast majority of these surgically recalcitrant cases. Qualifiers such as "limited" and "partial" typically precede the word "success" when describing the outcome of reconstructive procedures for the irradiated orbit.

20.2
Anatomic and Pathophysiologic Concepts

A number of factors including radiation beam quality, fractionation, total dose, volume treated, individual and tissue radiation sensitivity, and age and general health of the patient determine the degree of complications and deformity which may develop in the irradiated orbit. The structures of the eye are highly specialized with significant variability in their degree of radiation sensitivity (DUKE-ELDER 1972; REESE 1976; MERRIAM et al. 1972; HAYE et al. 1975) The less specialized bones of the orbitomaxillary complex and related orbital soft tissues including the socket, eyelids, nasolacrimal drainage system, and periorbital areas demonstrate similar variability in their sensitivity to radiation exposure. Unfortunately, radiation-related injuries suffered by these tissues may actually preclude normal function of the globe. In addition, they may be responsible for significant physical discomfort, corneal decompensation and ulceration, cosmetic deformity, and orbital asymmetry.

Before detailing the manifestations and response to radiation-induced injury of the varied orbital and adnexal soft tissues, pertinent anatomy and histology will be briefly reviewed. The highly specialized eyelids are basically composed of four layers. The outermost layer of the lid is composed of skin, with its superficially keratinizing surface epithelium and associated adnexal structures. The next layer, immediately deep to the skin, is the orbicularis oculi muscle. This muscle is directly responsible for normal eyelid closure. The third layer is composed of the tarsus with its enclosed meibomian glands and associated insertions of the levator muscle and underlying Müller's muscle. The final layer is the conjunctiva, a mucous membrane whose thin, nonkeratinizing epithelial surface lines the inner surface of the lids and anterior surface of a portion of the globe. The conjunctiva contains mucus-producing goblet cells which are essential to the maintenance of the qualitative integrity of the precorneal tear film.

Tears are drained from the surface of the eye and palpebral conjunctival surface by way of the puncta of the upper and lower eyelids. These small ostia in the medial aspect of the eyelids drain tears via the canaliculi to the lacrimal sac. The medial heads of the pretarsal portion of the orbicularis oculi muscle insert on the fascia of the lacrimal sac, creating the lacrimal pump mechanism. The lacrimal pump alternately generates negative suction pulling the tears into the sac, and positive pressure causing evacuation of the tears through the nasolacrimal canal to the nose and nasopharynx.

To understand the manifestations of radiation-related injuries to the normal orbital soft tissues, one must consider each one of these tissues individually. The myocutaneous tissues which compose the anterior or outer lamella of the eyelid are remarkably resilient. In almost no instance will radiation of these soft tissues contribute to eyelid malposition, dysfunction, or contracture. Cosmetic considerations may be significant since the irradiated skin may become depigmented and atrophic; diffuse telangiectasias may develop as well and, in rare instances, deep fibrosis and ulceration may be seen. Freshly grafted skin (less than 3 months old) appears to have extreme sensitivity to radiation and is associated with a significantly decreased rate of graft "take" (survival). The development of recurrent or secondary contracture is not unusual in these cases.

Acute anterior lamellar changes include loss of cilia, erythema, moist dermatitis, and ulceration (when the radiation doses exceed maximal skin tolerance). In those cases which manifest acute postradiation changes limited to loss of cilia and erythema, there is typically minimal, if any, permanent skin damage or loss of cilia. In contrast, radiation doses associated with moist desquamation usually cause some significant permanent changes. Histopathologically, the initial transient erythema results from

dilation of the vasculature with infiltration of the perivascular tissues. However, moist desquamation results from loss of cellular attachments to the basal epithelium and mitotic injury to the germinal cells. Ultimately, adjacent germinal cells divide to form a new basal layer which reepithelializes the desquamated areas (HAIK et al. 1983) In some cases, focal atrophy in areas of hyperkeratosis may occur, in addition to areas of pigment disturbance and misdirection of cilia (trichiasis). These misdirected lashes may become quite bothersome in terms of patient discomfort and increased risk of infection from chronic, recurrent conjunctival and corneal irritation. Additionally, in some cases the globe may be irreparably injured, leading to permanent loss of normal intraocular pressure and shrinkage (phthisis) of the globe itself.

In contrast to outer lamellar myocutaneous radiation injuries, which are, for the most part, transient and "benign" in nature, inner lamellar injuries are more significant in terms of eyelid function, malposition, and deformity. Inner lamellar tissues of concern include the palpebral (inner lid surface) conjunctiva and the fibrous tarsal plates. In these tissues, contracture may be profound. Acute conjunctival reaction typically includes erythema, hyperemia, and chemosis (conjunctival edema), This may result in hypersecretion and/or misdirection of tears and secondary epiphora (tearing). These reactive signs are usually transient and may be treated symptomatically with topical ocular anti-inflammatory and lubricant medications. With doses above 30 Gy, a more severe conjunctivitis and possible ulceration may develop, This corresponds to the moist dermatitis evident with corresponding radiation levels to the skin. In contrast to these acute effects, delayed conjunctival injury may include the development of persistent injection ("chronic" dilated vessels), telangiectasias and, possibly, necrosis (secondary scarring in these cases is particularly problematic.) "Chronic radiation vessels" usually do not develop in the palpebral and bulbar conjunctiva following radiation treatment unless doses greater than 30 Gy are used. Doses above 30 Gy are associated with the development of abnormal vessels with relatively anomalous vascular walls; these abnormal vessels are often responsible for secondary recurrent hemorrhage (HAIK et al. 1983).

With cumulative radiation doses over 60 Gy, significant permanent scarring and contracture of the conjunctiva may develop. These, cicatricial changes may include the development of symblepharon (adhesions between the conjunctival surfaces of the lid and globe) and loss of the normal conjunctival fornices. Contracture of this nature can lead to the development of entropion (inward rotation of the eyelid) and/ or trichiasis (inturned, misdirection of the eyelashes). Similarly, mucous membrane which is injured in the proximal lacrimal drainage system may result in permanent stricture of the puncta and canalicular system. In these cases, the conjunctiva may undergo degenerative metaplastic changes and keratin plaques may develop with loss of the normal glandular tissues. Associated loss of the conjunctival goblet cells and accessory lacrimal secretors may result in or contribute to contraction and loss of the normal fornices, compounding and exacerbating direct radiation-related scarring of this mucous membrane.

20.3
Surgical Considerations and Approaches for Radiation-Related Orbital Injuries

There are numerous techniques which may be employed to repair misdirected eyelashes, malpositioned eyelids, and contracted fornices. To rid misdirected lashes permanently, we employ the technique of lid margin incision and direct follicle cauterization. In our experience this technique is less deforming and more predictable than cryotherapy, electrolysis, hyfercation, or other methods of permanent epilation.

The surgical approach for correction of eyelid margin malposition must be individualized for each case since the pathophysiologic changes underlying the deformity determine the appropriate surgical technique. Marginal rotation procedures involving incision of a tarsal wedge or full-thickness tarsal plate are indicated and necessary on occasion. However, for many cases, resuspension and tightening of the limbs of the lateral canthal tendon is adequate (Fig. 20.3). For those cases with significant mucous membrane/ inner lamellar contraction, the use of autologous, mucous membrane grafts may be required. Full-thickness mucous membrane grafts are, in general, more successful than, split-thickness grafts in reconstructing conjunctival–inner lamellar defects regardless of whether radiation therapy has been employed. When mucous membrane grafts are necessary, we prefer to harvest autologous mucous membrane from the inner surface of the lip (Fig. 20.4).

For the repair of a ptotic upper eyelid, we use standard procedure approaches based on the degree of levator function as described by BEARD, BERKE, and others (BEARD 1976; ANDERSON and DIXON

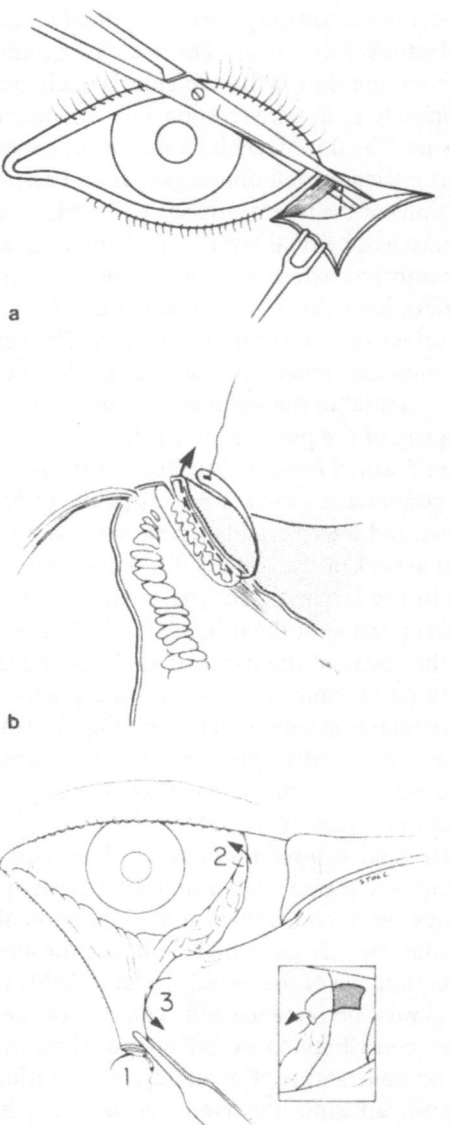

Fig. 20.3. a A skin-muscle flap is elevated and a lower limb lateral canthotomy is performed with inferior dissection of the deep tissue *(broken line)* to free the lateral lower lid septal attachments. b A number 4-0 proline suture on a small semi-circular needle is passed from deep to superficial tarsus along its lateral edge such that the needle traverses the entire height of tarsus, exiting at its most superior aspect. This suture is used to retract the lid and ultimately to resuspend it to the lateral orbital wall. c The lower limb of the lateral canthal tendon is reattached by passing a suture through full-thickness tarsus (1) as detailed in b. The suture is then passed to catch a bite of lateral orbital rim periosteum (2) followed by a septal tensing bite (3). [*Inset:* In cases with horizontal shortage of the, lower lid, the same procedure may be performed as detailed above; however, the tarsal resuspension suture can be attached to a periosteal flap which is elevated from the lateral orbital rim periosteum (2).] (WEISS et al. 1990)

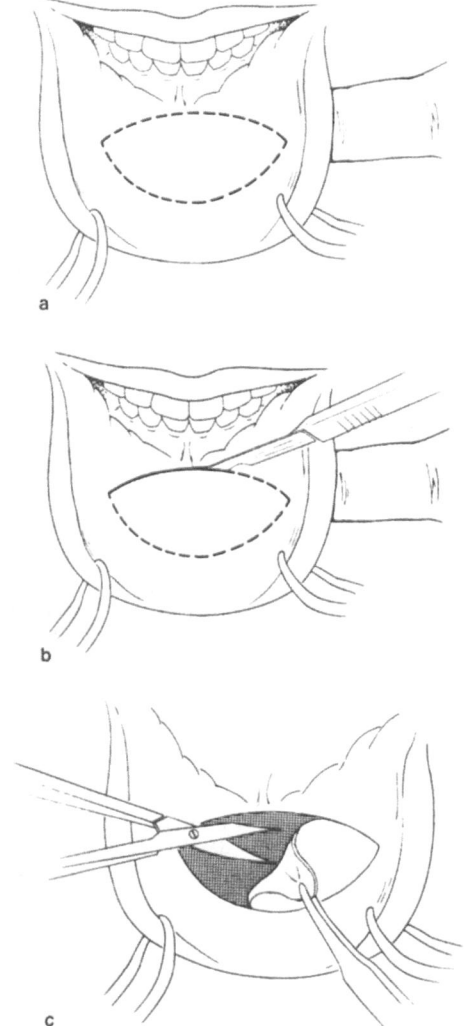

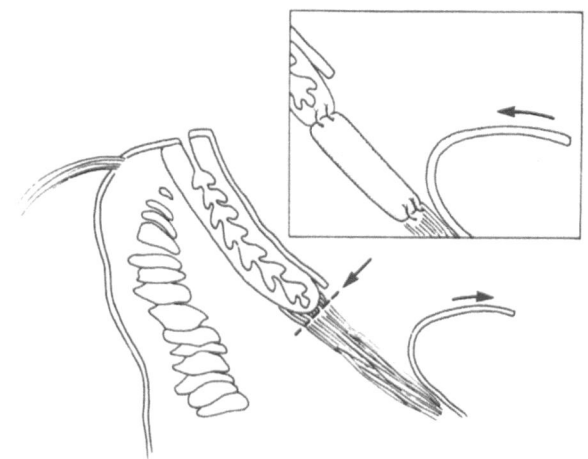

Fig. 20.5. Conjunctiva is dissected free and the lower eyelid retractors are detached from their tarsal insertion *(broken line)*. [*Inset:* The superior edge of an ear cartilage or other spacer material graft is sutured to the inferior tarsal border. A couple of anchoring stitches are placed inferiorly to attach the inferior edge of the cartilage/ spacer graft to the lower lid retractors in an effort to prevent the graft from dislodging.] Proper placement of this spacer material allows a foreshortened posterior lamella to be adequately and appropriately corrected. (WEISS et al. 1990)

Fig. 20.4. **a** The lower lip donor site is exposed by grasping it with towel clips and inverting it under tension over the assistant surgeon's finger. The donor tissue is delineated with methylene blue. **b** Mucous membrane is incised along the methylene blue line. **c** Harvest of the mucous membrane donor tissue is completed with further dissection. (WEISS et al. 1990)

1979; BERKE 1964; BEARD 1966; SMITH et al. 1969; WALKER et al. 1987). To reposition postradiation lower lid malposition (entropion, ectropion/retraction), we can usually attain good results by lateral canthal resuspension techniques, as previously mentioned (Fig. 20.3). Significant retraction due to outer lamellar cicatricial changes requires the use of full-thickness autologous skin. The best donor skin in terms of thickness and color is from an opposite eyelid. There is usually ample skin in the upper lid of elderly individuals; however, in younger patients, eyelid skin is taut and additional skin for grafting must be harvested from other sources. Autologous

donor sites, in our order of preference, include upper eyelids, posterior auricular, or supraclavicular areas. The techniques of harvesting and grafting these tissues are well known and described in the literature (WILKENS et al. 1987). For associated inner lamellar defects, autologous mucous membrane grafting with possible lower lid retractor extirpation, autologous ear cartilage or periosteal spacer grafting (Fig. 20.5), or forniceal reconstruction may be necessary (Fig. 20.6). Gore-Tex and other alloplastic spacers are useful to secure either mucous membrane or conjunctival amniotic membrane grafts to the conjunctival fornices. Typically, these spacers are anchored in place for one week (SCHMIDT et al. 1994). If there is inadequate tear production, however, mucous membrane grafts tend to contract, leading to suboptimal results. For some anophthalmic patients, when autologous mucous membrane grafts severely contract because of significant loss of the normal tear film following radiation therapy, we graft autologous skin or AlloDerm to line the anterior socket. AlloDerm®, an acellular matrix processed from cadaveric human skin, can be used to line the anterior socket because it inhibits wound contraction by reestablishing a dermal collagen matrix (TERNIO 2001, WALDEN et al. 2000, WAINRIGHT et al. 1996). This is our last choice approach since sockets with autologous skin invariably shrink as

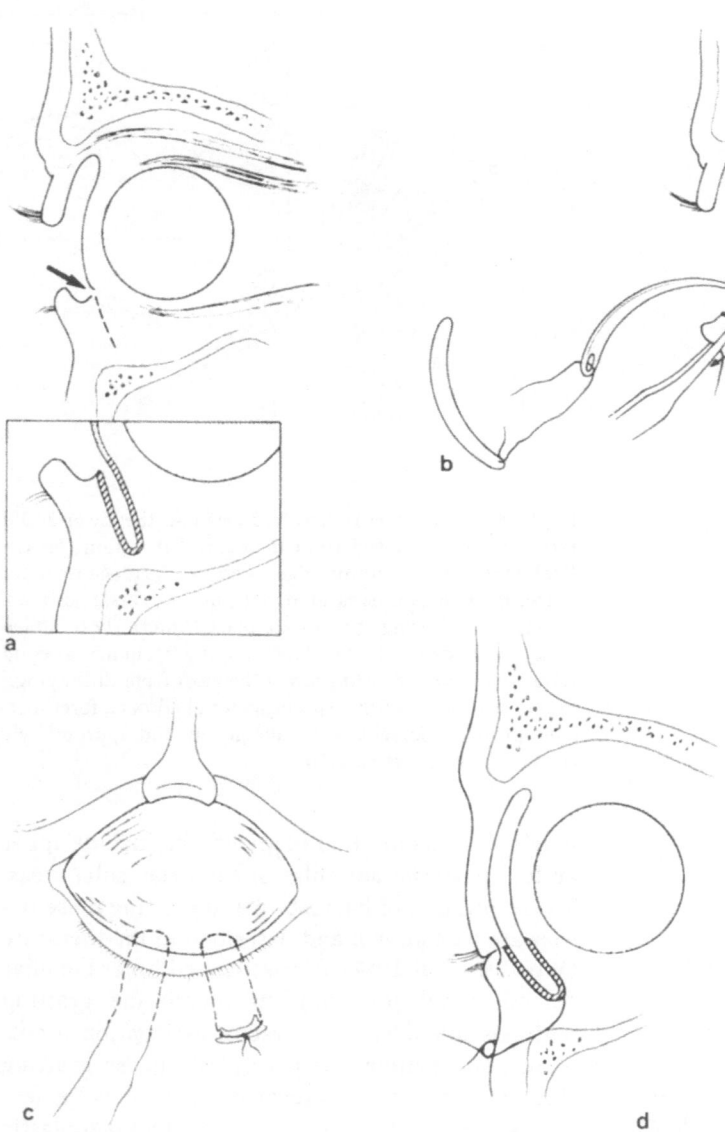

Fig. 20.6. a An expanded inferior fornix can be recreated by dissection of the contracted conjunctiva (mucous membrane) and underlying deep tissue. [*Inset:* Mucous membrane *(hatched line) is* grafted to the surfaces of the newly developed tissue planes.] **b** A comformer is sutured into the newly created forniceal space by passing the anchor sutures through the new apex such that they bite periosteum before exiting through skin-muscle. The periosteal bite serves to develop deep adhesions, assuring the creation of a deep fornix. **c** Anterior view demonstrating approximate relative position and spacing of the comformer/fornix anchoring sutures, and placement of cotton bolsters between skin and suture ties. **d** Lateral view of comformers sutured in place with properly positioned mucous membrane grafts and temporary intermarginal suture. (WEISS et al. 1990)

well. More significantly, these patients often suffer from a most annoying chronic socket discharge and they are unable to wear their prosthesis comfortably.

In addition to eyelid and eyelash difficulties, significant orbital deformities may result from radiation therapy as well. In the developing child, especially less than 1 year of age, destruction of the normal bone growth centers within the radiation fields may result in the well-recognized temporal fossa or orbitomaxillary complex deformity (Fig. 20.7). This is frequently seen in children who are treated during their 1st year of life for retinoblastoma. When this depression of the lateral orbitomaxillary complex develops, it is extremely difficult to address surgically. Similarly, significant deformity of the superior sulcus may develop from radiation-related atrophy of the normal eyelid and orbital fat. In these patients, there is a hollowness

of the normal superior sulcus and the globe itself may become enophthalmic or settle posteriorly relative to its normal axial position (Fig. 20.8).

A number of surgical approaches have been employed in an attempt to correct the orbitomaxillary complex deformity. These approaches include rotation of temporalis muscle to fill in some of the defect mechanically, free and vascularized autologous bone grafts, and numerous alloplastic implants. The nuances, complexities, and complications of these various surgical approaches are beyond the scope of this work. However, the fact that so many varied approaches have been developed attests to the fact that no single approach has met with consistent success. We are currently working with a malleable form of hydroxyapatite, an endogenous substance, which can be artificially supplied. This material is ideal because it is

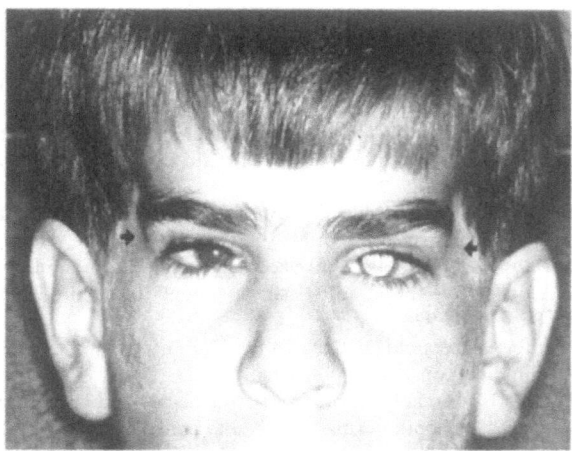

Fig. 20.7. Clinical photograph of a young boy who underwent bilateral radiation for retinoblastoma within the 1st year of life. Note the significant temporal fossa/orbitomaxillary complex deformity present bilaterally (*arrows*). Also of note, leukocoria or a "white pupil" is evident in the left eye from the residual, inactive intraocular tumor

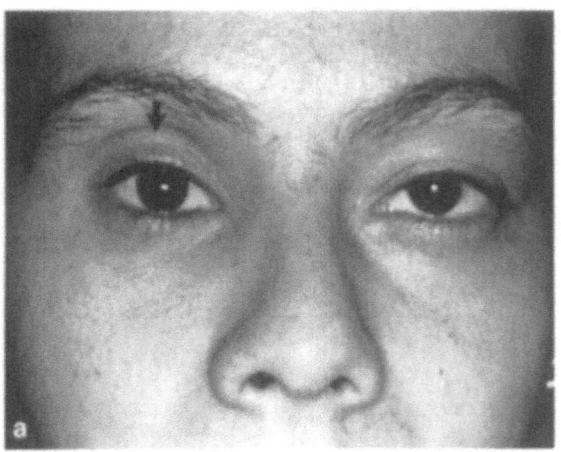

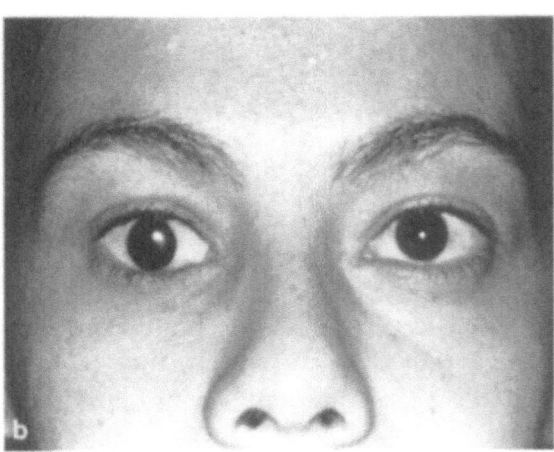

Fig. 20.8. a Clinical photograph of an anophthalmic patient demonstrating significant superior sulcus deformity (*arrow*). **b** Clinical photograph of the same patient after surgical repair of the superior sulcus deformity to improve cosmesis. (WEISS et al. 1990)

ultimately replaced by the individual's normal bone. This new approach shows great promise.

Finally, radiation-related injury to the nasolacrimal drainage outflow system is quite common in patients who receive radiation treatment of the medial canthal or naso-ethmoidal areas. For many of these patients, simple placement of a Crawford tube or similar stent in the lacrimal drainage apparatus will preclude contracture and dysfunction of the tear outflow system (Fig. 20.9). While many patients develop a radiation-related "dry eye" at least transiently, it is still wise to preserve the tear drainage system. While loss of the normal lacrimal drainage outflow canal from radiation-related cicatrization may not be associated with epiphora (tearing), for reasons just stated, these patients may develop significant, recurrent dacryocystitis from stasis of lacrimal fluids in the lacrimal sac. For those patients whose system cannot be recanalized because the simple placement of nasolacrimal stent tubes was not performed prior to radiation therapy, a complete conjunctival dacryocystorhinostomy is usually required. This involves the surgical implantation of permanent alloplastic drainage tubes. This is certainly a suboptimal approach since these integrated tubes have inherent problems and require chronic maintenance. Aside from routine intubation of the nasolacrimal drainage system with a spacer/stent tube, no real prophylaxis is indicated for these patients.

In conclusion, radiation-related injuries to the eyelids, orbits, and lacrimal drainage system may interfere with normal ophthalmic function and may be manifested by a wide variety of functional and cosmetic sequelae. Each of these problems can be addressed and improved if one understands the correct

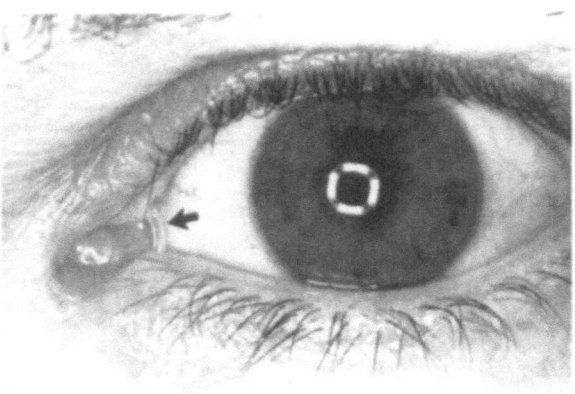

Fig. 20.9. Clinical photograph demonstrating Crawford nasolacrimal drainage stent tubes (*arrow*) which have been placed to preserve the integrity of the nasolacrimal drainage system of a patient prior to receiving therapeutic radiation therapy to the nasoethmoidal area

anatomic relationships and appropriate surgical techniques for repair of these damaged tissues.

Acknowledgments. This work was supported, in part, by grants from the St. Giles Foundation and Research to Prevent Blindness, Incorporated.

References

Anderson RL, Dixon RS (1979) Aponeurotic ptosis surgery. Arch Ophthalmol 97:1123-1128

Beard C (1966) The surgical treatment of blepharoptosis: a quantitative approach. Trans Am Ophthalmol Soc 64:401-487

Beard C (1976) Ptosis, 2nd edn. Mosby, St. Louis

Berke RM (1964) Blepharoptosis. In: Hughes WL (ed) Ophthalmic Plastic Surgery, 2nd edn. American Academy of Ophthalmology, Rochester, Minnesota

Duke-Elder S (1972) Non-mechanical injuries. In: DukeElder S (ed) System of ophthalmology: injuries. Henry Kimpton, London, 19, 2:934-1004

Haik BG, Jereb B, Abramson DH, Ellsworth RM (1983) Ophthalmic radiotherapy. In: Iliff NT (ed) Complications in ophthalmic surgery. Churchill Livingstone, New York, pp 449-485

Haye C, Jammett H, Dolfus MA (1965) L'Oeil et les radiations ionisantes. Masson, Paris, vol 1, 2

Lemp MA (1989) Diagnosis and treatment of tear deficiencies. In Duane TB (ed) Clinical ophthalmology. JB Lippincott, New York, pp 1-9

Lemp MA, Hamill J (1973) Factors affecting tear film breakup in normals. Arch Ophthalmol 89:103

Merriam GR Jr, Szechter A, Focht EF (1972) The effects of ionizing radiations on the eye. In: Vaeth JM, Darger, Basel G (eds) Frontiers of radiation therapy and oncology

Reese AB (1976) Tumors of the eye, 3rd edn. Harper & Row, Hagerstown, Md

Schmidt T, Kohler W (1994) Fornix reconstruction in ocular pemphigoid with Gore-Tex surgical membrane. Ophthalmologe 94:321-3

Smith B, NcCord CD, Baylis HI (1969) Surgical treatment of blepharoptosis. Am J Ophthalmol 68:92-99

Terino EO (2001) Alloderm acellular dermal graft: applications in aesthetic soft-tissue augmentation. Clin Plast Surg 28:83-99

Vantley GT, Leopold IH, Greg TA (1977) Interpretation of tear film breakup. Arch Ophthalmol 95:445

Walden JL, Garcia H, Hawkins H, Crouchet JR, Traber L, Gore DC (2000) Both dermal matrix and epidermis contribute to an inhibition of wound contraction. Ann Plast Surg 45:162-9

Wainwright D, Madden M, Luterman A et al. (1996) Clinical evaluation of an acellular allograft dermal matrix in fullthickness burns. J Burn Care Rehabil 17:124-136

Walker RR, McCord CD, Tanenbaum M (1987) Evaluation and management of the ptosis Patient. In: McCord CD, Tannenbaum H (eds) Oculoplastic surgery, 2nd edn. Raven New York, pp 325-376

Weiss RA, McCord CD, Ellsworth RM (1990) Reconstruction of the anophthalmic socket: lower eyelid malposition and canthal tendon laxity. In: Bosniak (ed) Advances in ophthalmic plastic and reconstructive surgery. Pergamon, New York, pp 192-208

Weiss RA, McCord CD, Ellsworth RM (1991) Orbital fractures. In: Shingleton (ed) Ophthalmic trauma. CV Mosby, St. Louis, pp 295-314

Wilkins RB, Kulwin DR, McCord CD, Tanenbaum M (1987) Techniques in oculoplastic surgery. In: McCord CD, Tannenbaum H (eds) Oculoplastic surgery, 2nd edn. Raven New York, pp 325-376

21 Effects of Ionizing Radiation on the Conjunctiva, Cornea, and Lens

H. J. Ingraham, E. D. Donnenfeld, D. H. Abramson

CONTENTS

21.1 Introduction

The human eye is exposed to a wide range of radiant energy aside from the visual spectrum, including ultraviolet, infrared, microwave, and ionizing radiation. Of these, ionizing radiation can cause some of the most significant and long-lasting ocular damage to the lens, conjunctiva, and cornea. Ionizing sources include cosmic (30 Mrem/year) and terrestrial sources (60 Mrem/year), as well as man-made sources (60 Mrem/year). These last include X-rays, radioactive isotopes, diagnostic and therapeutic radioactive sources, and release from nuclear power stations. Control of these man-made exposures with shielding of the globe, when possible, can minimize or eliminate the acute and chronic effects of radiation exposure.

The energy of ionizing radiation can be transmitted in a variety of ways, ranging from X-ray photons to heavy particles, and is dissipated in the same way regardless of how it is carried. Charged ions or radicals are created in the tissue; the depth of penetration is directly related to the wavelength of the ionizing source. Tissue destruction occurs through direct cell killing, DNA changes with the creation of abnormal or lethal mutations, direct blood vessel damage with secondary tissue necrosis, or through malignant transformation of the cell (Lerman 1980). The degree of tissue injury is related both to the intensity of the ionizing source and to the particular sensitivity of the species and the tissue concerned. As a general rule, increasing doses of ionizing radiation result in more severe effects with a shorter latency period. In the therapeutic use of ionizing radiation, damage to normal tissue is minimized through fractionation, a treatment that gives a therapeutically equivalent radiation dose by dividing it into daily sessions; this allows for cellular repair in normal tissues between doses.

The human eye is composed of two vital structures which allow light to enter the eye and focus on the photoreceptors of the retina (Fig. 21.1). These two anterior segment structures are the cornea and the lens. The cornea is a transparent, avascular structure, which functions as a watch crystal does on a watch. It allows light to pass through and provides structural support for the eye. Once the light has passed through the cornea, it next passes through the anterior segment to the lens. The lens is a biconvex, avascular, colorless, almost transparent structure, which also focuses the light so that it arrives on the retina.

The conjunctiva is a mucous membrane that covers the posterior surface of the lids and the anterior surface of the sclera. The conjunctiva is continuous with the skin at the lid margin and with the corneal epithelium at the limbus. Because the conjunctiva and the cornea are external structures of the human eye, they are directly exposed to external radiation. The cornea transmits electromagnetic radiation with wavelengths between 300 nm in the ultraviolet and 700 nm in the infrared spectra. Wavelengths

H. J. Ingraham, MD
Department of Ophthalmology, Geisinger Medical Center, Danville, PA 17822-2120, USA
E. D. Donnenfeld, MD
2000 North Village Avenue, Suite 402, Rockville Center, New York, NY 11570, USA
D. H. Abramson, MD
70 East 66th Street, New York, NY 10021, USA

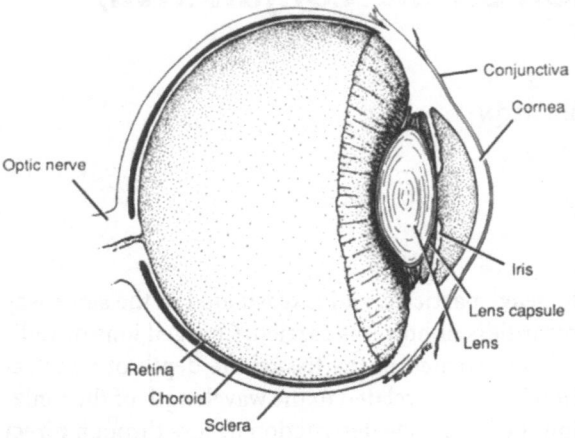

Fig. 21.1. Cross section of the eye, depicting both anterior segment structures and posterior pole structures

within this spectrum can pass through the cornea and interact with the lens. The effects of radiation on the conjunctiva, cornea, and lens range from insignificant to vision threatening. In an effort to understand these radiation effects, it is necessary first to be aware of the anatomy of these structures.

21.2
Anatomy

21.2.1
Conjunctiva

The conjunctiva can be divided into two geographic zones. The palpebral conjunctiva begins at the mucocutaneous junction of the lid, covers the entire undersurface of the eyelid, and is firmly adherent to the inner lid. The bulbar conjunctiva is attached to the orbital septum and the fornix, coats the external eye, and becomes contiguous with the corneal epithelium at the limbus.

The surface of the conjunctiva consists of nonkeratinized squamous epithelium, goblet cells, and a thin, vascularized substantia propria. The conjunctiva consists of two or more layers of epithelial cells, which are classified as superficial and basal. The superficial epithelial cells contain round or oval, mucous-secreting goblet cells. The mucous becomes an integral part of the tear film. The accessory lacrimal glands of Krause and Wolfring are located within the conjunctival stroma. These glands provide the basal aqueous tears necessary for baseline tear production. The conjunctiva is innervated by the ophthalmic division of the fifth cranial nerve, and is rich in lymphatic vessels.

21.2.2
Cornea

The cornea is a transparent and avascular structure that supports the anterior segment of the eye, providing protection and allowing the transmission of light. The cornea functions as a refracting surface, and is responsible for the majority of the refracting power of the eye: the remainder of the refracting power is provided by the lens. The average adult cornea is approximately 0.5 mm thick centrally and is 11.5 mm in diameter. The human cornea contains five distinct layers, beginning superficially with the corneal epithelium, which is contiguous with the conjunctival epithelium, continuing posteriorly to Bowman's membrane, stroma, Descemet's membrane, and ending with the endothelium. The corneal epithelium arises from stem cells located at the corneoscleral limbus, and is organized into five layers. The cornea is avascular; oxygen and nutrients are carried by the limbal vessels, and some oxygen is derived from the atmosphere. The cornea is innervated by the fifth cranial nerve. Three important factors contribute to corneal transparency. The first is the lack of blood vessels in the cornea. The second is the uniform structure of the cornea; the normal matrix of the cornea is composed of exactly replicating collagen fibrils. The final reason for the cornea's transparency is the relative deturgescence of the cornea maintained by the corneal endothelial pump. Damage to the endothelium results in edema of the cornea and corneal opacification. It is important to note that diseases of the cornea are extremely serious owing to the lack of regeneration of corneal tissue. This lack of regeneration results in scar formation and corneal opacification. This leads to visual impairment, which ranges from slight blurring to total blindness.

21.2.3
Lens

The lens is a biconvex, avascular structure located in the anterior segment of the eye. The lens is held in place by suspensory zonules, which connect to the ciliary body. The lens is bathed anteriorly by the aqueous humor and posteriorly by the vitreous. The lens contains a subcapsular epithelium, which is only present anteriorly, and is completely surrounded by a basement membrane. The lens nucleus composes the majority of the lens centrally, and is harder than the peripheral cortex. As part of the aging process, the lamellar fibers which are continually produced by the lens create a progressive thickening of the lens, hence making the lens less elastic, which results in decreased accommodation. The function of the lens is to focus the light rays that have been transmitted through the cornea onto the retina. A lack of transparency of the lens results in decreased visual acuity. The lens is composed of 55% water and approximately 35% protein. There are no pain fibers, blood vessels, or nerves in the lens.

The only abnormalities of the lens are opacification and dislocation. An opacity of the lens is a cataract. Cataracts vary markedly in density and are due to a variety of causes. Cataracts are characterized by lens edema, which causes a disruption of the normal lens fibers. Most cataracts are not visible to the casual observer, although when cataracts become more dense they can be observed as a whitening of the pupillary aperture.

The lens is a unique structure in that it is avascular and less capable than others of dispersing heat; in addition, the lens is derived from ectoderm, which matures inwardly. As it develops, the lens sheds its outer fibers inward toward the nucleus. Thus, the lens fibers are arranged in concentric rings similar to those of a tree. They record the history of damage to the lens contents.

21.2.4
Tear Film

The tear film, a watery saline solution secreted by the lacrimal glands, coats the anterior surface of the eye and creates a refractive surface for the cornea. The corneal epithelium and the conjunctiva are moistened by the tear film, which allows them to be maintained as a nonkeratinized epithelial structure.

The tears are a mixture of secretions from the major and minor lacrimal glands, the goblet cells within the conjunctiva, and the meibomian glands of the lids. The lacrimal glands are exocrine glands and produce a serous secretion. The major lacrimal gland is located in a shallow depression within the orbital portion of the frontal bone and is separated from the orbit by fibroadipose tissue. The small gland can be seen in the superolateral conjunctival fornix when the upper lid is retracted. A number of thin-walled ducts pass from the lacrimal gland downward, entering into the conjunctival fornix approximately 8 mm above the superior margin of the upper tarsus. The meibomian glands of the lid secrete a lipid, which floats on the surface of the tear film and provides stabilization. The goblet cells secrete mucin, which coats the corneal surface and allows interaction of the hydrophilic aqueous and the hydrophobic corneal epithelium.

The tear film is approximately 7–10 μm thick and covers the entire cornea and conjunctival epithelium. It functions to make the cornea a smooth optical surface by negating any epithelial irregularity. In addition, it wets the conjunctival and corneal epithelial surfaces to prevent damage and washes away foreign bodies. Finally, the tear film contains high levels of IgA, IgG and IgE, which inhibit the growth of microorganisms on the conjunctival and corneal surface. It is the interaction of the tear film on the conjunctiva and cornea, which maintains the integrity of these integral anatomical structures.

The lens, conjunctiva, and cornea of the human eye are exquisitely sensitive to ionizing radiation; the lens may be the most radiosensitive tissue in the body. In general, the susceptibility of a given tissue is determined by the mitotic activity of the cells and its ability to repair the damage done by a given dose. The conjunctiva consists of a stratified, nonkeratinizing epithelial layer with a relatively mitotically active basal layer, and an underlying fibrovascular tissue, the substantia propria. The cornea has a similar epithelium with underlying stroma and endothelium. The radiosensitivity of these tissues is thought to arise from the susceptibility of the relatively rapidly replicating basal epithelium. In contrast, the lens consists of fibers derived from the differentiation of an epithelium that is completely enclosed by its own basement membrane, the lens capsule. No exchange of cells takes place after embryogenesis; in adulthood, these epithelial cells line the equator of the lens, just within the enclosing lens capsule, and are relatively mitotically inactive. These cells have limited reparative capabilities, and unlike other tissues whose damaged or mutated cells can be sloughed, the lens is virtually a storehouse of radiation-induced damage.

21.3
Radiation Effects

21.3.1
Conjunctiva

Following a single dose of 500 cGy or more (MERRIAM et al. 1972) the conjunctiva becomes hyperemic and edematous, and develops a clear or mucopurulent discharge. After several days, significant chemosis may develop, which more often severely affects the lower fornix. Late changes may include significant scarring and shrinkage of tissue and the formation of adhesions between the conjunctiva of the lid and the globe, called symblepharon, leading to drying or limitation of movement of the eye. The conjunctiva, normally a mucous membrane, may become keratinized when tear production falls secondary to scarring and damage to the lacrimal gland. If a piece of radioactive material is embedded on the surface of the eye, necrosis of the conjunctiva and underlying sclera may follow. Blood vessel alterations in the form of dramatic telangiectasia are characteristic (Fig. 21.2). An epithelial carcinoma has been reported secondary to radiation-induced malignant transformation, but this is quite rare (KALT 1919). The conjunctiva may also be affected following total-body irradiation. A significant subconjunctival hemorrhage secondary to systemic thrombocytopenia is not unusual. These hemorrhages are usually self-limited, and not sight-threatening.

21.3.2
Cornea

The observed effects of ionizing radiation on the cornea arise from at least two different sources. The first is a direct toxic effect, which usually follows 1,000–2,000 cGy in a single dose (MacFAUL and BEDFORD 1970; MERRIAM et al. 1972), and the other effect is a secondary result of severe drying of the ocular surface. The main lacrimal gland will undergo

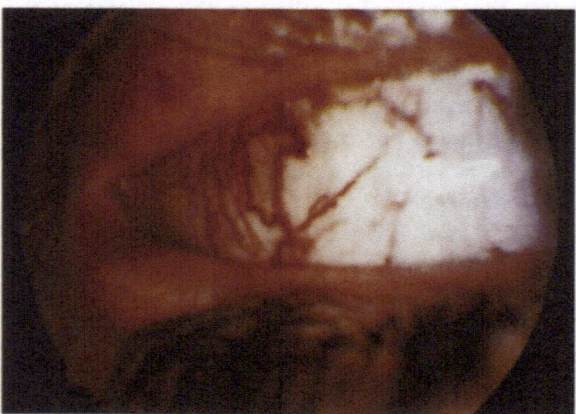

Fig. 21.2. Anterior segment photograph of a 28-year-old white woman's left eye 3 years after cobalt-60 plaque therapy for a ciliary body melanoma (8 mm in height x 15 mm in diameter). The plaque was in place for 2 weeks and delivered 40 Gy to the conjunctiva. Note the radiation vasculopathy of the conjunctiva

atrophy after a single dose of approximately 20 Gy. The conjunctiva, the secondary lacrimal glands in the eyelids, and the meibomian glands can all be injured at similar levels; significant xerosis may result (ROTH et al. 1976). When this occurs, the cornea acutely demonstrates a punctate epitheliopathy that progresses over days to weeks to punctate epithelial erosions and edema. If material becomes embedded in the cornea, perforation with exposure or loss of intraocular tissue may occur. Corneal sensation is often decreased for several weeks to months, but may persist longer, and results in neurotrophic complications. The lost epithelium tends to heal poorly, and initially, ulceration and secondary microbial infection may result. Later, vascularization, lipid infiltration, stromal thinning, and perforation may occur; the corneal surface may become keratinized in response to the hostile environment (LERMAN 1980; MERRIAM et al. 1972). Replacement of corneal tissue through penetrating keratoplasty or other surgical means is difficult owing to poor wound healing and a tendency to tissue necrosis. A report by FUJISHIMA et al. (1996) suggests that corneal stem cells may also be damaged by ionizing radiation, complicating wound healing still further.

21.3.3
Crystalline Lens

The human lens is uniquely susceptible to ionizing radiation. As previously mentioned, the arrangement of the lens does not allow for the removal of injured cells, and the avascular lens cannot disperse heat efficiently (HAM 1953; LIPMAN et al. 1988). The lens fibers arise from the lens epithelium, which is divided into the central, germinative, pre-equatorial and equatorial zones. The germinative epithelium, the most mitotically active zone, appears to be the primary target of ionizing radiation. This zone gives rise to abnormal cells that fail to differentiate properly, and eventually migrate posteriorly and centrally to form a posterior subcapsular cataract, the classic radiation-induced lesion. A radiation cataract can also assume a "doughnut" configuration with a clear central area surrounded by opacification, a sectorial distribution of clouding, or total opacification. These changes are seen commonly after beta irradiation. The first report of experimental production of a cataract in a laboratory animal was in 1897 (CHALU-PECKY 1897): the first description of radiation-induced cataracts in man was published by MEESMAN in 1926. In this report, and that by ROHRSCHNEIDER

(1928), cataracts appeared after latency periods of 5 and 9 years, and were described initially as fine subcapsular dots in the anterior cortex, with posterior granular, vacuolar deposits. These lesions can go on to significant or total lenticular opacification, recovery, or stabilization (ROTH et al. 1976). These reports in man and animals revealed a particular susceptibility of the young embryonic lens, presumably based on more active proliferation (LERMAN 1980). Typically, cataracts develop after a latency period of 1–20 years. Single doses of 2–5 Gy are cataractogenic (COGAN and DREISLER 1953; MERRIAM et al. 1972).

With the development and detonation of the atomic bomb, and the creation of the Atomic Bomb Casualty Commission and other agencies, extensive experience with the effects of ionizing radiation on human subjects became available. The formation of cataracts in scientists working on early cyclotrons has been noted, and a series of reports on survivors at Hiroshima and Nagasaki have been filed (COGAN et al. 1950; SINSKEY 1955; MILLER et al. 1967). Each study was limited by the uncertainty regarding the radiation dose for each person and by the difficulty in following up the survivors. The ionizing energy of the atomic bomb was carried by the full range of gamma rays, photons, neutrons, and other particles. Each has its own relative biological effectiveness (SALLMAN 1951; ROTH et al. 1976; LERMAN 1980) and calculation of the radiation dose was challenging. Radiation dose estimates have been made by comparing the degree of epilation among survivors (SINSKEY 1955). Most studies estimate radiation exposure by computing the relationship between the approximate distance of the subject from ground zero; the principle that the ionizing radiation dose decreases as the distance from the source increases is understood. The studies agreed on two major points: cataracts were often the only sign of radiation exposure, and the lens opacities were mostly posterior subcapsular in nature. With mild doses, a polychromatic "sheen" of the lens capsule was noted; with somewhat higher doses, a small posterior subcapsular plaque resulted. Those survivors closest to the blast had lens opacities, ranging from patches with an appearance reminiscent of a "doughnut" or "bivalve" through a dense posterior subcapsular plaque to complete opacification (MILLER et al. 1967).

The Chernobyl nuclear power plant accident in April 1986 provided additional experience with the effects of gamma and beta radiation exposure. In one study, 16 reactor workers or firemen were followed for 5–10 years after exposure to doses of 0.35–9 Gy. Five developed dense cataracts of the cortical or posterior subcapsular type, and 3 developed severely dry eyes, while 8 had no ocular changes. The authors could not differentiate between the effects of the deeply penetrating gamma radiation and the more superficial beta particles (JUNK et al. 1999).

Radiation-induced cataracts have also been documented in a number of therapeutic situations, including the use of plutonium-230 (GRIFFITH et al. 1985). The isotope was deposited hematogenously in the iris and ciliary body, or directly adjacent to the sensitive lens epithelium germinative zone, which resulted in subsequent cataract formation.

A number of authors have studied the histology of these acute and chronic lens changes in humans and animals. In the mitotically active germinative lens epithelium, mitotic arrest with nuclear fragmentation and degeneration has been noted (LERMAN 1980). Abnormal vacuolated cells, or polynucleated giant cells, are initially seen near the germinative zone and then migrate centrally and posteriorly (SALLMAN and LOCKE 1951). Along the posterior capsule, which has small nuclei and pale cytoplasm, the classic bladder cells of Wadl migrate centrally. The arrangement of the nuclei in the lens fibers, particularly in the nuclear bow region, is acutely disrupted (SALLMAN 1951; LIPMAN et al. 1988). Because this change does not require migration of damaged cells from the germinative zone, this presumably represents direct damage to the lens fiber cells and their nuclei (SALLMAN and LOCKE 1951). Late changes include "feathery" perpendicularly oriented lens fibers and posterior membrane whorls (HAYES and FISHER 1979).

The exact mechanism of this damage remains unclear. Evidence exists for oxidative damage and free radical formation causing DNA damage and protein cross-linkage (LERMAN 1980; LIPMAN et al. 1988). A variety of enzymes exhibit changes in their activity, which may be secondary to DNA mutations. Others postulate permeability changes in cell membranes, followed by alterations in Na^+/K^+ ATPase and calcium levels, followed by secondary accumulation of cellular water and resulting in opacification (LAMBERT and KINOSHITA 1967; MATSUDA et al. 1982; HIGHTOWER et al. 1983). Direct toxic lens cell injury with decreased zinc and increased iron and calcium concentrations has also been described in a rat model (AVUNDUK et al. 2000). Still others propose a combination of factors, such as the permeability changes following DNA and protein damage wrought by the ionizing source (SALLMAN and LOCKE 1951). In the avascular lens, where heat is inefficiently dissipated, the ionizing energy will also produce thermal effects; this complicates the mechanistic schema further (LIPMAN et al. 1988).

A number of substances have been examined in animal models for possible inhibition of radiation cataractogenesis. These include vitamin E, glutathione isopropyl ester, radio-protective drugs such as WR77913, and superoxide mimic TEMPOL (KOBAYASHI et al. 1993; LIVESEY et al. 1995; Ross et al. 1990; SASAKI et al. 1998). While these substances work in a variety of ways by preventing free radical damage, maintaining lenticular glutathione levels, or other unknown mechanisms, all share in common the need for treatment prior to radiation exposure to be effective. No compound has yet been identified which will reverse lenticular radiation damage when given after exposure.

21.3.4
Dry Eyes: Diagnosis and Treatment

The most common and potentially damaging effect of radiation on the external eye is dry eye syndrome. The tear film is a structure composed of three layers: lipid, aqueous, and mucin. Any deficiency or abnormality of any of these three layers will lead to a dry eye syndrome. This will cause a rapid break-up of the tear film, and dry spots will appear on the corneal and conjunctival epithelium. These changes may cause mild discomfort, pain, and corneal perforation, which may lead to enucleation.

Patient complaints associated with dry eyes include a dry, sandy, or scratchy sensation in the eyes, mild itching, distorted vision, blinking, excess mucus production, and burning. In mild cases of dry eyes, the ocular examination may appear to be remarkably normal.

As indicated in section 21.2.4, the tear film maintains a smooth refracting environment by negating any imperfections in the corneal surface. The tear film also covers the conjunctiva and corneal epithelium, and maintains its viability as a nonkeratinized squamous epithelium. In addition, the tear film contains the bactericidal properties of tear lysozyme and immunoglobulin and washes away noxious bacteria by pumping them from the lacrimal gland through the tear meniscus and out through the nasolacrimal duct. Any abnormality in the tear film predisposes the patient to an increased risk of infection and threatens the refractive ability of the corneal surface. The damaged corneal and conjunctival epithelium may be very difficult to appreciate without the use of dyes, such as Rose Bengal and fluorescein,

which stain damaged or defective conjunctival and corneal epithelium. Rose Bengal may also stain epithelium that is inadequately protected by the mucin layer of the tear film. The staining may provide the earliest clue to a dry eye.

In the later stages of keratitis sicca, corneal filaments may be seen attached to the corneal epithelium. These are composed of mucus coated with epithelium and are characteristically seen in more advanced cases of dry eyes. The other signs associated with a dry eye include a decrease in the tear meniscus of the lower lid and a decreased tear break-up time. The finding of excess particulate matter in the tear meniscus is a pathognomonic finding in dry eye.

One of the most difficult aspects of dry eye is the inability to quantify its severity. The Schirmer test is a simple screening test for the assessment of tear production; a wettable filter paper strip is placed in the inferior cul-de-sac. This can be done with anesthetic (Schirmer I) for the assessment of the basal tear production, or without anesthetic (Schirmer II) for the assessment of the reflex tear production. The filter paper is examined 5 min after its placement, and the extent of wetting is measured in millimeters. Although there are many false-positive and false-negative results associated with this test, it is generally considered the most reliable test of dry eyes. Schirmer I is felt to measure the tear production of the accessory lacrimal glands of Krause and Wolfring, while the Schirmer II measures the tear production of the major lacrimal glands (LAMBERTS et al. 1979). The development of many investigational tests for more accurate diagnosis of dry eye syndrome include the measurement of tear lysozyme, tear lactoferrin, tear osmolarity, and tear fluorophotometry. Other tests, including impression cytology, may be helpful in evaluating selected patients.

Treatment of the dry eye involves an accurate diagnosis by the physician and the attempt to supplement the tear film in an advantageous fashion. One of the most important aspects of patient education in respect to dry eyes is the necessity for informing the patient that this will be a chronic condition in which a cure is highly unlikely. In the early stages of the disease, the condition may cause corneal and conjunctival epithelial changes, which may be reversible. However, in the later stages, when corneal scarring and vascularization have occurred, the goal of treatment is to prevent progression of the disease.

Supplementation of tear production with tear substitutes is the core of dry eye therapy. Tear substitutes can be divided into three subgroups. The first subgroup consists of nonviscous tear preparations, which provide transient tear supplementation. These tear substitutes may be isotonic or hypotonic. Many patients obtain relief of the burning and stinging of the dry eye syndrome with the use of a hypotonic tear, which decreases the tear osmolarity. The second tear replacement is the use of a viscous tear substitute. Often the use of Celluvisc will provide patients who have more severe dry eyes with increased symptomatic relief; Celluvisc is a more viscous tear substitute and provides a longer contact time. The third subgroup of tear substitutes is made up of lubricating ointments, which are primarily composed of petrolatum and/or lanolin. These ointments provide the most prolonged contact time with the external eye; their advantage is a more stable lubricating environment. Their disadvantage is that the tear film is made markedly irregular by these ointments, and vision is significantly decreased. For this reason, most patients with dry eye begin therapy with ointments only at bedtime. If the signs and symptoms become more severe, ointments may be necessary during the day.

Research into the management of dry eyes has centered on the role of preservatives (LEMP 1987). Preservatives may cause significant side effects, such as epithelial breakdown and decreased epithelial healing, in patients with advanced disease whose tear production is negligible. The preservative concentration may build up significantly in the inferior cul-de-sac and create an environment in which the side effects may outweigh the advantages. For this reason, any patient who requires tear supplementation more often than every 4 h should be using a preservative-free artificial tear supplement. Another tear supplement involves the use of Lacriserts, which is a small piece of hydroxypropylmethyl cellulose. The hydroxypropylmethyl cellulose dissolves fully over a 6- to 12-h period in the inferior cul-de-sac, and is used in patients with moderate to severe dry eye. The advantage of this is prolonged tear supplementation; the disadvantages are that it tends to blur vision, it can create a foreign body sensation, or it may fall out.

Once a dry eye patient cannot be adequately controlled with tear supplementation, the role of tear preservation becomes paramount. Tear preservation can be performed in three distinct ways. The most widely used form of tear preservation is punctal occlusion. In punctal occlusion, the punctum, which allows the exit of tears to the nasolacrimal duct system, is closed. This can be done temporarily to assess its advantages, or it can be permanent. In effect, the tear drain out of the eye is closed. Temporary punctal occlusion may be performed with collagen inserts,

punctal plugs, suturing, or light cautery. With punctal occlusion, the available tear film and tear supplementation is maintained for a longer period of time. If punctal occlusion is effective, a permanent punctal occlusion may be performed with a Hyphercator tip. Argon laser treatment has also been found effective in punctal occlusion, particularly for controlled partial occlusion.

The use of moist chamber goggles has also been found effective in the management of dry eye patients (HAYES and FISHER 1979). In this technique, swimmer-type goggles are placed over the eye, creating a moist chamber which decreases evaporation. Moist chambers are extremely effective in dry and windy environments, in which evaporation is a major cause of tear loss. In more moderate cases of dry eyes, the simple use of eyeglasses or glasses with side panels may provide the same advantage without the poor cosmetic result. Finally, the supplementation of moisture in the environment can be extremely simple and a useful adjunct for the dry eye patient. In low-humidity environments the use of room humidifiers may increase moisture in the environment, thereby decreasing the evaporative loss. This technique is extremely helpful during the winter for patients who have forced-hot-air heating systems.

New medical advances may provide relief for selected dry eye patients. More advanced cases may undergo squamous metaplasia of the conjunctiva and the corneal surface. Some authors have reported that topical preparations of vitamin A may reverse conjunctival epithelial metaplasia and offer a new avenue for the treatment of more severe cases of dry eyes (WRIGHT 1985). In patients characterized by excessive mucus production and filament formation, the use of acetylcysteine 10% or 20% may decrease the tear viscosity. This may lead to a decrease in symptoms. Recent reports have addressed the use of oral tetracycline as an anti-inflammatory agent; tetracycline may stabilize the tear film and decrease the inflammatory leukocyte migration and macrophage activity, a concomitant problem in dry eye patients with lid disease.

Finally, surgical options must be examined for patients with severe dry eyes that are not responsive to medical therapy. The most common form of surgery performed is a small lateral tarsorrhaphy. In this technique, the lids are sutured together temporarily or cyanoacrylate adhesive is applied (DONNENFELD et al. 1991). Performance of a tarsorrhaphy means that the ocular surface is decreased and a significant decrease in tear evaporation results. In patients who are unresponsive to the temporary tarsorrhaphy, a conjunctival flap over the damaged cornea may be the only intervention that will prevent corneal stromal thinning and perforation. Patients with nonhealing epithelial defects of the cornea may also be managed with placement of an amniotic membrane graft with or without the addition of corneal limbal stem cells. These stem cells may come from the opposite eye if unaffected by the radiation, from living related donors, or from cadaveric sources (Tseng et al. 1998).

The dry eye associated with radiation is characteristically a moderate to severe dry eye, whose signs and symptoms require constant attention from the ophthalmologist. Every effort should be made to treat co-existing problems associated with dry eye, including blepharitis, exposure keratitis, trichiasis, lid malposition, and lagophthalmos. The radiation-induced dry eye patient may continue to show decreased tear film production for years after irradiation. For this reason, the patient must be given explicit instructions on the timing and dosage of tear substitutes.

21.3.5
Radiation-induced Cataracts

Radiation-induced cataracts (Fig. 21.3) are no different than senile cataract in their diagnosis. For this reason, the following information is generally applicable.

A cataract is a lens opacity. Cataracts may vary markedly in their symptoms and degree of density. The most important drawback of cataract formation is its effect on visual acuity. In general, as a cataract

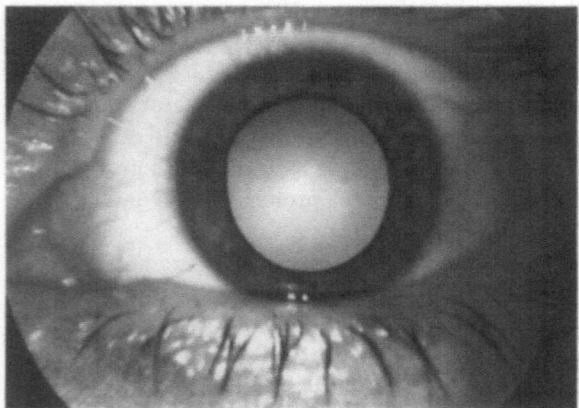

Fig. 21.3. Cataract of a 30-year-old white patient's right eye 3 1/2 years after iodine-125 plaque therapy for a choroidal melanoma anterior to the equator (7.2 mm in height × 12 mm in diameter). The plaque was in place for 1 week, and 100 Gy was delivered to the tumor apex

increases in density, visual acuity decreases proportionately. However, some patients whose dense cataracts are revealed by slit-lamp and direct ophthalmoscopy examination will maintain good visual acuity. For this reason, the most accurate way of measuring the impact of the cataract is by measuring visual acuity. Another major symptom of cataract formation is glare. The effects of glare induced by posterior subcapsular cataracts are most frequently seen in a patient who may have normal visual function under low-light conditions; however, under glare conditions, such as night driving, the patient may experience significant visual disability. One of the earliest symptoms of cataract formation is increasing myopia. This is due to a thickening and an increase in the index of refraction of the nucleus of the lens. The increased lens density may provide the patient with the ability to read without glasses and has been termed "second sight." Frequently, after the increase in myopia, vision may decline.

Cataracts are usually slowly progressive. However, some may progress more rapidly, over a period of weeks to months. In general, radiation-induced cataracts, which are posterior and subcapsular, progress more rapidly. At present, there are no preventative or curative medical treatments for cataracts. Occasionally, patients who have a central lens opacity may be helped by dilating drops, which enable the patient to see around the opacity.

21.3.5.1
Surgical Treatment of Cataracts

Cataract removal is indicated in two situations. The first and most common reason is a reduction in the patient's ability to perform the activities of daily living. There is no cut-off level of visual acuity that requires cataract extraction. Some patients may function well with lower levels of visual acuity, while others cannot function at all with even the most minor visual deficit. The second reason for cataract extraction is the threat to the integrity of the eye when the lens becomes hypermature and the protein released from the lens causes uveitis or secondary glaucoma.

Cataract surgery has changed and progressed markedly over the past 10 years, and it provides relatively rapid and safe visual rehabilitation for patients. In the past, the procedure of choice was intracapsular cataract extraction, in which the entire lens was removed through a 160–180° limbal incision. This technique was replaced by extracapsular cataract extraction, in which the anterior capsule, nucleus, and cortex were removed through a 140° limbal incision. The posterior capsule was left intact. The nucleus was delivered intact through the incision, while the cortex was removed using an irrigation and aspiration device. A variant of extracapsular cataract extraction, which is currently the favored technique, is phacoemulsification. For phacoemulsification, a 3-mm incision is made through the limbus and an ultrasonic fragmentation device is inserted into the eye. The lens nucleus is then removed in small pieces through the 3-mm incision. The advantage of phacoemulsification is the small incision and the possibility for more rapid visual rehabilitation. Adverse aspects of phacoemulsification include an increased risk of damage to the cornea from the ultrasonic tip.

Once the lens has been removed, the process of visual rehabilitation must be contemplated. At the time of cataract extraction, the majority of adult patients receive an intraocular lens, which replaces the patient's own crystalline lens. The intraocular lens may be made of polymethylmethacrylate (PMMA), silicon, acrylic compounds, or other materials, and in the extracapsular approach, or phacoemulsification, the implant is supported by the posterior capsule of the natural lens. The alternatives to intraocular lenses are cataract glasses or contact lenses. In general, patients who have radiation-induced cataracts can also expect to have radiation-induced dry eyes. For this reason, patients are often intolerant of or unable to wear contact lenses, making the aphakic contact lens a poor alternative. The powerful lenses used to correct refractive error with glasses following cataract extraction without an implant offer a variety of optical challenges to the patient, and are often poorly tolerated. This is particularly so if the cataract surgery is only necessary on one eye or if the opposite eye has an implant. The intraocular lens remains the best solution to postoperative visual rehabilitation.

The majority of cataract surgery today is performed on an ambulatory basis. Depending on the method of cataract extraction, the recuperation period may require several days to 2 months for complete healing. Recent advances in micro-surgical technique have made cataract extraction one of the most successful operations performed today, with a success rate of greater than 96%.

One subset of radiation-induced cataracts that deserves special mention is that of pediatric cataracts, or those that occur in children less than 8 years old. The pediatric cataract presents challenges in its surgical removal and for visual rehabilitation. The major difference between the surgery for adults and for children is that in children the soft nucleus can

simply be aspirated out through a limbal incision. Owing to its rapid opacification, the posterior capsule, which is left behind in adults, is generally removed, or a central opening created. The major short-term complication of pediatric cataract extraction is that children very often have a significant inflammatory reaction, which produces adhesions within the eye, later causing glaucoma.

The challenge after pediatric cataract surgery is visual rehabilitation. The pediatric eye is significantly smaller than the adult eye. In addition, the pediatric globe tends to undergo a myopic shift throughout the first 8 years of life. Good visual acuity must be restored as rapidly as possible to avoid amblyopia or a "lazy eye." In the past, the two main alternatives for visual correction were spectacles or contact lenses. In monocular cataracts, spectacle correction is not advised because of the disparity of the image created between the phakic eye and aphakic surgical glasses, which create a 25% magnification. Contact lenses in the pediatric age group are among the most challenging endeavors for the ophthalmologist and for the family. Frequent fittings are required, and lenses are often lost. The lens may produce vision-threatening ocular allergies and infections. In the best possible circumstances, contact lens fitting in a child requires an extremely devoted family, whose members are willing to learn how to insert and remove the contact lens, and multiple visits to the ophthalmologist. Attempts to avoid these difficulties with contact lenses have been known to lead to the performance of epikeratophakia.

In epikeratophakia, the contact lens size for the child is calculated and a dehydrated human cornea is carved and sewn onto the patient's eye. In this procedure, the epithelium grows over the donor cornea and the epikeratophakia cornea is incorporated into the patient's eye, producing a permanent contact lens. Visual success with this technique has been variable. These difficulties in visual rehabilitation, coupled with improvements in surgical technique and lens design, have led to a growing acceptance of intraocular lenses in the pediatric age group, particularly after the age of 2. The surgeon strives for an initial hyperopic correction, which will drift towards emmetropia as the eye grows. Careful preoperative assessment of patient cooperation will determine whether capsulotomy should be done during surgery, or later as a laser procedure. Risks of later lens decentration or dislocation are a continuing challenge.

Owing to the problems of visual rehabilitation in the pediatric monocular cataract, children under the age of 2 who develop monocular cataracts are subject to a significant risk of amblyopia or lazy eye. Cataract extraction with intraocular lens placement in infancy is also associated with a high risk of complications, including glaucoma, capsule opacification, and pupillary abnormalities (LAMBERT et al. 1999). Although the success rate for pediatric cataracts is not as high as that for adult cataract extraction, surgery in the age group 2–8 years is generally more successful and the visual prognosis and chance of restoring some binocular function or depth perception increases with age (HOSAL et al. 2000).

21.4
Summary

The conjunctiva, cornea, and lens of the human eye are exquisitely sensitive to ionizing radiation, and express the injury in two basic ways: dry eye and cataract. Of these, management of the dry eye clearly presents the more significant challenge to the clinician, and to the integrity of the globe. Radiation-induced cataracts may be treated with standard cataract extraction techniques.

References

Avunduk AM, Yardimci S, Avunduk MC et al (2000) A possible mechanism of X-ray-induced injury in rat lens. Jpn J Ophthalmol 44:88–91

Chalupecky H (1897) Über die Wirkung der Röntgenstrahlen. Zentralbl Prakt Augenheilkd 21:386–401

Cogan D, Dreisler K (1953) Minimal amount of X-ray exposure causing lens opacities in the human eye. Arch Ophthalmol 50:30–34

Cogan D, Martin S, Ikui H (1950) Ophthalmologic survey of atomic bomb survivors in Japan. Trans Am Ophthalmol Soc 48:62–87

Donnenfeld ED, Perry HD, Nelson DB (1991) Cyanoacrylate temporary tarsorrhaphy in the management of corneal epithelial defects. Ophthalmic Surg 22:591–593

Fujishima H, Shimazaki J, Tsubota K (1996) Temporary corneal stem cell dysfunction after radiation therapy. Br J Ophthalmol 80:911–914

Griffith T, Pirie A, Vaughn J (1985) Possible cataractogenic effects of radio-nuclides deposited within the eye from the bloodstream. Br J Ophthalmol 69:219–227

Ham W (1953) Radiation cataract. Arch Ophthalmol 50:618–643

Hayes B, Fisher R (1979) Influence of a prolonged period of low-dosage X-rays on the optic and ultrastructural appearances of cataract of the human lens. Br J Ophthalmol 63:457–464

Hightower KR, Giblin F, Reddy V (1983) Changes in the distribution of lens calcium during development of X-ray cataract. Invest Ophthalmol Vis Sci 24:1188–1193

Hosal BM, Biglan AW, Elhan AH (2000) High levels of binocular function are achievable after removal of monocular cataracts in children before 8 years of age. Ophthalmology 107:1647–1655

Junk AK, Egner P, Gottloeber P et al (1999) Long-term radiation damage to the skin and eye after combined beta and gamma radiation exposure during the reactor accident in Chernobyl. Klin Monatsbl Augenheilkd 215:355–360

Kalt (1919) Therapeutic use of X-rays and radium. Bull Soc Fr Ophthalmol 32:125

Kobayashi S, Kasuya M, Shimizu K et al (1993) Glutathione isopropyl ester (YM737) inhibits the progression of X-ray-induced cataract in rats. Curr Eye Res 12:115–122

Lambert B, Kinoshita J (1967) The effects of ionizing radiation on lens cation permeability, transport and hydration. Invest Ophthalmol Vis Sci 6:624–634

Lambert SR, Buckley EG, Plager DA et al (1999) Unilateral intraocular lens implantation during the first six months of life. J AAPOS 3:344–349

Lamberts D, Foster C, Perry H (1979) Schirmer test after topical anesthesia and the tear meniscus height in normal eyes. Arch Ophthalmol 97:1082

Lemp M (1987) Recent developments in dry eye management. Ophthalmol 94:1299–1304

Lerman S (1980) Radiant energy and the eye. Macmillan, New York, pp 279–302

Lipman R, Tripathi B, Tripathi R (1988) Cataracts induced by microwave and ionizing radiation. Surv Ophthalmol 33:200–210

Livesey JC, Wiens LW, VonSeggern DJ et al (1995) Inhibition of radiation cataractogenesis by WR-77913. Radiat Res 141:99–104

MacFaul P, Bedford M (1970) Ocular complications after therapeutic irradiation. Br J Ophthalmol 54:237–247

Matsuda H, Giblin F, Reddy V (1982) The effect of X-irradiation on Na-K ATPase and action distribution in rabbit lens. Invest Ophthalmol Vis Sci 22:180–185

Meesman A (1926) Beitrag zur Röntgen-Radium-Strahlenschädigung der menschlichen Linse Klin Monatsbl Augenheilkd 81:259–69

Merriam G Jr, Szechter A, Focht E (1972) The effects of ionizing radiation on the eye. Radiat Ther Oncol 6:346

Miller RJ, Fujino T, Nefzger M (1967) Lens findings in atomic bomb survivors. Arch Ophthalmol 78:697–704

Rohrschneider W (1928) Klinischer Beitrag zur Entstehung und Morphologie der Röntgenstrahlenkatarakt. Klin Monatsbl Augenheilkd 81:253–259

Ross WM, Creighton MO, Trevithick JR (1990) Radiation cataractogenesis induced by neutron or gamma irradiation in the rat lens is reduced by vitamin E. Scanning Microsc 4:641–649

Roth J, Brown N, Caterall M et al (1976) Effects of fast neutrons on the eye. Br J Ophthalmol 60:236–244

Sallman L, Locke B (1951) Experimental studies on early lens changes after roentgen irradiation. II. Exchange and penetration of radioactive indicators in normal and irradiated lenses of rabbits. Arch Ophthalmol 45:431–444

Sallman LV (1951) Experimental studies on early lens

changes after roentgen irradiation. I. Morphological and cytochemical changes. Arch Ophthalmol 44:149–164

Sasaki H, Lin LR, Yokoyama T et al (1998) TEMPOL protects against lens DNA strand breaks and cataract in the X-rayed rabbit. Invest Ophthalmol Vis Sci 39:544–552

Sinskey R (1955) The status of lenticular opacities caused by atomic radiation. Am J Ophthalmol 39:285–293

Tseng SCG, Prabhasawat P, Barton K et al (1998) Amniotic membrane transplantation with or without limbal allografts for corneal surface reconstruction in patients with limbal stem cell deficiency. Arch Ophthalmol 116:431–441

Wright P (1985) Topical retinoic acid therapy for disorders of the outer eye. Trans Ophthalmol Soc UK 104:869–874

22 Imaging of Tumors of the Eye and Orbit

A.-J. LEMKE and N. HOSTEN

CONTENTS

22.1 Introduction

Diagnosis of diseases affecting the eye and orbit with modern techniques has various meanings. Aspects of differential diagnosis are important in tumors or diseases of the retrobulbar space. but less important in tumors of the eyeball, because these tumors are usually well diagnosed by ophthalmoscopy and ultrasound. Determination of tumor staging may be performed in all pathologies of the eye and orbit using such imaging techniques as computed tomography (CT) and magnetic resonance imaging (MRI). Controllable tissue contrasts mean that the extent of the tumor and the infiltration of surrounding tissue can be evaluated exactly. Improved visualization techniques increasingly allow an integration of CT and MRI images into radiation planning systems. A precondition for this integration is the performance of images with isotropic voxels, i.e., the edges of the

A.-J. LEMKE
Universitätsklinikum Charité, Medizinische Fakultät der Humboldt-Universität zu Berlin, Campus Virchow-Klinikum, Klinik für Strahlenheilkunde, Augustenburger Platz 1, 13353 Berlin, Germany
N. HOSTEN
Zentrum für Radiologie, Ernst-Moritz-Arndt-Universität, Greifswald, Germany

voxels are equal in all three dimensions and they are cube-shaped. This requirement is met by using modern scanners and slice thicknesses between 0.3 and 0.5 mm. With a slice thickness of 0.3 mm, isotropic voxels are reached with a resolution of 512 to 512 pixels and a field of view of 150 mm or a resolution of 256 to 256 pixels and a field of view of 75 mm, respectively.

The cross-sectional imaging modalities, CT and MRI, have been improved drastically by the developments in scanner technique. The improvements of spatial resolution and soft tissue contrast in particular are very important for image quality in small fields of view imaging. Whether CT or MRI is used depends on the clinical question; the two methods have different indications.

The key to the correct differential diagnosis of orbital pathologies is the division of the orbit into several compartments. The assignment of orbital pathologies to a compartment reduces the number of differential diagnoses, because the frequency of a tumor entity differs rather with the compartment (ZONNEVELD et al. 1987; HOSTEN et al. 1992a).

22.2 Compartment Classification

The number of different pathologies found in each orbital compartment is lower than the total number of orbital diseases. Some changes seem to have an affinity for certain compartments. The first step in orbital diagnosis is the assignment of the detected pathology to the correct compartment (ZONNEVELD et al. 1987; HOSTEN et al. 1992a).

The division in orbital compartments is based on anatomical structures. The fibrous muscle conus (connecting the four extraocular muscles) divides the orbit into intraconal and extraconal compartments. The optic nerve traversing the intraconal compartment and the eye muscles are separate compartments. The outer border of the extraconal compartment is the bony orbit, and the subperiosteal compartment is the adjacent compartment. The lacrimal gland and the eye ball are each separate compartments. The ventral border of the extraconal compartment is the orbital septum, which determines the preseptal compartment containing the eyelids.

22.3
Pathologies of the Orbit

22.3.1
Intraconal Compartment: Optic Nerve

The optic nerve should be examined with the image plane at an angle of 10–20° to the orbitomeatal plane, using a thin-slice technique with 0.5–1.0 mm thickness. Those images can be reformated in a coronal and sagittal (parallel to the optic nerve) direction without loss of information. The transverse plane alone is not sufficient to evaluate the optic nerve, because the optic nerve has an S-shaped course along the sagittal plane and exits and enters a transverse plane. If thin slices are not available, transverse 5-mm slices are sufficient owing to reduction of partial volume effects. The center of the external acoustic canal and the lateral canthus are used as reference points.

On CT, the optic nerve complex appears hyperdense compared with the surrounding fatty tissue, but differentiation between nerve and nerve sheath is not expected in a healthy person.

On MRI, differentiation between nerve and nerve sheath is possible using T2-weighted images. In healthy individuals a small hyperintense ring (i.e., the subarachnoid space) delineates nerve and nerve sheath, both of which present with isointense signals. On T1-weighted sequences the optic nerve complex is hypointense and has strong contrast to the surrounding fatty tissue. Owing to the S-shaped course of the optic nerve some sequences should be performed parasagittally along the course of the optic nerve. Examination of both eyes is recommended, since subtle changes such as those found in neuritis might only be appreciated on comparison of both sides.

The determinant factor for differential diagnosis is the relation of the subarachnoidal space and the diameter of the optic nerve on coronal images. Widening of the optic sheath in both orbits will be expected in cases of increased intracranial pressure; enlargement of both optic nerves is a characteristic sign of symmetric optic gliomas in neurofibromatosis (SEILER et al. 1989).

Common pathologies of the optic nerve and the nerve sheath are optic neuritis, hemorrhage in fractures of the orbital apex, perineuritis in inflammatory pseudotumor, and optic glioma. Uncommon conditions are optic nerve sheath meningioma, sarcoidosis, metastases and hemangioblastoma.

Tumorous changes of the optic nerve are mainly attributable to optic gliomas, which are characterized by fusiform enlargement of the optic nerve and marked contrast enhancement (Fig. 22.1) (MAFEE et al. 1987). Optic nerve sheath meningiomas are quite rare tumors and characterized by a tubular enlargement of the optic nerve complex. Differentiation from perineuritic changes may be difficult since the characteristic calcifications are typically visible on CT but often invisible on MRI. Additionally, on CT a widening of the bony optic canal is visible as a sign of intracanalicular involvement.

Optic neuritis most frequently occurs as a manifestation of encephalomyelitis disseminata (GUTHOFF et al. 1988). The acute phase is characterized by a widening of the subarachnoid space and circumscribed contrast enhancement. Using optimized techniques, both findings are detectable on MRI and CT, but MRI has a markedly higher sensitivity. The characteristic sign for optic neuritis is a tubular enlargement of the nerve complex over the whole intraorbital course, while the nerve itself is not significantly enlarged. Infiltration of the surrounding tissue leads to the diagnosis of an inflammatory pseudotumor (ATLAS et al. 1987).

22.3.2
Intraconal Compartment: Other

The intraconal space refers to the muscle conus formed by the four straight extraocular muscles and septa connecting the muscles. The assignment to this compartment is best visualized on a coronal section. Small tumors can easily be assigned, whereas the origin of large tumors often cannot be determined (optic nerve or intraconal space).

The established CT examination technique for questions concerning the intraconal compartment consists of thin spiral CT with calculated coronal reformations.

The choice of the ideal surface coil for orbital MRI is determined by the limited penetration of coils with small diameters. Using a small coil with a diameter of 5 cm, a decrease of the signal intensity in the posterior portion of the orbit is visible and limits the diagnostic assessment. A compromise between the penetration depth of a coil and the spatial resolution has to be

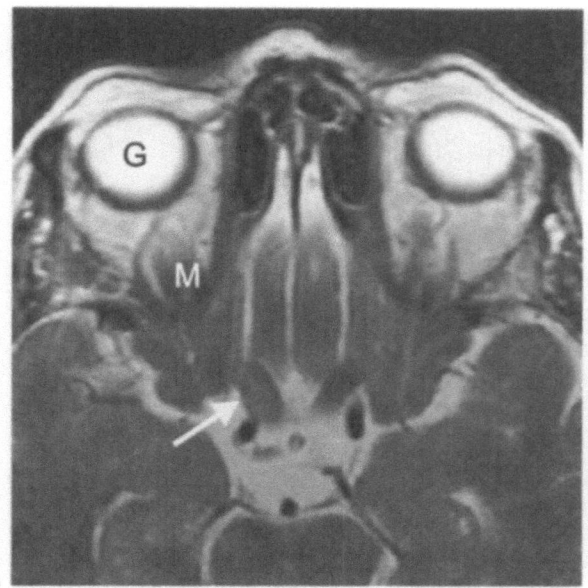 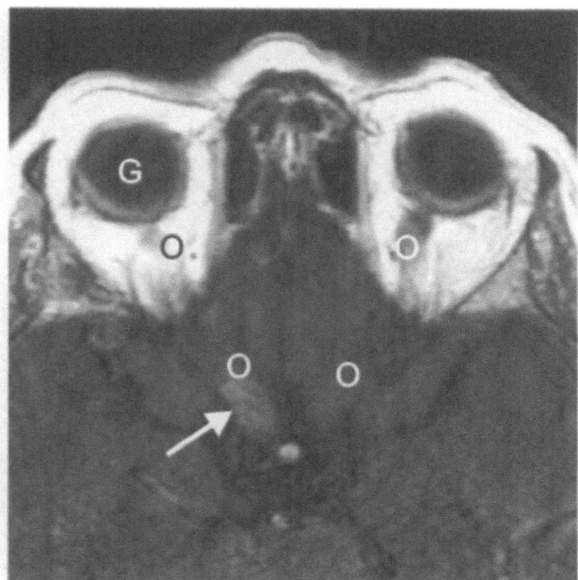

a   b

Fig. 22.1a, b. Optic nerve glioma (optic nerve). **a** MRI T2-weighted image, transverse orientation, edematous enlargement of the right optic nerve immediately ventral to the optic chiasm (*arrow*) **b** MRI T1-weighted image after administration of contrast medium, plain transverse orientation, marked contrast enhancement of the right optic nerve (*G* globe, *M* eye muscle, *O* optic nerve)

made. If comparison of the two eyes is necessary, either a larger surface coil has to be chosen to cover both eyes or both eyes have to be examined separately, which means the examination lasts longer because the coil has to be changed. The most important slice orientation is the coronal section, because it is the only orientation that is helpful in determining infiltration of the eye muscles and the optic nerve and the crossing of the fibrous conus. The initial detection of a mass is usually performed on plain T1-weighted sequences, because most masses are hypointense relative to the retrobulbar fat.

The most common tumors of the intraconal space are cavernous hemangioma, inflammatory pseudotumor and varix nodes. Less frequent are lymphangioma, neurofibroma, metastases and venous vascular changes (arteriovenous fistula). Lymphoma and capillary hemangioma are also found in the intraconal compartment, but an extraconal localization is more common. The differentiation between intraconal masses is difficult because most of the tumors are oval or round with sharp margins. On CT, nearly all tumors are hyperdense relative to fat; on MRI they have lower signal intensities on T1-weighted images and higher signal intensities on T2-weighted images than fat.

The cavernous hemangioma is the most common of all orbital tumors, and it has been well described by HARRIS and JAKOBIEC (1979). The tumor is well defined and septated. Although the typical appearance of cavernous hemangioma includes hypointense signals on T1-weighted images and hyperintense signals on T2-weighted images, partial thrombosis can lead to different signal intensities with conversion of the contrast. The strong contrast enhancement is caused by the sponge-like architecture of the tumor (Fig. 22.2) but can be missing in cases of total thrombosis. In contrast to cavernous hemangioma, lymphangiomas are not encapsulated. Histologically, they are composed of endothelial lacunas filled with serous fluid or blood (TUNC et al. 1999). Owing to their tendency to bleed, lymphangiomas have higher densities on CT than cavernous hemangioma.

The inflammatory pseudotumor of the orbit has been considered as a heterogeneous group of pathologies, which is characterized by inflammatory changes, and also reactive lymphatic hyperplasia and granulomatous changes. Pseudotumor has to be differentiated from infectious conditions of the orbit. The typical clinical appearance of the acute form of inflammatory pseudotumors includes severe pain on eye movement. Chronic courses of the disease are not uncommon (ATLAS et al. 1987). The extent of the disease and the pattern of involvement are not uniform. The range encloses diffuse attachments to the posterior wall of the eye, perioptic infiltrations and extensive intraconal masses (frozen eye). Involvement of several compartments is not rare, and involvement of the lacrimal gland and the eye muscles is possible.

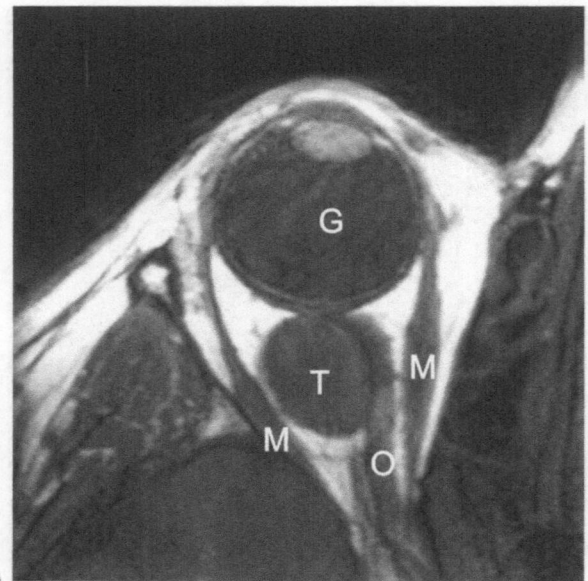 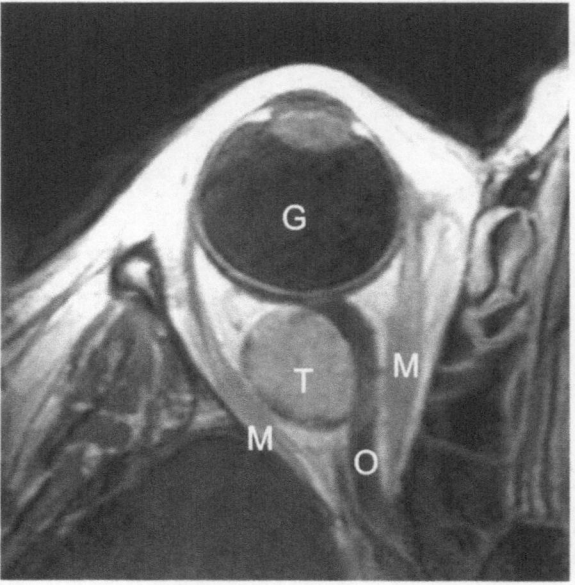

Fig. 22.2. Cavernous hemangioma (intraconal compartment). **a** MRI plain T1-weighted image, transverse orientation, well-defined intraconal mass, hypointense and homogeneous signal intensities, medial displacement of the optic nerve. **b** MRI T1-weighted image after contrast administration, transverse orientation, marked contrast enhancement of the whole mass with exception of a peripheral ring (*T* tumor)

On MRI, inflammatory pseudotumors have a low signal intensity on T1-weighted images (isointense compared to the extraocular muscles) and also on T2-weighted images. The best general view is obtained with coronal slices; involvement of the eye is best visualized on transverse or sagittal slices (Fig. 22.3).

On CT, the mass and the protrusion is seen. The density of the inflammatory pseudotumor corresponds to the density of the external eye muscles. A significant contrast enhancement is not found.

Common intraconal vascular changes are varix nodes and arteriovenous fistulas (rarely orbital, more commonly forwarded from a cavernous sinus fistula). The enlarged vessels are best seen in coronal slice orientation (LEMKE et al. 1994). Additional measurements can be performed during a Valsalva maneuver with adapted measure time.

22.3.3
External Eye Muscles

The diseases of the eye muscles are characterized by thickening of the muscle and/or the tendon. The diameter of the eye muscles is best measured by comparing both sides on coronal slices.

On CT, the eye muscles are well visible due to the natural contrast from the surrounding fatty tissue.

On MRI, the best slice orientation is the coronal; in addition to T1- and T2-weighted sequences,

multi-echo sequences are recommended to evaluate the inflammatory degree of the eye muscles changes in Graves' ophthalmopathy. On T1-weighted sequences the eye muscles are hypointense and the surrounding retrobulbar fat contributes a natural contrast agent due to its hyperintense signals on T1-weighted sequences. On T2-weighted sequences, the contrast is less pronounced and the muscles are slightly hyperintense relative to fat. The additional performance of transverse or parasagittal slices can be useful to evaluate the longitudinal section of the superior and inferior muscles.

The most common pathologies of the eye muscles are changes in the course of Graves' ophthalmopathy, myositis, and eye muscle changes in inflammatory pseudotumor of the orbit. Tumorous changes such as lymphoma and rhabdomyosarcoma are rare conditions.

The characteristic appearance of endocrine orbitopathy includes a symmetric enlargement of the straight eye muscles in both orbits, very frequently with involvement of the inferior and medial rectus muscles (Fig. 22.4) (LANGENBRUCH 1981). CT has no relevance in this field; only in late stages of the disease is a change of density visible owing to a fatty degeneration within the muscle bellies (DAICKER 1979). In contrast, MRI also enables control of therapy during treatment (HOSTEN et al. 1992b). Since structural changes of the eye muscles are only visible in late stages of the disease with T1-weighted images, T2-weight-

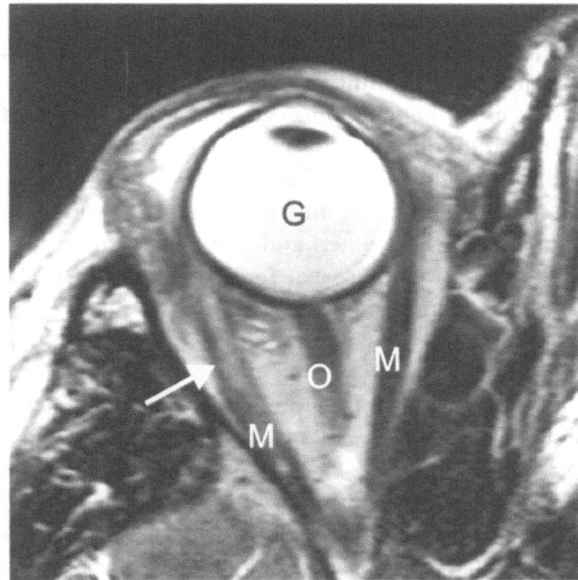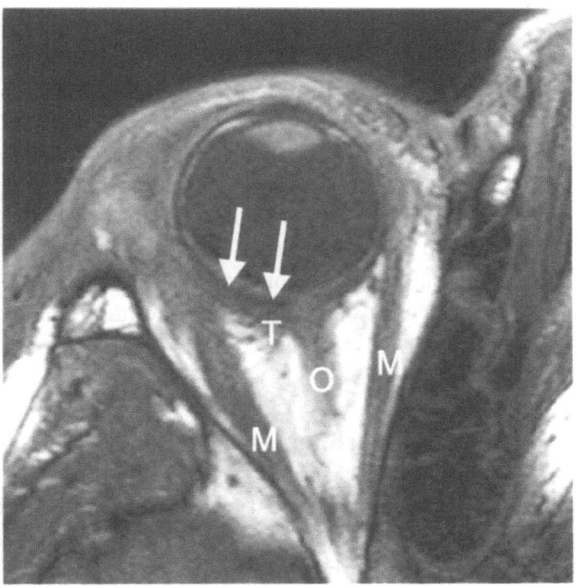

Fig. 22.3a, b. Inflammatory pseudotumor (intraconal compartment). **a** MRI T2-weighted image, transverse orientation, hyperintense area in the lateral rectus muscle (*arrow*) indicates inflammatory involvement. **b** MRI plain T1-weighted image, transverse orientation, diffuse retrobulbar mass in contact with the posterior eye wall (*arrow*)

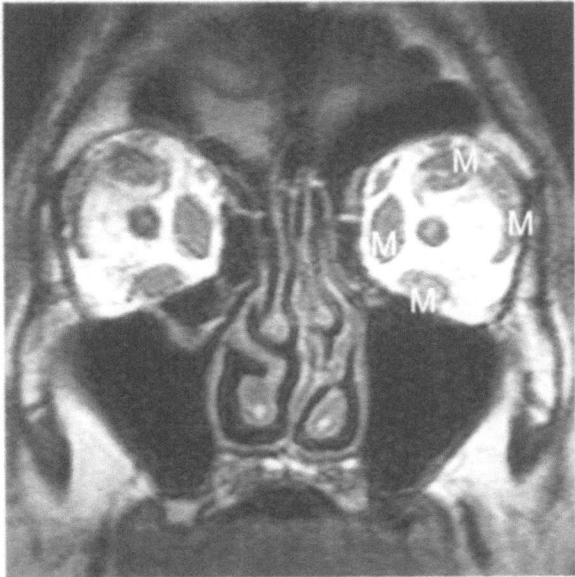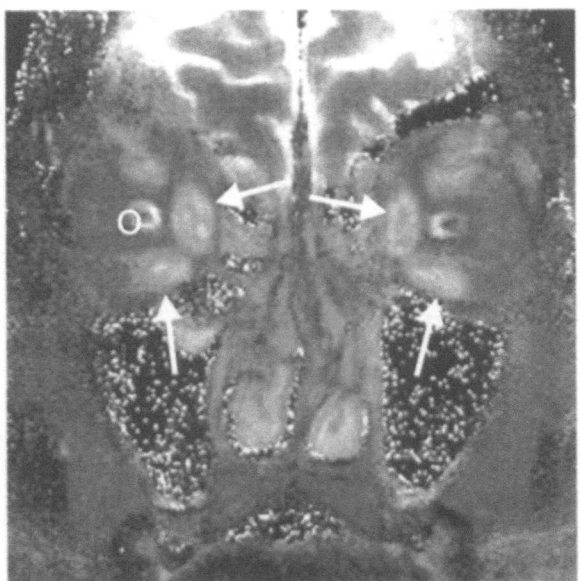

Fig. 22.4. Endocrine orbitopathy (eye muscle compartment). **a** MRI plain T1-weighted image, coronal orientation, enlargement of the medial and inferior straight eye muscles of both orbits. **b** MRI, calculated T2-weighted image, coronal orientation, hyperintense signal intensities of the enlarged eye muscles indicate acute inflammatory stage of endocrine orbitopathy (*arrows*)

ed sequences indicate inflammatory stages in an acute stage with hyperintense signal intensities. Quantification of the inflammatory changes is possible using calculated T2 times based on T2-weighted multi-echo sequences (HOSTEN et al. 1989).

Another inflammatory pathology of the eye muscles is unspecific myositis. Since neither CT nor MRI present significant changes in signal intensities in myositis compared with the normal appearance, morphological parameters have to be used for the differential diagnosis. Normally, the tendon and belly of the muscle are enlarged in myositis, while in endocrine orbitopathy only the muscle belly is enlarged (ROTHFUS and CURTIN 1984). The pattern of involvement is also different. Myositis is usually located in the lateral and medial muscles, and lymphomas are more often found in the superior rectus muscle.

The changes of muscles in inflammatory pseudotumors are comparable to those in unspecific myositis (ATLAS et al. 1987). The guiding findings are a characteristic clinical appearance with severe pain and accompanying intraorbital changes. Involvement of the eye muscles can also be solitary.

22.3.4
Extraconal Compartment

The extraconal compartment occupies only a small volume of the whole orbit and sheathes the muscle conus like a flexible pipe. A suitable imaging orientation in pathologies of this compartment is the coronal section, because it allows the best delineation from the eye muscles and the bony orbit.

The examination technique for CT and MRI does not differ from the technique used for the intraconal compartment.

The most frequent pathologies of the extraconal compartment are lymphoma and capillary hemangioma, followed less frequently by neurofibroma, rhabdomyosarcoma, and metastases (Fig. 22.5). The involvement of this compartment by tumors from neighboring compartments is possible, e.g., developmental tumors (dermoids or epidermoids) and branches of inflammatory pseudotumors.

Capillary hemangiomas are tumorous changes of early childhood and are characterized by unsharp tumor margins and infiltrative growth. On MRI, inhomogeneous signal intensities with hypointense signals on T1-weighted and very hyperintense signals on T2-weighted sequences are found. On CT, capillary hemangiomas are inhomogeneous and, owing to the vascular origin, markedly contrast enhancing.

In contrast, orbital lymphomas normally have a homogeneous parenchyma, and the signal intensities on T1- and T2-weighted images are equal to those of the eye muscles, with homogeneous and marked contrast enhancement. Tumor margins are mainly sharp, because the anatomical structures are respected. In contrast, the interface of the lymphoma with the retrobulbar fat is invariably serrated with small stripe-like extensions. The discrepancy between the often extensive size and only minimal displacement of other structures is characteristic and helps to differentiate lymphomas from other tumors. On CT, homogeneous densities and moderate enhancement is observed. Other possible orbital localizations of lymphomas are subconjunctival lymphomas, lymphomas of the lacrimal gland, and lymphomas of the eyelid (HOSTEN et al. 1991).

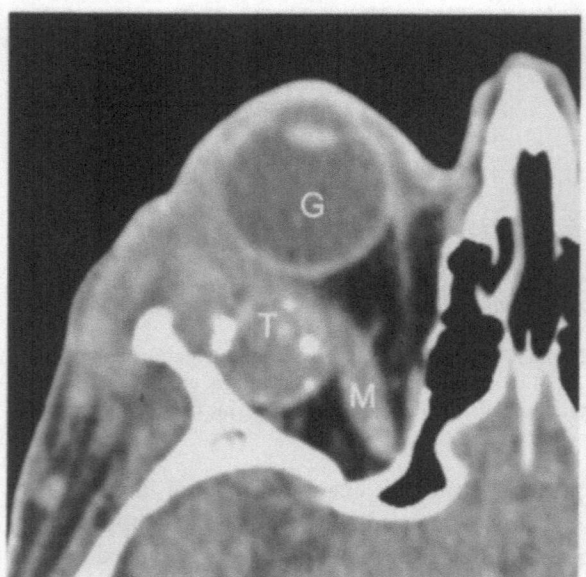 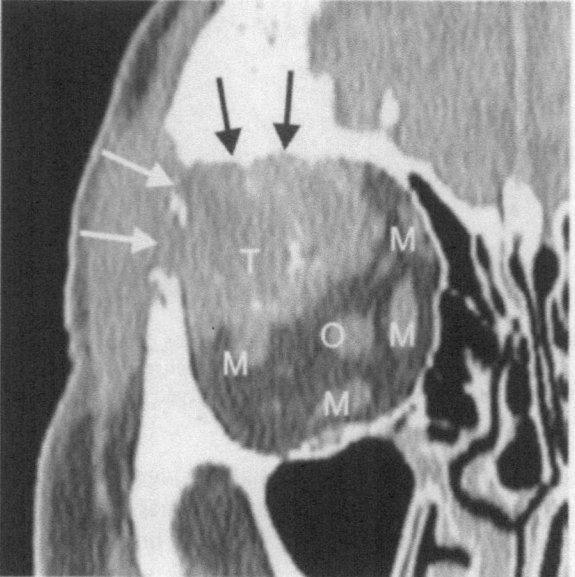

Fig. 22.5a, b. Metastasis from lung cancer (extraconal compartment). **a** CT, plain, transverse slice orientation, large extraconal mass posterior to the lacrimal gland with calcifications. **b** CT, coronal reformation of the transverse data set, medial and inferior displacement of the optic nerve and the external eye muscles, destruction of the bony orbit (*arrows*)

22.3.5
Subperiosteal Compartment

The subperiosteal compartment is defined as the small space between the periosteum and the bony orbit. Many changes from the surrounding structures of the orbit can simulate a subperiosteal mass.

The slice orientation of CT and MRI in masses of the subperiosteal compartment should be adapted to the localization of the mass. On MRI, the use of a larger surface coil is adequate to ensure an overview of both orbits. On CT, the examination protocol should include thin slices and the additional calculation of edge-enhanced images for good differentiation of the bony structures.

The most frequent pathologies of the subperiosteal compartment are musicales, orbital fractures, subperiosteal abscesses, tumors originating from the Para nasal sinuses, osteoma, metastases, dermoids, epidermoids and meningiomas. Less frequently occurring diagnose are fibrous dysphasia, Wegener's granulomatosis, plasmocytoma, cholesterol cysts and Paget's disease.

Frequent inflammatory changes of the subperiosteal compartment are mucoceles and abscesses. Both are characterized by high signals on T2- and low signal on T1-weighted sequences. Additionally, abscesses have strong contrast enhancement at the margins of the abscess, which is very small in mucoceles.

The group of orbital malformations includes dermoids and epidermoids. They are normally found within or in the neighborhood of bony structures. Often the closest neighbor is the crucial hint for this diagnosis. The usually fat-containing dermoids are hyperintense on T1-weighted sequences (Fig. 22.6), while the normally liquid-filled epidermoids are hypointense on T1-weighted and hyperintense on T2-weighted sequences. On CT, fat-equivalent densities are found in dermoids and water-equivalent densities in epidermoids.

Tumors originating from the bony orbit or the surrounding structures, or infiltrating the bony orbit, have a signal behavior or density like the respective tumors in the other region.

22.3.6
Lacrimal Gland

The normal lacrimal gland is almond shaped and covers the eye ball from craniolateral. The lacrimal gland consists of two lobes, the ventrocranial palpebral lobe and the dorsocaudal orbital lobe. Coronal sections are best suited to the depiction and evaluation of form and size of lacrimal gland pathologies. Transverse slices are needed in addition for the ventrodorsal extension of a mass.

On CT, thin transverse spiral CT slices with coronal reformations are appropriate for the evaluation

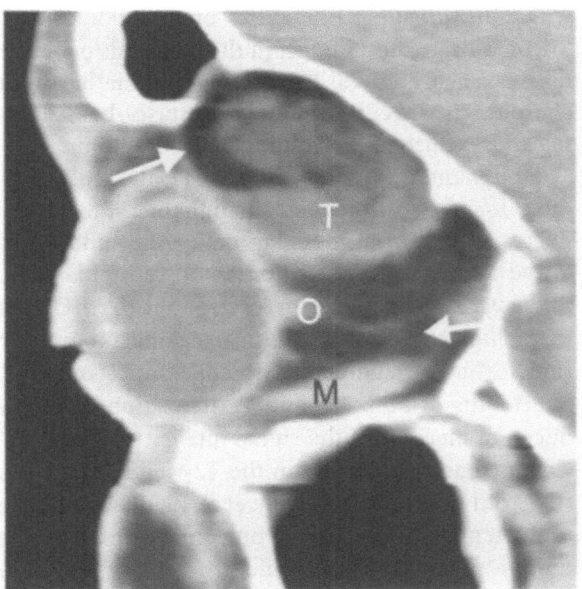
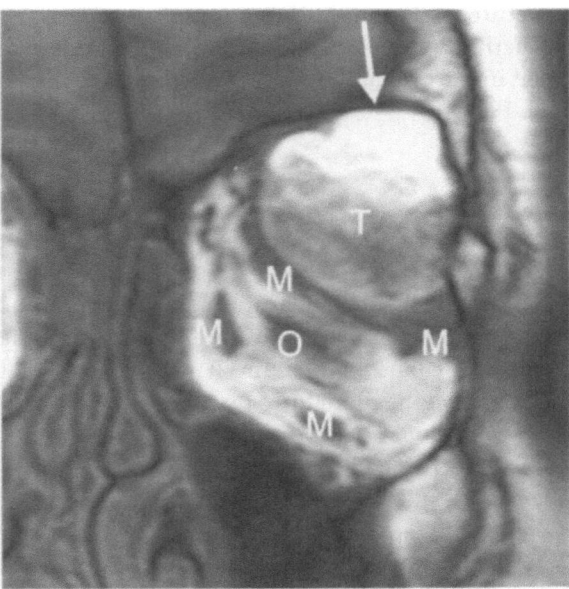

Fig. 22.6a, b. Dermoid (subperiosteal compartment). **a** CT, sagittal reformation of the transverse data set, large mass originating from the orbital roof and containing fat (*arrow*). **b** MRI plain T1-weighted image, coronal orientation, compression of the orbital structures (optic nerve, eye muscles), detection of both fat and soft tissue within the mass leading to the diagnosis of dermoid

of lacrimal gland masses. Using MRI with small surface coils, the structure of the mass can be examined more precisely. The normal lacrimal gland has a hypointense signal intensity on T1-weighted images and a hyperintense signal intensity on T2-weighted images compared with the surrounding fat.

Masses of the lacrimal gland can be subdivided into epithelial and nonepithelial types according to their origin. Pleomorphic adenoma and mixed tissue tumors are of epithelial origin, while lacrimal gland lymphomas and inflammatory pseudotumor are nonepithelial changes.

The inflammatory pseudotumor of the lacrimal gland often occurs in combination with inflammatory changes of the retrobulbar fat. It is clinically characterized by acute and severe pain and morphologically characterized by a retained lentiform shape of the enlarged lacrimal gland. A homogeneous enlargement of the lacrimal gland is observed in lacrimal lymphomas, with enlargement of both lobes and marked contrast enhancement. Lacrimal gland lymphoma can occur in both eyes, and such tumors often reach an enormous size. In contrast, epithelial masses of the lacrimal gland are characterized by an eccentric enlargement of the gland with a preference for the orbital lobe while the palpebral lobe remains normal. Pleomorphic adenomas and adenoid cystic carcinoma are characterized by inhomogeneous signal intensities on T1- and T2-weighted images (Fig. 22.7). In cases of carcinoma, an additional infiltration of the bony structures is found. MRI is superior to CT in the evaluation of homogeneity; both methods are equal in the evaluation of the tumor shape (LEMKE et al. 1996).

22.3.7
Globe

From outside in, the bulbar wall is composed of the sclera/cornea, the uvea, and the inner layer of the retina and ciliary epithelium. It is important that modern imaging modalities be used in the diagnosis of conditions affecting the globe, owing to questions concerning differential diagnosis, noninvasive tumor staging, and treatment planning (e.g., radiation therapy).

In the field of ocular MRI, the use of special surface coils with small diameters is recommended because of the required high resolution and high signal-to-noise ratio. The transverse plane is the initial slice orientation for tumor staging. For the evalua-

tion of the tumor extension, additional slices perpendicular to the largest tumor diameter are necessary. Intravenous contrast agent is used for better differentiation between tumor and subretinal fluid. The slice thickness should be selected depending on the clinical question; slice thicknesses of 1–2 mm are sufficient for diagnostic purposes. For the planning of radiation therapy, preparation of images with isotropic voxels (i.e., voxels with identical edges in all three dimensions) is performed. Using a field of view of 7.5 cm, and a resolution of 256 to 256 pixel, the criterion of isotropic voxel is reached using a slice thickness of 0.3 mm.

On MRI using T1-weighted sequences, the vitreous body has a hypointense signal intensity and the eye's wall has a slightly higher signal. The different layers of the eyeball are not distinguishable on plain images, but after contrast administration strong enhancement of the well-vascularized uvea and particularly of the retina is visible. The signal of the sclera remains nearly unchanged. On T2-weighted images the vitreous body has a hyperintense signal intensity owing to its high water content.

The importance of CT in the field of ocular imaging decreased with the increasing availability of MRI. Indications for CT are the localization of foreign bodies and the detection of calcified ocular masses (CHAR et al. 1984).

The most frequent changes in the eyeball, such as retinal detachment, scleritis, and uveitis, are usually not examined with MRI, because they are diagnosed with other imaging modalities or ophthalmoscopy. MRI has its greatest impact in the diagnosis of ocular masses, such as uveal melanoma (originating from choroid, iris and ciliary body), metastases, hemangioma and, exclusively in children, retinoblastoma.

Malignant melanoma of the uvea is the most common form of intraocular malignancy. Melanoma makes up 70% of intraocular malignant tumors, followed by metastatic carcinoma and retinoblastoma in the pediatric population (each about 10%). Owing to the high content of melanin, uveal melanomas are said to have a characteristic appearance on MRI. Shortening of both T1- and T2-relaxation times induces an increase of the signal intensities in the T1-weighted and a decrease in the T2-weighted images (GOMORI et al. 1986; PEYSTER et al. 1988). Among eye tumors, melanomas are the only ones to exhibit this unique signal behavior, which is used as the main differential diagnostic criterion between eye tumors (ADAM et al. 1990) (Fig. 22.8).

Owing to the linear correlation between signal intensity and melanin content, amelanotic and mixed

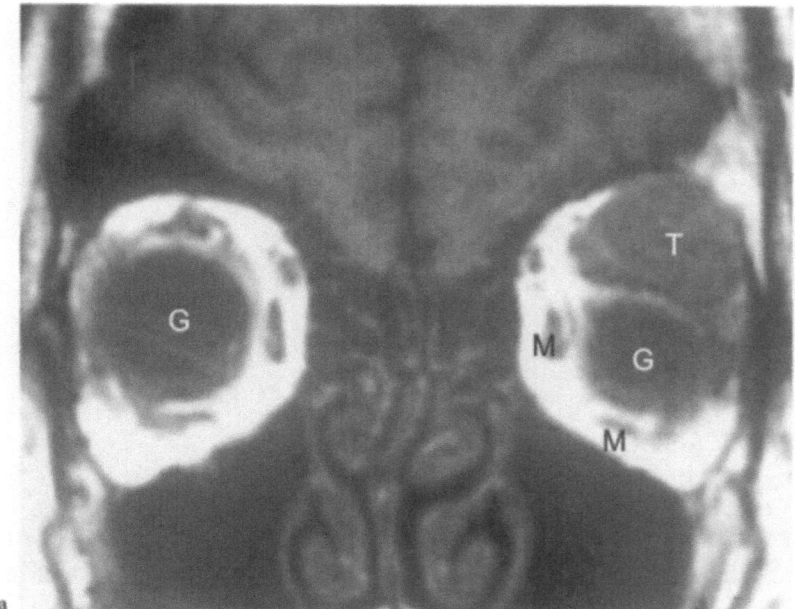

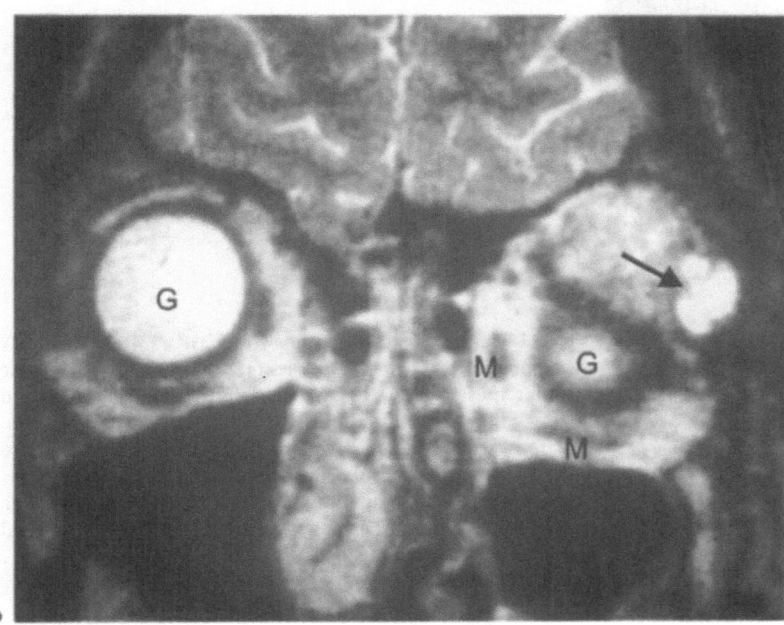

Fig. 22.7a, b. Lacrimal gland adenoma (lacrimal gland). **a** MRI plain T1-weighted image, coronal orientation, large mass of the orbital part of the left lacrimal gland. **b** MRI T2-weighted image, coronal orientation, detection of cystic area (*arrow*) within the tumor

pigmented melanomas have different signal intensities from typical melanomas and make the differential diagnosis harder (DE POTTER et al. 1994). Choroidal metastases, for example, have slightly hyperintense signal intensities on T1-weighted sequences and slightly hypointense signal intensities on T2-weighted sequences relative to the vitreous body. They are not distinguishable from poorly pigmented melanomas (LEMKE et al. 1999). Ocular hemangiomas have a characteristic MRI appearance with isointense signal intensities on T2-weighted sequences and slightly hyperintense signal intensities on T1-weighted sequences (STROSZCZYNSKI et al. 1998). Retinoblastomas are isointense on T1-weighted sequences and hypointense on T2-weighted sequences compared with the vitreous body. Up to now, MRI is still less sensitive than CT in the detection of typical calcifications (DE POTTER et al. 1996) (Fig. 22.9). In very small tumors such as small uveal melanomas, senile maculopathy, or uveal nevi, differential diagnosis is more difficult because the spatial resolution of MRI is limited. On plain MRI sequences, signal intensities do not make it possible to distinguish between serous retinal detachments and

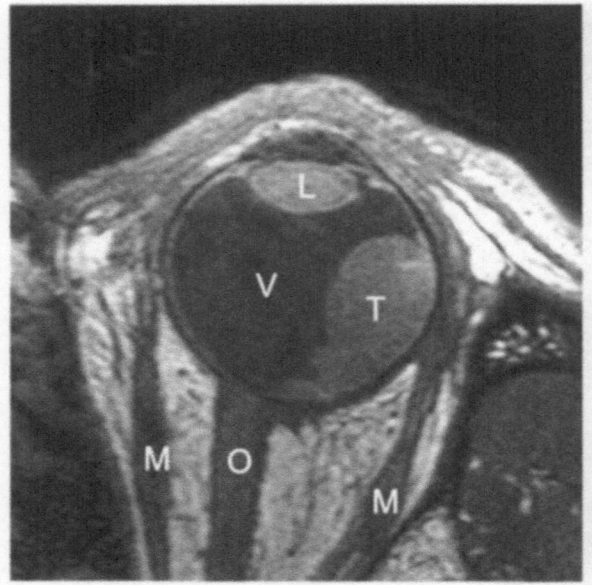

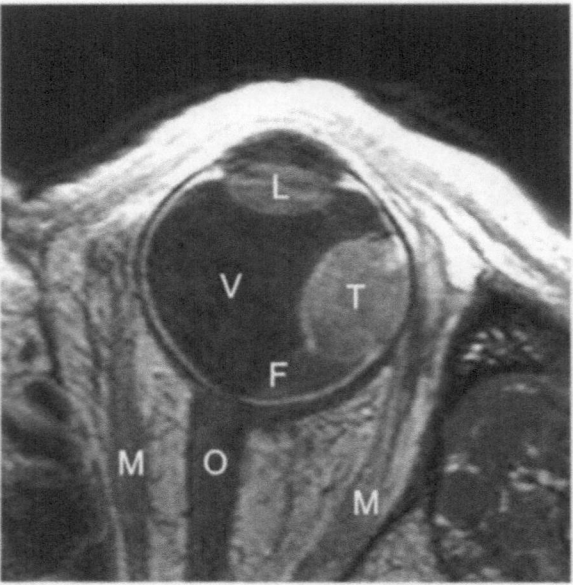

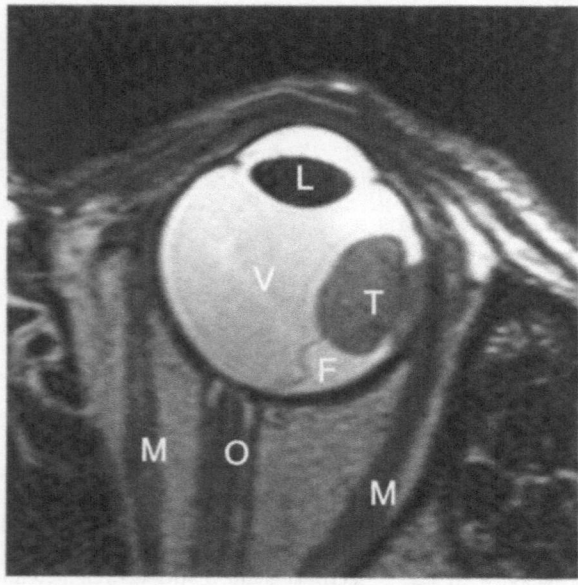

Fig. 22.8a–c. Uveal melanoma (globe). **a** MRI plain T1-weighted image, transverse orientation, slightly hyperintense ocular mass relative to vitreous body. **b** MRI T1-weighted image after contrast administration, transverse orientation, marked contrast enhancement of the uveal melanoma, no enhancement of the subretinal fluid. **c** MRI T2-weighted image, transverse orientation, mushroom-shaped melanoma with retinal detachment and subretinal fluid (*F* subretinal fluid, *L* lens, *V* vitreous body)

amelanotic melanomas or other intraocular tumors. After contrast administration, contrast enhancement is visible only in solid tumors and not in subretinal fluid (LEMKE et al. 1998).

22.3.8
Preseptal Compartment

Usually, preseptal changes of the upper or lower eyelid are clinically well examined (including percutaneous biopsy), so that imaging methods are not necessary for differential diagnosis but useful for the determination of the extent of the related mass. In particular, the detection of an intact or disrupted orbital septum (posterior border of the preseptal compartment) is relevant for therapy.

On MRI, sagittal slices and the use of a surface coil are recommended for the diagnosis of lid masses; relaxed closing of the eyes is helpful for a good image quality. The orbital septum is best visualized and evaluated by sagittal and transverse slices (HOFFMANN et al. 1998).

On CT, the contrasts are not sufficient for the evaluation of lid tumors; sagittal reformations of thin spiral CT datasets and the original transverse slices

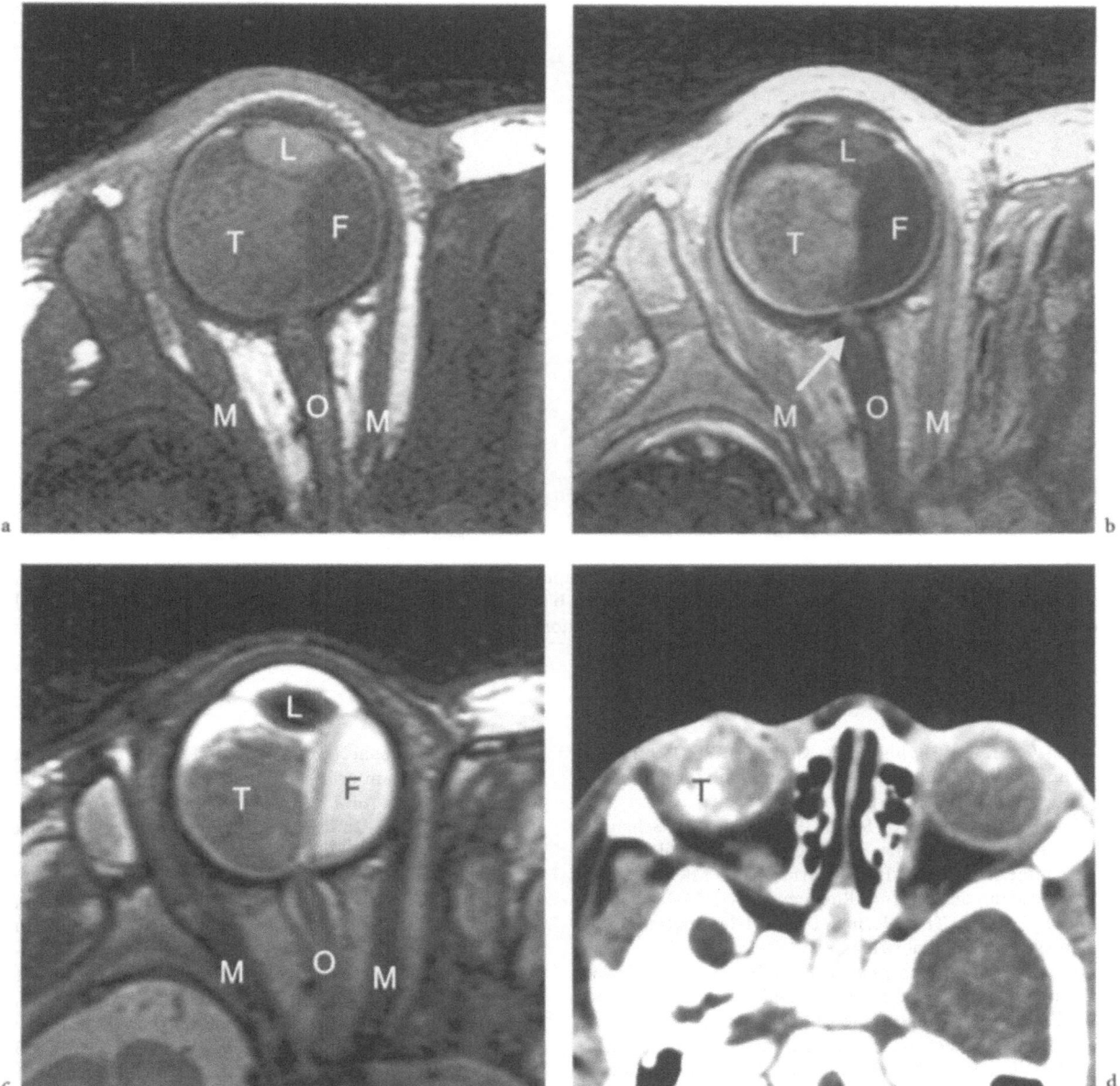

Fig. 22.9a–d. Retinoblastoma (globe). **a** MRI plain T1-weighted image, transverse orientation, nearly isointense ocular mass compared to vitreous body. **b** MRI T1-weighted image after contrast administration, transverse orientation, inhomogeneous contrast enhancement of the tumor, detection of optic infiltration (*arrow*). **c** MRI T2-weighted image, transverse orientation, subtotal retinal detachment with subretinal fluid. **d** CT, plain, transverse slice orientation, large calcified mass of the eye

lead to comparable results concerning the postseptal infiltration of a mass, although the septum itself is not visible on CT.

A number of masses can affect the preseptal compartment. The most common are benign masses, such as xanthelasma, and semimalignant basalioma. Less frequently, capillary Hemangioma, lymphomas, carcinomas and metastases occur (Fig. 22.10).

After clinical examination, most benign tumors are not further investigated with cut-plane modalities. In malignant tumors of the preseptal compartment the posterior extent of the mass is of interest, so that the integrity of the orbital septum has to be proven. Mainly on MRI, but also on CT, the detection of pre- and postseptal fat is helpful in the diagnosis of dorsal extension.

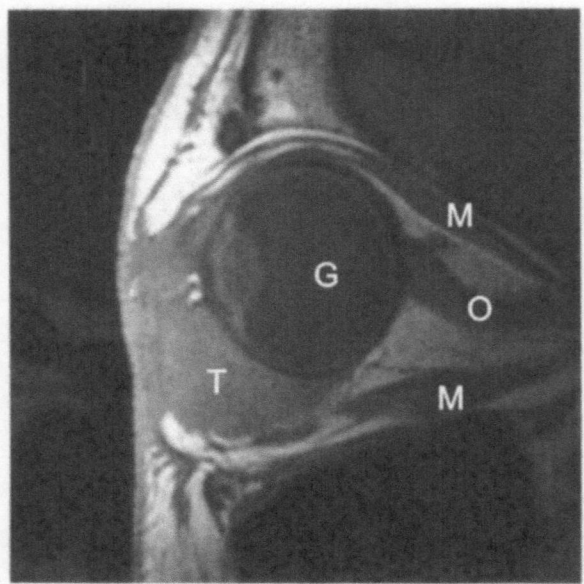
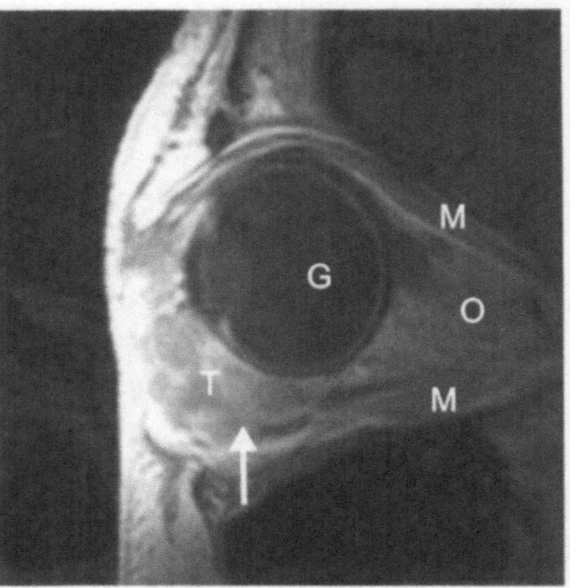

Fig. 22.10a, b. Carcinoma of the eccrine glands (preseptal compartment). **a** MRI plain T1-weighted image, sagittal orientation, slightly hyperintense and homogeneous mass of the lower lid. **b** MRI T1-weighted image after contrast administration, sagittal orientation, inhomogeneous contrast enhancement, destruction of the orbital septum (*arrow*)

References

Adam G, Brab M, Bohndorf K, Günther RW (1990) Gadolinium-DTPA-enhanced MRI of intraocular tumors. Magn Reson Imaging 8:683–689

Atlas SW, Grossman RI, Savino PJ, Sergott RC, Schatz NJ, Bosley TM, Hackney DB, Goldberg HI, Bilaniuk LT, Zimmerman RA (1987) Surface-coil MR of orbital pseudotumor. AJR Am J Roentgenol 148:803–808

Char DH, Hedges TRD, Norman D (1984) Retinoblastoma. CT diagnosis. Ophthalmology 91:1347–1350

Daicker B (1979) Das gewebliche Substrat der verdickten äußeren Augenmuskeln bei der endokrinen Orbitopathie. Klin Monatsbl Augenheilkd 174:843–847

De Potter P, Flanders AE, Shields JA, Shields CL, Gonzales CF, Rao VM (1994) The role of fat-suppression technique and gadopentetate dimeglumine in magnetic resonance imaging evaluation of intraocular tumors and simulating lesions. Arch Ophthalmol 112:340–348

De Potter PD, Shields CL, Shields JA, Flanders AE (1996) The role of magnetic resonance imaging in children with intraocular tumors and simulating lesions. Ophthalmology 103:1774–1783

Gomori JM, Grossman RI, Shields JA, Augsburger JJ, Joseph PM, DeSimeone D (1986) Choroidal melanomas: correlation of NMR spectroscopy and MR imaging. Radiology 158:443–445

Guthoff R, Terwey B, Bragelmann L (1988) Die Rolle der Kernspintomographie bei der Diagnose einer monosymptomatischen Neuritis nervi optici [Role of nuclear magnetic resonance imaging in the diagnosis of monosymptomatic optic neuritis]. Klin Monatsbl Augenheilkd 192:311–316

Harris GJ, Jakobiec FA (1979) Cavernous hemangioma of the orbit. J Neurosurg 51:219–228

Hoffmann KT, Hosten N, Lemke AJ, Sander B, Zwicker C, Felix R (1998) Septum orbitale: high-resolution MR in orbital anatomy. AJNR Am J Neuroradiol 19:91–94

Hosten N, Sander B, Cordes M, Schubert CJ, Schörner W, Felix R (1989) Graves ophthalmopathy: MR imaging of the orbits. Radiology 172:759–762

Hosten N, Schörner W, Zwicker C, Lietz A, Serke S, Huhn D, Felix R (1991) Lymphozytäre Infiltrationen der Orbita in MRT und CT. Lymphom, Pseudolymphom und entzündlicher Pseudotumor. Fortschr Röntgenstr 155:445–451

Hosten N, Schörner W, Lietz A, Kind A, Seiler T, Wollensak J, Wollensak H (1992a) Raumforderungen der Orbita: Moderne bildgebende Diagnostik. Aktuel Radiol 2:325–333

Hosten N, Schörner W, Lietz A, Wenzel KW (1992b) Der Krankheitsverlauf bei der endokrinen Orbitopathie (Magnetresonanztomographische Dokumentation). Fortschr Röntgenstr 157:210–214

Langenbruch K (1981) Die Computertomographie der Orbita bei der endokrinen Ophthalmopathie. Fortschr Röntgenstr 135:29–32

Lemke AJ, Hosten N, Neumann K, Wollensak J, Felix R (1994) Spiral-CT von orbitalen Raumforderungen: verbesserte Darstellungsmöglichkeiten durch frei rekonstruierbare Ebenen. Fortschr Röntgenstr 161:391–398

Lemke AJ, Hosten N, Grote A, Felix R, Wollensak J (1996) Differenzierung von Tränendrüsentumoren mit der hochauflösenden Spiral-CT im Vergleich zur Magnetresonanztomographie [Differentiation of lacrimal gland tumors with high resolution computerized tomography in comparison with magnetic resonance tomography]. Ophthalmologe 3:284–291

Lemke AJ, Hosten N, Bornfeld N, Bechrakis NE, Frenzel D, Richter M, Felix R (1998) Erscheinungsbild von Aderhautmelanomen in der hochauflösenden 1,5-T-MRT mit einer Oberflächenspule anhand von 200 konsekutiven Patienten [Appearance of choroidal melanoma on high resolution MRI using 1.5 T with a dedicated surface coil in 200 consecutive patients]. Fortschr Röntgenstr 169:471–478

Lemke AJ, Hosten N, Bornfeld N, Bechrakis NE, Schüler A, Richter M, Stroszczynski C, Felix R (1999) Uveal melanoma: correlation of histopathologic and radiologic findings by using thin-section MR imaging with a surface coil. Radiology 210:775–783

Mafee MF, Putterman A, Valvassori GE, Campos M, Capek V (1987) Orbital space-occupying lesions: role of computed tomography and magnetic resonance imaging. An analysis of 145 cases. Radiol Clin North Am 25:529–559

Peyster RG, Augsburger JJ, Shields JA, Hershey BL, Eagle R Jr, Haskin ME (1988) Intraocular tumors: evaluation with MR imaging. Radiology 168:773–779

Rothfus WE, Curtin HD (1984) Extraocular muscle enlargement: a CT review. Radiology 151:677–681

Seiler T, Bende T, Schilling A, Wollensak J (1989) Magnetische Resonanz-Tomographie in der Ophthalmologie. II. Stauungszeichen im Sehnerven [Magnetic resonance tomography in ophthalmology. II. Manifestations of edema of the optic nerve]. Klin Monatsbl Augenheilkd 195:72–78

Stroszczynski C, Hosten N, Bornfeld N, Wiegel T, Schueler A, Foerster P, Lemke AJ, Hoffmann KT, Felix R (1998) Choroidal hemangioma: MR findings and differentiation from uveal melanoma. AJNR Am J Neuroradiol 19:1441–1447

Tunc M, Sadri E, Char DH (1999) Orbital lymphangioma: an analysis of 26 patients. Br J Ophthalmol 83:76–80

Zonneveld FW, Koornneef L, Hillen B, de Slegte RG (1987) Normal direct multiplanar CT anatomy of the orbit with correlative anatomic cryosections. Radiol Clin North Am 25:381–407

23 Ultrasound Sonography in Intraocular Tumors

A. Walter, A. Hassenstein, G. Richard

CONTENTS

23.1 Introduction

Ultrasound is sound with a frequency beyond the range of human hearing (20000 Hz), which represents mechanical waves, i.e., a periodic movement of mass. Mundt and Hughes first described ultrasonography in 1956, and many technical improvements have been made since then.

In ophthalmology, the standardized A-scan sonography developed by Ossoinig (1974a, 1977, 1991), B-scan sonography, ultrasound biomicroscopy (UBM), and newer three-dimensional techniques and Doppler flowmetry are used.

The A-mode system derives its name from 'amplitude.' The A-echogram is one-dimensional. It indicates the exact location of the reflecting interface within the organs insonified by the ultrasound. The standard A-scan echography is based on a time-amplitude-modulated scanning procedure. It is used for quantitative echography, such as measurements of length or reflectivity, in intraocular structures. The most common applications of A-mode are measurements of the axial length of the globe and, lately, of corneal thickness. In A-scan echography, the initial peak corresponds to the anterior capsule and the second peak, to the posterior capsule of the lens. Normally, the vitreous does not show any reflectivity aside from small particles representing vitreous densities. At the posterior pole the retina and the sclera present a high reflective peak. The sclera is more reflective than the retina. The two structures can be differentiated in the case of separation such as might be caused by a retinal detachment.

In the B-mode technique (time–brightness method) the echoes are displayed as light dots of varying brightness (B = brightness). In this way a two-dimensional section through the tissue is obtained. The B-mode allows good evaluation of anatomical relationships. It provides us with the possibility of topographical visualization and localization of intraocular lesions and also kinetic characteristics.

In B-scan sonography the vitreous may show small reflectivities which represent a synchysis scintillans, vitreous hemorrhage, infiltrates in uveitis, or artifacts of a mature cataract or intraocular lens.

The frequency of A-scan and B-scan sonography is 8–12 MHz. The commercially available devices have a lateral resolution power of 2 mm and an axial resolution of 0.3 mm. For routine diagnostic conventional sonography both A-scan and B-scan sonography are performed.

The following tissue properties can be differentiated sonographically:

- Kinetic (dynamic) characteristics, such as motility and mobility of intraocular structures, e.g., aftermovements
- Anatomical characteristics, such as the delineation and shape of various tissues, e.g., the mushroom shape of choroidal melanoma and choroidal excavation
- Quantitative characteristics, e.g., relative strength of reflection, sound attenuation or shadow formation

Another possibility is the 'relative reflectivity' (dB difference). An echo signal is compared with a scleral echo. The difference (in decibels) of the amplifier control settings indicates the relative reflectivity of this structure. This method is often used to differen-

A. Walter, MD; A. Hassenstein, MD; G. Richard, MD
University Eye Hospital Eppendorf, Martinistrasse 52,
20251 Hamburg, Germany

tiate intraocular membranes. The most common use in ophthalmology is the localization and differentiation of intraocular structures and a quantification of lesions (GUTHOFF 1991; GUTHOFF et al. 1987, 1999).

Ultrasound biomicroscopy (UBM) is a new, high-resolution technique that has been available for only a few years (30–100 MHz). Because of its limited penetration depth of 3–8 mm, only the anterior globe can be examined by this technique. It provides high axial and lateral resolution of the tissue of up to 50 μm.

Doppler flowmetry is used for visualization of blood flow (velocity) and circulation, because of the color visualization at different frequencies. A major indication in intraocular tumors is hemangioma, in which a high velocity in the area of the tumor is typical.

The probe is either located on the conjunctiva under local anesthesia or on the upper lid in a closed eye. The examination is not painful or uncomfortable for the patient. There are no side effects known in routine sonography.

A survey of the anterior third of the orbit in relation to extraocular structures such as orbital bone, muscles and optic nerve is possible by ultrasound (OSSOINIG 1974b).

23.2
Benign Lesions

23.2.1
Hemangioma

Hemangioma may arise from the ciliary body, the choroid and the retina. Choroidal hemangiomas normally show a highly reflective surface and homogenous internal reflectivity with widening of the ocular coats. Sonographically, a hemangioma resembles a metastasis or disciform macular degeneration. Hemangiomas are often combined with serous retinal detachment and subretinal hemorrhage. The detachment of the sensory retina is typically close to the lesion, in contrast to the collateral retinal detachment in choroidal melanoma. The localization of focal choroidal hemangiomas is at the posterior pole, whereas diffuse choroidal hemangiomas occur more anteriorly, close to the ciliary body. In these cases UBM is useful for visualization and differentiation. The slow circulation of dilated blood vessels is not apparent echographically, but can be visualized by Doppler ultrasonography. The most suitable technique for determining blood velocity in the orbit is Doppler ultrasonography with false colors. Blues

represent flow directed away from the probe and reds, flow towards the probe. This method demonstrates the blood flow behavior and direction as long as the lesion is not thrombosed.

A-Scan sonography shows a high internal reflectivity of the lesion. B-Scan sonography reveals tumefaction of the choroid without choroidal excavation. Both B-scan and A-scan sonography can demonstrate calcifications in the tumors, which are highly reflected. At this stage a hemangioma cannot be differentiated from an osteoma or metastatic calcification of the choroid. Large hemangiomas may be firm or slightly compressible. (see Case Report in sect. 28.2.2, and Figs. 28.1a–c, 28.2a–e).

23.2.2
Osteoma

Osteoma is a well-differentiated benign tumor of bone. It is the most common bony tumor of the orbit. The tumor usually presents in the 2nd to 5th decades, predominantly in male subjects. The origin is unknown. Multiple osteomas may be associated with Gardner's syndrome (familial polyposis coli).

Clinically, osteomas present as orange to yellow lesions at the posterior pole involving the optic nerve head (Fig. 23.1a, b).

A-Scan sonography reveals a maximum of reflectivity in the area of the lesion. B-Scan sonography shows a unique and typical pattern. Because of the high density and reflectivity of osteomas, the sound beam is completely reflected. Ultrasound in osteoma demonstrates a high reflective layer within the sclera and orbital shadowing (Fig. 23.1c).

23.3
Malignant Lesions

23.3.1
Retinoblastoma

Retinoblastoma is the most common malignant intraocular tumor of childhood. The tumor arises from the sensory retina in young children, either as a sporadic genetic mutation or as a feature of known familial hereditary disease. Both eyes are affected in 30% of patients. Orbital involvement occurs along the optic nerve. The most common finding is leukokoria associated with loss of vision (Fig. 23.2a). In 60% of cases the patients first present while under 3 years old.

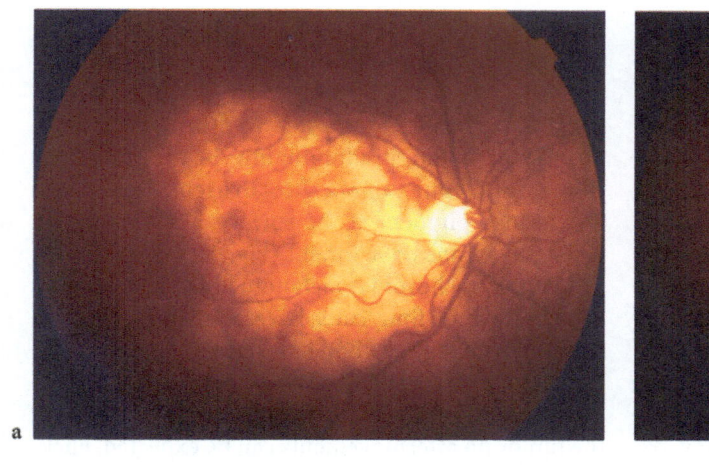

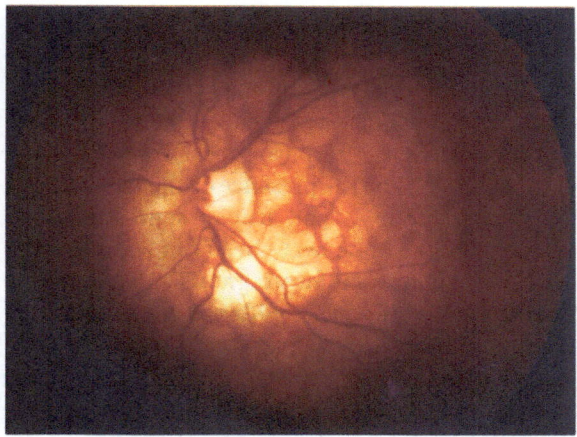

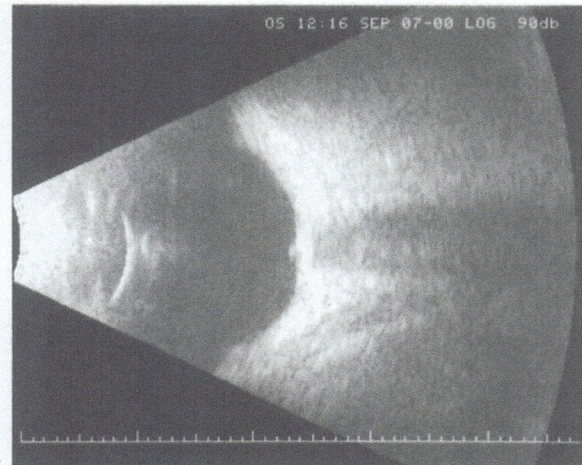

Fig. 23.1. a, b Biomicroscopy of osteoma (right and left eye) shows an orange-yellow geographic flat peripapillary lesion at the posterior pole without tumefaction. **c** Ultrasound (B-scan) reveals high-reflective sclera (osteoma) with orbital shadowing in osteoma

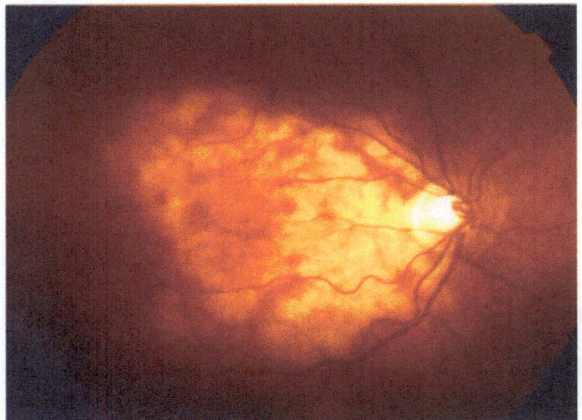

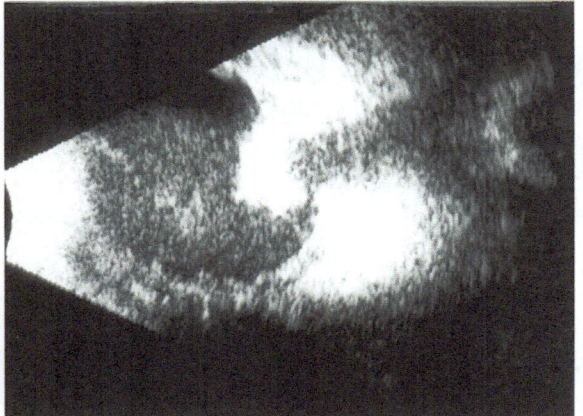

Fig. 23.2. a Biomicroscopy of a 3-year-old female patient with a diffusely growing retinoblastoma, presenting not only leukokoria, but also growth in the anterior chamber. **b** Ultrasound of the same patient demonstrates the typical pattern of intraocular calcification and orbital shadowing in retinoblastoma

The echographic cross section is characterized by a few areas of extremely high reflectivity caused by calcification within the tumor (Fig. 23.2b). B-Scan sonography demonstrates a mixed pattern of high and low reflectivity. A typical aspect is calcification, which is detected by the presence of shadowing (Fig. 23.2b). With both A- and B-scan sonography, involvement of the optic nerve head can be differentiated. This is important for prognosis and treatment. A perforation of the sclera with orbital invasion can be shown echographically.

Nuclear magnetic resonance tomography is an important additional imaging diagnostic tool for visualization of extraocular growth of the tumor. We use it to differentiate diffuse from exophytic and endophytic types of growth in retinoblastoma.

23.3.2
Choroidal Malignant Melanoma

Choroidal melanoma appears as a brownish, dark, prominent lesion, predominantly in the periphery (Fig. 23.3a). Some tumors show drusen-like deposits and orange pigment at the surface, and typically, a collateral serous detachment (Fig. 23.3a).

Malignant choroidal melanomas are histologically divided into four categories, namely spindle A, spindle B, mixed type and epithelioid type.

The internal structure of the tumor is best described by A-mode. Owing to the solid tissue nature of the tumor no aftermovements can be expected. Flickering spike complexes may be seen on the A-mode echogram. B-Mode Doppler devices, with a high reso-

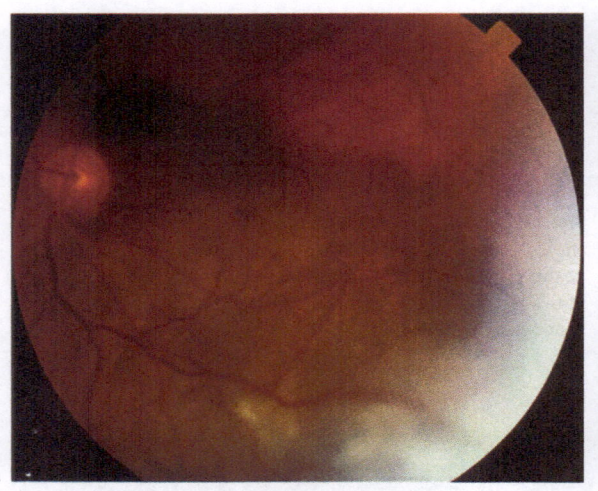

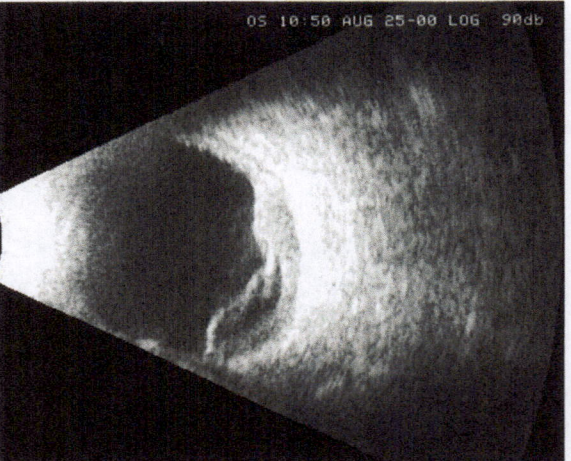

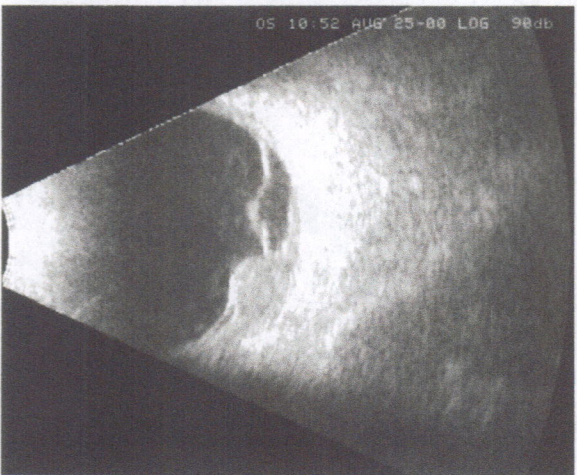

Fig. 23.3. a This 29-year-old male patient shows an expansive large choroidal melanoma of the posterior pole at the lower vessel arcade. The tumor is seen to be dark brown and gray, with a tumefaction. **b** Ultrasound of the same patient reveals the homogeneous tumor and a collateral serous detachment below the tumor (vertical scan). **c** Ultrasound (transverse scan) shows a detachment of the neurosensory retina nasal to the tumor and below the optic nerve head

lution power, can be used to visualize tumor vessel circulation. In A-scan sonography, choroidal melanoma shows a high reflective surface with a low to medium internal reflectivity (10–60% of the scleral spike). The tumor has a uniform internal structure and no after-movements. In some cases it is possible to visualize signs of vascularization by flickering spikes.

In B-mode echograms a melanoma appears as a biconvex area. The internal structure is relatively homogeneous and produces markedly fewer signals than the tumor surface or the sclera (Fig. 23.3b, c). The transverse and longitudinal diameters of the tumor, and its height including the choroidal excavation, if present, can be measured (Fig. 23.3b, c). Eventually, expansion of the tumor through Bruch's membrane can be identified by the highly specific sign of a mushroom shape (collar button). A widening of Tenon's space and a reduced scleral reflectivity at the tumor base are other signs of extraocular extension. An extraocular extension can be demonstrated more sensitively by B-scan sonography than by computed tomography and nuclear magnetic resonance imaging. A tumor lying beneath the sensory retina occasionally reflects the ultrasound more than a tumor beneath Bruch's membrane.

Sonography is important for planning the treatment of choroidal melanoma. For small tumors up to 2–3 mm in height a focal laser treatment by argon laser or transpupillary thermotherapy (TTT) might be sufficient. In the case of larger tumors the treat-ment of choice is ruthenium brachytherapy. The height of the tumor is measured and the brachytherapy dose calculated.

Ultrasound has proved very useful for follow-up after treatment and detection of recurrence.

References

Guthoff R (1991) Ultrasound in ophthalmologic diagnostics. Thieme, Stuttgart, pp 10–24

Guthoff R, Berger RW, Draeger J (1987) Ultrasonographic measurements of the posterior coats of the eye and their axial length. Graefe's Arch Clin Exp Ophthalmol 255:374–376

Guthoff R, Pauleikhoff D, Hingst V (1999) Bildgebende Diagnostik in der Augenheilkunde. Enke, Stuttgart, pp 138–184

Mundt GH, Hughes WF (1956) Ultrasonics in ocular diagnosis. Am J Ophthalmol 41:488–492

Ossoinig KC (1974a) Preoperative differential diagnosis of tumors with echography. IV. Diagnosis of orbital tumors. In: Blodi FC (ed) Current concepts in ophthalmology, vol 4. Mosby, St Louis, pp 313–341

Ossoinig KC (1974b) Quantitative echography – the basis of tissue differentiation. J Clin Ultrasound 2:33–46

Ossoinig KC (1977) Echography of the eye, orbit and periorbital region. In: Arger PH (ed) Orbit roentgenology. Wiley, New York, pp 224–269

Ossoinig KC (1991) Basics of clinical echo-ophthalmography. IV. Clinical standardization of equipment and techniques. In: Bock J, Ossoinig KC (eds) Ultrasonographia medica. Wiener Medizinische Akademie, Vienna, p 83

24 Radiation Techniques for the Treatment of Retinoblastoma and Orbital Tumors

W. E. Alberti, J. Schipper, R. H. Sagerman

CONTENTS

24.1
Introduction

External beam radiation therapy has been used successfully to treat primary and metastatic neoplasms of the globe and orbit. Depending upon tumor location and extent, adequate treatment with sparing of the lens can be accomplished but requires meticulous technique. Many field arrangements have been described for unilateral and bilateral disease. Isodose distributions for several of the more commonly employed techniques are presented for direct comparison. More recently, the development of 3D

W. E. Alberti, MD, Professor
Radiologische Klinik, Abteilung für Strahlentherapie und Radioonkologie, Universitäts-Klinikum, Hamburg-Eppendorf, Martinistrasse 52, 20246 Hamburg, Germany
J. Schipper, PhD
Adjunct Director Radiation Physics, Arnhem Radiotherapeutic Institute, Wagnerlaan 47, 6815 AD Arnhem, The Netherlands
R.H. Sagerman, MD, FACR, Professor
Professor, Department of Radiation Oncology, SUNY Upstate Medical University, 750 East Adams Street, Syracuse, NY 13210, USA

conformation irradiation techniques, intensity modulated irradiation, and linac based and gamma knife radiosurgery, which are increasingly more available, have begun to refine previously employed techniques. In addition, particle beam techniques and plaque brachytherapy employed predominantly in the treatment of melanoma have been applied to retinoblastoma, choroidal hemangioma, and age related macular degeneration. All of this techniques provide for better normal tissue sparing of ocular structures as exemplified in the treatment of tumors of the paranasal sinuses. Adequate discussion of these technical developments is beyond the scope of this chapter and the reader is referred to chapters 7 and 8 (particle beam) and chapters 4, 5, 6 and 25 (plaque) as well as Jones et al. (2000), Martel et al. (1997), Brizel et al. (1999), Daftari et al. (1997), Castro et al. (1997), Adams et al. (1999), Zografos et al. (1998).

This chapter is divided into two parts. Section 24.2 reviews the special considerations attending the treatment of retinoblastoma and its effects upon the eye during infancy and early childhood which led to the development of an accurate lens sparing technique. Section 24.3 compares various techniques which are generally applicable to orbital lesions.

24.2
Retinoblastoma

24.2.1
Historical Review

Hilgartner (1903) reported the first radiation treatment of a retinoblastoma. A child with bilateral disease received x-irradiation to both eyes. His face was protected with lead containing two openings which served as portals. After completion of irradiation, no active retinoblastoma was seen in the left eye and the tumors in the right eye regressed to two-thirds of the original size. The radiation dose was not reported, but was certainly very high as it was usual to give doses of 200 Gy until the 1930s.

In 1936, MARTIN and REESE in New York published a three-field technique using round nasal, anterior, and temporal portals of 2.5 cm diameter for orthovoltage irradiation. This technique allows for partial sparing of the anterior segment, thus avoiding some complications. The technique was used in many centers during the next three decades and was subsequently modified to use only the temporal and nasal fields. According to the recommendations of MARTIN and REESE (1936), the total dose was reduced from 200 Gy to 108 Gy, which was delivered over a long period.

MOORE (1930), in London, first used radon seeds which were sutured over the retinoblastoma foci. Subsequently STALLARD (1933) developed cobalt 60 applicators of varying size delivering a dose of 40 Gy to the summit of the tumor in 7 days.

From a study of the histologic sections of eyes treated with radon seeds, STALLARD (1936) determined that a dose of 35 Gy was effective in the treatment of retinoblastoma. Independently, the clinical experience of REESE et al. (1958) demonstrated that 35–45 Gy was sufficient to control the disease in most cases.

The lower total dose and the sparing of the anterior segment of the eye using the two-field technique of MARTIN and REESE greatly reduced the radiation damage to the eye and the surrounding structures.

24.2.2
Megavoltage Irradiation Techniques

Further improvement in results, with less radiation damage, was achieved with the introduction of megavoltage equipment in the 1950s and the development of appropriate radiation techniques. Megavoltage irradiation reduced the dose to the skin and bone and provided a better dose distribution with a sharper beam edge. At Stanford University, BAGSHAW and KAPLAN (1966) published results of irradiated bilateral retinoblastoma obtained with a precise technique using 4.5 MV photons from a linear accelerator. In principle, this first technique for megavoltage irradiation of the eye meets all major requirements for treating young patients with multifocal tumors of the retina:

1. The D-shaped field of 2.5×2 cm was contoured to spare the anterior segment and to irradiate only the posterior part of the eye from the proximal optic nerve to the lens.
2. An outboard lead collimator was positioned close to the patient to reduce the penumbra.
3. Positioning of the radiation field was achieved by means of a Comberg contact lens with five radiopaque markers to delineate the limbus.
4. The exit point on the child's head was located by means of a precisely aligned back pointer.
5. Irradiation was performed with a relatively brief, general anesthesia allowing complete immobilization of the patient and the treated eye(s).

Table 24.1. Megavoltage irradiation techniques, doses, and fractionations used for retinoblastoma in different centers

Center	Authors (year)	Irradiation technique	Year of introduction	Dose/fractionation
New York	McCORMICK et al. (1988)	Lateral beam technique (lat. electrons + oblique inferior + superior split beam wedged photons)	1984	44 Gy (22 fx, 4.5 wks)
Paris	HAYE et al. (1985)	1. Lateral electron D-shaped field for posterior tumors 2. Additional anterior field for anterior tumors	1963	40–50 Gy (20–25 fx, 4–5 wks) Lateral and anterior field weighted 4 : 1
Utrecht	SCHIPPER (1983)	Lateral collimated D-shaped field for 6 or 8 MV photons; fixation of the eye with a vacuum contact lens	1971	45 Gy (15 fx, 5 wks)
Harvard	WEISS et al. (1975)	Lateral and anterior field for 4 MV photons weighted 4.5 : 1; central divergent lens block	1975	42–45 Gy (14–16 fx, 4 wks)
Stanford	DONALDSON and EGBERT (1989)		1978	50–56 (25–28 fx, 5–5.5 wks)
Essen	ALBERTI et al. (1987)	Schipper technique	1982	40–50 Gy (16–20 fx, 4–5 wks)
London	Harnett et al. (1987)	Schipper technique	1987	40 Gy (20 fx, 4 wks)

Subsequently, many centers treating retinoblastoma patients developed radiation techniques for cobalt 60 units, betatrons, or linear accelerators. Table 24.1 gives an overview of the technique, dose and fractionation used in different centers. It is remarkable that only one technique (SCHIPPER 1983) fulfilled the technical criteria deemed so important by BAGSHAW and KAPLAN in 1966. BEDFORD et al. (1971) and SKEGGS and WILLIAMS (1966) used an anterior cobalt beam to treat the entire eye. The authors indicated that this technique had the advantage of treating the whole retina and vitreous and that one eye could be treated without irradiating the fellow eye. BEDFORD et al. (1971) defined the following indications for using this technique: large tumors (more than 13 mm in diameter), multiple tumors of any size spread over the retina, tumors with vitreous seeding, and tumors of any size near the optic disk.

A single, anterior portal, using 10–18 MeV electrons with a central block for the cornea and lens, was recommended for the treatment of retinoblastoma by GRIEM et al. (1968) and KÄRCHER et al. (1971). Two or more oblique 3- to 4-mm portals, covering the entire retina, were employed by HULTBERG et al. (1965). Eight oblique, anterior 8-mm portals had been used by ARMSTRONG (1974).

The disadvantages of all these techniques using anterior electron beams are:

1. Positioning of the lens block is critical and difficult even when using scleral sutures or contact lenses not fixed to the cornea. A slight geographic miss can result in rather high doses to the radiosensitive epithelial cells at the equator of the lens.
2. Protection of the lens and cornea results in a reduction in dose behind the lens block and the posterior retina, respectively.

In many centers, retinoblastoma is usually irradiated by a single lateral portal which should cover the entire retina and vitreous and spare the anterior segment of the eye. Efforts have been made by several authors to increase the dose in the retinal periphery, where most lateral approaches do not provide a full dose.

HAYE et al. (1985) use a lateral D-shaped 4×4 cm^2 field with 18–25 MeV electrons. The anterior border of the field is aligned at the bony orbital rim if the tumors are located at the posterior pole of the globe. Tumors anterior to the equator are irradiated with fields whose anterior border is aligned at the outer fleshy canthus. In this case, a second anterior field delivers 20% of the total dose. Delivering 50 Gy with this technique, the posterior pole receives the full dose while the remaining two-thirds of the retina receives only 30–40 Gy.

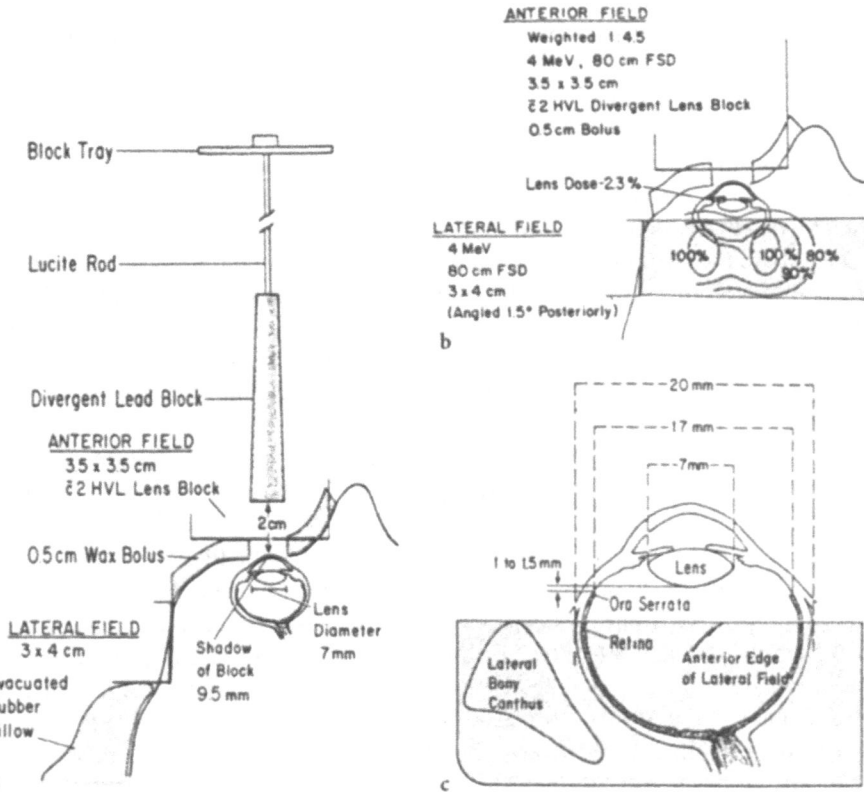

Fig. 24.1. a Clinical setup of the two-field technique: 3×4 cm lateral and 3.5×3.5 cm anterior field with a 2 HVL divergent lens block. **b** Computer-calculated isodose distribution for the two-field technique using 4MV photons. Fields are weighted 1 to 4.5 (anterior to lateral). *FSD*, focal skin distance. **c** Relationship of a single lateral field with the anterior beam edge at the bony lateral canthus to the anatomic structures of the eye (WEISS et al. 1975)

WEISS et al. (1975) developed a radiation therapy technique using a lateral and anterior field with a central divergent lens block. The fields are weighted 1 : 4.5 (anterior to lateral) (Fig. 24.1a,b). The computer-calculated isodose distribution for this technique, using 4 MV photons, showed an underdosage in the anterior retina, whereas the retina up to the equator is covered completely by the 80% and partly by the 90% isodose. This is true if the anterior border of the lateral field is aligned exactly at the bony lateral canthus (Fig. 24.1c); if not, the isodose curves are moved towards either the lens or the posterior pole. To ensure the necessary immobilization, treatment is performed under daily ketamine hydrochloride anesthesia using an individualized body cast and an evacuated rubber pillow as a head support.

McCORMICK et al. (1988) reported 170 children with retinoblastoma irradiated with two different techniques. They compared a lens-sparing technique, including an anterior electron beam with a contact lens-mounted lead shield (Fig. 24.2), with a modified lateral beam technique. The latter uses a lateral electron beam and superior and inferior, wedged lateral oblique split beam photons (Fig. 24.3).

DONALDSON and EGBERT (1989) use a beamsplitting technique with a 4 MV linear accelerator with a 3.5×7 cm^2 field blocked to 3.5×3.5 cm^2. Opposing lateral fields are used when both eyes are to be treated, and a single fields for uniocular treatment. In unilateral treatment, the opposite eye receives about 50% of the given dose. This technique covers the entire retina but the dose at the ora serrata is about 50%, increasing to 90% within 2–3 mm. The lens and the pituitary receive less than 10% of the given dose (Fig. 24.4). If tumors involve the ora serrata, the anterior border of the irradiation field can be brought 1–2 mm anteriorly to increase the dose to the peripheral retina. For optimal treatment, general anesthesia is necessary to guarantee immobilization and reproducibility of beam alignment.

24.2.3
Accurate Lens-Sparing Technique (Utrecht Method)

Requirements in the choice of an appropriate irradiation technique for the eye are high precision, simplicity, and reproducibility. All conditions are fulfilled by the precise irradiation technique for retinoblastoma developed by SCHIPPER (1980, 1983). This technique has been used in Utrecht since 1971 (SCHIPPER et al. 1985), in Essen since 1982 (ALBERTI

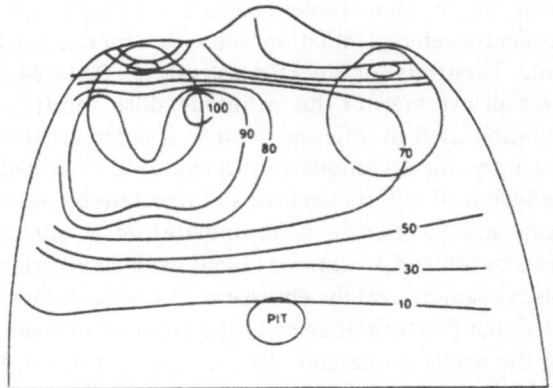

Fig. 24.2. Isodose curves for a patient treated with a "lens-sparing" technique, displayed over anatomy (McCORMICK et al. 1988)

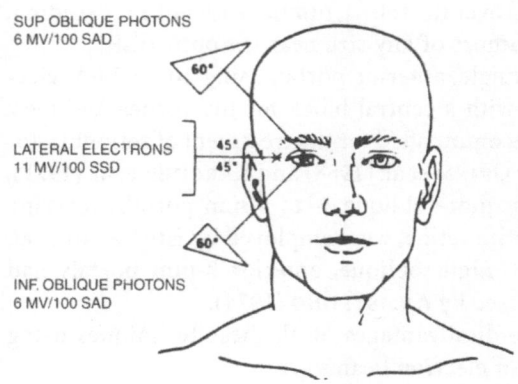

Fig. 24.3. Schematic representation of beam direction of the patient with unilateral disease ("lateral beam" technique) (McCORMICK et al. 1988)

et al. 1987), and in London since 1987 (HARNETT et al. 1987). Treatment is usually carried out with a 6-MV or 8-MV linear accelerator using a lateral D-shaped field of 26×32 mm^2 at the isocentric distance of 100 cm (Fig. 24.5). A smaller D-shaped field of 20×26 mm^2 is used in very young babies. The field covers the entire retina up to the ora serrata, the vitreous, and 10 mm of the anterior optic nerve. The lens and the sensitive anterior chamber are spared from the radiation field. Accurate alignment of the sharply collimated photon beam is achieved by magnetic fixation of the eye to the beam-defining collimator using a vacuum contact lens (Fig. 24.6).

Precise collimation of the small field is obtained by interposing precision-machined 11-cm-thick lead collimators in the beam. An exceptionally sharp beam results from the short collimator to center of eye distance (17 cm). Side scatter of the photon beam is less than 10% (see Fig. 24.8). The penumbra can be reduced to 1.5–2 mm.

OPPOSED PAIR, NORMALIZED TO d1/2 OF OPEN AREA

CENTERED AT ORA SERRATA

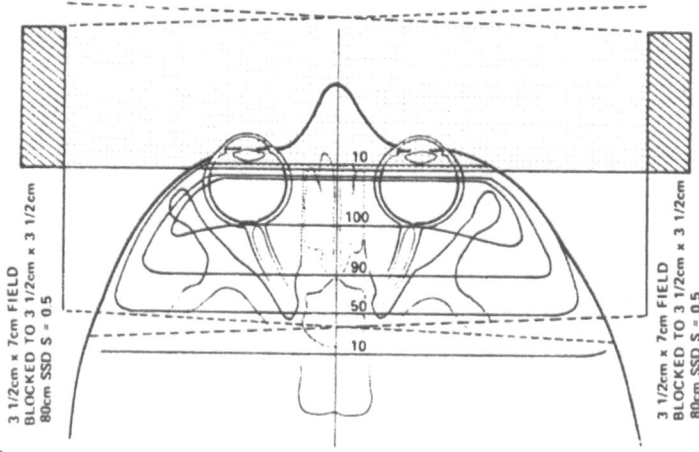

SINGLE FIELD NORMALIZED TO d3 OF OPEN AREA

CENTERED AT ORA SERRATA

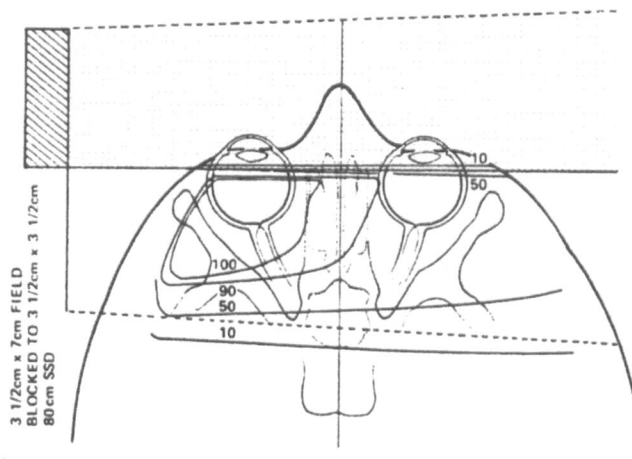

Fig. 24.4. a Beam-splitting technique for bilateral treatment using opposed lateral fields (effective field: 3.5 × 3.5 cm) with 4 MV photons. Anterior border of the treatment field located at the ora serrata, the dose is calculated at the midplane. **b** Isodose curves for unilateral treatment. The dose is calculated to a depth of 3 cm (DONALDSON and EGBERT 1989)

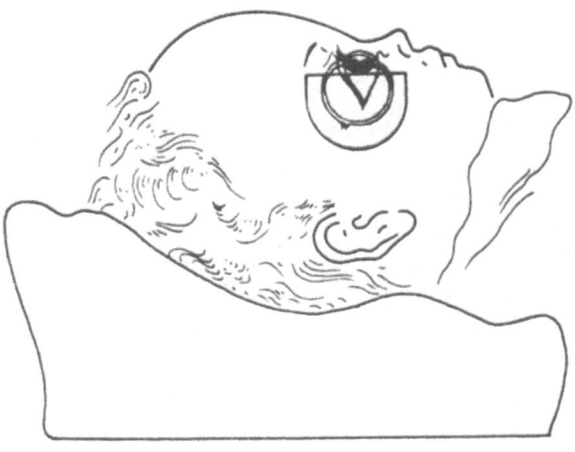

Fig. 24.5. Lateral, sharply collimated, D-shaped treatment field covering the entire retina and excluding the lens (SCHIPPER 1983)

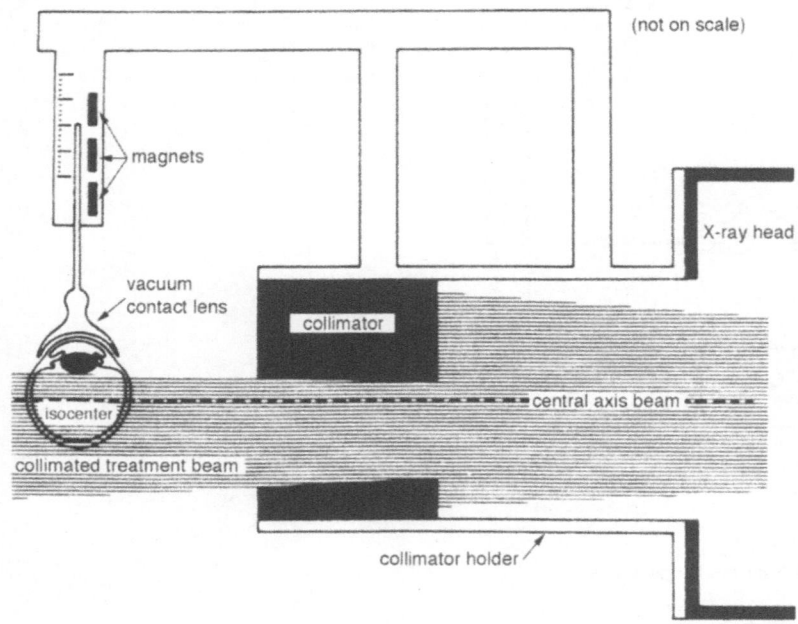

Fig. 24.6. Schematic representation of the radiation technique. Accurate alignment and positioning of the eye by indirect fixation of the eye to the beam-defining collimator (SCHIPPER 1983)

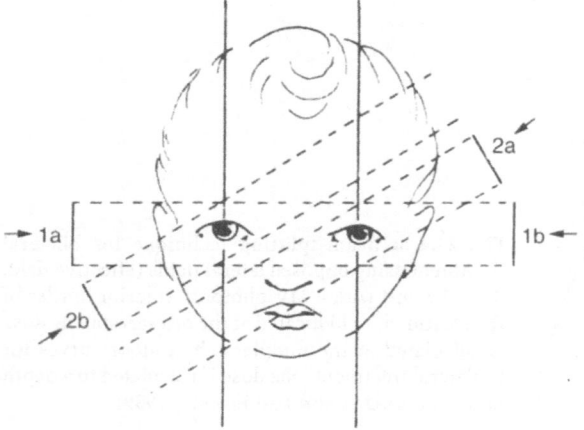

Fig. 24.7. Schematic representation of unilateral or bilateral irradiation of retinoblastoma. If the left eye is involved, treatment is performed by field 2a, sparing the second eye. If the right eye eventually is involved, a second field (2b) can be used without overlapping field 2a. Simultaneous irradiation can be performed using the opposing fields 1a and 1b (SCHIPPER 1983)

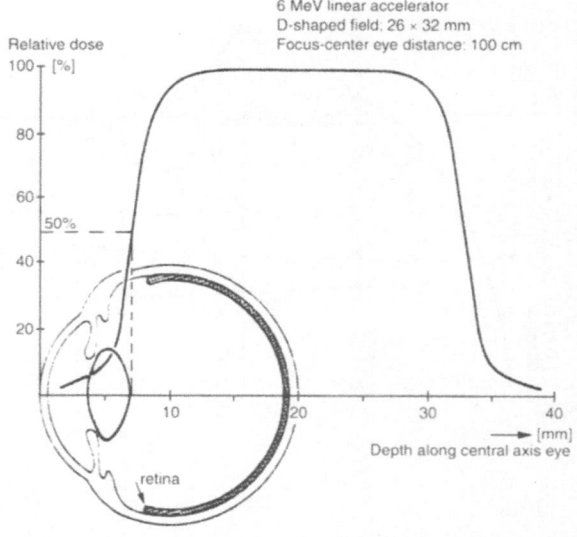

Fig. 24.8. Dose profile of a lateral D-shaped field of 26 × 32 mm along the axis of the eye (SCHIPPER 1983)

Seventeen- and 20-mm-diameter contact lenses are made from perspex and contain a steel cannula with a soft iron rod allowing magnetic fixation at the collimator holder. The axial dimensions of the eye(s) are measured by ultrasound for each patient. The A-scan allows determination of the distance between the front surface of the cornea and the anterior and posterior surfaces of the lens. The iron pin of the contact lens is magnetically coupled to a perspex millimeter scale on the collimator holder. The mea-

sured distance between the cornea and the anterior and posterior poles of the lens can be set up individually for each eye with the millimeter scale. The accurancy of beam positioning has been measured at ±0.3 mm. Beam divergence is not a problem as setup of the anterior edge of the field is performed for each eye individually. If tumor involves the ora serrata, it may be ,necessary to include the posterior portion of the lens. In this case the anterior border of the radiation field is moved anteriorly, i.e., the distance to be set up at the millimeter scale is reduced. The transparency of the contact lens allows visual confirmation of its central location on the eye and whether vacuum is achieved.

The center of the fixed eye is located at the isocenter of the accelerator. Therefore the radiation beam can be angled at any direction by rotation of the table or gantry without changing the position of the eye. The most frequent clinical situation is after one eye has been enucleated. In this case, the photon beam is aligned at a right angle, avoiding radiation exposure to the dental lamina of the contralateral maxilla. For unilateral treatment with both eyes present, the beam must be angled 35'-45' by rotation of the linac table. lf the contralateral eye later develops retinoblastoma, it can be irradiated by a parallel oblique beam without overlapping the first beam. Both eyes can be irradiated simultaneously with opposing lateral fields by fixing each eye alternately (see Fig. 12.8, this volume). The eye close to the collimator is always located at the isocenter (Fig. 24.7).

When both eyes are treated, the second perspex millimeter scale is attached to the aluminum T-bar. The distance between the two scales can be set individually and corresponds to the distance between the centers of the pupils. An 8-mm perspex scatterer, also mounted to the Tbar, is interposed in the beam to reduce the depth of dose buildup and to avoid an underdosage in the temporal retina. The scatterer is positioned at 4 or 2 cm from the skin for 6 and 8 MV photons, respectively. With TLD and film dosimetry, and a lucite phantom material, a dose distribution along the axis of the eye can be obtained which is quite favorable (Fig. 24.8).

The child is immobilized with halothane, a short-acting anesthetic. In the exceptional case of an older, more cooperative patient, the eye to be treated is anesthetized with a topical anesthetic. A vacuum pillow is used to position and fix the patient's Ihead during treatment.

24.2.4
Comparison of Results with the Utrecht Technique Versus Lateral or Anterior Field Techniques

With an anterior field, all normal ocular structures and a certain amount of brain are irradiated unnecessarily, and a cataract of varying density inevitably develops within about 18 months (McFAUL and BEDFORD 1970). Radiation complications led to enucleation in 10% (13/133) of eyes treated

conservatively; only nine eyes (6.8%) were removed because of uncontrolled disease (BEDFORD et al. 1971).

It is often stated that cataract surgery following irradiation of retinoblastoma is no longer a surgical problem. However, as pointed out by INGRAHAM et al. (Chap. 21, this volume), the main problem is not the removal of the cataractogenic lens, but the rehabilitation of vision in children with contaet lenses or appropriate glasses. The high percentage of serious complications related to the direct anterior field led the London retinoblastoma group to adopt the technique developed by SCHIPPER (1983) (HARNETT et al. 1987).

McCORMICK et al. (1988) analyzed clinical results obtained with their lens-sparing technique (Fig. 24.2) and the modified lateral beam technique (Fig. 24.3). For eyes with group I-III disease, the lens-sparing technique resulted in local control in 33% of eyes, compared to 83% of the eyes treated with the modified lateral beam technique ($P = 0.006$). Most of the failures could be successfully treated with coagulation and plaque therapy. Five eyes required enucleation; all had been treated with the lens-sparing technique. For eyes with group IV and V disease, no significant differenees were found between the two techniques in terms of local control or eventual need for enucleation. lt is remarkable that six cataracts developed in the 66 eyes treated with the lens-sparing technique. No cataracts were seen in 31 eyes treated with the lateral beam technique, indicating that longer follow-up is necessary.

MESSMER et al. (1990) compared elinical results in 127 eyes treated with two different megavoltage irradiation techniques between 1974 and 1988 in Essen. Seventy-four eyes were treated with a lateral beam technique and 53 with the Schipper technique. Significantly fewer new and recurrent tumors were found in those treated with the Schipper technique compared to those in whom the lateral beam was aligned, at the outer bony canthus (22% vs 48%). If the entire retina received the full radiation dose, no new or recurrent tumors occurred in the peripheral retina.

SCHIPPER et al. (1985) reported 39 children with retinoblastoma. Fifty-four of 73 affected eyes were treated with the precise megavoltage irradiation technique (SCHIPPER 1983). Eighteen eyes developed a clinically detectable cataract, exclusively in those lenses where more than 1 mm of the posterior portion was included in the treatment field.

It can be concluded that the Schipper technique, if properly applied, guarantees better results in terms of local control, especially in the retinal periphery, and low complication rates in the anterior segment of the eye.

24.3
Orbital Lesions

24.3.1
Materials and Methods

Isodose distributions were generated using an AECL Theraplan treatment planning computer for our Varian Clinac 4 linear accelerator with a source-axis distance (SAD) of 80 cm. All field sizes, or effective field sizes for "beam-split" fields, were 5 cm × 5 cm at 80 cm. All lead blocking was 5 HVL (half-value layers) thick. No tissue heterogeneity corrections were used. The normalization point was chosen to allow direct comparison of distributions.

24.3.2
Bilateral Fields

Bilateral fields are best suited to bilateral disease or disease in the medial aspect of the orbit. To spare the lens, the anterior field edge must be at, or behind, the posterior pole of the ipsilateral lens. Care must be taken to avoid divergence of the beam through the contralateral lens. This can be accomplished by doubling the field width and blocking the anterior half of the field (beamsplitting), or by angling the accelerator gantry some angle *(d)* below horizontal so that the anterior field edge is horizontal. The divergence angle, *d*, can be calculated by $d = \arctan(w/2\mathrm{SAD})$, where w = field width and SAD = source-axis distance.

Figure 24.9a shows "angled lateral" fields and Fig. 24.9b shows "beam-split lateral" fields on the Clinac 4 linear accelerator. Note the similarity of the isodose distributions to those of Fig. 24.4a, but the wider coverage at the optic canal necessary for soft tissue tumors. Figure 24.10 shows angled lateral fields for cobalt 60. Because of its larger penumbra, the co-

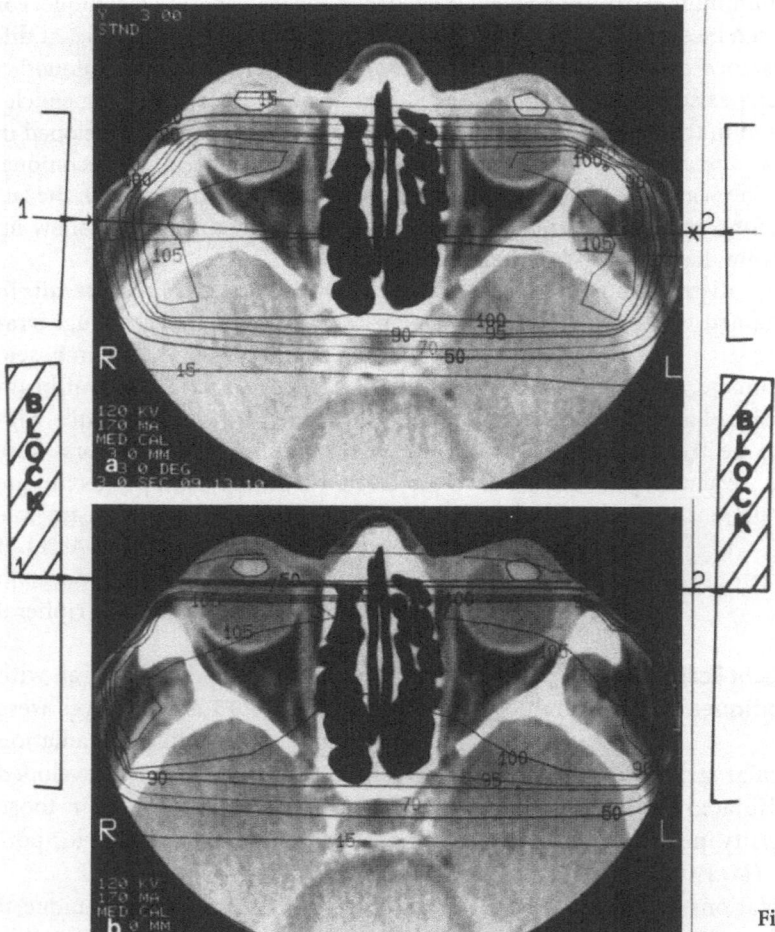

Fig. 24.9. a Angled lateral fields, 4 MV. **b** Beam-split lateral fields, 4 MV

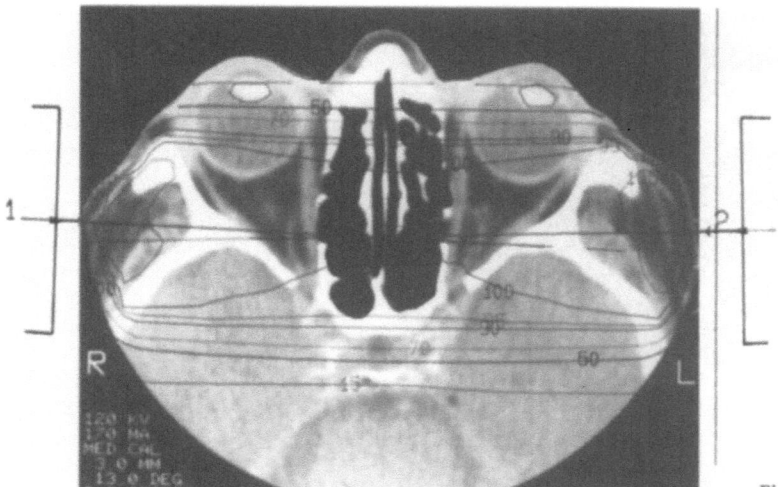

Fig. 24.10. Angled lateral fields for cobalt 60

balt 60 treatment significantly underdoses much of the globe and has a slightly higher lens dose.

This field arrangement should not be used when disease extends anterior to the equator of the globe. It is useful for diseases such as retrobulbar lymphoma, group I or II retinoblastoma, and orbital metastases.

24.3.3
Single Lateral Fields

In treatment of unilateral disease in the posterior/lateral orbit, a single field can be used instead of bilateral fields (Fig. 24.11). Setup is the same as for bilateral treatment. In most patients, the soft tissue canthus can be used as the anterior border of the field. In contrast to the lateral bony canthus, which approximates the equator of the globe, the lateral soft tissue canthus more closely approximates the posterior pole of the lens. More accurate lens localization is accomplished by computed tomography (CT), magnetic resonance imaging (MRI), and ultrasonography; CT and MRI produce images readily used for computer dosimetry. This is especially important in patients with proptosis.

Unilateral treatment results in a larger dose gradient across the ipsilateral orbit. When used in children, an asymmetric facial growth defect will result. Attempting to treat medially located disease with a single lateral field will cause a relatively high D max dose. Note that the dose to the contralateral orbit ranges from 50% to 70% in an adult patient. This may pose a problem if the opposite orbit replires treatment at a later date.

24.3.4
Single Anterior Fields

Single anterior fields are sometimes used to achieve quick palliation. By having the patient look directly into the collimator, with eyes wide open, some lens sparing can be achieved due to the inherent "dose buildup" (skin sparing) in megavoltage beams. As seen in Fig. 24.12a, there is minimal sparing of the lens and this should not be used if minimizing cataractogenesis is important.

Significant dose reduction in the lens can be achieved by adding a 1-cm-diameter round lens block (Fig. 24.12b). This results in a low dose cylindrical volume along the central axis. The dose distribution in the posterior orbit, off-axis, away from the block, looks much like that in Fig. 24.12a. This technique is most useful in treating anterior disease, such as conjunctival lymphomas not extending to the limbus. We favor the use of a hanging block technique as shown in Fig. 24.12c. A 1-cm-diameter lead block is threaded into a lucite rod of the same diameter. The rod is suspended from a tray in the collimator tray ring. This enables the use of a larger block that is easier to handle for a given "shadow diameter" on the patient, and a sharper blockedge penumbra than if the block were to be directly attached to the tray. Electron contamination from this small block is minimal.

24.3.5
Wedged Pairs

Adding a heavily wedged, lightly weighted, anterior field to a single lateral field decreases the dose gradi-

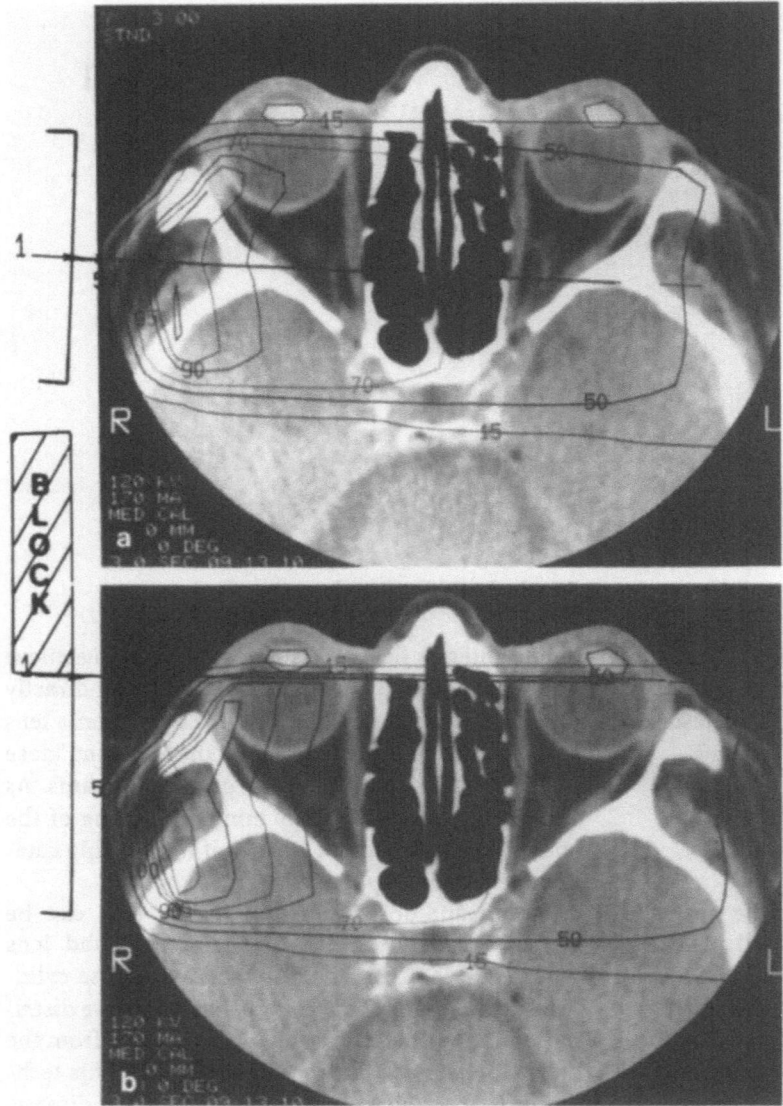

Fig. 24.11. a Single angled lateral field, 4 MV. b Single lateral field with half field block, 4 MV

ent across the orbit and brings the high dose region slightly more anteriorly.

Figures 24.13a and 24.13b show a lateral-to-anterior weighting of 3 : 1 for angled lateral and beam-split fields, respectively. Figures 24.14a and 24.14b show the result of weighting the lateral field at 4 : 1 for the same field arrangement. A 4 : 1 weighting with a 60° wedge is slightly under-wedged but provides a lower lens dose than 3 : 1 weighting. The dose to the contralateral orbit is slightly lower for a wedged pair than for a single lateral field (Fig. 24.11).

Wedged pairs can be used in similar situations as single lateral fields but provide better dose distributions when higher anterior and medial orbit doses are required.

24.3.6
Wedged Pairs with Lens Block

Figures 24.15a and 24.15b show how the addition of a small lens block in the anterior field modifies the distributions of Figs. 24.13b and 24.14b. A greater degree of lens sparing is provided, which is particularly important when higher doses are required, as for rhabdomyosarcoma. Note that the hanging anterior block-induced dose perturbation is significant only within ±5 mm of the central ray and the off-axis distributions look much like those in Figs. 24.13b and 24.14b. These distributions would not be appropriate when disease lies directly behind the lens in the posterior chamber or when the orbital mass would be shielded.

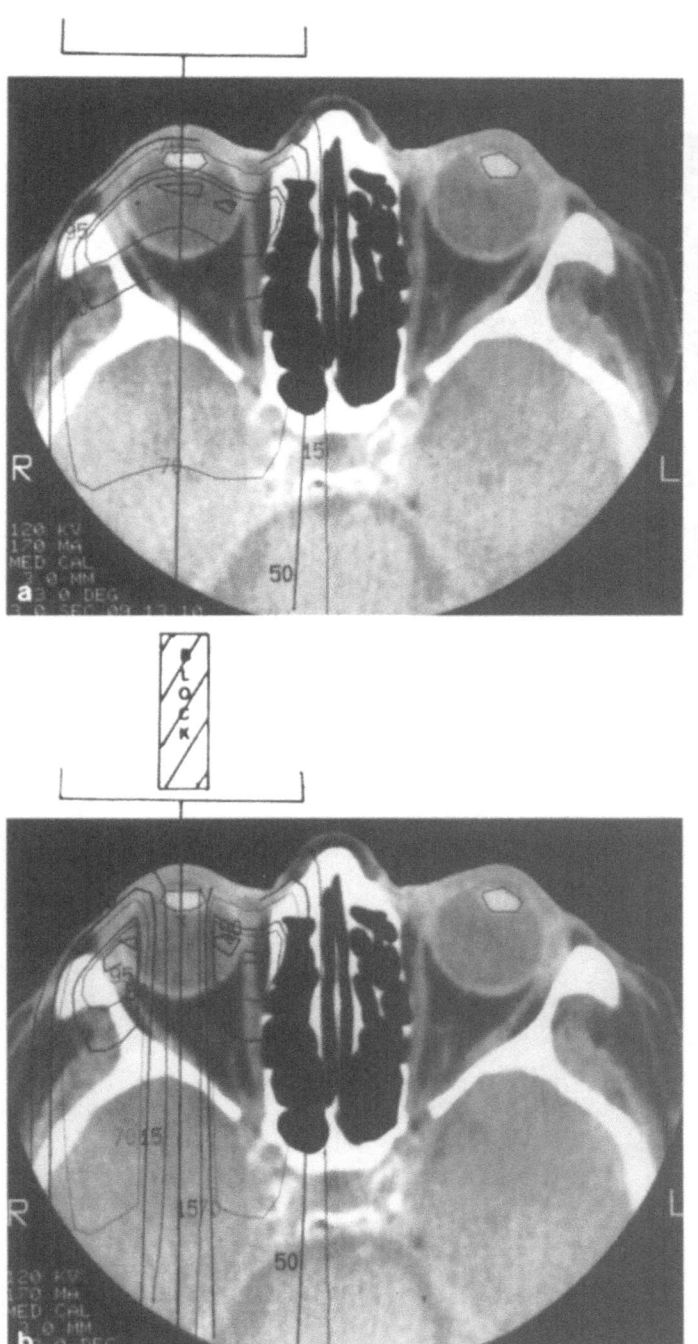

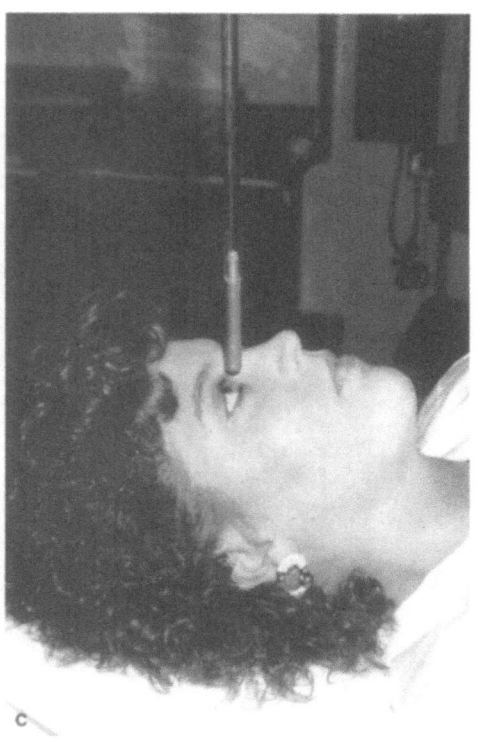

Fig. 24.12. a Single anterior field, 4 MV. **b** Single anterior field with 1-cm-diameter round lens block added, 4 MV. **c** 1-cm-diameter hanging lead block threaded into a lucite rod and suspended from collimator tray

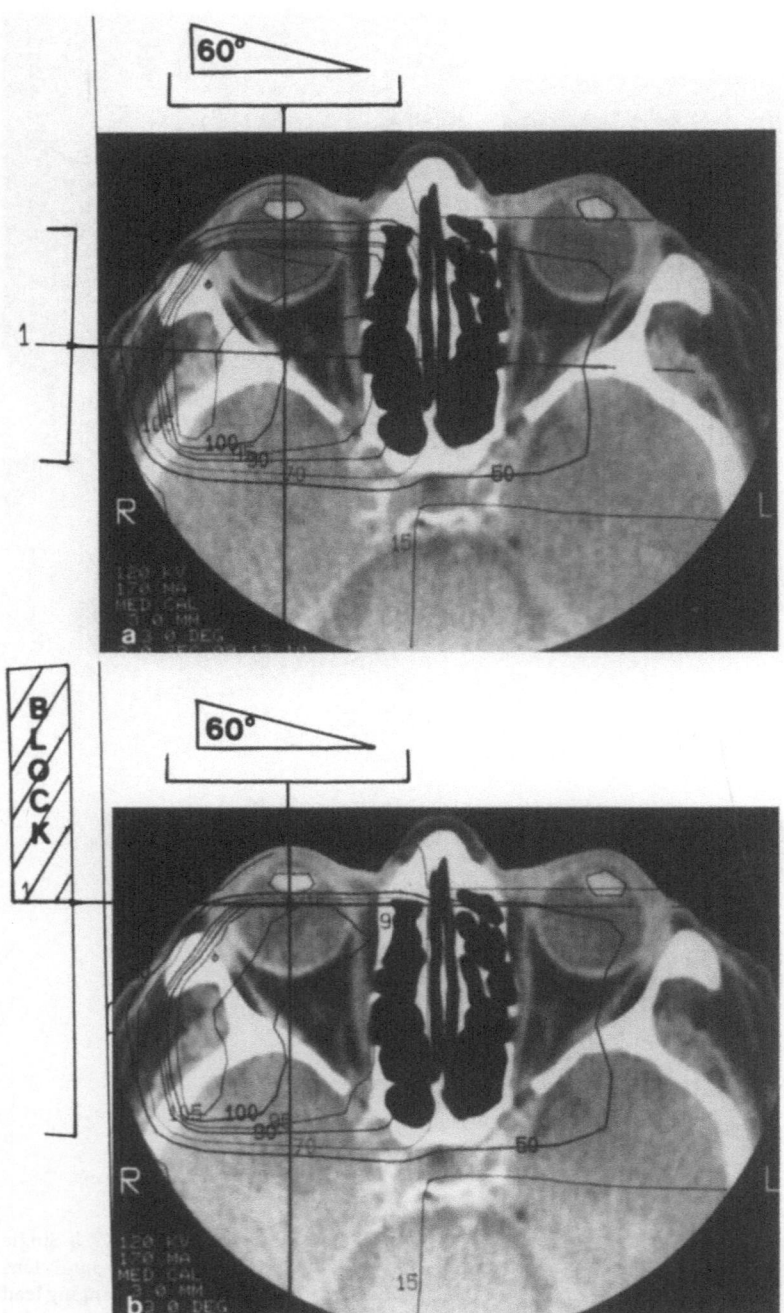

Fig. 24.13. a Lateral-to-anterior weighting of 3 : 1 for angled lateral fields, 4 MV. **b** Lateral-to-anterior weighting of 3 : 1 for beam-split fields, 4 MV

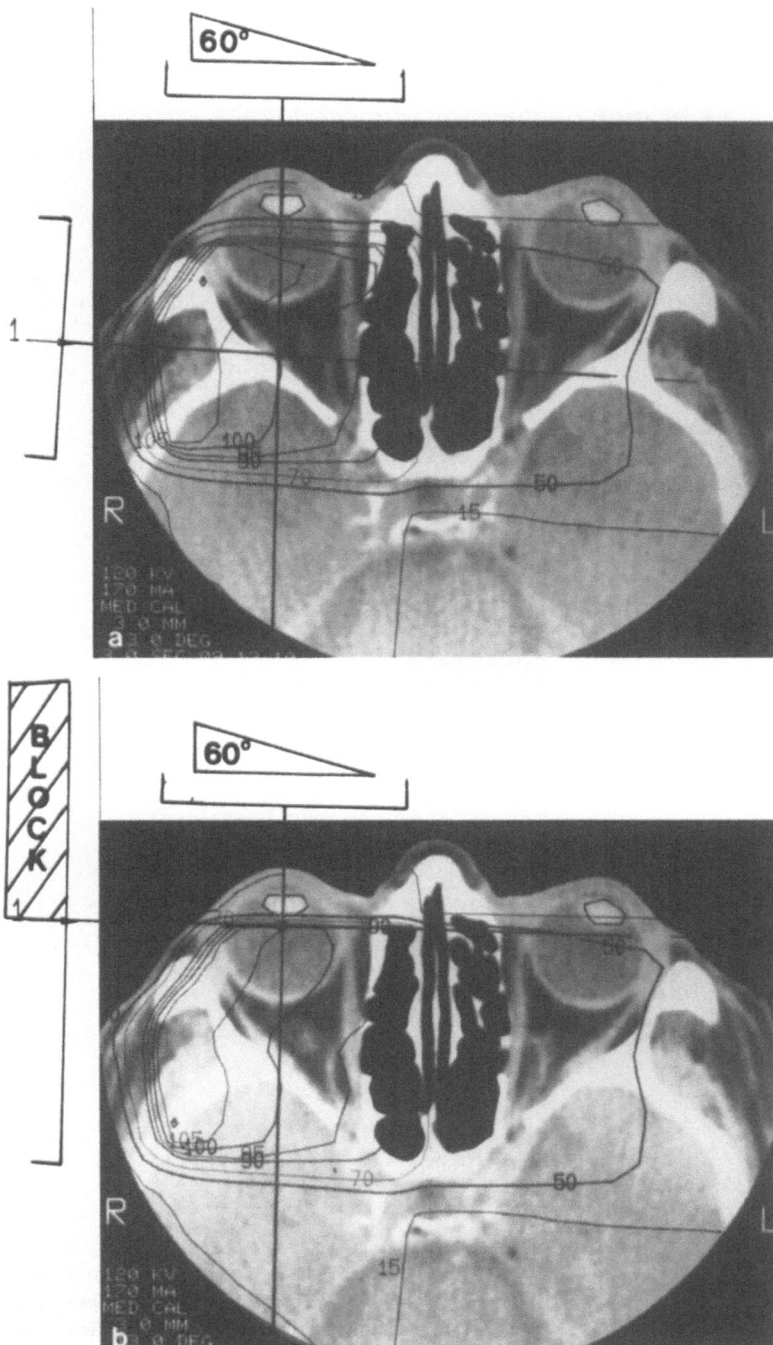

Fig. 24.14. a Lateral-to-anterior weighting of 4 : 1 for angled lateral fields, 4 MV. **b** Lateral-to-anterior weighting of 4 : 1 for beam-split fields, 4 MV

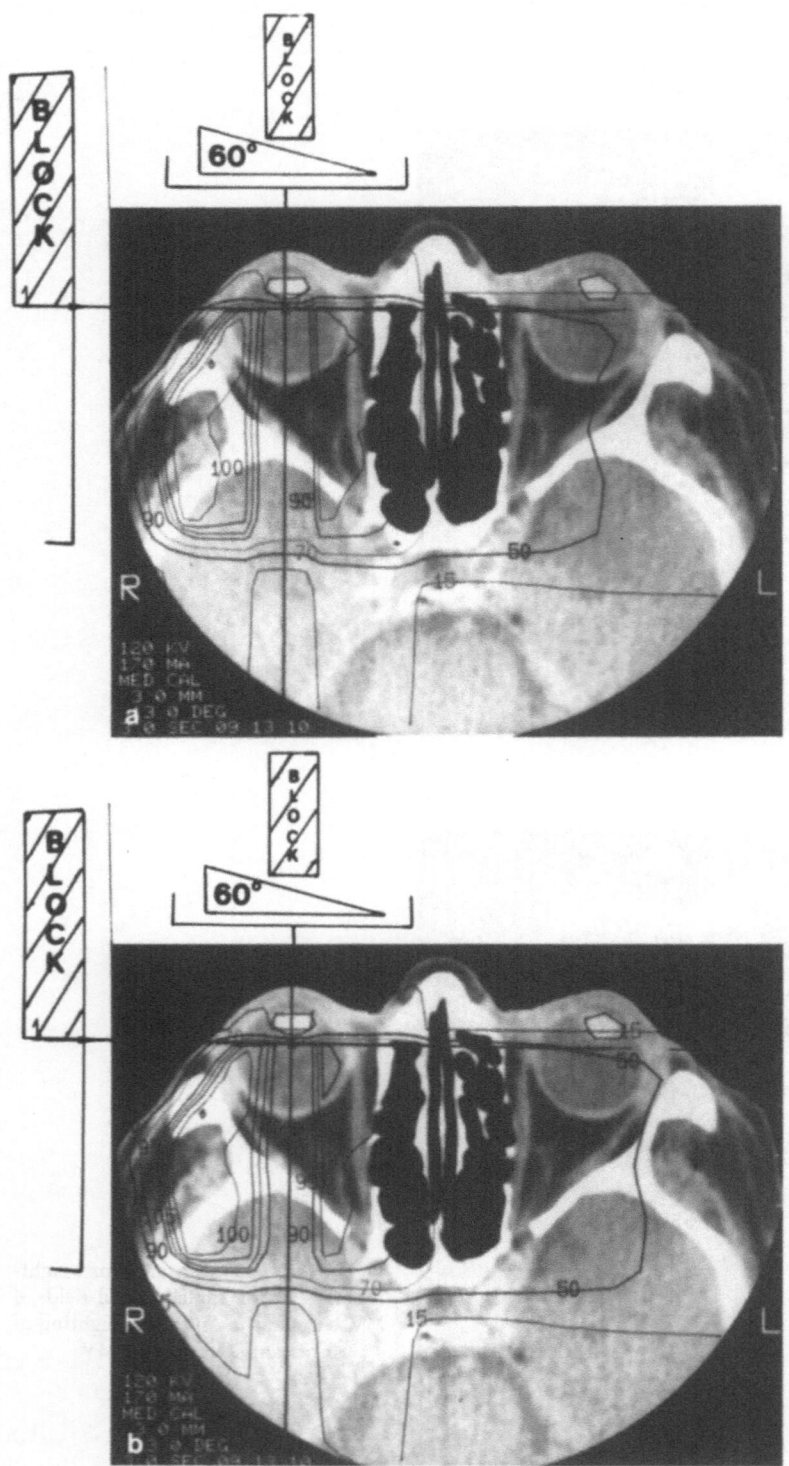

Fig. 24.15. a Lateral-to-anterior weighting of 3 : 1 for beam-split fields with addition of small lens block in the anterior field, 4 MV. **b** Lateral-to-anterior weighting of 4 : 1 for beam-split fields with addition of small lens block in the anterior field, 4 MV

24.3.7
Summary

Ingenuity and careful treatment planning with the aid of CT or MRI will allow design of an isodose distribution which best covers the tumor and spares critical structures. Lens-sparing external beam radiation therapy of the eye requires meticulous field placement and patient positioning. Cobalt 60 beams should be avoided due to their larger penumbra.

Beam splitting offers a sharper penumbra than does the edge of the field. Therefore, beam-split lateral fields, or a high precision technique, should be used when the high dose region needs to extend anteriorly, close to the lens. Nevertheless, there is still a finite width of 4 mm from the 10% to the 90% line, similar to that illustrated in Fig. 33.8. The lateral soft tissue canthus provides a reproducible setup landmark that is at, or slightly posterior to, the posterior surface of the lens, in most individuals.

Unless a wedge larger than 60° is available, 3 : 1 lateral-to-anterior weighting provides a more uniform distribution than 4 : 1 weighting in wedged-pair setups. If adequate tumor coverage is jeopardized when attempting to spare the lens, the patient has been done a disservice. Radiation-induced cataracts are now manageable by carefully applied, standard, surgical techniques. Impaired vision with tumor control is preferable to tumor recurrence with intact vision.

References

Adams JA, Paiva KL, Munzenrider JE, Miller JW, Gragoudas ES (1999) Proton beam therapy for age-related macular degeneration: Development of a standard plan. Medical Dosimetry 24 (4):233–238

Alberti W, Halama J, Wannenmacher M (1987) Tumoren im Kopfbereich. Tumoren des Auges und der Orbita. In: Scherer E (ed) Strahlentherapie. Radiologische Onkologie. Springer, Berlin Heidelberg New York, pp 412–453

Armstrong DI (1974) The use of 4–6 MeV electrons for the conservative treatment of retinoblastoma. Br J Radiol 47:326–269

Bagshaw MA, Kaplan HS (1966) Supervoltage linear accelerator radiation therapy. Radiology 86:242–246

Bedford MA, Bedotto C, MeFaul PA (1971) Retinoblastoma, a study of 139 cases. Br J Ophthalmol 55:19–27

Brizel DM, Light K, Zhou SM, Marks LB (1999) Conformal radiation therapy treatment planning reduces the dose to the optic structures for patients with tumors of the paranasal sinuses. Radiotherpy and Oncology 51:215–218

Castro JR, Char DH, Petti PL, Daftari IK, Quivey JM, Singh RP, Blakely EA, Phillips TL (1997) 15 years experience with helium ion radiotherapy for uveal melanoma. Int J Radiat Oncol Biol Phys 39(5):989–996

Daftari IK, Char DH, Verhey LJ, Castro JR, Petti PL, Meecham WJ, Kroll S, Blakely EA (1997) Anterior segment sparing to reduce charged particle radiotheraphy complications in uveal melanoma. Int J Radiation Oncol Biol Phys 39(5):997–1010

Donaldson SS, Egbert PR (1989) Retinoblastoma. In: Pizzo PA, Poplack DG (eds) Principles and practice of pediatrie oncology. JB Lippincott, Philadelphia

Griem ML, Ernest JT, Rozenfeld ML et al. (1986) Eye lens protection in the treatment of retinoblastoma with high-energy electrons. Radiology 90:351–352

Harnett AN, Hungerford IL, Lambert GD et al. (1987) Improved external beam radiotherapy for the treatment of retinoblastoma. Br J Radiol 60:753–760

Haye C, Schlienger P, Calle R et al. (1985) Traitement conservateur des tumeurs de la r6tine a l'Institut Curie. Bull Cancer (Paris) 73:87–98

Hilgartner HL (1903) Report of a case of double glioma treated by x-rays. Texas Medical J 18:322

Hultberg S, Walstam R, Asard PE (1965) Two special applications of high-energy electron beams. Acta Radiol Ther 3:287–295

Jones B, Errington RD (2000)British J of Radiology. Proton beam radiotherapy. 73:802–805

Kärcher KH, Heckenthaler W, Binder W, Dimopoulos J, Seitz W (1971) Indikation zur Strahlentherapie in der Ophthalmologie. Strahlentherapie 142:381–389

Martel MK, Sandler HM, Cornblath WT, Marsh LH, Hazuka MK, Roa WH, Fraass BA, Lichter AS (1997) Dose-volume complication analysis for visual pathway structures of patients with advanced paranasal sinus tumors. Int J Radiat Oncol Biol Phys 38(2):273–284

Martin HE, Reese AB (1936) Treatment of retinal gliomas by the fractionated or divided dose principle of roentgen radiation, a preliminary report. Arch Ophthalmol 16:733–761

McCormick B, Ellsworth R, Abramson D et al. (1988) Radiation therapy for retinoblastoma: comparison of results with lens-sparing versus lateral beam techniques. Int J Radiat Oncol Biol Phys 15:567–574

McFaul PA, Bedford MA (1970) Ocular complications after therapeutic irradiation. Br J Ophthalmol 54:237–247

Messmer EP, Sauerwein W, Heinrich T et al. (1990) New and recurrent tumor foci following local treatment as well as external beam radiation in eyes of patients with hereditary retinoblastoma. Graefes Arch Clin Exp Ophthalmol 228:426–431

Moore RF (1930) Choroidal sarcoma treated by the intraocular insertion of radon seeds. Br J Ophthalmol 14:145–152

Reese AB, Hyman GA, Tapley ND, Forrest AW (1985) The treatment of retionoblastoma by x-ray and triethylene melanine. Arch Ophthalmol 60:897–906

Schipper J (1980) Retinoblastoma. A medical and experimental study. Thesis, Utrecht

Schipper J (1983) An accurate and simple method for megavoltage irradiation therapy of retinoblastoma. Radiother Oncol 1:31–41

Schipper J, Tan KEWP, van Peperzeel A (1985) Treatment of retinoblastoma by precision megavoltage radiation therapy. Radiother Oncol 3:117–132

Skeggs DBL, Williams IG (1966) The treatment of advanced retinoblastoma by means of external irradiation combined, with chemotherapy. Clin Radiol 17:169–172

Stallard HB (1933) Radient energy as (a) a pathogenic, (b) a therapeutic agent in ophthalmic disorders. Br J Ophthalmol, Monograph Supplement 6

Stallard HB (1936) Glioma retinae treated by radon seeds. Br Med J 11:962–964

Weiss DR, Cassady JR, Petersen R (1975) Retinoblastoma: a modification in radiation therapy technique. Radiology 114:705–708

Zografos L, Egger E, Bercher L, Chamot L, Munkel G (1998) Proton beam irradiation of choroidal hemangiomas. Am J Ophthalmology 8:261–268

25 Brachytherapy in the Management of Retinoblastoma

J. E. Freire, L. W. Brady, C. L. Shields, J. A. Shields

25.1
Background

Among the different options for the treatment of retinoblastoma, plaque brachytherapy has become an important tool, as either the primary or the secondary modality, in selected cases.

At present, management of retinoblastoma requires a team of care providers: pediatrician, ophthalmic oncologist, medical oncologist, radiation oncologist, medical physicist, and anesthesiologist. Treatment modalities include surgery, laser photocoagulation, thermotherapy, chemotherapy, chemothermotherapy, cryotherapy, subconjunctival chemotherapy, plaque brachytherapy, and external beam radiotherapy (Shields and Shields 1999). A brief outline of these therapies is given below.

Enucleation is the most common surgical approach in advanced disease, being indicated in those patients who have no hope of functional useful vi-

J. E. Freire, MD
Department of Radiation Oncology, MCP–Hahnemann University Hospital, Philadelphia, Pennsylvania, PA 19102, USA
L. W. Brady, MD
Department of Radiation Oncology, MCP–Hahnemann University Hospital, Philadelphia, Pennsylvania, PA 19102, USA
C. L. Shields, MD
Thomas Jefferson University, Philadelphia and Ocular Oncology Service, Wills Eye Hospital, Ninth and Walnut Sts., Philadelphia, PA 19107, USA
J. A. Shields, MD
Thomas Jefferson University, Philadelphia and Ocular Oncology Service, Wills Eye Hospital, Ninth and Walnut Sts., Philadelphia, PA 19107, USA

sion and those who present with invasion of the optic nerve or choroid, and for painful eye as a result of neovascular glaucoma.

Laser photocoagulation using an argon, diode, or xenon laser beam helps to coagulate the blood supply to the tumors. The periphery of the tumor(s) is the laser target; the bulk of the tumor must be avoided because of the risk of releasing viable cells into the vitreous (Shields and Shields 1999).

Chemotherapy consists of six or more cycles of current therapeutic agents: vincristine, etoposide and carboplatin, with the purpose of reducing tumor volume and thus being able to apply other adjuvant forms of treatment. This modality is also called chemoreduction and has been described by Shields et al. (1997) and others.

Subconjunctival chemotherapy (Shields et al. 1999) with carboplatin has also been used with similar intent in a clinical trial that showed good responses; however, the result appeared to be of short duration, necessitating other focal therapies.

Thermotherapy (Shields et al 1999) promotes apoptosis when the temperature reaches between 42°C and 43°C; it is administered using ultrasound, microwaves, or infrared radiation and has shown satisfactory results.

Finally, ionizing radiation, in the form of either brachytherapy or external beam irradiation (teletherapy), is recommended to achieve better control in selected cases.

After the discovery of radium by Pierre and Marie Curie, enormous interest grew up among the medical and scientific community regarding the use of this newly discovered isotope and its application in the treatment of cancer. This motivation gave origin to a treatment modality that, owing to its use within or at a very short distance from the tumor, was labeled brachytherapy.

In the late 1920s, Foster-Moore and Scott (1929) inserted ^{222}Rn seeds directly into a retinoblastoma by piercing the sclera and were able to observe a tumor response; however, the final outcome is unknown. At present there is a risk of tumor seeding, with a consequent potential risk for metastases, when the affected eye is surgically invaded.

Since the 1920s, different radioisotopes have been used for the same purpose, including: ^{222}Rn, ^{60}Co, ^{106}Ru, ^{198}Au, ^{192}Ir, ^{103}Pd and ^{125}I. Iodine-125 is the preferred isotope in the United States, Canada and the United Kingdom, whereas ruthenium 106 is popular in Germany (Table 25.1).

In 1962, STALLARD pioneered the use of cobalt plaques for retinoblastoma. He treated 104 eyes and reported that 62 responded and could be preserved. Failures occurred in patients with tumor involving more than 50% of the retina. From 1970 through the early 1980s, the Wills Eye Hospital, in cooperation with Hahnemann University Hospital, used cobalt-60, ruthenium-106, and iridium-192 plaques before switching completely to iodine-125 (^{125}I). Comparative studies among these isotopes have clearly supported the benefits of iodine-125 (see chapter 5).

25.2
Radiation Considerations

The main reasons for using ^{125}I are its physical properties: a relatively long half-life of 59 days, 28 keV (kiloelectron volts) gamma ray energy, and a half-value layer (HVL) of 0.025 mm of lead, which makes shielding quite simple. All of this translates into adequate treatment, and also safety for the patient, surgeon and nursing and other staff close to the patient (FREIRE et al. 1997).

Cobalt-60, on the other hand, has gamma ray energy of 1.25 MeV and an HVL of 11 mm of lead, rendering it extremely difficult and cumbersome to

shield and place in the orbit. A ^{60}C plaque with less than 11 mm of lead would result in irradiation in both directions from the plaque, increasing the risk of complications in surrounding organs and tissues.

Furthermore, the thickness value layer (TVL) required to reduce transmission to 10% for ^{125}I is 0.1 mm of lead. Currently the plaque is made of a thickness of 0.3 mm of lead or, more commonly, 1.0 mm of gold. The TVL of ^{60}C would be 33.9 mm of lead.

The type of ^{125}I currently used is model 6711 (3 M Co. Medical Products Division, New Brighton, Minn.), which has a silver rod 3 mm in length and 0.5 mm in width; this is characterized by a more homogeneous isodose distribution than the old model 6702, which contained three ion-exchange resin spheres impregnated with ^{125}I. The silver rod is encased in 0.05-mm titanium foil with welded ends. The dimensions of the seed are 4.5 mm long and 0.8 mm wide (Fig. 25.1).

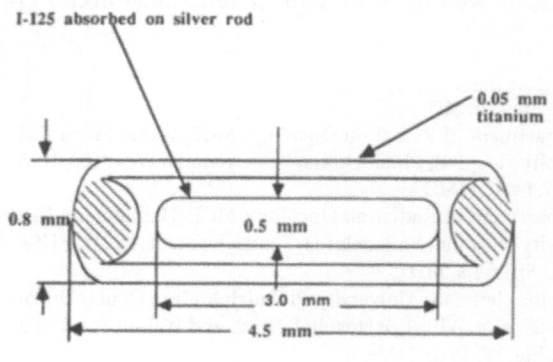

Fig. 25.1. Old and new iodine-125 seeds. The new seed model (6711) contains a cylindrical silver rod that has a more homogeneous distribution than the old model (6702) which has ion-exchange spheres at each end and a gold marker in the center

Table 25.1. Properties of important implant isotopes (*HVL*-half value layer thickness of lead to reduce transmission to 50%, *TVL* tenth value layer of lead to reduce transmission to 10%, *keV* kilo electron volt, *Pb* lead)

Isotope	Mean energy	Half-life	HVL Pb (mm)	TVL Pb (mm)
^{60}Co	1.25 MeV	5.26 years	11	33.9
^{226}Ra	1.03 MeV	1,626 years	16	28.9
^{137}Cs	662 keV	30.0 years	6.5	18.5
^{192}Ir	360 keV	74.2 days	3.1	7.1
^{222}Rn	1.03 keV	3.83 days	1.6	2.9
^{198}Au	412 keV	2.7 days	3.3	8.9
^{125}I	28 keV	59 days	0.025	0.38
^{103}Pd	22 keV	17 days	0.013	0.21
^{169}Yb	93 keV	32 days	1.6	3.1

Plaques are made of gold, for this is an inert metal that causes no allergic reaction, has an extended durability, resists sterilizing solutions well, and requires a thickness of 1 mm. The concave surface is a segment of a sphere with 12 mm radius, and the plaques range from 10 through 12, 15, and 18 to 20 mm, or occasionally 22 mm, in diameter. Plaques can be customized, according to tumor shape or location (Fig. 25.2). The ^{125}I seeds are glued to the concave surface using cyanoacrylic adhesive, and once this is dry the whole is soaked in sterilizing solution for several hours before the surgical procedure.

Planning for each plaque is done meticulously using Plaque Simulator software (Bebig, Berlin, Germany) for the proper calculation of doses to the tumor apex, base, optic disc, and fovea. The program also allows the arrangement of seed orientation for optimal final isodose distribution, number of seeds, and time of implant. We recommend a dose of 4,000 cGy (40 Gy) prescribed at the tumor apex. The treatment duration usually ranges from 48 h to 96 h, and the plaque is placed and removed in the operating suite under sedation and general anesthesia.

25.3
Technique

Plaque application in pediatric patients requires general anesthesia. The entire surgical procedure is carried out by the ophthalmologist and the team of radiation oncologist and radiation physicist.

The conjunctiva is opened through a peritomy, dissected, and the recti muscles identified and secured with loose silk sutures to allow easy rotation and mobilization of the globe. The actual tumor location is identified by using a transilluminator placed on the globe to cast a tumor shadow on the sclera, which is outlined with a special marker pen; the shadow is confirmed by indirect ophthalmoscopic globe depression. Then an inactive plastic or acrylic plaque, which is also known as a dummy plaque and is identical in shape and dimensions to the active plaque, is centered on the marks, and loose sutures are placed through the eyelets in the exact location. The dummy is then replaced by the active plaque, which is sutured to the sclera, and the conjunctiva is closed. A lead shield is taped over the patch before the patient leaves the operating suite.

The patient is kept in hospital for the whole of the time the implant is in place. This policy was decided on to allow better control of the treatment environ-

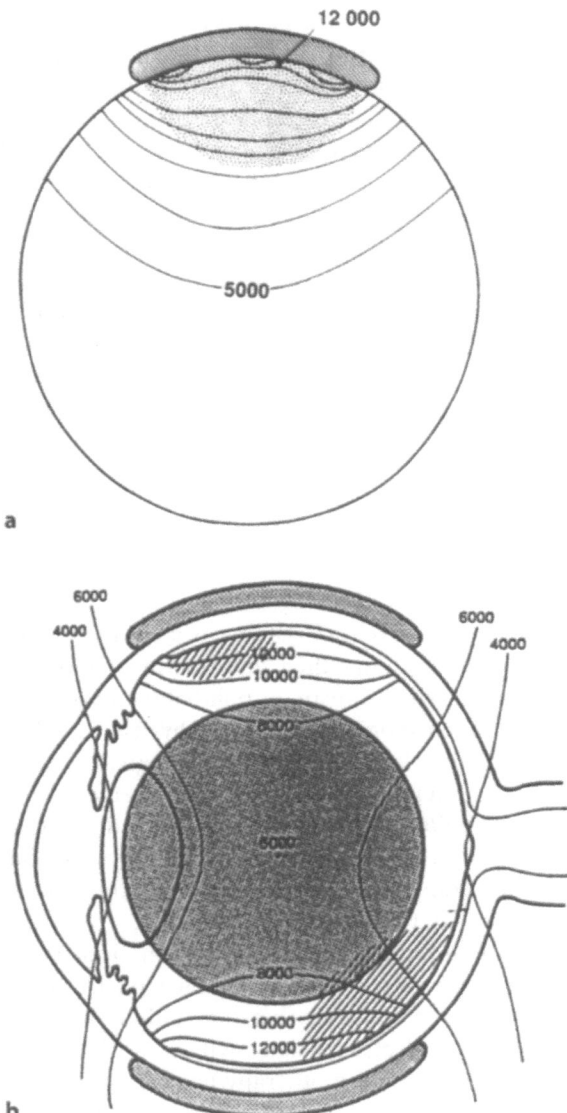

Fig. 25.3. a Isodose of single plaque on sclera. **b** Isodose of four-quadrant (SPOP) plaque technique (units: centigrays)

ment and to ensure optimal radiation safety. The family members stay with the pediatric patient, wearing a radiation badge and ring for monitoring. The patient and the room are monitored for radiation safety on a daily basis. After the calculated number of hours has elapsed the plaque is removed in the operating room under general anesthesia.

On extremely rare occasions, when other adjuvant therapies have failed to control the tumor and there is an isolated area that has been plaqued previously, and when vitreous seeds are conglomerated close to the retina and re-treatment with another plaque is feasible, the full dose of 4,000 cGy should be prescribed.

Another technique of plaque brachytherapy was described by AMENDOLA et al. (1989), whose purpose was to irradiate the entire globe while avoiding the side effects of external beam radiotherapy (EBRT). It consisted in placing two parallel opposed plaques and, after a calculated dose and time, repositioning the plaques at 90° from the previous location for another determined number of hours.

The dose to the mid-globe was 4,000–5,000 cGy, and the retina received approximately 15,000 cGy. The technique was called sequential pair opposed plaque therapy, or SPOP (Fig. 25.3). This program has considerable benefits and needs to be pursued.

Fig. 25.3. Photograph of different custom-designed plaques according to different tumor specifications

25.4
Results

Management of retinoblastoma is a complex problem, requiring more than one treatment modality and an experienced team of ophthalmic oncologist, radiation oncologist, radiation physicist, medical pediatric oncologist, and anesthesiologist.

Treatment modalities include, as described above, surgery and/or a combination of chemotherapy, laser therapy, cryotherapy, thermotherapy, plaque brachytherapy, and external beam radiotherapy (DE SUTTER et al. 1987; SHIELDS et al. 1999).

It is well known that retinoblastoma is sensitive both to ionizing radiation and to certain chemotherapeutic agents. However, there are limitations, toxicity, and side effects associated with these therapies.

External beam radiotherapy has been feared because of its effect on growing bone, which was more commonly seen decades ago with the use of low-energy orthovoltage machines with their greater bone absorption, which caused orbital hypoplasia that was cosmetically unacceptable and required plastic surgery. Currently, higher energy X-rays and electron beam radiation allow a more uniform distribution of the radiation dose in different tissues. Consequently, orbital hypoplasia is less likely to occur. With all this in mind, we recommend 6-MV photon-energy machines for retinoblastoma cases that require EBRT.

3-D Conformal treatment planning should be done in order to optimize the dose in the target volume and minimize irradiation to the surrounding tissues, as described by FREIRE et al. (2002).

Plaque brachytherapy is commonly used as a primary modality in selected, isolated, single tumors that are less than 8 mm in diameter and located away from the disc and foveola. Tumors with overlying vitreous seeds are also amenable to similar treatment, as are certain tumors recurrent after EBRT (HERNANDEZ et al. 1993; SHIELDS et al. 1992).

SHIELDS et al. (1994) reported their experience with 20 patients who were treated with plaque brachytherapy as a boost after external beam radiotherapy for large tumors which recurred locally. Tumor control was achieved in 16 (80%) of these patients, and each of the remaining 4 experienced a recurrence requiring enucleation. In fact, plaque brachytherapy was used as a secondary treatment to salvage the globe after prior failure, usually of EBRT, in 70% of cases, as described by FOSTER-MOORE and SCOTT (1929) and STALLARD (1962). With current modalities and varied combinations of adjuvant therapies, it is suggested that plaque therapy could be employed more commonly.

SHIELDS et al. (2001) also published results of tumor control and globe salvage in 89% with a mean dose to the apex of 41 Gy with ^{125}I plaques. In another series of 103 tumors treated with similar plaques, tumor control was achieved in 87% of patients (SHIELDS et al. 1993; SINGH et al. 1993).

In summary, plaque brachytherapy should be part of the therapeutic arsenal in the management of retinoblastoma. However, careful selection of patients is imperative, particularly among those in whom other therapeutic approaches have failed, provided that the recurrent tumor is localized and unifocal and away from the disc and fovea. The rate of tumor control is high, and follow-up should continue every 2 or 4 months during the first 2 years and every 6 months thereafter.

More studies and longer follow-up are necessary for better understanding of the effectiveness of the different treatment modalities and, hopefully, achievement of a significant improvement in the outcome of this debilitating and feared disease.

References

Amendola BE, Lamm FR, Markoe AM, et al (1990) Radiotherapy of retinoblastoma. A review of 63 children treated with different irradiation techniques. Cancer 66:21–26

Amendola BE, Markoe AM, Augsburger JJ et al (1989) Analysis of treatment results in 36 children with retinoblastoma treated with scleral plaque irradiation. Int J Radiat Oncol Biol Phys 17:63–70

De Sutter E, Havers W, Hopping W et al (1987) The prognosis of retinoblastoma in terms of globe saving treatment. A computer assisted study. I. Ophthalmic Pediatr Genet 8:77–84

Foster-Moore R, Scott RS (1929) Clinical and pathological report of bilateral glioma retinae. Proc R Soc Med 22:39–50

Freire JE, De Potter P, Brady LW et al (1997) Brachytherapy in primary ocular tumors. Semin Surg Oncol 13:167–176

Freire JE, Brady LW, Shields CL, Shields JA (2002) Eye. In: Perez CA, Brady LW (eds) Principles and practice of radiation oncology, 4th edn. Lippincott-Raven, Philadelphia (in press)

Hernandez JC, Brady LW, Shields CL, Shields JA (1993) Conservative treatment of retinoblastoma. The use of plaque brachytherapy. Am J Clin Oncol 16:397–401

Shields CL, Shields JA (1999) Recent developments in the management of retinoblastoma (review). J Pediatric Ophthalmol Strabismus 36:8–18

Shields CL, Shields JA, Minelli S et al (1993) Plaque radiotherapy in the management of retinoblastoma. Use as primary or secondary treatment. Ophthalmology 100:216–224

Shields CL, Shields JA, Needle M et al (1997) Combined chemoreduction and adjuvant treatment for intraocular retinoblastoma. Ophthalmology 104:2101–2111

Shields CL, Santos MC, Diniz W et al (1999) Thermotherapy for retinoblastoma. Arch Ophthalmol 117:885–893

Shields CL, Shields JA, Carter J, Othmane I, Singh AD, Micaily B et al (2001) Plaque radiotherapy for retinoblastoma: long term tumor control and treatment complications in 208 tumors. Ophthalmology 108:2116–2121

Shields JA, Shields CL (1992) Management and prognosis of retinoblastoma. In: Shields JA, Shields CL (eds) Saunders, Philadelphia, pp 377–392

Shields JA, Shields CL, Hernandez JC et al (1994) Plaque radiotherapy for residual or recurrent retinoblastoma in 91 cases. J Pediatr Ophthalmol Strabismus 31:242–245

Singh AD, Garway-Heath D, Love S et al (1993) Relationship of regression pattern to recurrence in retinoblastoma. Br J Ophthalmol 77:12–16

Stallard HB (1962) Doyle Memorial Lecture. The conservative treatment of retinoblastoma. Transophthalmol Soc UK 82:473–535

26 Physical Aspects of Eye Plaque Brachytherapy Using Photon Emitters

L. L. Anderson and S.-T. Chiu-Tsao

CONTENTS

26.1 Introduction

The current trend toward the use of ^{125}I seed rather than ^{60}Co applicators in the treatment of ocular tumors stems largely from the extent to which photons from the two radionuclides are attenuated differently by plaque material on the one hand and by intraocular tissue on the other. The much lower energies of ^{125}I photons from seeds in a rimmed gold plaque not only permit near-total elimination of radiation dose in orbital tissue adjacent to the plaque but also allow significant dose reduction to critical structures within the eye, relative to either ^{60}Co plaque or proton beam treatment (FAIRCHILD 1984). Although other photon-emitting radionuclides have been used in ophthalmic applicators (LUXTON et al. 1988a), we will focus attention here on the physical characteristics of ^{60}Co and ^{125}I applicators because they have been the most widely used and because they illustrate well the pertinent

L.L. ANDERSON, PhD
Attending Physicist, Department of Medical Physics, Memorial Sloan-Kettering Cancer Center, 1275 York Avenue, New York, NY 10021, USA
S.-T. CHIU-TSAO, PhD
Head, Physics Division Department of Radiation Oncology, Henry Ford Hospital, 2799 West Grand Boulevard, Detroit, MI 48202, USA

differences between "high energy" and "low energy" photons for this type of brachytherapy.

26.2 Radiation Sources

Because of the long (5.27 year) half life of ^{60}Co, it was feasible to make the radionuclide itself an integral part of the eye applicator. Its photon energies (1.17 and 1.33 MeV) are sufficiently high that, except for minor peripheral effects of oblique filtration (see Sect. 26.3.2), encapsulation by the applicator does not greatly modify the dose distribution. Further, it is evident from a review by MEISBERGER et al. (1968) that the total attenuation of photons from a point source in water is within 2 %–3 %, at a distance of 2.5 cm (one "eye diameter") of that arising only from the inverse square law. Clearly, from Fig. 26.1, the same statement may be made for other radionuclides emitting photons of moderately high energy. Sources of ^{192}Ir (0.37 MeV average gamma ray energy and 73.8 day half-life) and of ^{198}Au (0.42 MeV average gamma ray energy and 2.7 day half-life) have also been used in eye plaques. Since such nuclides may deliver significant dose to extraorbital tissue, attenuation by water at distances greater than 2 cm is also of interest and is seen (Fig. 26.1) to be less than about 15% at 10 cm.

For eye applicators using ^{125}I seeds, one is first interested in the dose distribution around the seed itself and then in the possible modifying effect of the plaque material. Since an up-todate review of ^{125}I seed design and single-seed dosimetry is included in Chaps. 1, 3, and 32 of a recently published book [INTERSTITIAL COLLABORATIVE WORKING GROUP (ICWG) 1990], only a brief summary will be provided here.

Photons from ^{125}I range in energy from 27.4 to 35.5 keV, with an average of 28.5 keV. The half life of ^{125}I is 59.6 days. Seeds containing ^{125}I are available (Medi-Physics, Inc., Amersham, Arlington Heights, IL) in two models (see Fig. 26.2), the 6711 and the 6702. Although both models use the same titanium

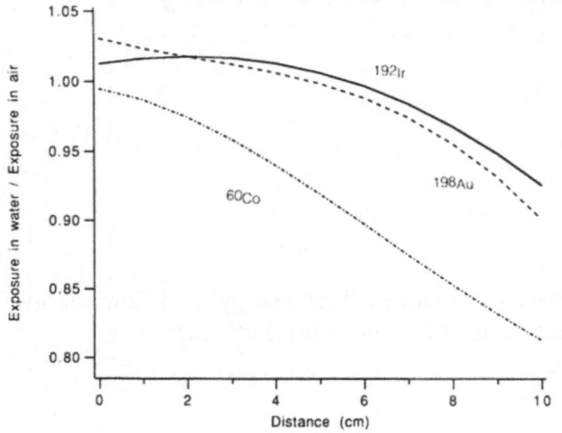

Fig. 26.1. Ratio of exposure in water to exposure in air as a function of distance from point sources of ^{60}Co, ^{192}Ir, and [198]Au, from a polynomial fit by MEISBERGER et al. (1968) to averaged experimental and calculated data

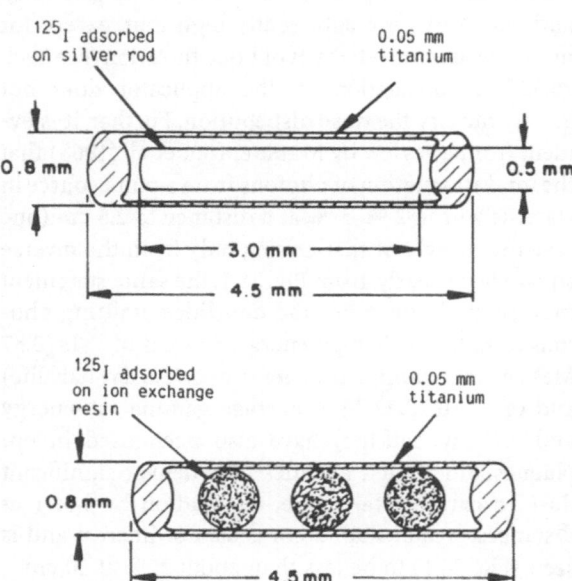

Fig. 26.2. Models 6711 (*above*) and 6702 (*below*) [125]I seeds shown in longitudinal cross-section. (Courtesy of Medical Products Division, 3M Company, New Brighton, MN)

shell, welded on both ends, the ^{125}I in the 6711 seed is deposited on the surface of a small silver wire, whereas that in the 6702 seed is adsorbed on two or more beads of ion exchange resin. As a result of photon absorption in the titanium capsule, especially in the welds, both seed models exhibit a high degree of anisotropy in photon emission, with only about 20% as many photons (per unit solid angle) emitted in the axial direction as along the transverse (perpendicular) axis. The anisotropy is exacerbated for the

6711 seed by photon absorption in the silver wire, which also adds 22 keV Ag fluorescent x-rays to the photon energy spectrum and lowers the average energy to 27.4 keV.

The calibration of ^{125}I seeds is based on exposure in air along the transverse axis. Seed strength is currently stated by the supplier in terms of "apparent" activity (in mCi), obtained by dividing the product of exposure rate and distance-squared by an exposure rate constant of $1.45 \text{ R cm}^2 \text{ mCi}^{-1} \text{ h}^{-1}$. In 1987, the American Association of Physicists in Medicine published a report (Task Group 32, 1987) recommending specification of brachytherapy source strength by the quantity "air kerma strength," defined as the product of air kerma rate (in free space) and distance-squared on the transverse axis, at distances from source center sufficiently large that the inverse square law is obeyed. Using the convention of the ICWG (1990) and substituting the symbol "U" for the units ($\text{cGy cm}^2 \text{ h}^{-1}$) of air kerma strength, we obtain the relationship between air kerma strength and apparent activity from the ^{125}I air kerma rate constant, 1.27 U mCi^{-1}.

The measured values of single-seed dose rate reported by the ICWG (1990) for ^{125}I seeds are lower by about 16% for the 6711 and 9% for the 6702 than values commonly used earlier, which had been based on relative data (dose rate times distance-squared) normalized to the product of the exposure rate constant and the "f" factor (in cGy/R) at a distance of 1 cm on the transverse axis. The latter product is, in fact, what one would expect to obtain in approaching zero distance from a point source, and recently measured water/air ratios (CHIU-TSAO et al. 1990) on the transverse axis do, in fact, appear to extrapolate to that value at zero distance, but values at 1.0 cm are lower by the percentages mentioned above. Table 26.1 presents a synthesis of TLD-measured and Monte Carlo-calculated dosimetry data for the model 6711, ^{125}I seed and Table 26.2 provides Monte Carlo-calculated data, which showed close agreement with TLD measurement results, for the 6702 seed (CHIU-TSAO et al. 1990). The x-axis in each table corresponds to the longitudinal axis of the seed and the y-axis to the transverse (perpendicular) axis of the seed. Greater detail is provided at "Intraocular" distances than at larger distances. Since each value tabulated is the product of distance-squared and dose per unit apparent activity, variation with distance is primarily the result of scattering and absorption by water. Secondarily, the fact that the source is not a point source leads to decreasing values as the source is approached (i.e., the "extended source effect").

Table 26.1. Distance-squared times dose rate per unit apparent activity (cGy cm^2 h^{-1} mCi^{-1}) for ^{125}I model 6711 seed in water

y (cm) \ x (cm)	0.0	0.1	0.2	0.3	0.4	0.5	0.6	0.8	1.0	1.2	1.4	1.6	1.8	2.0	2.5	3.0	3.5	4.0	5.0	6.0	8.0	10.0
0.0	–	–	–	0.284	0.288	0.308	0.330	0.375	0.430	0.446	0.450	0.450	0.430	0.410	0.360	0.321	0.285	0.253	0.196	0.152	0.090	0.052
0.1	–	–	–	0.926	0.670	0.562	0.522	0.504	0.514	0.509	0.501	0.496	0.470	0.443	0.382	0.337	0.297	0.261	0.201	0.154	0.091	0.053
0.2	–	–	–	1.112	0.964	0.842	0.743	0.634	0.597	0.570	0.552	0.540	0.508	0.476	0.405	0.352	0.308	0.269	0.205	0.157	0.092	0.053
0.3	1.049	1.087	1.195	1.157	1.068	0.971	0.879	0.754	0.682	0.633	0.602	0.581	0.544	0.507	0.427	0.367	0.318	0.277	0.210	0.160	0.093	0.054
0.4	1.087	1.117	1.180	1.175	1.119	1.049	0.969	0.842	0.757	0.692	0.649	0.615	0.575	0.535	0.448	0.382	0.329	0.285	0.214	0.162	0.094	0.054
0.5	1.104	1.128	1.173	1.186	1.145	1.089	1.032	0.913	0.823	0.748	0.691	0.647	0.602	0.559	0.466	0.395	0.339	0.292	0.218	0.165	0.095	0.054
0.6	1.110	1.132	1.171	1.180	1.157	1.116	1.063	0.963	0.878	0.798	0.733	0.677	0.627	0.581	0.482	0.407	0.348	0.299	0.222	0.167	0.096	0.056
0.8	1.103	1.128	1.150	1.164	1.151	1.126	1.091	1.015	0.940	0.866	0.798	0.728	0.668	0.617	0.510	0.428	0.363	0.311	0.230	0.172	0.098	0.056
1.0	1.080	1.106	1.127	1.132	1.127	1.108	1.085	1.028	0.962	0.894	0.822	0.757	0.697	0.643	0.532	0.445	0.376	0.321	0.236	0.176	0.099	0.057
1.2	1.048	1.072	1.095	1.097	1.094	1.081	1.061	1.014	0.960	0.894	0.830	0.766	0.710	0.659	0.546	0.458	0.387	0.329	0.241	0.179	0.101	0.057
1.4	1.011	1.033	1.053	1.060	1.054	1.046	1.027	0.986	0.936	0.883	0.821	0.767	0.714	0.664	0.555	0.465	0.394	0.335	0.245	0.181	0.102	0.058
1.6	0.970	0.987	1.003	1.014	1.005	0.995	0.983	0.947	0.904	0.855	0.808	0.758	0.710	0.663	0.556	0.470	0.398	0.339	0.248	0.183	0.103	
1.8	0.927	0.940	0.950	0.959	0.954	0.945	0.934	0.903	0.869	0.829	0.787	0.743	0.698	0.655	0.554	0.471	0.400	0.341	0.250	0.185	0.104	
2.0	0.884	0.892	0.898	0.903	0.902	0.894	0.886	0.863	0.833	0.799	0.761	0.722	0.682	0.641	0.549	0.468	0.400	0.342	0.251	0.186	0.104	
2.5	0.778	0.781	0.783	0.784	0.785	0.781	0.775	0.760	0.740	0.714	0.687	0.656	0.626	0.597	0.522	0.453	0.390	0.336	0.249	0.186	0.104	
3.0	0.679	0.680	0.680	0.680	0.679	0.677	0.673	0.662	0.649	0.632	0.611	0.590	0.567	0.543	0.483	0.425	0.372	0.323	0.242	0.182	0.104	
3.5	0.590	0.590	0.590	0.590	0.588	0.587	0.585	0.577	0.567	0.556	0.541	0.523	0.505	0.487	0.439	0.392	0.346	0.304	0.232	0.176	0.101	
4.0	0.511	0.511	0.511	0.510	0.509	0.508	0.506	0.500	0.493	0.484	0.475	0.462	0.448	0.433	0.395	0.356	0.319	0.282	0.219	0.168	0.098	
5.0	0.383	0.382	0.382	0.382	0.381	0.380	0.379	0.376	0.372	0.366	0.360	0.354	0.347	0.337	0.312	0.286	0.260	0.235	0.188	0.148	0.089	
6.0	0.285	0.285	0.285	0.285	0.284	0.284	0.283	0.281	0.279	0.275	0.272	0.268	0.263	0.258	0.243	0.226	0.208	0.191	0.157	0.126	0.079	
8.0	0.159	0.159	0.159	0.158	0.158	0.158	0.158	0.157	0.156	0.155	0.153	0.152	0.150	0.148	0.142	0.135	0.127	0.119	0.102	0.085		
10.0	0.088	0.088	0.088	0.088	0.088	0.088	0.088	0.088	0.087	0.087	0.086											

Table 26.2. Distance-squared times dose rate per unit apparent activity (cGy cm² h⁻¹ mCi⁻¹) for ^{125}I model 6702 seed in water

y (cm) \ x (cm)	0.0	0.1	0.2	0.3	0.4	0.5	0.6	0.8	1.0	1.2	1.4	1.6	1.8	2.0	2.5	3.0	3.5	4.0	5.0	6.0	8.0	10.0
0.0	-	-	-	0.498	0.489	0.476	0.473	0.494	0.501	0.505	0.517	0.528	0.530	0.514	0.472	0.439	0.414	0.373	0.298	0.232	0.137	0.076
0.1	-	-	-	1.039	0.720	0.610	0.567	0.565	0.566	0.558	0.560	0.561	0.560	0.539	0.492	0.453	0.423	0.380	0.301	0.234	0.137	0.076
0.2	-	-	-	1.243	1.052	0.905	0.794	0.685	0.642	0.611	0.601	0.594	0.589	0.565	0.511	0.466	0.430	0.385	0.305	0.235	0.138	0.077
0.3	1.103	1.144	1.208	1.225	t.167	1.069	0.965	0.829	0.752	0.698	0.660	0.632	0.615	0.590	0.530	0.479	0.438	0.390	0.308	0.237	0.138	0.077
0.4	1.156	1.165	1.195	1.205	1.186	1.146	1.070	0.939	0.847	0.782	0.730	0.690	0.658	0.620	0.548	0.490	0.446	0.396	0.311	0.238	0.138	0.077
0.5	1.186	1.186	1.190	1.196	1.184	1.161	1.131	1.017	0.918	0.846	0.798	0.746	0.701	0.657	0.570	0.501	0.452	0.401	0.314	0.241	0.139	0.077
0.6	1.t89	1.185	1.186	1.186	1.179	1.170	1.142	1.069	0.972	0.893	0.837	0.794	0.742	0.691	0.594	0.517	0.460	0.405	0.317	0.242	0.139	0.077
0.8	1.184	1.179	1.180	1.184	1.170	1.158	1.155	1.104	1.041	0.962	0.899	0.847	0.796	0.746	0.636	0.547	0.480	0.418	0.322	0.243	0.139	0.077
1.0	1.180	1.177	1.175	1.172	1.163	1.147	1.131	1.100	1.053	1.008	0.942	0.887	0.836	0.780	0.667	0.575	0.498	0.432	0.327	0.246	0.139	0.077
1.2	1.146	1.144	1.143	1.141	1.139	1.128	1.113	1.081	1.048	1.006	0.965	0.912	0.853	0.803	0.686	0.592	0.513	0.443	0.333	0.248	0.139	0.077
1.4	1.110	1.110	1.109	1.108	1.106	1.104	1.090	1.060	1.031	0.999	0.961	0.914	0.861	0.810	0.700	0.605	0.523	0.453	0.338	0.252	0.139	0.077
1.6	1.075	1.075	1.074	1.071	1.070	1.067	1.061	1.036	1.009	0.982	0.947	0.901	0.857	0.812	0.705	0.613	0.529	0.460	0.343	0.254	0.139	
1.8	1.044	1.043	1.041	1.038	1.036	1.032	1.027	1.008	0.982	0.953	0.923	0.886	0.844	0.804	0.705	0.617	0.533	0.462	0.347	0.256	0.141	
2.0	1.015	1.014	1.012	1.008	1.003	0.996	0.990	0.971	0.948	0.924	0.896	0.867	0.832	0.793	0.700	0.614	0.534	0.463	0.347	0.257	0.141	
2.5	0.090	0.908	0.905	0.903	0.898	0.894	0.889	0.877	0.862	0.844	0.824	0.799	0.774	0.749	0.672	0.596	0.522	0.453	0.342	0.256	0.139	
3.0	0.810	0.809	0.806	0.804	0.801	0.798	0.795	0.786	0.775	0.761	0.743	0.723	0.703	0.682	0.625	0.560	0.496	0.433	0.332	0.249	0.138	
3.5	0.717	0.717	0.715	0.714	0.711	0.710	0.706	0.699	0.690	0.679	0.666	0.649	0.633	0.617	0.568	0.515	0.458	0.406	0.315	0.241	0.134	
4.0	0.632	0.632	0.632	0.630	0.629	0.628	0.625	0.619	0.611	0.601	0.590	0.579	0.566	0.552	0.511	0.466	0.420	0.376	0.295	0.227	0.128	
5.0	0.484	0.484	0.482	0.482	0.481	0.480	0.477	0.473	0.468	0.461	0.453	0.446	0.437	0.428	0.403	0.375	0.342	0.310	0.251	0.197	0.115	
6.0	0.365	0.365	0.363	0.363	0.362	0.361	0.360	0.357	0.353	0.349	0.346	0.341	0.334	0.328	0.3 tO	0.290	0.270	0.247	0.203	0.163	0.099	
8.0	0.200	0.200	0.200	0.200	0.200	0.199	0.199	0.197	0.196	0.194	0.192	0.190	0.187	0.185	0.177	0.170	0.160	0.148	0.125	0.105		
10.0	0.108	0.108	0.108	0.108	0.108	0.106	0.106	0.106	0.105	0.105	0.104											

Of practical interest is the ratio of the dose times distance-squared at 2.5 cm to the dose times distance-squared at a typical seed-to-tumor apex distance of, say, 0.6 cm. On the transverse axis, this ratio is 0.70 for the 6711 seed and 0.76 for the 6702 seed. It illustrates roughly the maximum dose reduction to normal eye tissue that may be associated with the use of ^{125}I rather, than [60]Co. A somewhat greater reduction might be achieved using [103]Pd seeds (20.9 keV average photon energy and 17 day half life), for which the same ratio would be about 0.38.

26.3
[60]Co Eye Applicators

26.3.1
[60]CO Plaque Design

Ophthalmic applicators for retinoblastoma incorporated ^{60}Co soon after that radioisotope became available. Designed by G.S. Innes, H.B. Stallard and associates at St. Bartholomew's Hospital, London, after 1948 (INNES 1962), these applicators were produced initially by the United Kingdom Atomic Energy Authority, Harwell, and subsequently by Amersham International, plc. In the basic design, the radioactive cobalt was distributed in one or more rings within a 0.5 mm thick platinum sheath having an 11 mm innersurface radius of curvature and lugs on either side for suturing to the eye. It was assumed that the source diameter should be equal to or greater than the diameter of the tumor base and that the tumor height, on the average, would be twothirds of the base diameter. Treatment design depth, therefore, was the thickness of the sclera, taken to be 1.5 mm, plus twothirds of the source diameter. Four circular applica-

tors were provided, as shown in Fig. 26.3, with source diameters of 5, 7.5, 10, and 15 mm (Amersham designations CKA 1-4). In addition, three sizes of D-shaped (CKA 5-7) and four sizes of crescent-shaped (CKA 8-11) sources were made available for treating tumors close to the ciliary body and optic nerve, respectively. The design source strength for each applicator was that necessary to produce a total (exposure) dose of 4000 R in 6 days at the design depth. Applicators were manufactured with slightly greater source strengths, anticipating a 3 year use period before reactivation would be required.

26.3.2
[60]CO Plaque Dosimetry

The original specification (INNES 1962) of design source strength implied the dose rate only at one point (i.e., at the design depth) on each plaque axis. For the 5 mm plaque, MAGNUS (1967) calculated the dose rate at other axial points by multiplying the design depth dose rate, as originally given, by the inverse ratio of distance-squared. The distance used in these calculations was that between a given axial point and the "effective center" of the cobalt ring cross-section (the circular line source thus defined divided the cobalt ring's surface into two equal surfaces and its thickness in half). In addition, the calculated dose rate was reduced by an exponential tissue attenuation factor for which the exponent was the product of an attenuation coefficient based on a half-value layer of 16.7 cm and the (axial) distance to the plaque surface (rather than to the cobalt ring); the resulting attenuation factor at 25 mm was 0.902. The same method was applied to the calculation of axial dose rates for the other (CKA 2-4) circular applicators, with the inverse square factors for a central disk

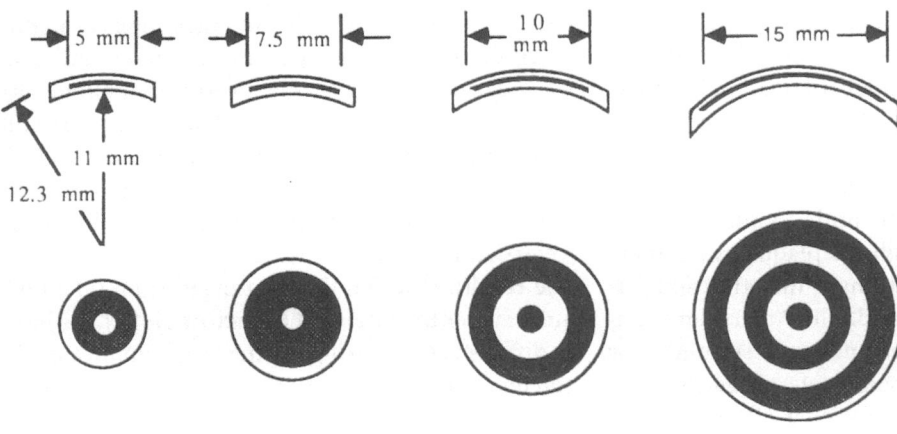

Fig. 26.3. Circular ^{60}Co applicators CKA 1-4, showing distribution of the active source within the spherical platinum sheath

or ring of ^{60}Co weighted according to the proportion of source strength involved.

Subsequently, MAGNUS et al. (1968) reported the results of similar calculations for plaques having the D-shaped or crescent-shaped sources (CKA 5–11). Although the crescent-shaped sources were calculable by the inverse square method used in the earlier paper, the D-shaped sources did not possess rotational symmetry and a simplified model was invoked, substituting two larger diameter quarter rings of ^{60}Co for the top and bottom of the "D" and two opposed quarter rings of smaller diameter for the middle part.

The above calculation conformed to the data of INNES, except for the tissue attenuation correction (which made no allowance for scattering buildup). With regard to the original determinations of design source strength, it implicitly assumed accuracy in source dimensions, in the exposure rate constant, and in any correction for platinum filtration. None of these computational details had been mentioned in the INNES article.

Isodose measurements using radiographic film in a paraffin phantom were subsequently reported by MAGNUS et al. (1969) for the circular plaques CKA 1–4. The dose rates measured on the plaque axis agreed with the earlier calculations for plaques CKA 3 and CKA 4. They were, however, about 20% higher than calculated for the CKA 1 and CKA 2 applicators, indicating that the design source strengths as originally specified were also in error. Film measurements of contact dose on the back (convex) side of applicators CKA 3 and CKA 4 indicated 6-day exposures of 23000 and 22000 R, respectively. For the crescent-shaped plaques, RASSOW et al. (1970) reported similar isodose measurements with film and introduced a more general calculational method (involving integration over the ^{60}Co source surface) for obtaining dose rate along the plaque axis. The new calculation was no longer linked to the original specification of design source strength and design depth. It did include scattering buildup, as well as exponential attenuation in tissue, a platinum filtration correction, and an implied exposure rate constant of 12.4 R cm^2 mCi^{-1} h^{-1}. Satisfactory agreement was obtained between measurement and calculation in both symmetric and asymmetric planes through the plaque axis. No extension of the new calculations to the other applicators (CKA 1–7) was reported. The Amersham catalog for 1973 listed new design source strengths for all ophthalmic applicators and referenced the CKA 1–4 measurements of MAGNUS et al. (1969).

Isodose contours were both measured (using film in Perspex phantom) and calculated by CASEBOW (1971) for all 11 ophthalmic applicators. The calculation, performed by computer, evaluated the dose at each point as the integral over a half-ring representation of each ^{60}Co source component. It assumed an exposure rate constant of 13.2 R cm^2 mCi^{-1} h^{-1} and did not address the question of tissue attenuation. For D-shaped and crescent-shaped applicators, both measurements and calculations were performed in the asymmetric as well as the symmetric plane through the plaque axis. Agreement between measurement and calculation within the "body of the eye" was generally within 0.5 mm, i.e., within the accuracy of film positioning, whereas calculations overestimated the dose at the edge of the applicator (due to failure to account for oblique filtration by platinum) and close to the applicator surface (due to the ring approximation of source segments). The calculated results were used to tabulate new values of design depth corresponding to original values of design activity; it would have been more appropriate to compute new values of design activity for the original design depths, which were predicated on the 2/3 ratio of tumor height to tumor base width.

For the circular applicators CKA 1–4, CHAN et al. (1972) accounted approximately for oblique filtration in platinum by representing each ^{60}Co segment by many uniformly filtered line sources in dose calculations employing the Sievert integral, with an exposure rate constant of 13.0 R cm^2 mCi^{-1} h^{-1}. They also used film and LiF thermoluminescent dosimeters for dose measurements in polystyrene phantom, obtaining fair (about ±10%) agreement with calculated results. Depth dose results of the line source calculation were tabulated, based on the original values of design source strength.

Isodose data for all the applicators were calculated by BEDDOE (1975), using an exposure rate constant of 13.2 R cm^2 mCi^{-1} h^{-1} and including (in an unspecified manner) the effects of tissue attenuation. An allowance of 5.5% was made for (nonoblique) attenuation by the platinum case. These data were still based (as were the CASEBOW and the CHAN et al. data) on the original design source strengths, although the changed design source strengths in the Amersham catalog were acknowledged in a footnote. The resulting design depths ranged from 0.1 to 0.8 mm smaller than those of CASEBOW (1971), the larger differences occurring for the larger applicator diameters and attributed to the inclusion of tissue attenuation.

Published calculations of dose rate from ^{60}Co eye plaques generally either ignored tissue attenuation and scattering or took both into account in a manner that assumed an infinite medium and resulted in minimal correction because of the well-known compensation of exponential attenuation by scattering buildup. However, in the usual treatment situation, with the applicator near the back of the eye, there is relatively little scattering material beyond the tumor and attenuation may predominate. Monte Carlo calculations for a ^{60}Co point source 2.42 cm from the surface of a cylindrical water phantom 18 cm in diameter have indicated that the dose within the "eye" at distances greater than 5 mm from the source is 5%–10% lower than that in an infinite phantom (CHIU-TSAO et al. 1986). These results are not greatly different from those of MAGNUS (1967), who took account of attenuation but not scattering buildup.

In 1984, Amersham International, plc, began limiting regular production of ophthalmic applicators to the four circular models (CKA 1–4) and changed the design to a "dish" distribution of ^{60}Co, in which source material was distributed uniformly within spherical segments of the same outer dimensions as in the earlier ring design. At the same time, they made available isodose contours, normalized to 4000 rads in 6 days at the originally specified design depths, for both ring-type and dish-type applicators (see Fig. 26.4).

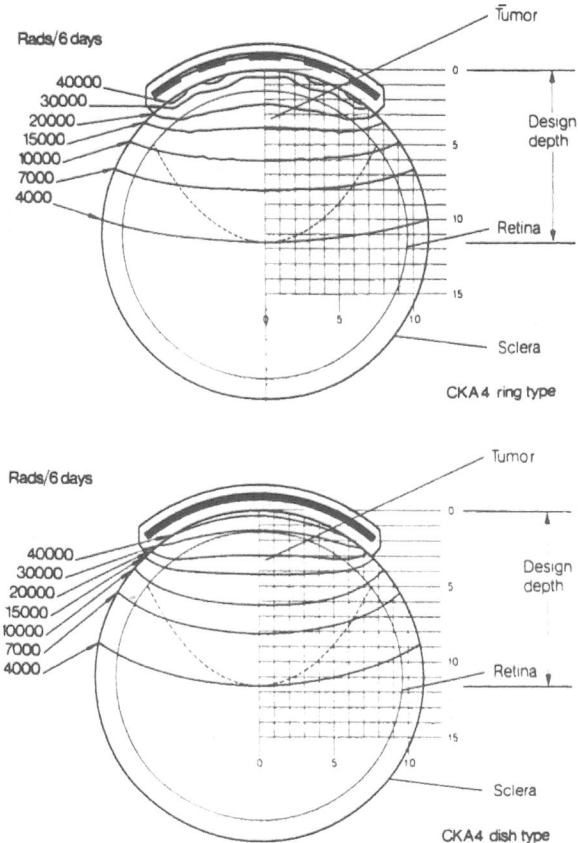

Fig. 26.4. Isodose contours for the CKA 4 (15 mm source diameter) ^{60}Co eye applicator, both the ring type, now discontinued, and the dish type. (Courtesy of Amersham International, plc, Arlington Heights, IL)

26.4
^{125}I Eye Applicators

26.4.1
^{125}I Plaque Design

In contrast to the development of ^{60}Co for eye tumor brachytherapy, where a standard set of applicators introduced at the outset was widely adopted and persisted for many years, the use of ^{125}I seeds to treat ocular tumors has been characterized by custom design and local fabrication of plaques, no doubt because of the relatively short half life of ^{125}I and the need to procure a new source complement, at least, for each treatment. The potential of ^{125}I for treating ophthalmic tumors, with effective shielding of nearby structures, was recognized early by SEALY et al. (1976), who reported treating two eyelid tumors and an anterior choroidal melanoma with seeds mounted in custom applicators incorporating metal shields to limit dose to the lens and the cornea. The plaque

fabrication technique they developed for intraocular tumors (SEALY et al. 1980) involved forming gold sheet over a 2.5 cm hemispherical brass dye machined to the required size. Edges were formed wherever it was necessary to protect normal structures and peripheral suture holes were drilled. Seeds were arranged in the plaque in sufficient number and strength to achieve the desired dose (in 6 days) at the tumor apex. After the seeds were individually cemented to the plaque, the array was covered with self-curing liquid acrylic which, as it hardened, was given the proper curvature by pressure from a 2.5 cm diameter metal ball. Seeds were recovered after use by soaking in chloroform.

A similar approach has been followed by others. PACKER and ROTMAN (1980) described custom plaques made from 0.4 mm 24-carat gold sheet, shaped and polished by a jeweler or in a dental laboratory. These plaques were bordered by a 160° lip of about 1 mm, drilled with multiple holes to provide spacing options for three suture points (two were found to provide inadequate stability). Seeds were glued into position, using leaded gloves and a lead-glass shield, and a smooth surface over them was formed with a commercially available acrylic material that required about 24 h to set. The thickness and composition of gold alloy used is selected as much for rigidity as for shielding, since 0.2 mm pure gold is sufficient to reduce the number of ^{125}I photons by a factor of more than 3000.

HARNETT and THOMSON (1988) have reported using plaques in the form of flat-bottomed circular dishes of 9-carat (37.5%) gold, 0.4 mm thick, with filler material of epoxy resin rather than acrylic. [125]I seeds are placed only around the periphery (next to the rim) and a concave inner surface is achieved by pressure against the resin with a 25 mm ball. The result is a rather thin plaque 1.7 mm thick over the seeds and only 0.9 mm thick in the center.

A more recent development in ^{125}I plaque design is the use of a molded plastic insert with troughs for seed placement in standard patterns. An example is the so-called COMS plaque designed for the Collaborative Ocular Melanoma Study (EARLE et al. 1987). Circular COMS plaques are currently available in five diameters, from 12 to 20 mm in 2 mm intervals, with silicone seed carrier inserts providing troughs for as many as 8, 13, 13, 21, and 24 ^{125}I seeds in roughly concentric circles. Trough pattern and dimensions are shown for the 14 mm plaque in Fig 26.5. The trough depth (1.25 mm) places at least 1 mm silicone spacer between each ^{125}I seed and the sclera. Because the lip surface is cylindrical about the plaque central axis, lip height increases with plaque diameter and ranges from 2.5 to 3.3 mm. Seeds are inserted with the carrier supported on a hemispherical stand and held in place when the carrier is covered by the metal (77% gold) plaque. The carrier is secured to the plaque peripherally with three drops of silicone adhesive, which is allowed to cure for 24 h before the assembly is gas sterilized. The carrier is reusable if care is used in its removal. For each diameter, a dummy plaque for placing sutures is a silver replica of the actual plaque's rim and flange, with either a clear acrylic contoured disk or (if preferred) an open space in the center.

LUXTON et al. (1988a) have described the design and fabrication of gold alloy eye plaques with radially oriented grooves, in the plaque itself, to hold either ^{125}I seeds or ^{192}Ir seeds. The radial pattern was chosen to permit closer spacing than a circular pattern and, therefore, a lower individual-seed strength for a given total seed strength (with potentially fewer complications from regions of very high dose). Cast

in a plaster mold, each plaque is a section of a spherical shell 25 mm in diameter and 1.5 mm thick. In use, no plastic covering is applied over the seeds and the gold plaque is in direct contact with the sclera.

KAROLIS et al. (1989) have reported the design of a ^{125}I plaque of 1 mm stainless steel, with a 1.6 mm thick acrylic insert having machined spherical surfaces and into which trenches were milled to accommodate individual seeds. Since the insert is tight fitting and made secure to the plaque with only silicone grease, assembly (under sterile conditions) takes only a few minutes. The plaque incorporates a stepped-diameter removable disk at its center to facilitate equally rapid disassembly. Both the plaque and the opencenter template have a five-hole suturing flange. Two sizes (10 and 15 mm diameters) have been constructed. The 1 mm thickness of steel atten-

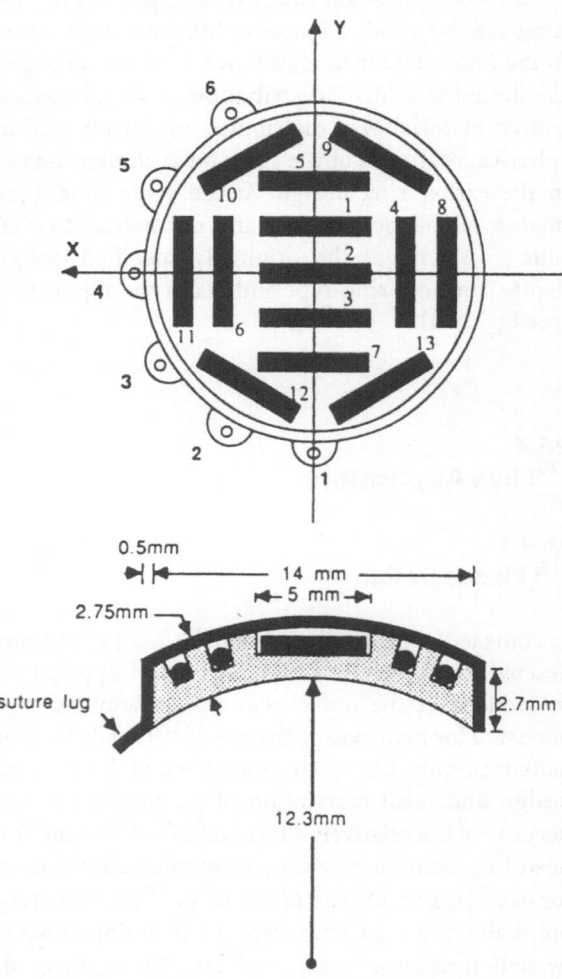

Fig. 26.5. One of the five ^{125}I plaques used in the Collaborative Ocular Melanoma Study, showing the gold backing design and the arrangement of seeds in troughs within the silicone seed carrier insert

uates ^{125}I photons by more than a factor of 10. Reduction of the plaque radial thickness to 2.1 mm is anticipated by using a gold alloy instead of stainless steel (KAROLIS et al. 1990).

In a third-generation design described by SCHELL et al. (1989), 0.3 mm gold alloy sheets are formed into plaques having a 12.5 mm radius of curvature and the plaques themselves, with dummy seeds cemented to the concave surface, are used to mold removable inserts from self-curing acrylic; the insert is partially cured in contact with a 25.4 mm diameter steel ball, to shape its concave surface. Plaque rims are sufficiently high that this procedure leaves 1 mm of acrylic material between a seed trough bottom and the concave surface. Although mold production requires 24 h for curing, plaque assembly with the completed mold takes only 10 min. Plaque diameters range from 9 to 17 mm and plaque replicas (open in the center) are provided to assist placement by transillumination.

26.4.2
[125]I Plaque Dosimetry

Because ^{125}I seeds used with eye plaques are variable with respect both to strength and to position on the plaque, clinical dose calculations have generally invoked reference data for individual seeds rather than for the plaque as a whole. Dosimetric studies of ^{125}I plaques have focused, therefore, on the effect of the plaque on the dose distribution from an installed seed. Perhaps the first study of this kind was that of WEAVER (1986), in which a capsule of LiF TLD powder was deployed at depths of 0.5, 0.97, and 1.5 cm in a plastic phantom directly opposite a square array (0.5 cm on an edge) of four Model 6702 ^{125}I seeds abutting the phantom surface. The dose measured with an eye-plaque-type gold alloy sheet (4 × 6 × 0.03 cm) serving as backing material for the seed array was, on average, about 8% lower than that measured with a paraffin slab (20 × 20 × 4 cm) backing. Measurements with either gold-plus-paraffin backing or no backing at all gave comparable results. On the basis of these data, the author introduced a routine correction factor of 0.92 to be applied to clinical calculations of ^{125}I eye-plaque dose rate.

A comparable study has been reported on the effect of the gold plaque on dose distribution in acrylic phantom along the transverse axis of a Model 6711 ^{125}I seed (LUXTON et al. 1988b). With the seed mounted on top of a hemispherical simulated eye projecting from a horizontal phantom surface, six 3 × 1 mm diameter LiF TLDs monitored the dose in phantom

at distances 2–18 mm below the center of the seed under conditions of (a) full scatter, i.e., with a mating block installed to surround completely the seed with acrylic, (b) no scatter, i.e., with the mating block omitted, and (c) with only a gold plaque (1.5 mm thick, 18 × 12 mm chord length) installed above the seed. Corrected to water phantom and for the inhomogeneities of the TLDs themselves, the measured dose with the gold plaque in place, relative to that with full scatter, varied from 1.02 ± 0.03 at 2 mm to 0.90 ± 0.03 at 18 mm distance from the seed. For no backscatter, the same ratio was consistently lower by a few percent, varying from 0.98 ± 0.03 to 0.86 ± 0.03 over the range of distances.

In contrast to the above results, HARNETT and THOMSON (1988) found that the gold backing used in their foil design had no effect on the dose in WTI (a water substitute material) at distances of 3–10 mm along the central axis from the seed plane of a simulated plaque (six 6702 ^{125}I seeds arranged on the periphery of a 10 mm diameter circle). Their measurements were performed with TLDs in the form of 7 LiF disks 4.5 mm in diameter and 0.8 mm thick.

Further contrasting results were obtained by WU et al. (1988), who used 1 mm LiF cubes in thermoluminescent dosimetry along the transverse axis of a 6711 ^{125}I seed in solid water phantom, with actual water providing backscattering from the (upper) side of the seed away from the TLD measurement points. The exposures were conducted at one distance at a time, with and without a gold shield (1.6 × 2.6 × 0.1 cm) between the seed and the backscattering water. Ratios of the dose measured with the shield in place to the dose without the shield ranged from 1.065 ± 0.032 at 1 mm distance to 0.997 ± 0.005 at 10 mm distance. The authors suggest that fluorescent x-rays generated in the gold shield may account for the observed dose enhancement near the source.

A more extensive set of measurements was undertaken by CYGLER et al. (1990) in an effort to find reasons for the disparities among the data mentioned above. They observed the response of a silicon diode in a water tank to a 6702 ^{125}I seed taped to the outside surface of the tank in the region of a mylar window 0.1 mm thick. The diode-sensitive volume was 2.5 mm in diameter, 0.06 mm thick, and 0.5 ± 0.2 mm behind the front face, which permitted measure-ments as close as 1.0 ± 0.3 mm to the center of the seed. Data were obtained to 30 mm on the seed's transverse axis under backscattering conditions which included (a) air only, (b) water, in the form of a plastic bag filled with water held against the tank wall over the seed, (c) a gold sheet 110 × 60 × 0.1 mm, and (d) a silver disk 25 mm in diameter and 0.25 mm thick. In the distance range 1–30 mm, the ratio of diode response (for a given backing) to that with the water backing varied roughly from 1.0 to 0.90 for the air backing, 1.09 to 0.90 for the gold backing, and 1.26 to 1.05 for the silver backing. The strong enhancement with the silver backing (with which K-shell flurorescence is possible from ^{125}I photons) suggests that the smaller enhancement seen with gold backing was also due to fluorescent x-rays, in this case 10 keV L-shell x-rays. A comparison of these results with those of other investigators is shown in Fig. 26.6. The authors conclude that clinical calculations for ^{125}I seeds in gold plaques should include a 10% reduction in dose for distances greater than 10 mm and that there is fluorescent x-ray enhancement of dose very close to the source.

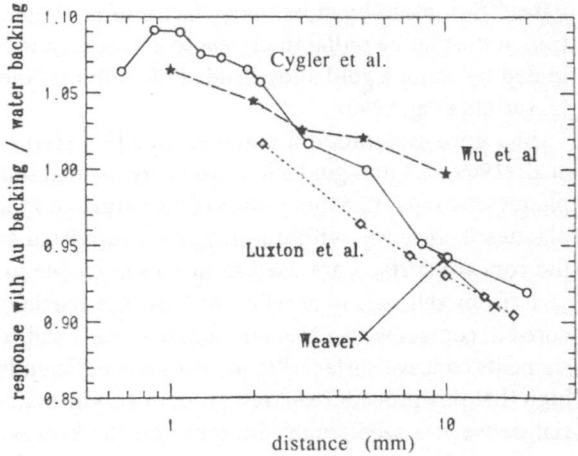

Fig. 26.6. Comparison of various experimental results for the ratio of the dose from an ^{125}I seed with a gold backing to that with a water backing. All measurements were made with TLD except those of CYGLER et al. (1990), who used a silicon diode. (Redrawn from CYGLER et al. 1990)

26.5
Treatment Planning and Evaluation

Planning ^{60}Co plaque applications, as originally conceived (INNES 1962), required choosing a plaque diameter equal to or greater than the tumor base diameter and consulting a depth dose table (appropriately decayed to reflect the current strength of the source) to determine treatment time as the quotient of prescribed dose and dose rate at tumor apex. Then, if the tumor height were indeed two-thirds the source diameter, the intersection of the treatment isodose contour with the inner scleral surface would provide a margin around the tumor base ranging from 2 mm wide for the (CKA 1) 5 mm plaque to 6 mm wide for the (CKA 4) 15 mm plaque. Except for the CKA 1 plaque, these margins are probably in excess of those needed to accommodate placement uncertainty and/ or possible extension of disease.

Seed plaques allow greater flexibility in tailoring the source loading to the needs of the individual patient and, for ^{125}I seeds, the lip (or rim) of the metal plaque, together with the less isotropic dose distribution from source elements, may result in scleral treatment dose margins that are smaller by 1–2 mm for the larger tumors than those seen with ^{60}Co plaques. The degree to which the source distribution may be customized, of course, depends on the number of seeds used and thus (for a given total strength) on the individual seed strength. Some investigators have indicated a preference for a closer spacing of seeds having smaller individual strengths, in order to reduce either the total seed cost (PACKER et al. 1987) or the dose levels in the immediate vicinity of seeds (LUXTON et al.

1988a). A policy of fewer, higher-strength seeds not only affords greater placement flexibility but also simplifies loading and dose calculations; it does, however, make it more imperative to take anisotropy into account in the dose calculation (SCHELL et al. 1989).

Planning an ophthalmic plaque of ^{125}I seeds requires first the ophthalmologist's estimate of tumor height (apex to outside of sclera) and maximum base dimension. In addition, the desired dose rate at the apex must be known; for melanoma, it is typically 100 Gy in 1 week, or 0.595 Gy/h. If a circular plaque is to be used, its diameter is selected to be larger than the maximum base diameter by a standard margin, e.g., 4 mm, and isodose rate contours are plotted for a symmetric arrangement of uniform strength seeds. The required seed strength is determined by multiplying the ratio of the apex dose rate desired to that calculated, by the strength used for the calculation, and increasing the result by an appropriate factor to allow for decay during treatment.

The development of treatment planning computer programs that permit dose assessment at a number of intraocular points has taken place after the widespread acceptance of ^{125}I plaques as an alternative to ^{60}Co applicators (GOITEIN and MILLER 1983; KEPKA et al. 1988; LING et al. 1989). For the most part, these programs do not require direct localization of the plaque on the eye, but rather assume that the plaque is centered over the tumor during treatment. The dimensions and relative positions of both tumor and pertinent eye features are derived initially from pretreatment information supplied by the ophthalmologist, i.e., both A-scan and B-scan ultrasound data, a fundus diagram based on examination by indirect ophthalmoscopy and wide-angle fundus photography, and, in some cases, CT images.

A planning program developed mainly (but not exclusively) for the protocol and plaque design of the COMS has been reported by ASTRAHAN et al. (1990). For plaque files containing the seed-carrier-insert slot coordinates and other parameters of standard COMS plaques, loading is specified (after seed type and strength have been selected) simply by "clicking" the mouse either to add a seed to an empty slot or to remove a seed from a full slot. Custom plaque designs are created by manipulating peripheral points spaced initially at 15° intervals. Plaque position on the eye may be specified interactively, "dragging" its center to a desired location, or by electing automatic centering on the tumor. The eye is displayed on the screen in a solid-surface projection, scaled from dimensional data entered by the user, or (during animated rotations) as a wireframe outline. Dose distributions are calculated as described by LUXTON et al. (1988a) and displayed as isodose surfaces, tabulations in a plane, or dose values at individual points. Attenuation of primary (unscattered) photons by a COMS plaque lip is taken into account, if desired, by applying the appropriate attenuation factor (zero for ^{125}I) if a straight line from the dose calculation point to a source point passes through the plaque; the authors point out that the (neglected) scattering contribution to the penumbra region is unknown. A representative isodose display is shown in Fig. 26.7. Comparisons of different loading patterns (e.g., uniform vs peripheral) are facilitated by dose-volume histogram calculations as well as by the versatility in dose distribution display.

The use of magnetic resonance imaging both in plaque localization for planning and in verification of placement for dose calculation has been described by HOUDEK et al. (1989). For planning, continuous 3 mm thick cuts suffice to define the extent of the tumor and its position in the globe. In postimplant scans with a loaded (6711 ^{125}I seeds) plaque in place, the plaque image is hypointense and the plaque position in relation to the tumor is clearly discerned.

26.6
Discussion

For a given configuration of source material, the dose distribution from a ^{60}Co ophthalmic applicator is not

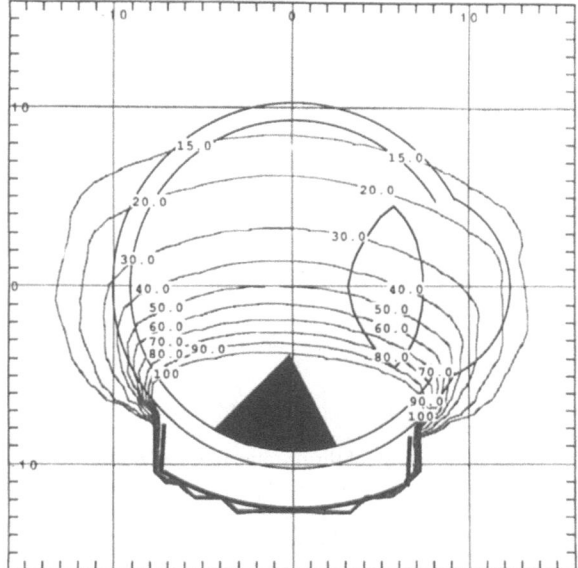

Fig. 26.7. Isodose contours generated by the specialized treatment planning program described by ASTRAHAN et al. (1990), showing the attenuation of ^{125}I seed primary photons by the lip of the 14 mm COMS eye plaque (see Fig. 26.5) with all but the three center positions loaded. For a uniform seed strength of 2.95 mCi, a 100 Gy dose is delivered to the tumor apex at 5 mm from the inner sclera in about 7 days

significantly (<5%) different from the dose distribution for other "high energy" photon applicators such as ^{192}Ir (LUXTON et al. 1988a). Comparisons of interest between ^{125}I and ^{60}Co, for a given dose to a tumor apex at, say, 5 mm from the surface of the plaque concern (a) the relative doses delivered to the adjacent sclera, and (b) the relative doses delivered to the opposite side of the eye. With respect to the first question, it has been shown that the maximum scleral dose (relative to apex dose), although dependent on the spatial distribution of source strength, depends very little on whether the sources are ^{125}I or one of the high energy photon types (LUXTON et al. 1988a).

The issue of dose to the opposite side involves, as well, the question of whether the comparison is made under full scattering conditions (approximated by anterior or equatorial plaque position) or minimal scattering conditions (posterior plaque position). For point sources at the back of a simulated eye in head phantom, Monte Carlo calculations (see Fig. 26.8) have indicated that the dose diminution from lack of full scattering material anteriorly is 10% at the surface for both ^{60}Co and ^{125}I but that the effect persists in some measure all the way back to the source for ^{60}Co and only about 1 cm back in the case of ^{125}I (CHIU-TSAO et al. 1986). For dose normalization at 5 mm from the source, these point source data suggest

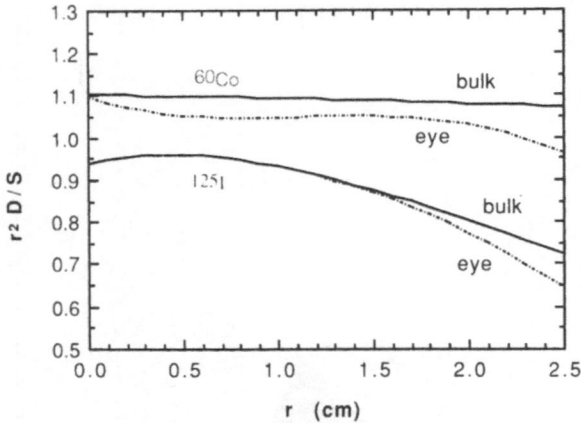

Fig. 26.8. Comparison of the product of dose (D) and distance squared per unit air kerma strength (S) as a function of the distance (r) from point sources of ^{60}Co and ^{125}I in full phantom (*bulk*) and in head phantom (*eye*) at the back of a simulated eye. (Redrawn from CHIU-TSAO et al. 1986)

that ^{125}I, relative to ^{60}Co, reduces dose to the opposite side of the eye by a factor of 0.74–0.78 (for low and high scattering conditions on the eye side of the plaque, respectively). The same comparison, involving an ^{125}I plaque of 12 Model 6711 seeds and a CKA 4 ^{60}Co applicator, results in a reduction factor of about 0.69 (LUXTON et al. 1988a), in close agreement with the single-seed estimate for the 6711 in Sect. 26.2.

As we have seen, the use of few seeds rather than many in a ^{125}I plaque involves considerations of flexibility and convenience on the one hand and concerns about scleral dose hot spots on the other. Since the maximum dose to the sclera depends on many other plaque design factors as well, a comparison of few versus many seeds can be made most readily at arbitrarily fixed distances d_s of seed center to sclera and d_a of seed center to apex. In an idealization of scleral/apex dose ratios, one can approximate the many-seed case by a uniform distribution of source strength within a circle of radius R and the few-seed case by a single seed in the center of the circle plus a "background-contributing" uniform distribution outside the single seed's smaller-area circle of radius R, such that the number of seeds, n, is equal to R^2/R_1^2. Densely packed seeds, each seed occupying an area of 3.6 mm^2, would fill an approximate circle of radius $R = (3.6\, n/\pi)^{1/2}$, and the estimate of scieral/apex dose ratio is given by

$$\frac{D_{\text{sclera}}}{D_{\text{apex}}} = \frac{\ln\left(1 + \dfrac{3.6n}{\pi d_s^2}\right)}{\ln\left(1 + \dfrac{3.6n}{\pi d_a^2}\right)}. \tag{26.1}$$

For loosely packed seeds in a circle of radius R, an individual seed at the center may be considered to occupy a circle of radius $R_1 = (R^2/n)^{1/2}$. The dose at the nearest scleral point, i.e., along the plaque axis, is delivered partly by the continuous-source region outside R_1, representing all the other seeds, and partly by this seed, for which the contribution is diminished by a factor f_s representing the extended source effect appropriate for the particular distance d_s. For this model, the scleral/apex dose ratio is

$$\frac{D_{\text{sclera}}}{D_{\text{apex}}} = \frac{\ln\left(\dfrac{1 + \dfrac{R^2}{d_s^2}}{1 + \dfrac{R^2}{nd_s^2}}\right) + f_s \dfrac{R^2}{nd_s^2}}{\ln\left(1 + \dfrac{R^2}{d_a^2}\right)} \tag{26.2}$$

The above expressions have been evaluated (see Table 26.3) for a range of numbers of seeds at $d_s = 1$ mm, representative of the plaque design in which the seeds themselves may touch the sclera, and $d_s = 2$ mm, which approximates more closely the COMS plaque design; the table includes ratios representing both small tumors ($d_a = 5$ mm) and large tumors ($d_a = 10$ mm). It is apparent from these results that for a given total source area and when compared to ten seeds loosely packed, dense packing affords a substantial reduction in relative sceral dose for $d_s = 1$ mm but only a moderate reduction for $d_s = 2$ mm. The higher values of maximum scleral dose for fewer seeds are, of course, associated with smaller high-dose areas.

Of the dose perturbations by a gold plaque, as seen in Fig. 26.6, enhancement near the plaque by fluorescent x-rays would appear to have a deleterious effect on the scleral/apex dose ratio, and diminution beyond 1 cm by scattered photon absorption may be seen as a beneficial reduction of the ratio of opposite-side dose to apex dose. As CYGLER et al. (1990) have pointed out, however, a seed carrier insert may absorb the 10 keV fluorescent photons and account for our failure to observe any gold-related enhancement with the COMS plaque, which has a silicone insert (CHIU-TSAO et al. 1988). The lesson to be learned from the disparate data on perturbations by the gold backing is that any correction to be applied should be based on measurements (or, perhaps, on Monte Carlo calculations) performed for the plaque design actually used clinically.

Several ^{125}I plaque designs (EARLE et al. 1987; LUXTON et al. 1988a; KAROLIS et al. 1989, 1990; SCHELL et al. 1989) involve "trenches" or "troughs" to define candidate locations for the seeds relative to

Table 26.3. Ratio of maximum scleral dose to tumor apex dose for densely packed vs loosely packed ^{125}I seeds in idealized plaque geometry (see text)

Seed packing	Seeds n	R (mm)	R_1 (mm)	$d_a = 5$mm		$d_a = 10$mm	
				$d_s = 2$mm $f_s = 0.85$	$d_s = 1$mm $f_s = 0.67$	$d_s = 2$mm $f_s = 0.85$	$d_s = 1$mm $f_s = 0.67$
Dense	20	4.8	–	2.9	4.9	9.2	15.4
	40	6.8	–	2.4	3.7	6.7	10.2
	60	8.3	–	2.2	3.2	5.5	8.1
Loose	4	4.0	2.0	3.6	7.9	11.9	26.3
	7	–	1.5	3.3	6.4	11.1	21.4
	10	–	1.3	3.3	6.0	10.9	19.9
	4	10.0	5.0	4.1	11.3	9.5	26.1
	7	–	3.8	3.0	7.1	6.9	16.5
	10	–	3.2	2.6	5.5	6.0	12.9

one another, thus permitting a relatively straightforward approach to optimization if seed strength is chosen large enough that strategically selected slots can remain empty. The extent to which radiation field shaping by this method might be useful has not yet been fully explored. If the number of "unique" candidate locations is sufficiently small (e.g., uniformly spaced slots in concentric circles) the possibility also arises of more accurate dosimetry' since it should then be feasible to provide for each such location a separate, measurement-based lookup table that would take into account the effect of plaque metal on the dose distribution from a seed in that particular position.

If the seed troughs are inset in the metal itself (LUXTON et al. 1988a) or even in a partially absorbing seed-carrier insert (e.g., as in the COMS plaque), the possibility also exists of useful collimation of ^{125}I photons; this possibility was recognized by SEALY et al. (1980), and edge collimation by the plaque rim is an integral feature of the design described by HARNETT and THOMSON (1988), in which all the seeds are located on the periphery. Any sparing of normal tissue by collimation, of course, increases the need for accurate plaque placement to avoid underdosing the tumor. If imaging techniques are to be used for effective verification of plaque placement, they must have greater accuracy than the placement procedure itself, and it is encouraging to note progress in this direction (HOUDEK et al. 1989). Methods being explored to permit reducing the radiation dose to normal eye tissue include combining plaque therapy with another treatment modality, such as hyperthermia (FINGER et al. 1985; COLEMAN et al. 1986; ASTRAHAN et al. 1988; FINGER et al. 1989).

References

Astrahan M, Liggett P, Petrovich Z, Luxton G (1988) A 500 kHz localized current field hyperthermia system for use with ophthalmic plaque radiotherapy. Recent Results Cancer Res 107:93–98

Astrahan MA, Luxton G, Gabor J, Kampp TD, Liggett PE, Sapozink MD, Petrovich Z (1990) An interactive treatment planning system for ophthalmic plaque radiotherapy. Int J Radiat Oncol Biol Phys 18:679–687

Beddoe AH (1972) Exposure distributions from ^{60}Co ophthalmic applicator. Br J Radiol 45:157

Beddoe AH (1975) Isoexposure curves for ^{60}Co ophthalmic applicators. Australas Radiol 19:145–151

Casebow MP (1971) The calculation and measurement of exposure distributions from ^{60}Co ophthalmic applicators. Br J Radiol 44:618–624

Chan B, Rotman M, Randall GJ (1972) Computerized dosimetry of ^{60}Co ophthalmic applicators. Radiology 103:705–707

Chiu-Tsao ST, O'Brien K, Sanna R et al. (1986) Monte Carlo dosimetry for ^{125}I and ^{60}Co in eye plaque therapy. Med Phys 13:678–682

Chiu-Tsao ST, Anderson LL, Stabile L (1988) TLD dosimetry for ^{125}I eye plaque. Phys Med Biol 33 [Suppl 1]:128

Chiu-Tsao ST, Anderson LL, O'Brien K, Sanna R (1990) Dose rate determination for ^{125}I seeds. Med Phys 17: 815–825

Coleman DJ, Lizzi FL, Burgess SEP et al. (1986) Ultrasonic hyperthermia and radiation in the management of intraocular malignant melanoma. Am J Ophthalmol 101:635–642

Cygler J, Szanto J, Soubra M, Rogers DWO (1990) Effects of gold and silver backings on the dose rate around an ^{125}I seed. Med Phys 17:172–178

Earle J, Kline RW, Robertson DM (1987) Selection of iodine ^{125} for the collaborative ocular melanoma study. Arch Ophthalmol 105:763–764

Fairchild RG (1984) New radiotherapeutic techniques in nuclear ophthalmology. Sem Nucl Med 14:35–45

Finger PT, Packer S, Svitra PP, Paglione RW, Anderson LL, Kim JH, Jacobiec FA (1985) Thermoradiotherapy for intraocular tumors. Arch Ophthalmol 103:1574–1578

Finger PT, Packer S, Paglione RW, Gatz JF, Ho TK, Bosworth JL (1989) Thermoradiotherapy of choroidal melanoma: clinical experience. Ophthalmology 96:1384–1388

Goitein M, Miller T (1983) Planning proton therapy of the eye. Med Phys 10:275–283

Harnett AN, Thomson ES (1988) An iodine-125 plaque for radiotherapy of the eye: manufacture and dosimetric considerations. Br J Radiol 61:835–838

Houdek PV, Schwade JG, Medina AJ et al. (1989) MR technique for localization and verification procedures in episcieral brachytherapy. Int J Radiat Oncol Biol Phys 17:1111–1114

Innes G (1962) The application of physics in the treatment of ocular neoplasms. In: Boniuk M (ed) Ocular and adnexal tumors. CV Mosby, St. Louis, p 142

Interstitial Collaborative Working Group: Anderson LL, Nath R, Weaver KA et al. (1990) Interstitial brachytherapy: physical, biological and clinical considerations. Raven, New York

Karolis C, Amies C, Frost RB, Billson FA (1989) The development of a thin stainless steel eye plaque to treat tumours of the eye up to 15 mm in diameter. Australas Phys Eng Sci Med 12:172–177

Karolis C, Frost RB, Billson FA (1990) A thin I-125 seed eye plaque to treat intraocular tumors using an acrylic insert to precisely position the sources. Int J Radiat Oncol Biol Phys 18:1209–1213

Kepka AG, Johnson PM, Kline RW (1988) The generalized geometry of eye plaque therapy. Med Phys 15:375–379

Ling CC, Chen GT, Boothby JW et al. (1989) Computer assisted treatment planning for ^{125}I ophthalmic plaque radiotherapy. Int J Radiat Oncol Biol Phys 17:405–410

Luxton G, Astrahan MA, Liggett PE, Neblett DL, Cohen DM, Petrovich Z (1988a) Dosimetric calculations and measurements of gold plaque ophthalmic irradiators using iridium-192 and iodine-125 seeds. Int J Radiat Oncol Biol Phys 15:167–176

Luxton G, Astrahan MA, Petrovich Z (1988b) Backscatter measurements from a single seed of ^{125}I for ophthalmic plaque dosimetry. Med Phys 15:397–400

Magnus L (1967) Tiefendosisberechnung für die ^{60}Co-Augenapplikatoren CKA 1–4 (nach Stallard). Strahlentherapie 132:379–386

Magnus L, Göbbeler T, Strötges (1968) Tiefendosisberechnung für die ^{60}Co-Augenapplikatoren CKA 5–11 (nach Stallard). Strahlentherapie 136:170–177

Magnus L, Göbbeler T, Rassow J, Strötges W (1969) Isodosenmessungen an den Kobalt-60-Augenapplikatoren (nach Stallard): die Isodosen bei den Applikatoren CKA 1–4. Radiol Clin Biol 38:213–227

Meisberger LJ, Keller RJ, Shalek RJ (1968) The effective attenuation in water of the gamma rays of gold 198, iridium 192, cesium 137, radium 226, and cobalt 60. Radiology 90:953–957

Packer S, Rotman M (1980) Radiotherapy of choroidal melanoma with iodine-125. Ophthalmology 87:582–590

Packer S, Fairchild RG, Salanitro P (1987) New techniques for iodine-125 radiotherapy of intraocular tumors. Ann Ophthalmol 19:26–30

Rassow J, Strüter H-D, Magnus L, Göbbeler T (1970) Isodosenmessungen an den Kobalt-60-Augenapplikatoren (nach Stallard): allgemeine Berechnung der Tiefendosis für kreisförmige Flächenaktivitäten und die Messung der Isodosen für die Applikatoren CKA 8–11. Radiol Clin Biol 39:32–46

Schell MC, Weaver KA, Phillips TL, Char DH, Quivey JM, Barnett C, Ling CC (1989) Design of iodine-125 eye plaques for radiation therapy. Endocurietherapy/ Hyperthermia Oncology 5:83–90

Sealy R, le Roux PLM, Rapley F, Hering E, Shackleton D, Sevel D (1976) The treatment of ophthalmic tumours with low-energy sources. Br J Radiol 49:551–554

Sealy R, Buret E, Cleminshaw H et al. (1980) Progress in the use of iodine therapy for tumours of the eye. Br J Radiol 53:1052–1060

Task Group 32: Nath R, Anderson L, Jones D, Ling C, Loevinger R, Williamson J, Hanson W (1987) Specification of brachytherapy source strength, AAPM Report No. 21. American Institute of Physics, New York

Weaver KA (1986) The dosimetry of ^{125}I seed eye plaques. Med Phys 13:78–83

Wu A, Sternick ES, Muise DJ (1988) Effect of gold shielding on the dosimetry of an ^{125}I seed at close range. Med Phys 15:627–628

27 Radiosensitivity of Ocular and Orbital Structures

R. H. Sagerman and W. E. Alberti

CONTENTS

27.1
Introduction

Radiation therapy carries a love-fear relationship in the management of tumors of the eye and orbit, and of nearby structures. Its ability to control tumors with preservation of function and cosmesis earns respect, but it is feared because it is known to have caused disfigurement, loss of vision, and structural necrosis. The authors believe that judicious use of irradiation as primary treatment or as an adjunctive therapy is well established and that many strong contrary opinions are based upon adverse clinical circumstances and an unfortunate choice of technical radiotherapeutic variables. Clinically, it is important to know the nature of the tumor, its location and extent in relation to the sensitive structures of the eye, the tumor control results and adverse consequences of each applicable therapy, and what best suits an individual patient's circumstances. Technically, the radiation oncologist must choose between several varieties of external beam therapy and

brachytherapy, the dose-time fractionation scheme, the size and direction of fields, and the use of shielding blocks, always balancing the best tumor control probability against the risk of radiation damage while knowing what treatment is available to salvage a tumor recurrence or a complication. While many situations are readily dealt with by simple techniques because dose, volume, and results are well known and can be handled in most departments, others require techniques and knowledge that can best be found in the interdisciplinary setting where radiation oncology works closely with ophthalmologic oncology and large numbers of patients are seen. When critical structures must be exposed to tolerance doses, the radiation oncologist must ensure the use of a meticulous technique.

It was not long after Roentgen's discovery of X-rays before Chalupecky (1897) published his study of its effects upon the structures of the eye. The high radiosensitivity of the eye was documented by Birch-Hirschfeld (1904), and Amman (1906) was the first to report a radiation-induced cataract. Rubin and Casarett (1968) summarized what was known of ocular radiation effects.

In this chapter we will deal primarily with radiation effects upon the retina and optic nerve. Radiation effects upon the skin are noted in Chap. 17, effects upon the lids, conjunctiva, tear formation, and the lens in Chap. 21, and effects upon the lacrimal gland and the nasolacrimal duct in Chap. 20. An overview and scoring system developed at a Late Effects Consensus Conference have been presented in Gordon et al. (1995) and Pavy et al (1995). Gordon and O'Brien (1999) provide a current review of the management of radiation effects on the eye and orbit.

R.H. Sagerman, MD, FACR
Department of Radiation Oncology, SUNY Upstate Medical University, 750E. Adams Street, Syracuse, NY 13210, USA
W.E. Alberti, MD
Universität Hamburg, Martinistrasse 52, 20246 Hamburg, Germany

27.2
Skin, Eyelids

The skin of the eyelids reacts to irradiation as does skin in other parts of the body, with erythema followed by dry and moist desquamation and, depending upon the interplay between high doses and tumor extent, leading to necrosis or the inability of the tissues to cover a defect. Erythema can be observed early – usually within 2–4 weeks – with a single dose of 6 Gy of 200–250 kVp X-rays. This is usually transient and disappears rapidly. Moist desquamation is more common with doses of 50–60 Gy in 5–6 weeks and is often seen during the course of daily irradiation of basal cell or squamous cell carcinoma of the eyelids, especially when the lesion has broken the skin. Healing is usually visible 2–4 weeks later, leaving no significant scar or deformity unless there has been sufficient damage secondary to the tumor or previous surgery. However, concomitant infection, trauma, or a high dose of irradiation delivered in a few fractions may lead to severe scarring, resulting in ectropion or entropion. With doses of 45 Gy/15 fractions/3 weeks to 60 Gy/30 fractions/6 weeks, the lid looks best, and may appear virtually normal, 6–12 months after treatment. Slowly progressive changes leading to thinning of the skin, hypopigmentation, and fine telangiectasis then appear and progress for 1–2 years before stabilizing. These changes are particularly important at the lateral and medial canthi and in the mid-portion of the lower lid. Although obstruction of the nasolacrimal duct leading to epiphora has often been attributed to irradiation, we have seen this only when the duct has been damaged by tumor or surgery; we have not seen obstruction develop with conventionally fractionated irradiation at 60–65 Gy even when treating postoperatively and after tumor recurrence (see Fig. 20.2a, b, Chap. 20).

Epilation may be incomplete or complete, depending on the dose-fractionation scheme, and this can occur with as little as 10 Gy in a few days; permanent epilation begins at 30 Gy/3 weeks and is more likely at conventionally fractionated doses exceeding 50 Gy. Radiation therapy has been used to produce epilation in patients with trichiasis to prevent corneal ulceration and perforation.

The tarsus, the fibrocartilaginous plate in the lids, is quite resistant to irradiation but can undergo late atrophy and thinning with doses above 40–50 Gy; this does not usually lead to any functional impairment.

Very little is known about the radiation tolerance of the meibomian glands. Experiments with rabbit eyelids show that the meibomian glands tolerate a dose of approximately 40 Gy (13 fractions/4 weeks)(HARTZLER et al. 1984).

27.3
Lacrimal Apparatus

The lacrimal apparatus secretes and drains lubricating fluid for the eye. The secretory mechanism consists of the lacrimal gland, several auxiliary glands, and mucin-secreting goblet cells. The major lacrimal gland lies lateral to and above the outer canthus; the accessory glands are located predominantly in the superior-lateral conjunctiva and in the upper lid. The majority of patients tolerate doses in the range of 30–40 Gy to the entire orbit without developing severe symptoms of a dry eye (PARSONS et al. 1983, 1991; SAGERMAN 1975; WHARAM et al. 1987). Atrophy of the gland is said to develop with a single dose of 20 Gy, but is more likely to occur with doses of 50–60 Gy in 5–6 weeks (MERRIAM et al. 1972). Tolerance to irradiation and avoidance of the dry eye syndrome are heavily dependent upon the interplay between the lacrimal gland secretions and those of the auxiliary glands, and the dose to the cornea; the latter is discussed fully in Chap. 21. In this regard, it is critical to estimate the dose to the various structures. For example, we have delivered 60 Gy at 2 Gy/fraction to the lacrimal gland through an unblocked anterior field in the treatment of orbital rhabdomyosarcoma; a dry eye syndrome developed only in those eyes in which the lids had been sutured together, the tumor/chemosis was so great as to close the eye, or trauma or infection injured the eye months later. Approximately 90% of these children have maintained satisfactory tear production for more than 10 years. We believe this is due to the preservation of (a) the majority of function in the accessory lacrimal glands (estimated dose <30 Gy/6 weeks) and (b) the integrity of the corneal epithelium (SAGERMAN 1975). In contrast, PARSONS et al. (1994c) report 0% severe dry eye syndrome at ≤30 Gy but 100% at ≥57 Gy.

27.4
Conjunctiva, Cornea, and Lens

Detailed anatomic and physiologic appraisals of the effects of irradiation upon these structures are presented by INGRAHAM et al. (Chap. 21) and WEISS et al. (Chap. 20) elsewhere in this volume.

Cataracts are an unwanted complication of irradiation, but development of a dose–effect curve is complicated by the gathering of data with many variables, including dose and fractionation, and underlying disease processes. The dose quoted is often only an estimate of the lens dose derived from isodose curves or even in vitro study, but the dose to the lens may vary widely when lateral fields or anterior fields with blocks are employed. Even a half-field-blocked lateral field may deliver a widely varying dose, depending upon the accuracy of repetitive set-ups, as millimeter variations in position cause large variations in dose. SCHIPPER et al. (1985) delivered 45 Gy to the retina in 15 fractions in 5 weeks to 73 eyes in 39 children with retinoblastoma. Cataracts developed in 18 eyes, but only when more than 1 mm of the posterior lens was in the field; 8 Gy/15 fractions was the lowest cataractogenic dose. Lens dose variation and treatment techniques for retinoblastoma are reviewed in Chap. 24.

Homogeneous doses in a narrow dose range at the low end of the scale (~8–15 Gy) are incidentally delivered to the lenses with total-body irradiation in single or fractionated doses, albeit with graft-vs-host disease and chemotherapy as confounding factors. DEEG et al. (1984) gave 10 Gy (single fraction) to 105 patients or 12–15.75 Gy (usually as 2–2.25 Gy/day in 6–7 days) to 76 patients with hematologic cancers, while 96 patients with anaplastic anemia were conditioned with chemotherapy only. Eighty-six patients developed cataracts, with incidences of 80%, 18% and 19% for the three groups, respectively (P<0.00005). All cataracts were diagnosed between 300 and 2,000 days after transplantation. However, there were only 2 surviving patients without a cataract 6 years after transplantation.

27.5
Sclera

The sclera is resistant to radiation, and no radiation damage is clinically evident after external beam irradiation even at high doses (>60 Gy). Damage can occur after plaque brachytherapy, in which the sclera necessarily receives a very high dose. Thinning of the sclera is often observed in the high dose area under the plaque. LOMMATZSCH (1968, 1973) reported necrosis of the sclera in animal experiments and in patients with 1,000 Gy from radioactive plaques (see Chap. 18). TARR and CONSTABLE (1981) described scleral ulceration after single doses of 20–52 Gy from a strontium-90 plaque. Deep scleral ulceration should be repaired with a scleral patch graft to prevent endophthalmitis.

27.6
Iris

A transient, early iritis can develop with a single dose of 10–20 Gy, but more severe, persistent, anterior uveitis has been observed with doses of 30–40 Gy in 3–4 days and 70–80 Gy in 6–8 weeks (ELLSWORTH 1969; MERRIAM et al. 1972). The coexistence of a corneal ulcer exacerbates and prolongs this process, and healing may take several months. A varying degree of iris atrophy and rubeosis iritis can occur.

Localized atrophy has been observed following beta radiation with surface doses >170–250 Gy (TARR and CONSTABLE 1981).

27.7
Retina

The human retina and choroid are intrinsically linked anatomically and physiologically, and radiation retinopathy usually develops because of their combined injury. The retina used to be considered radioresistant because of the paucity of clinical problems directly attributable to its being radiated, but more recent studies have shown it to be far more sensitive than previously thought. STALLARD (1933) was the first to describe radiation retinopathy after radium seed implantation for hemangioma and retinoblastoma. Since then, an extensive literature has developed describing retinopathy after external beam photon therapy, proton beam therapy, and plaque brachytherapy (BEDFORD et al. 1970; BROWN et al. 1982; CHAR et al. 1977; DE SCHRYVER et al. 1971; FOERSTER et al. 1986; GRAGOUDAS et al. 1987; HAYREH 1970; KINYOUN et al. 1984; LOMMATZSCH 1983; McFAUL and BEDFORD 1970; MERRIAM et al. 1972; NOBLE and KUPERSMITH 1984; PARSONS et al. 1983, 1994b; PERRERS-TAYLOR et al. 1965; SHUKOVSKY and FLETCHER 1972; STALLARD 1966; THOMPSON et al. 1983; WARA et al. 1979). Clinical changes have been observed in the retina at 35 Gy/3 weeks in a few eyes and DUKE-ELDER (1972) reported vesicle formation at 30 Gy. However, a significant increase in complications occurs with doses >50 Gy/5 weeks (ELLSWORTH 1969; PARSONS et al. 1983; REESE et al. 1949).

Chronic radiation damage to the retina is usually the result of disruption of the vascular supply and is primarily a form of micro-occlusive vascular disease. The vascular lumens are narrowed or obliterated, and abnormal vascular permeability occurs; secondary ischemia leads to infarction of the nerve fibers. Exudates and hemorrhage then occur, which may be associated with occluded ghost vessels, vascular sheathing, microaneurysm formation and increased tortuosity (retinotelangiectasis), and gross new vessel formation. Major occlusions of both the arterial and the venous circulation may occur. Typically, radiation retinopathy occurs between 6 months and 3 years after treatment, but can occur much later (BROWN et al. 1982; MERRIAM et al. 1972).

Retinal edema, reflecting early capillary incompetence, is an early clinical finding in radiation retinopathy; later it is characterized by capillary microaneurysms, intraretinal hemorrhage, cotton-wool spots, hard exudates, and telangiectatic and sheathed vessels. Vitreous hemorrhage, retinal detachment, and optic nerve atrophy occur in later stages. Histologic studies have shown thickening and hyaline degeneration of the vessel walls with areas of occlusion. In trypsin-digest preparations, E.R. Simpson and D. Payne (personal communication, 1992) have shown no preferential loss of mural cells or endothelial cells in the capillary walls of early radiation microangiopathy; both cell types were affected equally. New vessel formation occurs in an attempt to improve the local circulation. Further bleeding can occur from these thin-walled, endothelial tubes. After the initial reaction subsides, changes in the retinal pigment epithelium may be seen. This usually occurs in the area of the tumor as a diffuse salt-and-pepper pigmentation, or in an area of retinal detachment.

The neural elements of the retina are more radioresistant than the vasculature. Histologic examination reveals atrophy and thinning of the retina and a loss of ganglion cells. These neural changes are thought to be secondary to vascular occlusions, similar to the changes observed in eyes with severe arteriolar sclerosis and hypertension (EGBERT et al. 1980; HOWARD 1966). Advanced radiation retinopathy is illustrated in Fig. 27.1 and the fluorescein angiographic appearance is shown in Figs. 27.2.

The threshold dose of retinal damage is not known. PERRERS-TAYLOR et al. (1965) reported significant late retinal and choroidal changes in 20% of patients following a dose of 15–21 Gy/8 days to 27–31 Gy/24 days; the latent period was 2–4 years, but there was no reported loss of visual acuity. Histology from peripheral regions of the retina in eyes receiving 60 Gy in 20 fractions of 3 Gy each (D beam technique) revealed disruption and fragmentation of the elastic core of Bruch's membrane in the choroid, despite relative preservation of capillary wall integrity (E.R. Simpson and D. Payne, personal communica-

tion, 1992). SHUKOVSKY and FLETCHER (1972) reported retinal damage in 7 of 15 patients 2–3.5 years after 68 Gy in 6 weeks. CHAN and SHUKOVOSKY (1976) reported that 2 of 22 patients with 60 Gy developed blindness. MERRIAM et al. (1972) suggested that 30–35 Gy would produce retinal changes (threshold dose) and that retinopathy would develop within a few months in 85% of eyes radiated to 70–80 Gy. ELLSWORTH (1977) reported vascular changes after 35 Gy, 45 Gy, and 80 Gy in 10%, 66%, and almost 100% of retinoblastoma patients, respectively; the fraction size was 300–350 cGy, given thrice weekly, for most of these children. SCHIPPER et al. (1985) reported three patients with retinal vascular necrosis following 45 Gy/15 fractions/5 weeks, although all three eyes retained useful vision.

PARSONS et al. (1983) reviewed the ocular effects in 74 patients whose eye(s) were irradiated for tumors near (nasopharynx, sinuses) or involving the orbit. ^{60}Co Irradiation or 2 MeV was employed, and 70 of the patients were treated through anterior and lateral fields. Loss of vision due to retinal injury occurred in 1 of 14 patients receiving ≤50 Gy, and Cytoxan was given in that case. In contrast, only 1 patient (treated with a split course technique) of 13 escaped visual loss when the dose was >50–70 Gy. Concomitant chemotherapy and large fraction size were judged to be important factors increasing the risk of injury. PARSONS et al. (1983) concluded that the risk of retinal damage increased rapidly between 50 and 60 Gy and recommended using 170- to 200-cGy fractions.

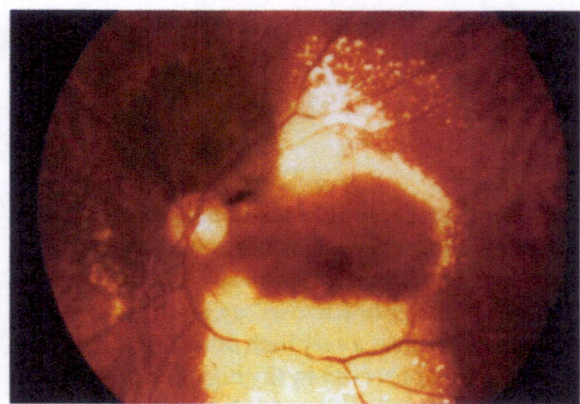

Fig. 27.1. Advanced radiation chorioretinopathy following ^{60}Co teletherapy for choroidal melanoma. Widespread vasculopathy, exudation, optic pallor and retinal hemorrhage have involved tumor and nontumor retina. The treated choroidal melanoma is superior to the optic nerve. (Photograph courtesy of E. Rand Simpson, MD, FRCS and David Payne, MD, FRCP of the Ontario Cancer Institute/Princess Margaret Hospital, Toronto, Ontario, Canada)

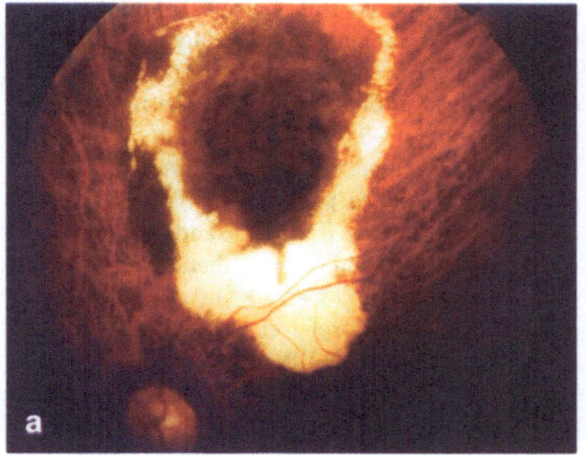
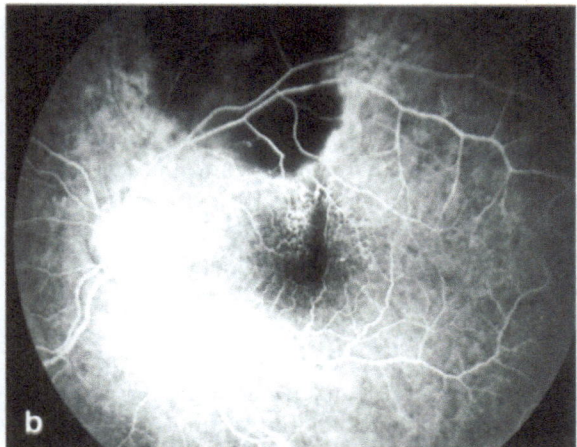
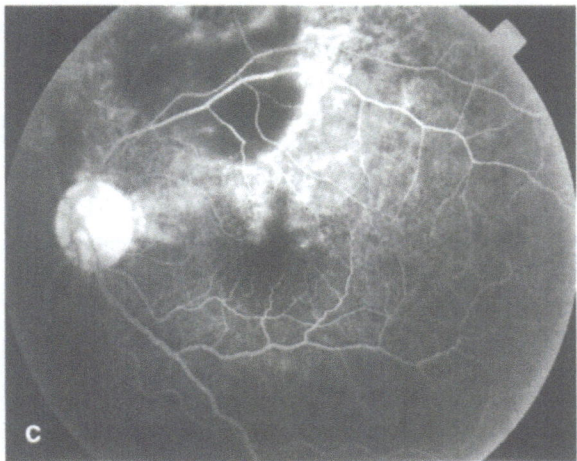

Fig. 27.2a–c. Radiation retinopathy 3 years after proton beam treatment of a choroidal melanoma. **a** The tumor is now surrounded by exudate (yellow-white). Telangiectatic capillaries from radiation (**b**) are leaking dye in the late pictures (**c**). Corrected visual acuity is still 20/20. (Photograph courtesy of William V. Delaney Jr. MD)

WARA et al. (1979) analyzed visual loss in eight patients in whom an inherently normal eye was irradiated because of tumor extension from the sinuses (4), nasopharynx (3), or pituitary gland. Four were treated with a 4-MV linear accelerator, two with ^{60}Co, and one with a 1-MeV X-ray unit. Retinopathy developed after a latent period of 1–4 years in seven patients and at 7 years in the eighth. The retinal doses were estimated to be 4,644, 4,860, 4,860, 4,923, 5,500, 5,789, 6,480, and ~7,975 cGy; fraction size never exceeded 200 cGy, and was ≤180 cGy in all four eyes receiving ≤50 Gy.

The importance of fraction size has been emphasized by many authors, all concluding that fractionated doses ≤2 Gy are safer than those ≥2.5 Gy (ARISTIZ-ABAL et al. 1977; HARRIS and LEVENE 1976; NAKISSA et al. 1983; WARA et al. 1979). Severe retinopathy developed in four patients, and three became blind, receiving 40 Gy/10 fractions/2 weeks through opposed lateral fields for Graves' ophthalmopathy (KINYOUN et al. 1984). PARKER and WITHERS' (1988) analysis of this

event indicated that the daily midplane, central axis dose was >350 cGy and the total dose >35 Gy.

PARSONS et al (1994b) reviewed 68 retinae in 64 patients receiving fractionated external beam irradiation followed for 3–26 years (mean 9 years). Twenty-seven eyes in 26 patients had developed retinopathy resulting in visual acuity of ≤20/200 by a mean of 2.8 years after the treatment. Retinopathy did not occur below 45 Gy but rose with higher doses. There was a trend to increased risk at lower doses when chemotherapy was given.

Radiation retinopathy should be viewed as a spectrum of evolving disease in the injured eye. Reports should specify the nature of the observed injury (since rates may be over- or undervalued relative to the criteria chosen) to facilitate comparisons between series and are quite sensitive to the time of follow-up. E.R. Simpson and D. Payne (personal communication, 1992) retrospectively analyzed 79 cases consisting of two patient groups with posterior segment choroidal melanoma treated with ^{60}Co teletherapy at the Ontario Cancer Institute/Princess Margaret Hospital. These patients were generally selected for treatment if plaque therapy was considered impractical or as an alternative to enucleation. The dose was changed from 60 Gy to 75 Gy in the early 1980s because of an impression that retinopathy was not eliminated at the lower dose. All patients were treated with 3 Gy fractions and 42 received 60 Gy in 20 fractions while 30 received 75 Gy in 25 fractions. Median follow-up for patients receiving 60 Gy was 58 months and for patients receiving 75 Gy, 45 months.

The development of nonproliferative (without neovascularization) and proliferative (presence of neovascularization) radiation retinopathy was observed with reference to time of onset and degree of involvement for both patient groups.

Nonproliferative retinopathy (presence of one or all of edema, microinfarcts, hemorrhages, microaneurysms, telangiectasia, pigmentation alteration, and vascular sheathing) developed as early as 4 months and was present in 50% of cases by 10 months. All patients (79 eyes) developed nonproliferative retinopathy by 25 months. There appeared to be no significant difference between the two treatment groups in time of onset or degree of involvement.

Proliferative radiation retinopathy (presence of neovascularization) did not become apparent before 12 months and was present in only 50% of patients by 48 months (75 Gy) and 65 months (60 Gy). There was no statistical difference between the patient groups for these comparisons.

No promising or successful treatment exists for this progressive, severe retinopathy. Spontaneous resolution of microvascular abnormalities was described in a 34-year-old patient with bilateral radiation retinopathy (NOBLE and KUPERSMITH 1984). CHAUDHURI et al. (1981) reported a fairly successful treatment of optic disc and retinal new vessel formation with argon laser photocoagulation for 4 months. PARSONS et al. (1983) suggested laser photocoagulation and noted that neovascularization had not progressed after 3 years in some patients. THOMPSON et al. (1983) reported a successful control of recurring vitreous hemorrhage.

Experimental studies in rabbits and minipigs provide an important avenue to study radiation effects (ALBERTI and EL-HIFNAWI 1993a, b). Animal experimental studies have noted no changes in visual cells with a dose of 30 Gy (HAMBERGER et al. 1964; POPPE 1942). BROWN et al. (1955) reported edema, hemorrhages, microaneurysms, and papilledema within 2.5 h after an exposure of 100 Gy, followed by destruction of all the rods in 8 h, in monkeys. At doses of 40–60 Gy,

definite effects on the rods were seen. Rod degeneration resulted in monkeys after a single dose of 60 Gy (CIBIS and BROWN 1955). BIEGEL (1955) reported slight changes in the periphery of the retina with a single dose of 36–45 Gy in rabbits. CIBIS et al. (1955) reported that a single dose of 20 Gy produced rod degeneration in guinea pigs and rabbits and a single dose of 55 Gy destroyed the rods and produced atrophy of the choroid and retina. Others reporting these changes include BAILEY and NOELL (1958), BURNST (1958, 1969), CAVAGGIONI et al. (1969), DEVI et al. (1968), DONEGAN (1956), NEWELL et al. (1960), and WINTER et al. (1958). It appears that the threshold for impairment of rod function in the experimental animal is ~20 Gy single dose and that extensive destruction results after a single dose of 50 Gy. The cones and ganglion cells are much more resistant.

The addition of chemotherapy may potentiate radiation retinopathy (BROWN et al. 1982; CHAN and SHUKOVSKY 1976; FISHMAN et al. 1976; WILSON et al. 1987). These authors reported that the latent period for developing injury was shorter, and the risk of developing blindness was higher, in eyes treated with chemotherapy than in eyes receiving only radiation therapy. GRIFFIN and GARNICK (1981) reviewed the toxicity of many chemotherapy agents upon the various structures of the eye when it was given alone or in conjunction with irradiation. Ocular toxicity from chemotherapeutic agents was also reviewed by VIZEL and OSTER (1982), and the importance of drug-radiation interactions has been noted by ALBERTI (1991), PARSONS et al. (1991), and WILSON et al. (1987), among many.

R.M. ELLSWORTH (personal communication, 1992) has followed patients irradiated for orbital rhabdomyosarcoma for many years. Although they were treated by irradiation alone (1961–1975) or by irradiation plus chemotherapy (1975–present) and were not randomized, and the radiation dose was ~60 Gy in the earlier group and 40–55 Gy in the latter, he estimated the incidence of retinopathy at ~30% vs ~50% in the two groups, respectively.

27.8
Optic Nerve

Radiation optic neuropathy occasionally develops in patients receiving high-dose irradiation for tumors of the optic nerve, the base of the skull, the pituitary gland, and the paranasal sinuses and has been reported by many authors (FITZGERALD et al. 1981;

GOLDSMITH et al. 1992; NAKISSA et al. 1983; PARSONS et al. 1983; ROSS et al. 1973; SHUKOVSKY and FLETCHER 1972). It may be secondary to vascular damage and retinal degeneration (McFAUL and BEDFORD 1970; MERRIAM et al. 1972). Following irradiation of pituitary gland tumors, optic neuropathy may actually be part of a more extensive delayed radionecrosis of the central nervous system (ARISTIZABAL et al. 1977; GHATAK and WHITE 1969; HARRIS and LEVENE 1976; MARTINS et al. 1977). It can follow local plaque therapy as well as photon and proton beam external beam irradiation of intraocular malignancies (BROWN et al. 1982; CASSADY et al. 1969; EGBERT et al. 1978, 1980; ELLSWORTH 1977; FOERSTER et al. 1986; GRAGOUDAS et al. 1987; LOMMATZSCH 1983; McFAUL 1977; SHIELDS et al. 1982).

The clinical characteristics of radiation optic neuropathy have been described by BROWN et al. (1982), KLINE et al. (1985), and SHUKOVSKY and FLETCHER (1972). PARSONS et al. (1983) divided radiation optic neuropathy into two different clinical groups: (a) injury at the distal end of the nerve with ischemic neuropathy, disc pallor, edema, and hemorrhages around or on the disc and (b) more proximal injury producing retrobulbar optic neuropathy without detectable changes around the disc. The onset of optic neuropathy may be heralded by the appearance of a "wreath-like" circinate peripapillary retinal edema, which may last for several months (Fig. 27.3). This classical appearance of radiation-induced optic neuropathy usually subsides, only to reveal a rapidly progressive optic atrophy (E.R. Simp-

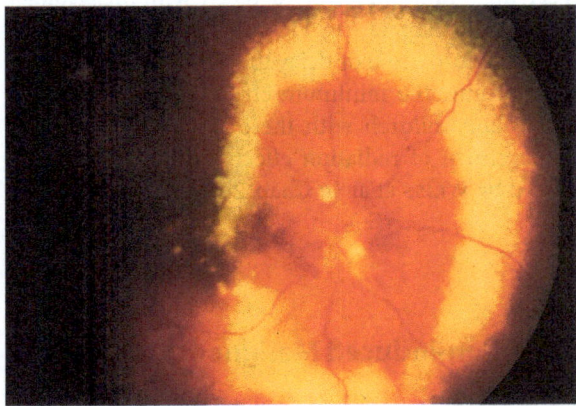

Fig. 27.3. Radiation induced optic neuropathy. Circinate peripapillary exudation in a wreathlike distribution can be characteristic following radiation insult and may disappear as optic atrophy develops. (Photograph courtesy of E. Rand Simpson, MD, FRCS and David Payne, MD, FRCP of the Ontario Cancer Institute/Princess Margaret Hospital, Toronto, Ontario, Canada)

son and D. Payne, personal communication, 1992). Usually, there is a sudden loss of vision; the loss may be complete or partial, and may progress over months. Residual vision may be limited to light perception or finger counting. When both eyes are radiated, visual loss may be unilateral or bilateral, and bilateral loss may occur discordantly. Acute signs due to disc swelling include hard peripapillary exudates, hemorrhages, and subretinal fluid, and BROWN et al. (1982) observed "cotton-wool spots." Nerve head ischemia, with areas of nonperfusion, are seen with fluorescein angiography.

Careful ophthalmic and radiographic examinations are necessary to establish a diagnosis of optic neuropathy. KLINE et al.'s (1985) diagnostic criteria include acute loss of vision, visual field defects indicating optic nerve or chiasmal dysfunction, absence of optic disc edema, onset of symptoms within 3 years of radiation therapy, and no evidence of visual pathway compression with high-resolution computed tomography. Optic neuropathy may develop from several months to several years after irradiation, with a peak at 1–1.5 years. BROWN et al. (1982) report a shorter latency after brachytherapy (12 months, range 3–22 months) than after external beam irradiation (19 months, range 5–36 months), but this may be related to the higher doses with brachytherapy (mean 125 Gy vs 55 Gy, range 35–230 Gy vs 36–70 Gy). KLINE et al. (1985) reported four cases of optic neuropathy with doses from 46 to 63.4 Gy in 25–47 fractions and suggested that optic nerve deficits secondary to tumor or surgery present prior to the initiation of radiotherapy may contribute to an increased risk of injury.

Radiation optic neuropathy rarely occurs following the usually employed courses of radiotherapy for retinoblastoma (~35 Gy/3 weeks or 45 Gy/5 weeks, thrice weekly; 46–60 Gy/4.5–6 weeks, 5 fractions per week, 1.8–2 Gy per fraction). EGBERT et al. (1978) reported one patient with optic neuropathy who had received 47 Gy/5 weeks and then 49 Gy/5 weeks for recurrence. ABRAMSON et al. (1982) reported a 24% incidence of enucleation due to radiation complications after second and third courses of external beam irradiation for retinoblastoma with total doses ranging from 54–165 Gy. Because there were so many treatment failures resulting in death or enucleation, they suggested that there would have been a much higher incidence of radiation complications had more eyes been salvaged. HARRIS and LEVENE (1976) noted 18% optic nerve damage with 2.5 Gy or more per fraction, as against no damage with 2 Gy per day (total dose of 42–70 Gy). The incidence of optic nerve damage was 12.5% with 2 Gy fractions, in contrast to 22% with 2.5-Gy fractions for patients with pituitary adenoma treated with 50 Gy (ARISTIZABAL et al. 1977).

PARSONS et al. (1983) observed 12 eyes with optic neuropathy in 74 patients treated for tumors around the eye. Among long-term survivors, 8% (2 of 24) developed optic neuropathy after receiving 60–73 Gy, 1.65–1.9 Gy per fraction. However, with similar total doses, 41% (7 of 17) showed such damage when the fraction size was >1.95 Gy. In a subsequent paper, PARSONS et al. (1994a) evaluated the effect of total dose and fraction size in 215 optic nerves in 131 patients. Anterior ischemic neuropathy developed in 5 at a median time of 30 months and retrobulbar neuropathy in 12 nerves at a median of 28 months. No injuries were seen in 106 nerves treated with total doses of less than 59 Gy. At a dose of 60 Gy or greater, neuropathy developed in 11% when the fraction size was less than 1.9 Gy but was 47% when it was ≥1.9 Gy. KINYOUN et al. (1984) observed optic neuropathy in four patients (three blind) treated for Graves' ophthalmopathy with a daily dose of ~3.5 Gy × 10 fractions.

The incidence of optic nerve injury after plaque therapy is related to the dose, the dose rate, the energy of the nuclide, and the size and location of the tumor. LOMMATZSCH (1983) noted 9.8% complete optic atrophy and 3.8% partial atrophy following ^{106}Ru/^{106}Rh plaque radiotherapy for posterior uveal malignant melanoma with a follow-up of 6–16 years. FOERSTER et al. (1986) reported complication rates of 1.1% from beta irradiation (^{106}Ru/^{106}Rh), but could not find a relation between the dose and complications. Among 128 patients with proton beam-irradiated uveal melanomas, only two developed optic neuropathy and one optic papillopathy (GRAGOUDAS et al. 1987; see also MUNZENRIDER, Chap. 6). FISHMAN et al. (1976) and MARGILETH et al. (1977) observed optic nerve atrophy in patients receiving prophylactic cranial irradiation (24 Gy) along with systemic and intrathecal chemotherapy.

GOLDSMITH et al. (1992) reviewed 49 patients irradiated at the University of California, San Francisco after biopsy or partial resection of a meningioma adjacent to the anterior visual pathway and followed for more than 18 months. The mean dose was 53.59 Gy (range 45.0–59.4 Gy) delivered in 30 fractions (range 28–45 fractions) over 44 days (range 35–61 days). Only 1 patient developed optic neuropathy, 23 months after receiving 54 Gy in 30 fractions of 1.8 Gy over 43 days with 6-MV photons through a three-field technique (vertex + opposing lateral fields). Prior

surgery and embolization may have been contributing factors. The authors analyzed 35 cases of radiation optic neuropathy and developed a formula for the optic ret:

$$\text{Optic ret} = DN^{-0.53}$$

They found only three cases of radiation optic neuropathy in patients receiving ≤890 optic ret and recommend this as the ceiling for a low risk. Interestingly, the linear quadratic model did not provide a satisfactory discriminant. Recent experience with radiosurgery provides support for this dose. TISHLER et al. (1993) reported no visual complications (0/35 patients) at a dose of less than 800 cGy, but 24% (4/17 patients) 2h3n when any part of the optic apparatus received more than 800cGy.

27.9
Orbit (See also Chap. 20)

Orbital and facial deformity remains a well-known late effect of irradiation in children treated for retinoblastoma and rhabdomyosarcoma (ELLSWORTH 1969; REESE et al. 1949; SAGERMAN et al. 1969, 1972). Although the "saddle-nose deformity" produced by the contralateral oblique nasal field and kilovoltage irradiation is no longer seen, the hypoplasia of bony and soft tissue produced by megavoltage beams remains and the deformity is worse the younger the child when treated and the greater the fraction size and total dose. The deformity is relatively minimal for children aged 5–8 years receiving a tumor dose of 40–60 Gy with megavoltage beams (see Chap. 11, Fig. 11.2g). Continuing efforts are being made to avoid or delay the use of irradiation and to determine the minimum effective dose for infants and young children with these cancers. The current management of radiation effects on the orbit is discussed by WEISS et al. in Chap. 20.

27.10
Radiation-induced Malignancies

Second malignancies occur most frequently in children with bilateral or hereditable retinoblastoma; this subject is reviewed in Chap. 11. They are not common after irradiation for other tumors of the eye or when the orbit is irradiated incidentally, even with doses far greater than those used for retinoblastoma (SCHLIENGER et al. 1985).

ABRAMSON et al. (1984) reported that 98% of patients who developed a second malignancy had the bilateral form of retinoblastoma. The majority of these second cancers are osteosarcomas, and other mesenchymal sarcomas form the second largest group. Epithelial malignancies are not common (SAGERMAN et al. 1969; WHITE et al. 1985). The common denominator for these cancers is the genetic abnormality at chromosome 13 band q14. This explains the approximately equal incidence of second cancers in children with bilateral retinoblastoma who have never received irradiation and in those who have. However, about two-thirds of second tumors occur in the radiation field for those irradiated, while two-thirds appear in tissues which would not have been in the field in those not irradiated (ABRAMSON et al. 1984).

SAGERMAN et al. (1969) described a dose–response relationship for radiation-induced neoplasia in these children, and ALBERTI and HALAMA (1987) reported a higher risk in children receiving 55 Gy than in those receiving a lower dose. ABRAMSON et al. (1984) concluded that the risk was not increased among those receiving a second or third course of irradiation. Although it seems likely that higher doses increase the risk, the complex interplay of dose, fractionation, and the very limited survival of these children with second malignancies precludes establishment of a threshold dose, if there is one. The problem is compounded further by the increased incidence of second malignancies in those treated with both irradiation and chemotherapy (DRAPER et al. 1986; SCHIPPER and ALBERTI 1985) and by latency; the cumulative risk at 10, 20, and 30 years was 6%, 19%, and 38% vs 20%, 50%, and 90% in the reports of ABRAMSON et al. (1984) and SMITH et al. (1989), respectively. The cumulative risk has also been reported as 4.3% at 12 years and 8.4% at 18 years (DRAPER et al. 1986), 11% at 35 years (KOTEN et al. 1988), and 48% in those receiving more than 55 Gy vs 5% for those receiving a lower dose of orthovoltage irradiation at 16 years (ALBERTI and HALAMA 1987). Careful lifetime follow-up of these patients is imperative if these second cancers are to be discovered as early as possible so that aggressive multimodal treatment may improve their prognosis (SMITH et al. 1989; SMITH and DONALDSON 1991).

In contrast to retinoblastoma, children with orbital rhabdomyosarcoma, who also have a long survival, have demonstrated a low incidence of second cancers despite consistently applied high doses of 60 Gy (SAGERMAN et al. 1968) and chemoradiotherapy at 40–55 Gy (WHARAM et al. 1987). To the best of our knowledge, none of the 33 children reported by SAGERMAN et al. (1972, 1974) has developed a second cancer (R.M. ELLSWORTH, personal communication, 1992). HEYN et al. (1986) reported only one second malignancy (acute myeloblastic leukemia) among the 50 children treated according to the Intergroup Rhabdomyosarcoma Study I protocol. Only one of the 53 cases of postradiation soft tissue sarcoma reported from the Armed Forces Institute of Pathology occurred in a child with rhabdomyosarcoma (a 12-year-old girl treated for rhabdomyosarcoma of the infraorbital ridge) (LASKIN et al. 1988).

Although the risk of developing second cancers will be relatively small, larger numbers of these children will have to be followed for many more years before the true incidence can be established. A recent analysis of 1,770 patients, with 9,877 patient-years of follow-up, identified 22 cases of second malignancy occurring at a mean of 7 years after treatment for rhabdomyosarcoma (HEYN et al. 1993). The orbit was the primary site in 5 patients, and all had received chemoradiotherapy. The second malignancies were acute nonlymphoblastic leukemia (2), leiomyosarcoma (1), adrenocortical cancer (1), and fibrillary astrocytoma (1). The patient with leiomyosarcoma was alive with a very short follow-up; the other 4 died about 2 years after developing the second cancer. HEYN et al. (1993) attribute the preponderance of second malignancies in children with head and neck primary rhabdomyosarcoma (15 of 22) to the better tumor control and longer survival in these patients than in those with other primary sites, and to the use of combined modality treatment rather than chemotherapy or radiotherapy alone.

27.11
Summary

The development of dose vs risk of damage relations for the various structures of the eye is complicated by patient factors (e.g. hypertension, diabetes), the effects of the disease process or tumor being treated, the segment of the eye involved, the size and location of the tumor, and many technical radiotherapeutic factors, not all of which have been precisely specified in many reports. Perhaps the "purest" data are derived when the eye is intrinsically normal and irradiated incidentally, but great efforts are made to exclude or block all or part of the eye whenever possible so that precise dosimetric reconstruction is difficult. In addition, radiation changes in the posterior chamber may not be visible because of changes anteriorly, or they may not bother the patient and will therefore not be investigated. The development of the dry eye syndrome is complicated by the interplay of tear production by the lacrimal gland, which we routinely try to spare, but the quantity and quality of the tears from the auxiliary glands, in conjunction with the minimization of keratoconjunctivitis with megavoltage irradiation through an anterior field with the lids open, may be even more important. Animal studies are important and useful, but more carefully reported data from human experience are necessary to refine our knowledge and produce useful guidelines.

References

Abramson DH, Ellsworth RM, Rosenblatt M, Tretter P, Jereb B, Kitchin D (1982) Retreatment of retinoblastoma with external beam irradiation. Arch Ophthalmol 100:1257–1260

Abramson DH, Ellsworth RM, Kitchin D, Tung G (1984) Second nonocular tumors in retinoblastoma survivors. Are they radiation-induced? Ophthalmology 91:1351–1355

Alberti W (1991) Effects of radiation on the eye and ocular adnexa. In: Scherer E, Streffer C, Trott KR (eds) Radiopathology of organs and tissues. Springer, Berlin Heidelberg New York, pp 269–282

Alberti W, El-Sayed El Hifnawi (1993a) Morphologic changes after iodine-125 plaque irradiation of rabbit eyes. In: Alberti W, Sagerman R (eds) Radiotherapy of intraocular and orbital tumors. Springer, Berlin Heidelberg New York, pp 387–398

Alberti W, El Hifnawi ES (1993b) Morphologic changes after fractionated external beam therapy of minipig eyes. In: Alberti W, Sagerman R (eds) Radiotherapy of intraocular and orbital tumors. Springer, Berlin Heidelberg New York, pp 399–414

Alberti W, Halama J (1987) Tumoren des Auges und der Orbita. In: Scherer E (ed) Strahlentherapie, Radiologische Onkologie. Springer, Berlin Heidelberg New York, pp 412–467

Amman E (1906) Zur Wirkung der Roentgenstrahlen auf das menschliche Auge. Korrespondenz-Blatt fur Schweizer Ärzte 15

Aristizabal S, Caldwell WL, Avita J (1977) The relationship of time–dose fractionation factors of complications in the treatment of pituitary tumors by irradiation. Int J Radiat Oncol Biol Phys 2:667–673

Bailey NA, Noell WK (1958) Relative biological effectiveness of various qualities of radiation as determined by electroretinograms. Radiat Res 9:459

Bedford MA, Bedotto C, McFaul PA (1970) Radiation retinopathy after the application of a cobalt plaque. Br J Ophthalmol 54:505–509

Biegel AC (1955) Experimental ocular effects of high-voltage radiation from betatron. AMA Arch Ophthalmol 54:392–406

Birch-Hirschfeld A (1904) Die Wirkung der Roentgen und Radiumstrahlen auf das Auge. Graefes Arch Ophthalmol 59:229–310

Brown CD, Cibis PA, Pickering JE (1955) Radiation studies on the monkey eyes. Arch Ophthalmol 59: 249–256

Brown GC, Shields JA, Sanborn G, Augsburger JJ, Savino PJ, Schatz NJ (1982) Radiation optic neuropathy. Ophthalmology 89:1489–1493

Burnst VV (1958) The roentgen sensitivity of various protions of the eye of young axolotl (Siredon mexicanum). AJR Am J Roentgenol 80:1015–1030

Burnst VV (1969) Destructive effects of strictly local irradiation of the eye of the adult axolotl (Siredon mexicanum). Radiat Res 39:26–35

Cassady JR, Sagerman RH, Tretter P, Ellsworth RM (1969) Radiation therapy in retinoblastoma. Radiology 93:405–409

Cavaggioni A, Peracchia G, Rosati G (1969) Electrical activity of the ganglion cells in irradiated retinas. Radiat Res 39:658–704

Chalupecky H (1897) Über die Wirkung der Röntgenstrahlen auf das Auge und die Haut. Zentralbl Augenheilkd 21:234

Chan RC, Shukovsky LJ (1976) Effects of irradiation on the eye. Radiology 120:673–675

Char DH, Lonn LI, Margolis LW (1977) Complications of cobalt plaque therapy of choroidal melanomas. Am J Ophthalmol 84:536–540

Chaudhuri PR, Austin DJ, Rosenthal AR (1981) Treatment of radiation retinopathy. Br J Ophthalmol 65:623–625

Cibis PA, Brown DVL (1955) Retinal changes following ionizing radiation. Am J Ophthalmol 40:84–88

Cibis PA, Noell WK, Eichel B (1955) Ocular effects produced by high intensity x-radiation. Arch Ophthalmol 53:651–663

Deeg HG, Flournoy N, Sullivan KM et al (1984) Cataracts after total body irradiation and marrow transplantation: a sparing effect of dose fractionation. Int J Radiat Oncol Biol Phys 10:957–964

DeSchryver A, Wachmeister L, Baryd I (1971) Ophthalmologic observations on long-term survivors after radiotherapy for nasopharyngeal tumours. Acta Radiol 10:193–209

Devi SK, Riley EF, Burns CA (1968) Electron-retinographic responses of the rabbit after x-irradiation. Invest Ophthalmol 7:219–226

Donegan J (1956) Ocular effects of body ^{60}Co irradiation. Am J Ophthalmol 42:309

Draper GJ, Sanders BM, Kingston JE (1986) Second primary neoplasms in patients with retinoblastoma. Br J Cancer 53:661–671

Duke-Elder S (1972) System of ophthalmology, vol 14, part 2: Injuries: nonmechanical injuries. Mosby, St Louis, pp 985–999

Egbert PR, Donaldson SS, Moazed K, Rosenthal AR (1978) Visual results and ocular complications following radiotherapy for retinoblastoma. Arch Ophthalmol 96:1826–1830

Egbert PR, Fajardo LF, Donaldson S, Moazed K (1980) Posterior ocular abnormalities after irradiation for retinoblastoma: a histopathological study. Br J Ophthalmol 64:660–665

Ellsworth RM (1969) The practical management of retinoblastoma. Trans Am Ophthalmol Soc 67:462–534

Ellsworth RM (1977) Retinoblastoma. Mod Probl Ophthalmol 18:94–199

Fishman ML, Bean SC, Cogan DG (1976) Optic atrophy following prophylactic chemotherapy and cranial radiation for acute lymphocytic leukemia. Am J Ophthalmol 82:571–575

Fitzpatrick CR, Enoch JM, Temme LA (1981) Radiation therapy in and about the retina, optic nerve and anterior visual pathway; psychophysical assessment. Arch Ophthalmol 99:611–623

Foerster MH, Bornfeld N, Schulz U, Wessing A, Meyer-Schwickerath G (1986) Complications of local beta radiation of uveal melanomas. Graefes Arch Clin Exp Ophthalmol 224:336–340

Ghatak NR, White BE (1969) Delayed radiation necrosis of the hypothalamus. Arch Neurol 21:425–430

Goldsmith BJ, Rosenthal SA, Wara WM, Larson DA (1992) Optic neuropathy after radiation therapy for subtotally and non-resected meningiomas. Radiology 195:71–76

Gordon KB, O'Brien JM (1999) Management of radiation effects on the eye and orbit. Front Radiat Ther Oncol 32:127–144

Gordon KB, Char DH, Sagerman RH (1995) Late effects of radiation on the eye and ocular adnexa. Int J Radiat Oncol Biol Phys 34:1123–1139

Gragoudas ES, Seddon JM, Egan K et al (1987) Long-term results of proton beam irradiated uvea melanomas. Ophthalmology 94:349–353

Griffin JD, Garnick MB (1981) Eye toxicity of cancer chemotherapy: a review of the literature. Cancer 48:1539–1549

Hamberger A, Rosengren BOH, Tengroth B (1964) Radiation studies on retina. Acta Ophthalmol (Copenh) 42:951–956

Harris JR, Levene MB (1976) Visual complications following irradiation for pituitary adenomas and craniopharyngiomas. Radiology 120:167–171

Hartzler J, Neldner KH, Forstot L (1984) X-ray epilation for the treatment of trichiasis. Arch Dermatol 120:620–624

Hayreh SS (1970) Post-radiation retinopathy. A fluorescence fundus angiographic study. Br J Ophthalmol 54:705–714

Heyn R, Ragab A, Raney RB et al (1986) Late effects of therapy in orbital rhabdomyosarcoma in children. A report from the Intergroup Rhabdomyosarcoma Study. Cancer 57:1738–1743

Heyn R, Haeberlen V, Newton WA, Ragab A, Raney RB, Tefft M, Wharam M, Ensign LG, Maurer HM (1993) Second malignant neoplasms in children treated for rhabdomyosarcoma. J Clin Oncol 11:262–270

Howard GM (1966) Ocular effects of radiation and photocoagulation. Arch Ophthalmol 76:7–10

Kinyoun JL, Kalina RE, Browser SA, Mills RP, Johnson RH (1984) Radiation retinopathy after orbital irradiation for Graves' ophthalmopathy. Arch Ophthalmol 102:1473–1476

Kline LB, Kim JY, Ceballos R (1985) Radiation optic neuropathy. Ophthalmology 92:1118–1126

Koten JW, der Kindren DJ, Otter WD (1988) Editorial reply. N Engl J Med 318:581–582

Laskin WB, Silverman TA, Enzinger FM (1988) Post-radiation soft tissue sarcomas. An analysis of 53 cases. Cancer 62:2330–2340

Lommatzsch P (1968) Morphologische und funktionelle Veränderungen des Kaninchenauges nach Einwirkung von Betastrahlen auf den dorsalen Bulbusabschnitt. Graefes Arch Klin Exp Ophthalmol 176:100–125

Lommatzsch P (1973) Experiences in the treatment of malignant melanoma of the choroid with ^{106}Ru/^{106}Rh beta ray applicators. Trans Ophthalmol Soc UK 93:119–132

Lommatzsch P (1983) β-Irradiation of choroidal melanoma with ^{106}Ru/^{106}Rh applicators. Arch Ophthalmol 101:713–717

Margileth DA, Poplack DG, Pizzo PA, Leventhal BG (1977) Blindness during remission in two patients with acute lymphoblastic leukemia. Cancer 39:58–61

Martins AN, Johnston JS, Henry JM (1977) Delayed radiation necrosis of the brain. J Neurosurg 47:336–345

McFaul PA (1977) Local radiotherapy in the treatment of malignant melanomas of the choroid. Trans Ophthalmol Soc UK 97:421–427

McFaul PA, Bedford MA (1970) Ocular complications after therapeutic irradiation. Br J Ophthalmol 54:237–247

Merriam GR, Szechter A, Focht EF (1972) The effects of ionizing radiations on the eye. Front Radiat Ther Oncol 6:346–385

Nakissa N, Rubin P, Strohl R, Keys H (1983) Ocular and orbital complications following radiation therapy of paranasal sinus malignancies and review of literature. Cancer 51:980–986

Newell FW, Choi O, Book NA, Harper PV, Simkus A (1960) Focal ionizing radiation of the posterior ocular segment. Am J Ophthalmol 50:1215–1225

Noble KG, Kupersmith MJ (1984) Retinal vascular remodelling in radiation retinopathy. Br J Ophthalmol 68:475–478

Parker RG, Withers HR (1988) Radiation retinopathy. JAMA 259:43

Parsons JT, Fitzgerald CR, Hood CI, Ellingwood KE, Bova FJ, Million RR (1983) The effects of irradiation on the eye and optic nerve. Int J Radiat Oncol Biol Phys 9:609–622

Parsons JT, Bova FJ, Fitzgerald Cr, Hood I, Mendenhall WM, Million RR (1991) Tolerance of visual apparatus to conventional therapeutic irradiation. In: Gutin PH, Leibel SA, Sheline GE (eds) Radiation injury to the nervous system. Raven, New York, pp 283–302

Parsons JT, Bova FJ, Fitzgerald CR, Mendenhall WM, Million RR (1994a) Radiation optic neuropathy after megavoltage external-beam irradiation: Analysis of time-dose factors. Int J Radiat Oncol Biol Phys 30:755–763

Parsons JT, Bova FJ, Fitzgerald CR, Wendenhall WM, Million RR (1994b) Radiation retinopathy after external-beam irradiation: analysis of time-dose factors. Int J Radiat Oncol Biol Phys 30:765–773

Parsons JT, Bova FJ, Fitzgerald CR, Wendenhall WM, Million RR (1994c) Severe dry-eye syndrome following external beam irradiation. Int J Radiat Oncol Biol Phys 30:775–780

Pavy JJ, Denekamp J, Letscher J, Littbrand B (1995) Late effects toxicity scoring: the SOMA scale. Radiother Oncol 35:268–270

Perrers-Taylor M, Brinkley D, Reynolds T (1965) Choriodoretinal damage as a complication of radiotherapy. Acta Radiol 3:431–440

Poppe E (1942) Experimental investigations of the effects of roentgen rays on the eye. Thesis, Oslo

Reese AB, Merriam GR, Martin HE (1949) Treatment of bilateral retinoblastoma by irradiation and surgery. Am J Ophthalmol 32:175

Ross HS, Rosenberg S, Friedman AH (1973) Delayed radiation necrosis of the optic nerve. Am J Ophthalmol 76:683–686

Rubin P, Casarett GW (1968) Organs of special sense: the eye and the ear. In: Rubin PH, Casarett GW (eds) Clinical radiation pathology. Saunders, Philadelphia, pp 662–719

Sagerman RH (1975) The role of diagnostic radiology and radiation therapy in the management of soft tissue sarcomas in children. Cancer 35:946–949

Sagerman RH, Cassady JR, Tretter P (1968) Radiation therapy for rhabdomyosarcoma of the orbit. Trans Am Acad Ophthalmol Otol 72:849–854

Sagerman RH, Cassady JR, Tretter P, Ellsworth RM (1969) Radiation induced neoplasia following external beam therapy for children with retinoblastoma. AJR Am J Roentgenol 105:529–535

Sagerman RH, Tretter P, Ellsworth RM (1972) The treatment of orbital rhabdomyosarcoma of children with primary radiation therapy. AJR Am J Roentgenol 114:31–34

Sagerman RH, Tretter P, Ellsworth RM (1974) Orbital rhabdomyosarcoma in children. Trans Am Acad Ophthalmol Otol 78:602–605

Schipper J, Alberti W (1985) Letter to the editor. Ophthalmology 92:60a–62a

Schipper J, Tan KEWP, van Peperzeel HA (1985) Treatment of retinoblastoma by precision megavoltage radiation therapy. Radiother Oncol 3:117–132

Schlienger P, Calle R, Haye C, Vilcoq JR (1985) Sarcomes osseux et tumeurs malignes de la retine. Bull Cancer 72:16–24

Shields JA, Augsburger JJ, Brady LW, Day IL (1982) Cobalt plaque therapy for posterior uveal melanomas. Ophthalmology 89:1201–1207

Shukovsky LJ, Fletcher GH (1972) Retinal and optic nerve complications in a high dose irradiation technique of ethmoid sinus and nasal cavity. Radiology 104:629–634

Smith LM, Donaldson SS (1991) Incidence and management of secondary malignancies in patients with retinoblastoma and Ewing's sarcoma. Oncology 5:135–148

Smith LM, Donaldson SS, Egbert PR, Link MP, Bagshaw MA (1989) Aggressive management of second primary tumors in survivors of hereditary retinoblastoma. Int J Radiat Oncol Biol Phys 17:499–505

Stallard HB (1933) Radiant energy as (a) a pathogenic, (b) a therapeutic agent in ophthalmic disorders. Br J Ophthalmol [Monogr Suppl] 6 (whole issue)

Stallard HB (1966) Radiotherapy for malignant melanoma of the choroid. Br J Ophthalmol 50:147–155

Tarr KH, Constable IJ (1981) Radiation damage after pterygium treatment. Aust J Ophthalmol 9:97–101

Thompson GM, Migdal CS, Whittle RJM (1983) Radiation retinopathy following treatment of posterior nasal space carcinoma. Br J Ophthalmol 67:609–614

Tishler RB, Loeffler JS, Lunsford LD, Duma C (1993) Tolerance of cranial nerves of the cavernous sinus to radiosurgery. Int J Radiat Oncol Biol Phys 27:215–221

Vizel M, Oster MW (1982) Ocular side effects of cancer chemotherapy. Cancer 49:1999–2002

Wara WM, Irvine AR, Neger RE, Howes EL, Phillips TL (1979) Radiation retinopathy. Int J Radiat Oncol Biol Phys 5:81–83

Wharam M, Beltangady M, Hays D et al (1987) Localized orbital rhabdomyosarcoma. An interim report of the Intergroup Rhabdomyosarcoma Study Committee. Ophthalmology 94:251–254

White L, Ortega JA, Ying KL (1985) Acute nonlymphocytic leukemia following multimodality therapy for retinoblastoma. Cancer 55:496–498

Wilson WB, Perez GM, Kleinschmidt-Demasters BK (1987) Sudden onset of blindness in patients treated with oral CCNU and low-dose cranial irradiation. Cancer 59:901–907

Winter FC, Reinhardt PR, Madden J (1958) Ocular effects of high intensity g-radiation in the cat. Am J Ophthalmol 46:114–122

28 Angiographic Diagnosis of Intraocular Tumors

A. Hassenstein and G. Richard

CONTENTS

28.1 Fluorescein Angiography

Fluorescein angiography (FAG) of the fundus is one of the main steps in investigation of the circulation of the retina and choroid. Fluorescent molecules are used to visualize the bloodstream. Each molecule is excited with short-wavelength light, and this is followed by the issuance of light of a longer wavelength; this phenomenon is called fluorescence. The light is not reflected, but is changed in quality. Physically, the incoming light elevates the electrons to a higher level, and the resulting energy is transmitted by a light with longer wavelength. The maximum absorption of fluorescein is at 490 nm, in the blue part of the spectrum. The issuing light has a maximum wavelength at 530 nm, in the green part of the spectrum. Most, 70–85%, of the fluorescein is attached to serum proteins, mainly albumin, in the blood. The remaining fluorescein is called "free" fluorescein. The zonulae occludentes of the retinal endothelium forms the "inner blood–retina barrier," which is not permeable to fluorescein. Any leakage of fluorescein out of the retinal vessels is pathologic.

The choroidal vessels are not permeable to fluorescein, but the choriocapillaris has multiple fenes-trations and is permeable to free fluorescein, which penetrates the intercellular part of the retinal pigment epithelium (RPE). The tight junctions of the RPE are not permeable to free fluorescein and are called the "outer blood–retina barrier." Leakage of fluorescein through the RPE is pathologic.

The injected fluorescein reaches the eye via the ophthalmic artery, following the short posterior ciliary arteries to the choroid, and through the central retinal artery to the retinal circulation. The retinal circulation follows the choroidal circulation 1 s later.

Choroidal filling is segmental, patchy, or diffuse. Choroidal fluorescence depends on the fundus pigmentation. Because of the quick filling of the choriocapillaris, delineation of the choroidal filling is not possible except in pathologic hypoperfusion of the choroid such as occurs in choroidal infarction (Elschnig spot). Late fluorescence of the optic nerve head is normal.

The dark foveal presentation is due to the lack of vessels within the foveolar avascular arcade and to the high concentration of xanthophyll in the neuroretina (Guthoff et al. 1999; Hassenstein and Richard 1998; Richard 1998; Rohrbach and Lieb 1998).

28.1.1 Technique

Serial photographs are taken with a fundus camera with a high-energetic flash and locking filter. The focus of the camera is the central 30–50°. The first picture is taken in red-free light. The first essentials for good-quality angiograms are dilated pupils and clear media. After injection of the fluorescein (5% concentration, 5 ml), pictures are taken in quick series. In the early phase, which is especially important for diagnosis, photographs are taken every second. Late photographs are taken starting 5–10 min later. Today, photographs are transferred to a computer so that digital processing for better contrast is possible, and the photographs are available immediately.

There are only minor side effects with FAG. Sometimes nausea occurs and there may be a yel-

A. Hassenstein, G. Richard
University Eye Hospital Eppendorf, Martinistrasse 52, 20251 Hamburg, Germany

lowish coloration to the skin and the urine. Allergic reactions, such as anaphylactic bronchospasm and shock, are rare.

Four phases of the circulation are described:
1. Prearterial phase: filling of the choroid, no fluorescein in the retinal circulation
2. Arterial phase: 1 s later, from beginning until complete filling of retinal arteries
3. Arteriovenous phase: complete filling of retinal arteries and laminar flow in retinal veins
4. Venous phase: complete filling of retinal veins and clearance of the retinal arteries

28.1.2
Intraocular Tumors

In cases of malignant intraocular tumors, such as choroidal melanoma, the tumor vessels always show patchy leakage because of a pathologic endothelium and endothelial fenestrations.

28.2
Indocyanine Green Angiography

Indocyanine green (ICG) angiography was developed to allow for better overall visualization of the choroidal circulation. Indocyanine is an organic substance with maximum of absorption at 805 nm and a maximum fluorescence at 835 nm, in the near infrared spectrum. It bonds even more strongly to proteins (98%) than to fluorescein (60–80%). The dye cannot penetrate the choroidal vessels because of the high attachment to the high-molecular albumin. It is now possible to visualize the choroidal vessels without the choriocapillaris; this is important in the differential diagnosis of choroidal tumors.

The main indications for ICG angiography in intraocular tumors are choroidal hemangioma, choroidal melanoma, and metastasis. ICG angiography is an additional diagnostic tool to FAG, especially in cases of primary choroidal tumors (GUTHOFF et al. 1999; RICHARD 1998; ROHRBACH and LIEB 1998). It is similar to FAG in that a modified fundus camera that allows maximum infrared transmission is used. One disadvantage of ICG angiography is the low contrast of the photographs.

Typical angiographic findings are found in benign lesions such as melanocytoma and choroidal hemangioma, and in malignant lesions such as choroidal melanoma and metastatic tumors.

28.2.1
Melanocytoma

Melanocytoma of the optic disc is a rare melanotic change that is usually seen in dark-skinned people. The pigmented lesion most often remains stable and is located in the lower half of the optic disc, but may also be prominent and cover the entire optic nerve head. Melanocytomas are considered to be a variation of the nevus. They are characterized clinically by a dark brown color and are composed histologically of round or oval cells, each with a small, round, uniform nucleus. As melanocytoma and melanoma are easily confused, it is important to remember that 50% of the melanocytomas observed occur in black-skinned races. In contrast, only 1% of melanomas are seen in these races; choroidal melanomas occur predominantly in fair, blond, or red-haired Caucasians.

Patients with melanocytoma of the optic disc do not usually have any symptoms; only occasionally does the tumor increase in size and result in secondary visual disturbances. Approximately 30% of the patients have an afferent pupillary defect (Marcus Gunn) in the affected eye. This might be due to compression of nerve fibers by melanocytes resulting in visual field defects. Neither an individual vessel network in the tumor nor leakage is present (RICHARD 1998; RICHARD et al. 1998).

28.2.2
Choroidal Hemangioma

The choroidal hemangioma is a benign lesion postulated to arise from a vascular malformation. Solitary hemangiomas typically occur in the 4th to 5th decade. Hemangiomas are classified as diffuse (often Sturge-Weber syndrome), and solitary, and microscopically as cavernous and capillary. It is very rare for them to show growth.

The solitary tumefaction is typically located at the posterior pole and is amelanotic or red to orange in color (Fig. 28.1a). There is typically an exudative serous retinal detachment surrounding the tumor, but there is no peripheral collateral retinal detachment such as is seen in choroidal melanoma. Histologically, the hemangioma consists of cavernous choroidal spaces separated by thin connective tissue septa. The leading symptom is a painless and slow visual deterioration, depending on the localization. In case of a central localization there might be worsening hyperopia.

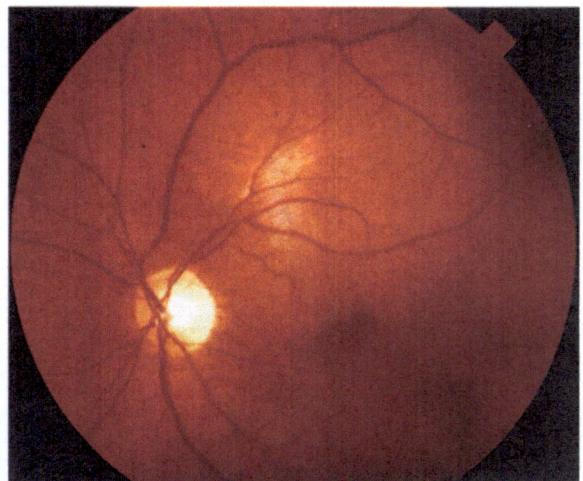

Fig. 28.1. a Biomicroscopy of an orange tumefaction superotemporal to the optic nerve head with serous retinal detachment involving the macula of the left eye (visual acuity 0.2). **b** Fluorescein angiography (FAG) of the same patient demonstrates pooling of dye in serous detachment and a patchy hyperfluorescence within the tumefaction. **c** FAG (left eye) after laser treatment shows a hypofluorescent scar superotemporal to the optic nerve head and no pooling (visual acuity 0.8)

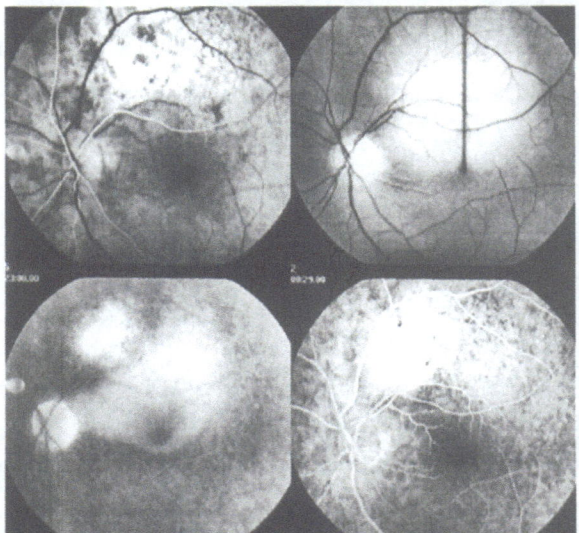

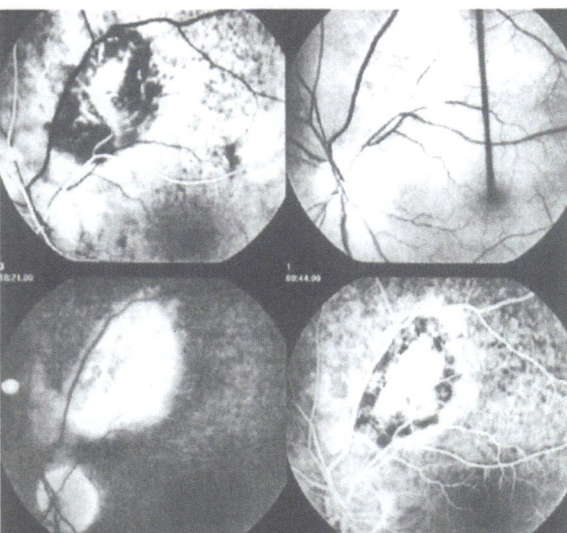

The diagnosis is made on the basis of medical history (age), symptoms, clinical appearance, FAG and ICG angiography, and high-frequency color ultrasonography.

In FAG, hemangiomas show hyperfluorescence in early phases and leakage in the late phase, but there is no pathognomonic pattern (Fig. 28.1b, c)

Treatment is only necessary in cases in which they cause symptoms, which are usually secondary to serous detachment causing visual deterioration, especially with a posterior localization. The treatment of choice is laser coagulation for small lesions and radiation for diffuse lesions. Laser coagulation produces a retinochoroidal adhesion and resolution of subretinal fluid (RICHARD 1998; RICHARD et al. 1998) (Fig. 28.1b, c). The visual acuity of the patient whose eye is shown in Fig. 28.1a–c increased from 0.2 to 0.8 after laser treatment.

Case Report. A 44-year-old patient presented with visual deterioration to 0.6 in 1 week in the right eye. Biomicroscopy showed a slightly prominent lesion close to the optic nerve head in the superonasal quadrant and an accompanying serous detachment reaching the macula (Fig. 28.2a). This detachment caused visual deterioration and worsening hyperopia. FAG revealed a patchy hyperfluorescence in the early arterial phase and fluorescein pooling in the serous retinal detachment (Fig. 28.2b). ICG angiography revealed an irregular hyperfluorescent lesion and leakage (Fig. 28.2c). High-frequency color ultrasound showed a high vascular velocity typical for hemangioma within the tumor at the posterior pole (Fig. 28.2d). Laser treatment of the right eye, starting at the edge of the tumor and continuing to the center, was performed. The visual acuity increased to 1.0 after the last laser treatment. Neither

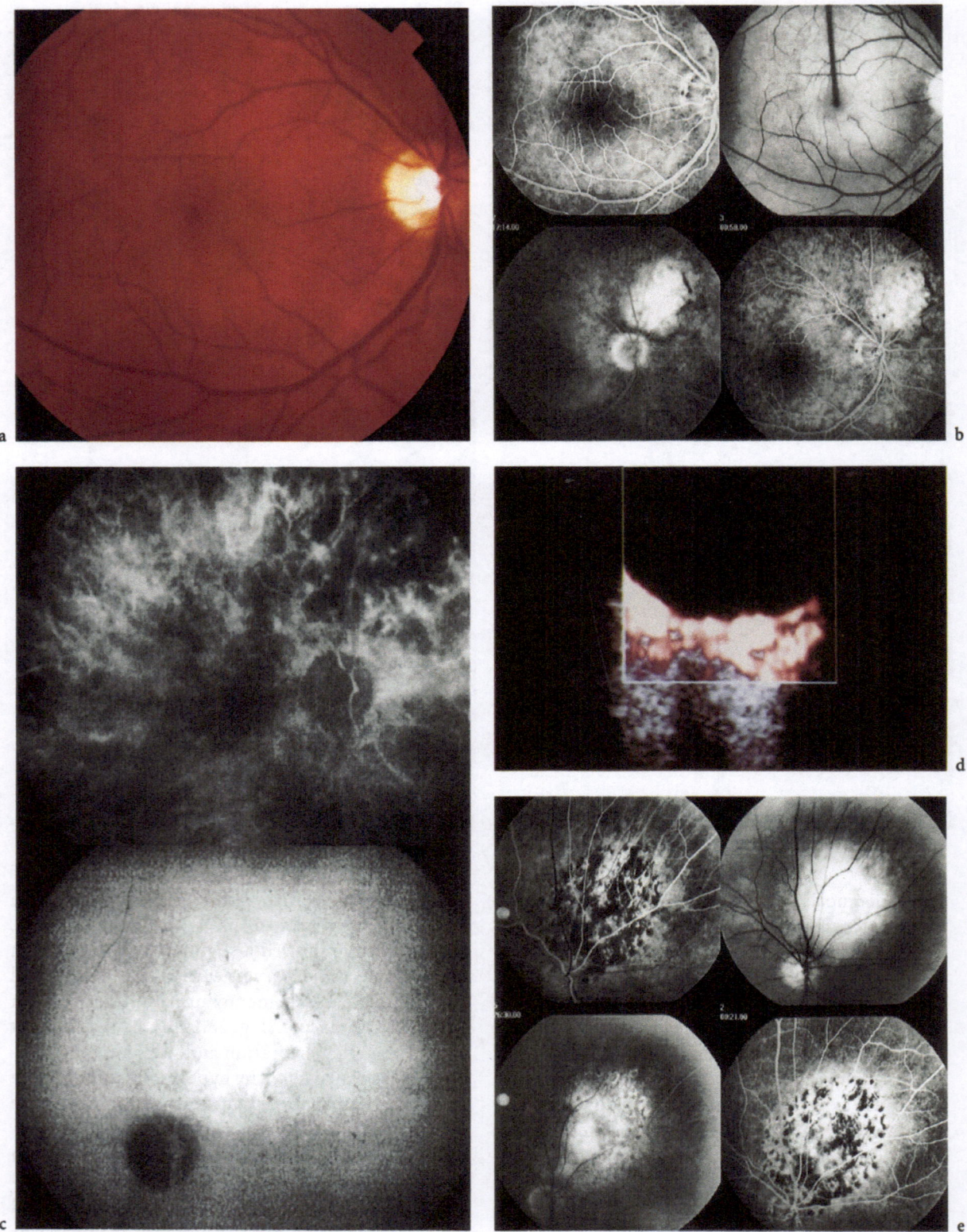

Fig. 28.2. a Biomicroscopy shows slight serous retinal detachment of the macula. Visual acuity was 0.6 in the right eye. **b** FAG demonstrates a patchy hyperfluorescence of the superonasal tumor and pooling within the retinal detachment. **c** Indocyanine green angiography shows an irregular, hyperfluorescent lesion and leakage. **d** High-frequency ultrasound demonstrates a highly vascular circulation within the tumor, indicating a hemangioma. **e** FAG after laser treatment. The retinal detachment resolved and the spotted laser scars are visible

leakage nor pooling was seen in the post-treatment FAG (Fig. 28.2e). The serous retinal detachment was confirmed by OCT (optical coherence tomography) at admission and its resolution, after laser treatment.

28.2.3
Malignant Choroidal Melanoma

Choroidal melanoma is the most common primary malignant intraocular tumor of adults. The incidence is 0.5–1 per 100,000 inhabitants. It usually occurs in older patients (6th to 7th decade) without gender preference. The tumor is usually unilateral. The etiology is unknown. Histopathologically, the tumor is composed of choroidal melanocytes. Choroidal melanomas are predominantly located at the posterior pole. Approximately 10% of blind and painful eyes contain choroidal melanoma.

Clinically, the tumor appears as a dark prominence, mostly in the periphery. The color of the tumor is typically dark brown, possibly with an orange-red pigmentation (Fig. 28.3a). In rare cases the tumor may appear amelanotic. In case of malignant melanoma the fundus shows an exudative retinal detachment collaterally (at 6 o'clock). Most choroidal tumors grow endophytically (towards the vitreous). With rapid and progressive growth, the tumor may penetrate Bruch's membrane and the retinal pigment epithelium, resulting in the classic collar-button appearance. Bruch's membrane resists penetra-

tion by the tumor, resulting in the "mushroom" appearance. In about 25% of cases the retina is infiltrated by tumor cells.

Complications resulting from local growth include subretinal and vitreous hemorrhage, extensive accompanying exudative retinal detachment, and choroidal foldings. Long-term complications include secondary glaucoma, cataract, and severe panuveitis caused by tumor cells.

Diagnostic evaluation includes FAG, ICG angiography, and ultrasonography.

Fluorescein Angiography. In the early phase the angiogram shows an irregular fluorescein pattern or an individual tumor vessel network. In the later phases there is increasing hyperfluorescence. In the case of orange pigmentation, hemorrhage, or necrosis, blockade of the underlying choroid may be found. A typical appearance is that of punctate hyperfluorescence with leakage, which is called "starry sky." Most often an irregular patchy pattern of fluorescence is found (Fig. 28.3b).

The diagnosis is made on the basis of medical history, findings at biomicroscopy, FAG and ultrasonography.

The treatment of choroidal melanoma is laser coagulation when the tumors are small and flat, and ruthenium brachytherapy for larger lesions. Enucleation may be unavoidable in the case of very large tumors. The differential diagnosis of choroidal melanoma includes choroidal nevi and metastatic tu-

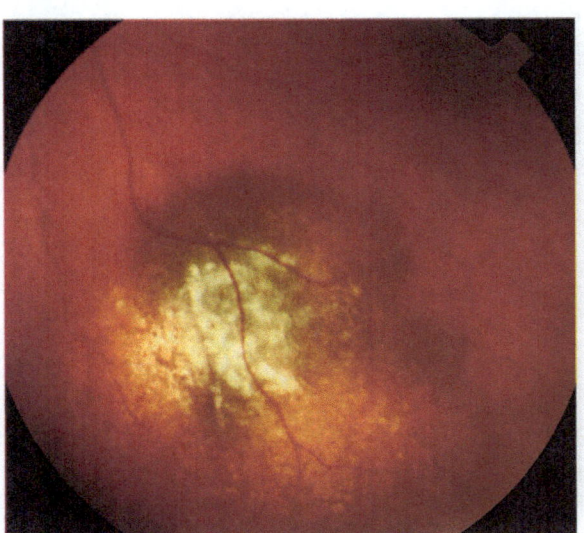
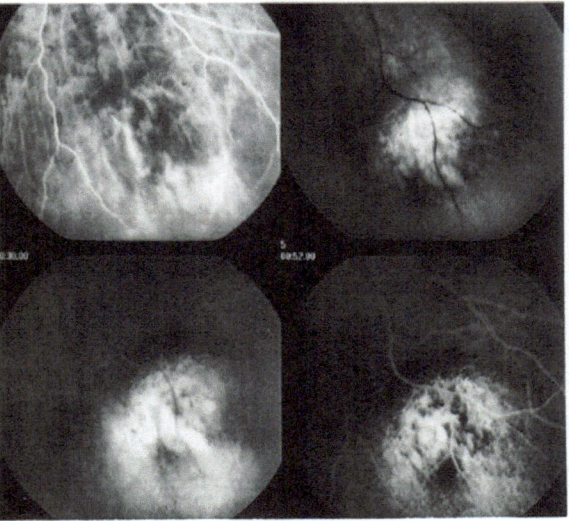

Fig. 28.3. a In this 61-year-old female patient, a choroidal melanoma was suspected at the periphery. Biomicroscopy shows a dark brown tumor and yellowish spots similar to drusen. This appearance may also be seen in choroidal nevi. **b** FAG shows early filling of the underlying choroidal vessels and leakage in the late phase

mors (GUTHOFF et al. 1999; RICHARD 1998; RICHARD et al. 1998; ROHRBACH and LIEB 1998).

28.2.4
Metastatic Tumors to the Uvea

Metastatic tumors are the most common intraocular tumors. The uvea is involved in 80–90% of cases. The leading symptom is painless visual de-

terioration. Metastatic tumors reach the uvea via the bloodstream. The mean age of patients is 60 years, and the most common primary tumor sites are breast, lung, thyroid, and kidney. Carcinomas are predominant, but leukemia may manifest itself in the choroid in children. Metastases present as white to yellow masses in the choroid, usually at the posterior pole (Figs. 28.4a, 28.5a). The masses do not normally cause hemorrhage or vitreous infiltration. The tumor looks similar to amelanot-

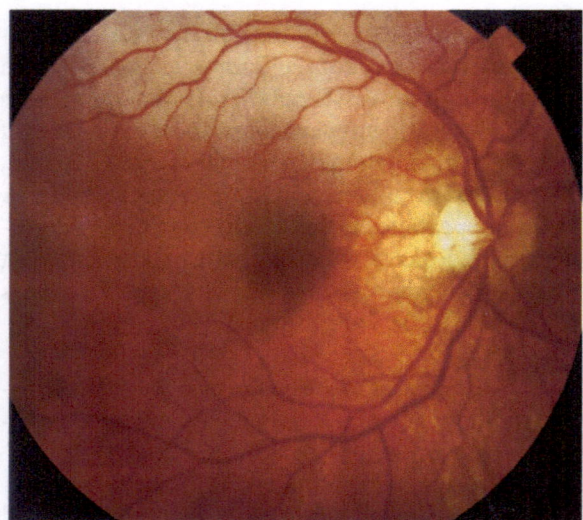
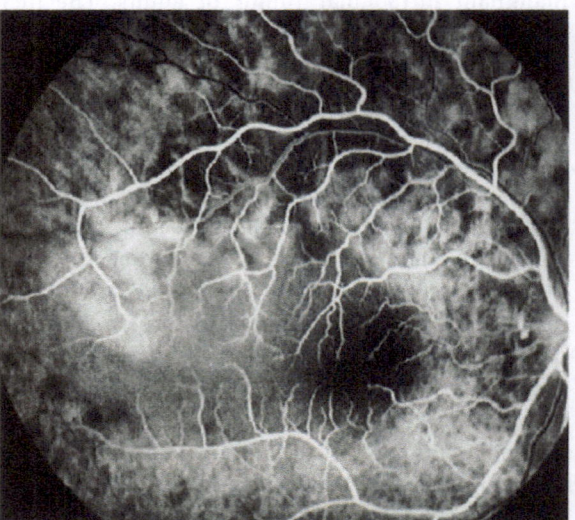

Fig. 28.4. a Biomicroscopy of a 36-year-old female patient suffering from metastatic breast carcinoma. The visual acuity in both eyes was 1.0. Biomicroscopy reveals a macular serous detachment in both eyes (right eye is shown). **b** FAG demonstrates the typical flecked appearance of the retinal pigment epithelium (leopard skin) and fluorescein pooling (right eye)

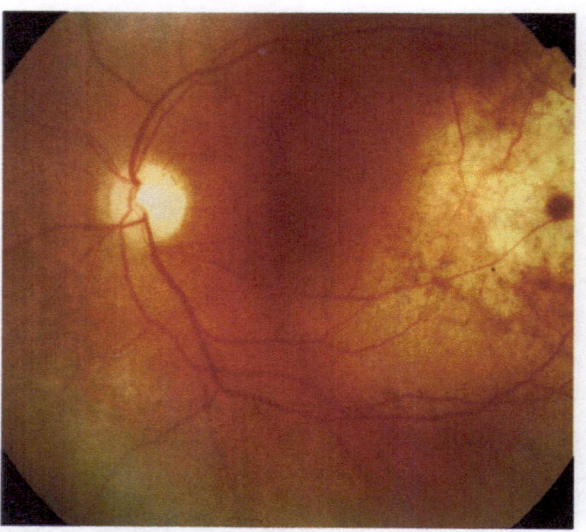
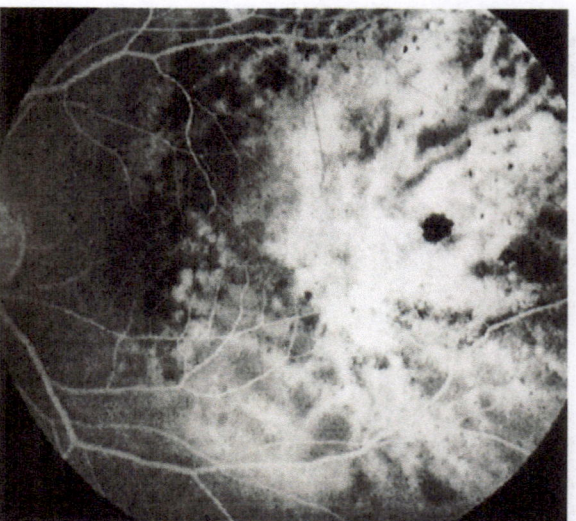

Fig. 28.5. a This 51-year-old female patient was suffering from breast carcinoma with bilateral metastatic tumors of the uvea. Biomicroscopy demonstrates yellowish prominent tumors with the vessel arcade (left eye is shown). **b** FAG (left eye) demonstrates a prominent area of hyperfluorescence at the temporal side of the vessel arcade, which is due to leakage. The patchy pattern is typical for metastatic tumors of the uvea

ic choroidal melanoma. A typical sign is a flecked appearance of the retinal pigment epithelium [leopard skin (Figs. 28.4b, 28.5b)] covering the tumor. In contrast to choroidal melanoma, metastases are normally flatter and sometimes multifocal or diffuse. Retinal detachment is rarely observed, but metastatic tumors of the choroid are often bilateral.

Fluorescein Angiography. Angiography shows flecky and patchy hyperfluorescence (leopard skin) in the area of the tumor. Hyperfluorescence with pinpoints is visible in the late phase (Fig. 28.4b, 28.5b).

Treatment is indicated in the presence of visual deterioration or other symptoms. Concomitant treatment of the primary tumor site or of other metastases may be necessary. While systemic chemotherapy may be effective in the treatment of choroidal metastasis, laser coagulation and radiotherapy, either external beam or plaque brachytherapy, are most often employed successfully (GUTHOFF et al. 1999; RICHARD 1998; RICHARD et al. 1998; ROHRBACH and LIEB 1998).

References

Guthoff R, Pauleikhoff D, Hingst V (1999) Bildgebende Diagnostik in der Augenheilkunde. Enke, Stuttgart

Hassenstein A, Richard G (1998) Geschichte und Entwicklung der Fluoreszenzangiographie. Ophthal Chir 10:75–84

Richard G (1998) Fluorescein and ICG angiography, textbook and atlas, 2nd edn. Thieme, Stuttgart, pp 142–153

Richard G, Soubrane G, Yannuzzi LA (1998) Fluorescein and ICG angiography. Textbook and atlas, 2nd rev edn. Thieme, Stuttgart, p 316 ff

Rohrbach JM, Lieb WE (1998) Tumoren des Auges und seiner Adnexe. Textbuch und Atlas. Schattauer, Stuttgart

Subject Index

List of Contributors

DAVID H. ABRAMSON, MD, FACS
Clinical Professor of Ophthalmology
The New York Hospital - Cornell Medical Center
70 East 66th Street
New York, NY 10021
USA

W. E. ALBERTI, MD
Professor, Radiologische Klinik
Abteilung für Strahlentherapie und Radioonkologie
Universitäts-Klinikum Hamburg-Eppendorf
Martinistrasse 52
20246 Hamburg
Germany

LOWELL L. ANDERSON, PhD
Attending Physicist
Department of Medical Physics
Memorial Sloan-Kettering Cancer Center
1275 York Avenue
New York, NY 10021
USA

LUTHER W. BRADY, MD
Hylda Cohn/American Cancer Society
Professor of Clinical Oncology, and
Professor, Department of Radiation Oncology
Hahnemann University Hospital
Broad & Vine Sts., Mail Stop 200
Philadelphia, PA 19102
USA

JEFFREY A. BOGART, MD
Department of Radiation Oncology
SUNY Upstate Medical University
750 E. Adams St.
Syracuse, NY 13210
USA

SOU-TUNG CHIU-TSAO, PhD
Head, Physics Division
Department of Radiation Oncology
Henry Ford Hospital
2799 West Grand Boulevard
Detroit, MI 48202
USA

CHUNG T. CHUNG, MD, FACR
Department of Radiation Oncology
SUNY Upstate Medical University
750 E. Adams Street
Syracuse, New York 13210
USA

BERTIL DAMATO, MD
Liverpool Ocular Oncology Centre
Royal Liverpool University Hospital
Prescot Street
Liverpool L7 8XP
UK

SARAH S. DONALDSON, MD
Professor, Department of Radiation Oncology
Stanford University Medical Center
300 Pasteur Drive
Stanford, CA 94305
USA

ERIC D. DONNENFELD, MD
2000 North Village Avenue, Suite 402
Rockville Centre
New York, NY 11570
USA

EMMANUEL EGGER, PhD
Division of Radiation Medicine
Paul Scherrer Institute
5232 Villigen-PSI
Switzerland

PAUL T. FINGER, MD, FACS
The New York Eye Cancer Center
115 E. 61st Street
New York, NY 10021
USA

J. E. FREIRE, MD
Department of Radiation Oncology
MCP Hahneman University Hospital
Broad & Vine Sts.
Mail Stop 200
Philadelphia, PA 19102
USA

PETER J. FITZPATRICK, MB, BS, FRCP, FRCR
Physician-in-Chief
CTRF Nova Scotia Cancer Treatment
and Research Center
5820 University Avenue
Halifax, Nova Scotia B3H 1V7
Canada

GUDRUN GOITEIN, MD
Division of Radiation Medicine
Paul Scherrer Institute
5232 Villigen-PSI
Switzerland

RUSSELL S. GONNERING, MD
Professor of Ophthalmology
Medical College of Wisconsin
Division of Oculoplastics
Clinical Professor of Ophthalmology
University of WisconsinEye Institute
925 N. 87th Street
Milwaukee, WI 53226
USA

SEUNG S. HAHN, MD
Associate Professor, Department of Radiation Oncology
SUNY Upstate Medical University
750 East Adams Street
Syracuse, NY 13210
USA

GEORGES F. HATOUM, MD
Department of Radiation Oncology
SUNY Upstate Medical University
750 East Adams Street
Syracuse, NY 13210
USA

ANDREA HASSENSTEIN, MD
University Eye Hospital
University Hamburg
Martinistrasse 52
20246 Hamburg
Germany

NORBERT HOSTEN, MD
Professor, Zentrum für Radiologie
Ernst-Moritz-Arndt-Universität
Institut für diagnostische und interventionelle Radiologie
Friedrich-Löffler-Strasse 23
17487 Greifswald
Germany

HERBERT J. INGRAHAM, MD
Department of Ophthalmology
Geisinger Medical Center
North Academy Avenue
Danville, PA 17822-2120
USA

MOHSEN ISAAC, MD
Department of Radiation Oncology
SUNY Upstate Medical University
750 East Adams Street
Syracuse, NY 13210
USA

JAN LEI IWATA, Pharm.D., DO
Clinical Instructor of Ophthalmology
Medical College of Wisconsin
Division of Oculoplastics, Eye Institute
925 N. 87th Street
Milwaukee, WI 53226
USA

HANNEKE G. JOURNÉE-DE KORVER, PhD
Department of Ophthalmology
Leiden University Medical Center
P.O. Box 9600
2300 RC Leiden
The Netherlands

JAN E. E. KEUNEN, MD
Department of Ophthalmology
Leiden University Medical Center
P.O. Box 9600
2300 RC Leiden
The Netherlands

ARNE-JÖRN LEMKE, MD
Klinikum Charité, Campus Virchow-Klinikum
Med. Fakultät der Humboldt-Universität zu Berlin
Strahlenklinik und Poliklinik
Augustenburger Platz 1
13353 Berlin
Germany

PETER K. LOMMATZSCH, MD
Professor
Goldschmidtstrasse 30
04103 Leipzig
Germany

I. ROSS McDOUGALL, MB, ChB, PhD
Professor, Stanford University Medical Center
300 Pasteur Drive
Stanford, CA 94305
USA

BIZHAN MICAILY, MD
Department of Radiation Oncology
Hahnemann University Hospital
Broad & Vine Sts., Mail Stop 200
Philadelphia, PA 19102
USA

JOHN E. MUNZENRIDER, MD
Department of Radiation Oncology
Massachusetts General Hospital
Harvard University Medical School
Cox Building, Room 341
Boston, MA 02114
USA

J. A. OOSTERHUIS, MD
Professor
Prinsenweg 57
2242 EB Wassenaar
The Netherlands

ZBIGNIEW PETROVICH, MD, FACR
Department of Radiation Oncology
University of Southern California
School of Medicine
Los Angeles, CA
USA

GISBERT RICHARD, MD
Professor of Ophthalmology
Director of the University Eye Hospital
University Hamburg
Martinistrasse 52
20246 Hamburg
Germany

SHARI B. RUDOLER, MD
Thomas Jefferson University
Bodine Center for Cancer Treatment
111 S. 11th Street
Philadelphia, PA 19107-5098
USA

ROBERT H. SAGERMAN, MD, FACR
Professor, Department of Radiation Oncology
SUNY Upstate Medical University
750 East Adams Street
Syracuse, NY 13210
USA

JAN SCHIPPER, PhD
Adjunct Director Radiation Physics
Arnhem Radiotherapeutisch Institut
Wagnerlaan 47
6815 AD Arnhem
The Netherlands

CAROL L. SHIELDS, MD
Associate Professor at Thomas Jefferson University
Attending Surgeon, Ocular Oncology Service
Wills Eye Hospital
Ninth and Walnut Sts.
Philadelphia, PA 19107
USA

JERRY A. SHIELDS, MD
Professor at Thomas Jefferson University
Department Chairman and
Director, Ocular Oncology Service
Wills Eye Hospital
Ninth and Walnut Sts.
Philadelphia, PA 19107
USA

ANDREAS WALTER, MD
University Eye Hospital
University Hamburg
Martinistrasse 52
20246 Hamburg
Germany

ROBERT A. WEISS, MD
Clinical Associate Professor
Departments of Ophthalmology and
Visual Science, and Neurosurgery
The University of Illinois at Chicago
Director of Oculoplastic and Reconstructive Surgery,
and Ophthalmologic Oncology, Chicago Eye Institute
and Advocate Illinois Masonic Medical Health Systems
3982 North Milwaukee Avenue
Chicago, IL 60641
USA

CORNELIA WERSCHNIK, MD
Klinik und Poliklinik für Augenheilkunde
Martin Luther University Halle
Magedburger Strasse 8
06112 Halle
Germany

A. Youssef, MD
Department of Radiation Oncology
MCP Hahneman University Hospital
Broad & Vine Sts.
Mail Stop 200
Philadelphia, PA 19102
USA

LEONIDAS ZOGRAFOS, MD, PhD
Chef de Clinique
Hôpital Ophtalmique Jules Gonin
15 avenue de France
1004 Lausanne
Switzerland

MEDICAL RADIOLOGY
Diagnostic Imaging and Radiation Oncology

Titles in the series already published

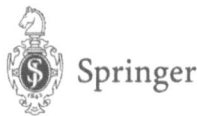

Springer

MEDICAL RADIOLOGY
Diagnostic Imaging and Radiation Oncology

Titles in the series already published

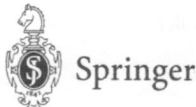
Springer